MW00399184

Psychological Problems
of the Child in the Family

PSYCHOLOGICAL
PROBLEMS
OF THE CHILD
IN THE FAMILY

SECOND EDITION

EDITED BY

Paul D. Steinhauer

AND

Quentin Rae-Grant

Basic Books, Inc., Publishers   *New York*

Library of Congress Cataloging in Publication Data
Main entry under title:

Psychological problems of the child in the family.

  First ed. published in 1977 under title:
Psychological problems of the child and his family.
  References: p. 682
  Includes index.
    1. Child psychiatry. 2. Mentally ill children—
Family relationships. 3. Child psychopathology.
I. Steinhauer, Paul D., 1933–   II. Rae-Grant,
Quentin. [DNLM: 1. Adolescent psychiatry.
2. Child psychiatry. 3. Family therapy. WS 350 P9746]
RJ499.P7683   1983   618.92'89   82-72960
ISBN 0-465-06676-3

First edition published as
Psychological Problems of the Child and His Family
Copyright © Macmillan of Canada 1977
Copyright © 1983 by Basic Books, Inc.
Printed in the United States of America
Designed by Vincent Torre
10 9 8 7 6 5 4 3

The editors would like to dedicate this book to

Drs. E. James Anthony, Leon Eisenberg,

and the late Hyman S. Lippman,

whose example and friendship

have had such an influence on their careers

in academic child psychiatry,

and to their colleagues in the

Canadian Academy of Child Psychiatry

CONTENTS

PART III

Common Syndromes in Child Psychiatry

Contents

PART IV

Psychological Crises for Child and Family

PART V

Principles of Intervention

Contents

CONTRIBUTORS

HARVEY ARMSTRONG, M.D., F.R.C.P.(C)., Dip. Child Psychiat. Associate Professor of Psychiatry, University of Toronto; Clinical Director, Metropolitan Toronto Adolescent Crisis Unit; Director of Psychiatry, Sioux-Lookout Zone Hospital.

GEORGE AWAD, M.D., F.R.C.P.(C). Associate Professor of Psychiatry, University of Toronto; Senior Staff Psychiatrist, Family Court Clinic.

GRAHAM BERMAN, M.D., F.R.C.P.(C). Assistant Professor of Psychiatry, University of Toronto; Staff Psychiatrist, Hospital for Sick Children, Toronto.

ELSA A. BRODER, M.D., F.R.C.P. (C). Assistant Professor of Psychiatry, University of Toronto; Staff Psychiatrist, C. M. Hincks Treatment Centre, Toronto; Consultant, Probation and Aftercare, Ministry of Community and Social Services of Ontario.

ROBERT P. CARR, M.D., F.R.C.P.(C)., Dip. Child Psychiat. Assistant Professor of Psychiatry, University of Toronto, Staff Psychiatrist, Hospital for Sick Children, Toronto.

CLIVE CHAMBERLAIN, M.D., F.R.C.P.(C). Associate Professor of Psychiatry, University of Toronto; Clinical Director, Thistletown Regional Centre.

DAVID DICKMAN, M.D., F.R.C.P.(C). Assistant Professor of Psychiatry, University of Toronto; Staff Psychiatrist, Hospital for Sick Children, Toronto.

ROSE GEIST, M.D., F.R.C.P.(C)., Dip. Child Psychiat. Staff Psychiatrist; Hospital for Sick Children, Toronto; Consultant to Gastroenterology and Lecturer in Psychiatry, University of Toronto.

BENJAMIN GOLDBERG, M.D., C.M., F.R.C.P.(C), F.A.A.M.D. Director of Treatment, Training, and Research, Children's Psychiatric Research Institute, London, Ontario; Clinical Professor of Psychiatry, University of Western Ontario.

SUSAN GOLDBERG, Ph.D. Associate Professor of Psychiatry and Psychology, University of Toronto; Research Scientist, Hospital for Sick Children, Toronto.

HARVEY GOLOMBEK, M.D., F.R.C.P.(C). Head of Preventive Studies, C. M. Hincks Treatment Centre, Toronto; Associate Professor of Psychiatry, University of Toronto; Senior Psychiatric Consultant, Etobicoke Board of Education.

MILADA HAVELKOVA, M.D., F.R.C.P.(C). Associate Professor of Psychiatry, University of Toronto; Staff Psychiatrist, Hospital for Sick Children, Toronto; Senior Psychiatrist, West End Creche, Child and Family Centre; Consultant, Bruce Grey Children's Services, Owen Sound.

WILLIAM HAWKE, M.D. Special Lecturer in Psychiatry, University of Toronto; Professor Emeritus of Pediatrics, University of Toronto; Honorary Consultant, Hospital for Sick Children, Toronto.

ERIC HOOD, M.B. Ch.B., F.R.C.P.(C). Assistant Professor of Psychiatry, University of Toronto; Staff Psychiatrist, Clarke Institute of Psychiatry, Toronto.

SIMON KREINDLER, M.D., F.R.C.P.(C). Assistant Professor of Psychiatry, University of Toronto; Staff Psychiatrist and Psychiatric Consultant to Child Abuse Team, Hospital for Sick Children, Toronto.

MARSHALL KORENBLUM, M.D., F.R.C.P.(C). Dip. Child Psychiat. Lecturer in Psychiatry, University of Toronto; Staff Psychiatrist and Head, Adolescent Clinical Investigation Unit, C.M. Hincks Treatment Centre; Consultant, Sunnybrook Medical Centre.

ARLETTE M. L. LEFEBVRE, M.D., F.R.C.P.(C), Dip. Child Psychiatry. Staff Psychiatrist and Consultant to Plastic Surgery and Burns Unit, Hospital for Sick Children, Toronto; Assistant Professor, University of Toronto.

SAUL V. LEVINE, M.D., C.P., F.R.C.P.(C). Head, Department of Psychiatry, Sunnybrook Medical Centre, University of Toronto; Professor of Psychiatry, University of Toronto.

BRIAN MCCONVILLE, M.D., F.R.C.P.(C). Professor and Chairman, Division of Child Psychiatry, Department of Psychiatry, Queen's University, Kingston, and Clinical Director, Beechgrove Regional Children's Centre, Kingston.

DOUGLAS MCGREAL, M.D. Associate Professor of Pediatrics, University of Toronto; Neurologist, Hospital for Sick Children, Toronto.

FREDA MARTIN, M.D., F.R.C.P.(C). Associate Professor of Psychiatry, University of Toronto; Chief of Service, Child and Family Study Centre, Clarke Institute of Psychiatry.

KLAUS MINDE, M.D. Professor of Psychiatry and Pediatrics, University of Toronto; Director of Psychiatric Research, Hospital for Sick Children, Toronto.

DAVID N. MUSHIN, M.B. B.S., F.R.A.N.Z.C.P., F.R.C.P.(C), Dip. Child Psychiatry. Clinical Director, Department of Child Psychiatry, and Chairman, Division of Psychiatry, Queen Victoria Medical Centre, Melbourne, Victoria, Australia.

DAN OFFORD, M.D., F.R.C.P.(C). Professor of Psychiatry, McMaster University, and Research Director, Child and Family Centre, Chedoke-McMaster Hospitals, Hamilton, Ontario. President, Canandian Academy of Child Psychiatry.

EDWARD H. PAKES, M.D., F.R.C.P.(C), F.A.P.A. Assistant Professor of Psychiatry, University of Toronto; Senior Staff Psychiatrist, Hospital for Sick Children, Toronto.

NAOMI I. RAE-GRANT, M.B.B.S., F.R.C.Psych., F.R.C.P.(C). Professor of Psychiatry, McMaster University, Hamilton, Ontario. Clinical Director, Child and Family Centre, Chedoke-McMaster Hospital.

QUENTIN RAE-GRANT, M.B., Ch.B., D.P.M., F.R.C. Psych., F.R.C.P.(C). Professor of Child Psychiatry and Pediatrics and Vice-Chairman of Department of Psychiatry, University of Toronto; Psychiatrist-in-Chief, Hospital for Sick Children, Toronto; President, Canadian Psychiatric Association.

BONNIE ROBSON, M.D. Staff Psychiatrist, C.M. Hincks Treatment Centre, Toronto; Assistant Professor of Psychiatry, University of Toronto; Co-Chairperson, Training Committee, Division of Child Psychiatry; worked with Social Work Department, Toronto Board of Education, in citywide program of group counseling in elementary and secondary schools for children who have experienced separation.

PAUL D. STEINHAUER, M.D., F.R.C.P.(C). Professor of Psychiatry and Director of Training in Child and Adolescent Psychiatry, University of Toronto; Senior Staff Psychiatrist, Hospital for Sick Children, Toronto; first President of the Canadian Academy of Child Psychiatry.

MICHAEL THOMPSON, M.D. Associate Professor of Psychiatry, University of Toronto; Executive Director, West End Creche, Child and Family Clinic.

JAMES J. VANLEEUWEN, M.D., F.R.C.P.(C). Associate Professor of Psychiatry, University of Toronto; Senior Staff Psychiatrist, Hospital for Sick Children, Toronto.

PREFACE

Preparing an introductory text presents an intriguing series of challenges. The writing must be basic enough to be readily comprehensible, while it must present the subject matter in an authoritative and comprehensive way. It must order a large number of facts and key concepts in a language and manner that are clear, organized, and sequential. Highly technical terms and concepts must be so introduced that even readers new to the field can relate them to their own experience or to concrete illustrations supplied by the text. If it is to succeed in its task, it is not enough that it be read and memorized; it must be understood and even enjoyed.

Psychological Problems of the Child in the Family is intended to present the basic principles of child and adolescent psychiatry while meeting the preceding criteria. It covers the subject area of child and adolescent psychiatry from biological, developmental, psychoanalytic, and systems perspectives. Even more important, it attempts to integrate these conceptual approaches so that readers from a variety of disciplines are guided toward a practical approach in dealing with and understanding patients and their families.

Throughout the text, children are viewed both as individuals with their own internal network of drives and defenses and as members of a family and social system. An integration of these inner (intrapsychic) and outer (familial and social) aspects of the child's reality is continually kept in focus. Emphasis is placed on the process of development and on the effects of blocks and deviations in the development of the child's personality and functioning.

In response to the changing emphases and new research, a number of new chapters have been added to this second edition. These include: Issues of Attachment and Separation: Foster Care and Adoption; Alternative Family Styles; Classification and Epidemiology in Child Psychiatry: Status and Unresolved Problems; Infant Psychiatry; Convulsive Disorders and Other Neurological Conditions Commonly Associated or Confused with Psychiatric Illness; Disorders Commonly Appearing First During Adolescence; The Child with Physical Handicaps; The Effects of Marital Breakdown; and Prevention. In addition, most chapters from the first edition have been almost completely rewritten to bring them up to date with advances in the field, to improve the referencing, to separate theory from clinical experience from proven fact, and to present clearly and fairly major areas of unresolved controversy in the field. As in the first edition, each chapter contains a number of annotated suggestions for further reading, but a single list of references serves the entire text.

As editors, we have tried throughout to minimize the use of jargon. Past experience has shown us that this text is likely to be read by students and practitioners of medicine and of the allied health and mental health professions. Each of these professions has its own technical vocabulary, which, to members of other professions, sounds like jargon. Except for a few necessarily technical sections in the chapters on psychosis, psychopharmacology, and neurological disorders, familiarity with psychiatric or medical terminology is not needed to understand and follow the text. When technical terms are used, they are clearly defined either at the point of their introduction or in the extensive glossary of medical and psychiatric terms at the end of the book. Key concepts are illustrated by schematic diagrams and brief clinical vignettes.

Throughout the text, the classification system outlined in the *Diagnostical and Statistical Manual of Mental Disorders* (3rd edition), usually abbreviated herein as DSM-III (American Psychiatric Association 1980), has been used. This system was selected as it is the classification used most commonly in North America, and whenever a diagnosis is followed by a number in parentheses, it is to DSM-III that it refers.

The editors would like to express their appreciation to their fellow authors for the spirit in which they cooperated in the preparation of this edition and to their colleagues in the Division of Child Psychiatry at the University of Toronto, whose knowledge, experience, and friendship were so generously shared with us. In addition, we would like to thank the following people, whose assistance was crucial to the preparation of the text: (in alphabetical order) Wilma Aranha, John Rae-Grant, Elizabeth Steinhauer, Shelley Tepperman, and John Gordon White, whose hard work, loyalty, attentiveness to detail, and ability to retain their creativity and sense of humor in the midst of chaos did as much to preserve our sanity as to complete the text; Pat Follett, whose unflappability was matched only by her skill as a typist; and Jo Ann Miller and Linda Carbone at Basic Books, whose professionalism did so much to improve the quality of the text.

P.D.S. and Q.R.-G.

PART I

The Child and the Family

1   *Klaus Minde and Bonnie Robson*

Normal Child Development

Introduction and Historical Review

Child psychiatry as a medical specialty has both an educational and a clinical mandate. As a consequence, its practitioners assess and treat those children who have difficulties in meeting the normal expectations that their families or society at large place on them. In addition, however, child psychiatrists and other mental health professionals also attempt to assemble knowledge about children's emotional needs and provide it to those who assist children in their growth and development.

The following chapters describe a great number of psychiatric syndromes and abnormal behavioral manifestations in children of various ages. They also show how specific constitutional and environmental forces influence the behavior of children and their families. Yet common to all chapters is the awareness that disturbed children show deviations, for whatever reason, in some aspect of their social, cognitive, or emotional development.

It follows then that one cannot begin to understand psychological problems in children without an adequate appreciation of their normal development. How do children change as they grow up? What are the determinants of these changes? This chapter will investigate these issues in two ways. First, some general developmental principles are discussed. These will allow us to see the features common to various theories of human development. They also provide an opportunity to describe some of the internal and external forces that produce developmental change in children. Then the effects of particular developmental principles on specific aspects of a child's development at different ages are illustrated.

Until relatively recently in the history of western culture, childhood was not considered important. For example, until the seventeenth century, children were seen as "little adults." Parents and teachers did not regard the child, once past infancy, as having specific educational or emotional needs. Toward the end of the seventeenth century, through the more systematic observation of individual children by educators and parents, the particular nature of childhood began to be recognized. Children came to be seen as "innocent," yet "primitive" and "irrational," in need of safeguarding from pollution by the temptations of adult life. In many respects these concepts proved beneficial for younger children, for example, by reducing the amount of heavy work they were permitted to do. But children were considered in need of protection not only from the corrupting influences of the outer world but also from their own primitive psychic forces. These forces, including many basic biological drives, were seen as a potential source of damnation, very much in need of containment. Society took upon itself the mandate of "civilizing" children by taming the essentially "savage" and "bestial" aspect of their natures. This led to the creation of an educational system that saw as its prime responsibility the task of suppressing such potentially dangerous impulses.

Confirmation for this "predeterminist" concept of development seemed to come from biology. Here scientists claimed that "ontogeny recapitulates phylogeny" (i.e., the development of the individual repeats that of the species), which meant that each human embryo, in the course of intrauterine development, passes through each stage of the evolutionary process. Starting as a single cell, the embryo proceeds up the evolutionary ladder, its structure resembling at one point that of a reptile and finally that of a mammal. This theory was seen as further proof of the close association between humans and animals. It contributed to the philosophical rationale for seeing humans as always having, lurking beneath the surface, a bit of the beast that needed to be tamed, and for viewing all children as endowed with the sins and failures of their phylogenetic ancestors.

Various scientific advances during the past fifty years have called the predeterminist position into question. There was, for example, the recognition that the physical or psychological characteristics that an individual inherits (i.e., the genotype) may not be identical with the psychological and physical characteristics that the individual shows (i.e., the phenotype). The phenotype was seen to reflect the genetic base after its modification by the environment. Thus scientists came to accept that the genetic constitution contributed the potential for development, but that throughout the process of growth and maturation environmental forces continually influenced the outcome.

Nevertheless, significant questions remained about how development, in fact, proceeded. One group of investigators (Baer 1970) felt that any change in the behavior or ability of children, such as those changes occurring in their physical growth, was a continual process that varied little over time. These theorists also maintained that the learning of complex behav-

4

iors was based on the forming of simple connections in response to experience, just as was the case in the learning of basic tasks.

On the other hand, a considerable body of opinion and evidence, derived both from Anna Freud's psychoanalytic discoveries (1963, 1965) and Piaget's cognitive developmental theory (1953), stressed that development proceeded in clearly defined stages. This "stage," or "epigenetic," concept of development was based on the observation that certain groups, or "segments," of behavior routinely occurred together. For example, children begin to show stranger anxiety usually around the time they recognize the differences between strange and familiar faces. The epigenetic theory further implies that these behavioral segments are routinely followed by other specific behaviors or functions. In the case of stranger anxiety, the next step would be that children develop an ability to visualize and hence remember their mothers even when they are not physically present. This allows children to become more independent and to explore areas when their mother could or would not follow them. This in turn would facilitate new learning and increased competence. Development, therefore, was seen as proceeding in an orderly, steplike manner through a series of stages, each representing a higher level of function than its predecessor.

While still acknowledging that individual development is biologically influenced, epigenetic theory suggests that a group of behaviors would occur only if its more elementary precursors had been mastered. It also assumes that some environmental influences are more significant at some allegedly "critical" times in a child's development than at other times. For example, theorists felt that the absence of the biological mother during the first years of life would necessarily produce a psychologically deviant older child and adult. This notion has since been replaced by the recognition that while children need stable, predictable relationships with their caregivers, these can be provided by people other than the biological parents. It has also been recognized that there is no special or critical period in human development. Developmental blocks and distortions may occur at any level, causing either temporary or permanent developmental arrest. Alternatively, positive environmental experiences may help to unblock or assist in reactivating developmental progress. Life often provides second chances.

Current State of Knowledge

In summary, child development is a complex process. Proponents of various emotional and cognitive theories have tried in different ways to conceptualize and explain general laws that govern the development of children. How does one begin to integrate and make sense of so many different and, at times, conflicting theoretical attempts to explain a child's development?

While the following three principles may not be accepted by every expert in child development, they do represent a consensus of most contemporary scientists.

First, scientists recognize that no single concept of development does justice to all the phenomena that we observe in a developing organism. Some functions, such as body and cell growth, occur continuously throughout development. The acquisition of other functions, such as the use of language or particular ways of thinking, proceeds in stages. Because of this, there is a lower age limit for the appearance of most developmental phenomena; this limit is primarily determined by the maturation of the central nervous system. For example, no amount of stimulation will lead to speech within the first six months of life. On the other hand, verbal stimulation during this period does play an important role in preparing the ground for the later acquisition of language. What is not yet known is whether there are upper time limits for the acquisition of a given ability, such that if the appropriate stimuli are not provided within a given interval the ability will never appear. Despite the assumption by some that this is true, convincing evidence in the area of human development has not yet been provided.

Second, most scientists believe that the child is an important shaper of the environment. Children do not merely react to their environment; the environment reacts to them as well. Parents have their own needs, and whether or not their particular infant meets these needs will affect the parents' response and therefore the environment in which the child grows. An active, exploring, aggressive infant may prove a delight to parents who value such qualities but may arouse anxiety, frustration, and annoyance in parents who would have preferred a more passive and nonchallenging child. The first parents might have had equal trouble accepting the passive child whom the others would have found much easier to enjoy. Thus parental feelings and responses will be influenced by the degree to which the child meets their preexisting needs. The more these are satisfied, the easier parents will find it to accept and value their child, and the greater will be their ability to provide the environment their child needs for optimal growth.

Another consequence of this principle suggests that a specific developmental level can be reached by different routes. As each new level allows for extensive reorganization of behavior, past tendencies may not persist in present psychological functioning. For example, the feelings and behavior of a person who, because of doubts and anxieties, avoids marrying until the age of forty may, by age forty-five, be indistinguishable

6

from those of someone who married without obvious conflict at twenty.

This principle also makes it difficult to predict accurately the final outcome of a child's development, because reaching a particular stage such as adolescence can provide a second chance by permitting a revision of earlier adaptations to life. For example, the boy who at age ten was unpopular because he lacked athletic abilities may, in adolescence, be admired for his success in heterosexual relationships, and thereby gain the confidence, self-esteem, and poise he needs for social success.

Only persistent and recurrent deviant transactions between children and their environment will produce predictable later abnormalities. These abnormal transactions can be due to a severe defect in the child's integrative mechanism (e.g., childhood schizophrenia or severe brain damage) or to very abnormal environmental forces such as severely neglecting or battering parents.

The third principle is that development is not a phenomenon that affects only one particular sphere of life, such as emotions or intelligence, but is the sum total of various interlocking forces that embrace changes in biological, intellectual, emotional, and social behavior. These forces constantly interact and influence their mutual progression. Therefore, all areas of development should be examined in any assessment of possible emotional and intellectual deviations in either children or adults. Table 1.1 may help the reader by demonstrating the synchronized emergence of some developmental functions in children and adolescents. In the table, a number of age-dependent phases are arbitrarily established, and the levels of functioning along biological, cognitive, language, social, and emotional parameters usually achieved within each phase are summarized and correlated.

Patterns of Child Development

The preceding section stressed that the adequacy of an individual's development must be assessed from various parameters. The most important of these will be outlined here. Then specific age-related developmental phases will be examined and their manifestations in a child's behavior and ability will be described. To illustrate this process in more concrete terms, the example of two normal, healthy, but very different boys will be used. We will observe how each boy appeared at particular ages, how his personality took shape as his development proceeded. Let us introduce them now as they appear at age eleven. We will return to them later when examining each developmental level in more detail.

TABLE 1.1

Age and Development Correspondences

At completion of	Biological	Language	Cognitive	Personal Social	Psychological
2 months	Develops eye, head control. —Looks at rattle in hand. —Chin and chest held up. Real binocular color vision.	Impassive face —considerable crying.	Basic reflexes: sucking, grasping, tracking object in field of vision.	Number of feedings reduces from 7–8 to 5–6. Spontaneous reflex smiling (12 hours). Unselected social smile at human voice (14 days). Smiles at face in motion (5 weeks). Smiles at face with some detail, e.g., eyebrows and eyes (2 months).	1. Primary caregiver's bond to the child forming: caregiver responsive to child's needs. 2. Infant aware of this responsiveness: develops sense of predictability of surroundings— begins to develop sense of security. 3. Infant biased toward the familiar from birth—settles into routine of home.
6 months	Vision: depth perception. Sits bending forward, uses hands for support, bears weight when put in standing position, but cannot stand without holding on. Reaches and grasps toy —transfers toy from hand to hand.	When talked to smiles, squeals, and coos. Consonants begin to be interspersed with vowellike cooing. Cooing changes to babbling resembling one-syllable utterances.	Coordination of basic reflexes, e.g., can look at toy, reach for it, grasp it, mouth it. Grasps for rattle, but if hidden forgets it. —Unable to retrieve rattle if even partly hidden from view. —Significance of above: part is not yet indicative of the whole.	Smiles selectively to mother's face. Plays with feet "Teething."	Begins to distinguish between self and others. With discriminatory vision able to distinguish visually faces and people. Reacts to the strange, unfamiliar with apprehension: "makes strange."

TABLE 1.1 *(continued)*

At completion of	Biological	Language	Cognitive	Personal Social	Psychological
8–9 months	Sits well. Pulls self to feet at railing. Plays with 2 toys: picks up pellet with thumb and index finger.	Reduplication (more continuous repetitions) utterances can signal emphasis and emotions.	Recognizes top and bottom of baby bottle as belonging to same object. —Presented with bottom will rotate it to get nipple.	Taking fine solids and rusks, feeds self cracker. Smiles only to whole familiar face.	Links good things (warmth, food) with the familiar: —Links security with caregivers. Has developed special *attachment bonding* with significant adults. —Anxious or disturbed when separated from them.
15 months	Crawling, climbing stairs. Walks alone. Toddler builds tower with 2 cubes. —Puts 6 cubes into cup and imitates vertical stroke.	Says Dada, Mama, and a vocabulary of between 3 and 20 words. Responds to "Give it to me," "Show me your eyes." Little ability to join words into spontaneous phrases. Pronoun "I" and "mine" understood.	*Object permanence.* —Hidden object can now be removed to new hiding place and child will follow the progression, searching appropriately. —Significance: object has permanence, independent of child's perception.	Toilet regulated during day, carries and hugs doll, assists and cooperates in dressing.	Demonstrates a sense of self separate from mother. —Begins to individuate, i.e., do things adults used to do for child. —Seems to enjoy separateness. *Rapprochement Phase* (15–18 months)— Returns to close, intense relationship with primary caregiver. —Appears more vulnerable to separation than previously. —Attachment bonding at its peak. *Transitional object:* Behaves as if favorite toy or security blanket can protect him

TABLE 1.1 *(continued)*

At completion of	Biological	Language	Cognitive	Personal Social	Psychological
					or her from harm. —Object appears a substitute for contact with primary caregiver.
3 years	Runs, rides tricycle, up and down stairs alone with alternating feet, tiptoes, jumps 12 inches, stands on one foot momentarily. Builds tower 6–7 cubes. Draws a circle; copies a plus sign and a zero.	Vocabulary 1000 words, 80% of utterances intelligible even to strangers. Grammatical complexity roughly that of colloquial adult language. Gives full name and sex.	True symbolic play. —Continues exploration of the world. —Objects seen as entities and named. —Child begins to group objects together, naming the whole group.	Puts doll to bed, feeds self well, puts on socks, unbuttons, asks for toilet during day, begins to want to play with peers. Interested in difference between boys and girls.	Parents expect some obedience and socialization. —Child establishes "self" by opposing will of parents: the "terrible twos." By age 3, child subjects will to wishes of parents. —Often experiences anger at having to give up own wishes. —Fear of punishment, imaginary dangers, and monsters common; fears physical injury through play —May defend against these dangers via imaginary playmate or animal who, while ferocious and larger than life, is subject to child's whims.
6 years	Hops on one foot, stands on alternate feet with eyes closed for 10 seconds, jumps	Language well established. —Deviations from adult norm tend to be more in	Builds on objects to form concepts and on concepts to form classes of concepts.	Ties shoelaces. Can walk to school by self, crosses road at lights safely, plays	Acceptance of parents' morals and wishes. Child "identifies" with parent of same sex, taking

TABLE 1.1 *(continued)*

At completion of	Biological	Language	Cognitive	Personal Social	Psychological
	12 inches high landing on toes, can throw a ball. Copies a triangle (age 6) and a diamond (age 7).	style than grammar. Can name values of coins, all colors. Can give description of pictures.	—Continues grouping, regrouping, naming and exploring.	cooperatively with peers. Can play simple game by rules without adult supervision.	on that parent's values, sex-role behavior. —Conscience and value system develop. Child increasingly behaves as if controlled and regulated by own internal standards and ideals. —Not as influenced by external punishment or reward.
8–10 years	Can tap either foot on floor and right or left finger on table at same time maintaining rhythm for 20 seconds. By age 10, good fine-motor control. Can balance on board, standing with arms out in front, palms down, eyes open.	Good understanding of general language and its rules. —For example, knows plural of man is men. —gives 3 rhyming words for "map" or "cat" within 30 seconds. By age 10–11, can express self in abstract concepts. —For example, can name 10 wild animals in one minute.	By age 9, can group objects in 2 categories simultaneously. For example, bead is both red and wooden. —This is still a building process on reflexes and grouping. True abstract reasoning (i.e., the ability to go beyond the concrete and envision changes without visual props) does not occur until adolescence.	Uses knife at table, combs and brushes hair. Catches a baseball, plays complicated games by rules.	School involves: accepting rules and regulations; adapting to others; competing with others; possibility of defeat, ridicule, humiliation; persisting at task even if unpleasant until it is complete. Child's self-image and self-esteem are cemented by sense of own accomplishments and feedback from others.

Bill is an average sixth-grade student who prefers gym and math and plays hockey on the team his father helps coach. Bill has six equally close friends and is popular. He has never been in any real trouble, but recently was caught with three friends on the roof of the recreation center. His father got angry and hit him, but that was the last of it. Recently Bill has been interested in his appearance and accompanies his mother to shop for jeans and T-shirts. All his friends dress alike. They play football and hockey, listen to rock music, and kid one another about girls.

Kristian, called Krissie by his mother, is a tall, lean, blond boy. He is a top sixth-grade student, bright, attentive, and well liked by his teachers. His art teacher is especially encouraging of his talent, although Krissie is modest and thinks art is "sissy." He is proud of his ability in electronics, however. He dreams of being a space pilot and reads science fiction avidly at a tenth- or eleventh-grade level. Krissie and Peter are constant friends who build model cars and airplanes together and even "play" with their car collections at times, even though they feel it is babyish.

BASIC DEVELOPMENTAL PARAMETERS

Biological Development

All aspects of development are predicated upon the continuing growth and maturation of the body, particularly that of the central nervous, musculoskeletal, and endocrine systems. The readiness to learn and the accessibility to specific environmental influences are highly contingent on biological maturation. Thus no amount of training or stimulation prior to an organ's maturational readiness will allow coordination and motor skills, bowel and bladder control, or specific cognitive, language, or emotional achievements to come about. The interrelationships between these different developmental parameters were first expressed by Gesell and his group (Pasamanick and Knobloch 1966) who correlated stages of biological maturation with the emergence of various developmental skills on significant numbers of children. Table 1.1 summarizes their findings. Recent work has documented that even man's biological development is significantly influenced by the social environment. For example, children who receive little social stimulation for extended periods may fall behind in their physical as well as their intellectual growth. Children are also genetically endowed with specific temperamental dispositions. These determine the style with which a child will interact with his caregivers and other facets of his environment. Table 1.2 summarizes nine specific temperamental traits as they were described by Thomas and associates (1963).

It should be stressed, however, that the notion of temperament is potentially much more complex than some writers make it out to be. Thus virtually all temperamental measures employed at present are based on reports by parents. This does not help us distinguish subjective elements of parental "judgment" of the child from the purely constitutional component of temperament. As a result, it should be understood that parental

TABLE 1.2
Basic Temperamental Traits

1. Activity Level	Describes the level, tempo, and frequency of motor behavior, ranging from hypoactive to hyperactive.
2. Rhythmicity	Describes the rhythmicity of repetitive biological functions such as sleeping and waking, eating and appetite, bowel and bladder functioning. Ranges from regular (establishment of pattern) to irregular (failure to establish even a partial pattern).
3. Approach and Withdrawal	Describes the child's initial reaction to any new stimulus, be it food, people, places, or procedures.
4. Adaptability	Describes the child's sequences of responses to a new or altered situation; deals with the ease or difficulty with which the initial response can be modified by parents or others.
5. Intensity of Reaction	Describes energy content of the response, irrespective of its direction, ranging from mild to intense in either a positive or negative sense.
6. Threshold of Responsiveness	Refers to the level (quantity) of extrinsic stimulation required to produce a discernible response, regardless of the nature or quality of the stimulus.
7. Quality of Mood	Deals with the amount of pleasant, joyful, and friendly behavior versus unpleasant, crying, and unfriendly behavior.
8. Distractibility	Refers to the effectiveness of external environmental stimuli in interfering with, or in altering the direction of, the ongoing behavior.
9. Attention Span and Persistence	Attention span refers to the length of time a particular activity is pursued. Persistence refers to the child's continuing with an activity in spite of obstacles either external (e.g., environmental interferences) or internal (e.g., limitation of ability related to the activity).

SOURCE: This table summarizes data from A. Thomas, et al. *Behavioral Individuality in Early Childhood* (New York: New York University Press, 1963).

reports of a child's temperament are not truly objective measures. Also, different temperaments may be more or less adaptive in specific situations depending on family structure or social class.

Despite this difficulty, the concept of temperament has been extremely useful to the average clinician, as it has made it possible to understand and explain some of the difficulties parents or other adults have with children and/or with each other in a much more interactive perspective. It has had further clinical implications since it has been established that children with certain temperamental clusters (e.g., an irregularity of feeding and sleeping, or high intensity of reaction and a low adaptability or attention span) tend to have far more difficulties in negotiating specific developmental tasks than do children with a more placid and easygoing temperament (Graham, Rutter, and George 1973; Rutter et al. 1964).

Cognitive Development

"Cognitive development" includes three different perspectives of the child. The first refers to how children think at different ages, compared to adults' perception of the world. The second sees children as essentially social beings. Thus it examines children's ability to learn new and ever more complex things as a reflection of their environment or culture, and focuses on the primary mechanisms that allow this transmission of knowledge, mainly language and other facets of interpersonal relationships. The final perspective tries to assess children less as action-oriented organisms than by observing their developing abilities to listen, watch, or feel.

All these functions must be considered in trying to judge a child's state of cognitive development. It is equally clear that some of these functions, such as the development of language or interpersonal relationships, will also be important modifiers of a child's emotional well-being. This again illustrates how intimately interconnected various parameters of human development are, and how consequently laws governing one facet of development are often equally applicable to others. For example, Piaget and his pupils have clearly documented that while the rate of cognitive development may vary, the structure of the child's thinking changes according to a predetermined sequence, and hence is dependent on maturational forces (Piaget and Inhelder 1958). This means that an adult can do nothing to shape a child's developmentally appropriate, idiosyncratic view of the world and that the child's "thoughts" and thinking are a reflection of his or her stage of mental evolution. As in most evolutionary processes, thinking, language, and perceptions progress from a concrete to a more abstract level. They also move, as we shall see, from a more self-centered to an other-oriented view of the world.

Emotional Development

Traditionally, emotions have been equated with feelings and hence the relative happiness or unhappiness of an individual. At the same time, intelligence and the ability to reason were seen as the hallmark of man's superiority over other species, while feelings were seen as philogenetically older and hence more primitive phenomena. Studies examining the emotional development of children have only been done in the more recent past. Before that children's feelings were seen as arising primarily from biological needs such as hunger, cold, or other specific frustrations. For example, early psychoanalysts saw an infant's happiness as depending primarily on the availability of the mother's breast, while later stages of emotional development were seen as reflections of the child's experiences surrounding toilet training or rivalry with the parents. Today there is very good evidence that the emotional development of children is much more complex than has been previously recognized. Thus we know that all human beings are both in need of and capable of communication with others from birth onward and that emotions play a crucial role in establishing and/or maintaining interpersonal relationships (Fraiberg, 1959; Lewis, 1981). For example, it has been shown that infants as young as six days of age prefer their mother's breast to that of another woman (MacFarlane 1975). They also like to look at faces much more than at pictures, prefer the human voice to any other sound, and within the following four weeks have developed a good spectrum of differentiated expressions of emotions such as fear, delight, wariness, or anxiety (Emde and Robinson 1981).

As much of the early behavioral repertoire of infants, such as smiling or crying, is directed primarily at the source of their comforts, the resulting attachment between them and their caregivers serves to make the rearing of a healthy baby a generally pleasurable task.

Soon after the initial six months of life, during which much of the infant's emotional behavior is dominated by motivations derived from biological needs, infants become increasingly aware of the difference between familiar phenomena and those that are strange or unfamiliar. Thus faces that are new or have unusual features (such as a beard) may evoke fear or at least caution in the infant. At around the same time (between six and ten months), infants also begin to distinguish clearly between themselves and others. Thus they can now potentially grasp that they need others to survive and that others may not automatically be available when they want them. While this realization may make the child anxious and upset, the same cognitive achievement also helps the infant "understand" that mothers or fathers who go away normally come back when they are needed, and that waiting and/or postponing a perceived wish or need will usually pay off. As caregivers increasingly begin to demand that the child accept the frustrations and discomforts that come from modifying urgent biological demands for rapid and total gratification (e.g., hunger, thirst, elimination), the attachment bond developed during the early months of life serves as the vehicle on which much future social and emotional development is based. If the child's caregivers quickly satisfy the child's need for physical and emotional comfort and are responsive to his or her behavioral leads and cues during this period, they will assist in the initial formation of stable interpersonal bonds between child and family. When a good fit between child and parents exists, the parents' dependable responsiveness to the infant's needs leads to the development of security and trust, first between child and parents and later by the process of generalizing between the child and others at school or work (Winnicott 1964).

It follows that later on children will want to pattern themselves on (i.e., identify with) the parents and the parents' standards of good and bad, right and wrong, will increasingly become the children's. At age two or three,

15

these standards feel as if they are an echo of the parents' true voices within the children. Later, as parental expectations become integrated within the children's own personality, the children shun misbehaving not just to avoid offending others but to escape the internal censor of what they are becoming increasingly aware of as their developing conscience. Thus by this time the children's biological drives or wishes are opposed both by environmental restrictions (pressure from parents and others) and, increasingly, by the growing inner voice of conscience. These often conflicting demands of inner wishes and outside restrictions normally generate a certain degree of anxiety within children, who, in response, usually develop a series of defense mechanisms. Such defenses may take, among others, the form of denying the discrepancies between one or the other demand, or of becoming very preoccupied by the need to fulfill the parents' wishes, as shown by a longing for routines and other caregiving rituals. Most children develop defenses sufficient to keep them relatively free of anxiety and to allow continuing development without significantly restricting the scope of enjoyment of their lives. Yet in some children the defenses developed prove inadequate to the task, so that the children constantly fear lest instinctual drives, escaping from their precarious controls, erupt and expose them to the threat of punishment or rejection. In still other children the use of defense mechanisms in response to this threat is so excessive or inappropriate that the children's behavior and personality are dominated by these abnormal manifestations of defense, and are then seen as psychological symptoms. (See chapter 12.)

Superimposed on this basic struggle are a number of major tasks the growing child must negotiate in moving toward emotional maturity (Erikson 1959). For example, children must achieve a stable and integrated self-concept and adequate self-esteem in order to feel that finding out new things and experimenting are basically useful and pleasurable tasks worth the risk of possible failure; they must develop healthy attitudes toward authority; they must gradually but successfully negotiate the process of individuation in order to achieve a degree of emotional independence from the immediate family and to be free to relate intimately to others; psychosexual development must proceed, allowing the adoption of an appropriate gender identity and healthy attitudes toward their own sexuality. The process by which these are achieved will be discussed in more detail later in the chapter.

Personal-Social Development

It should be clear by now that there is a major overlap between development in the emotional and in the personal-social spheres, as all children are struggling to contain their biological demands in response to various social forces. While social forces are usually transmitted through individuals such as parents, peers, or teachers, their expression commonly reflects the more general customs of the local culture. A good example is the differ-

16

ence in the degree of emotional expressiveness permitted in Anglo-Saxon and Latin cultures. Likewise there are vast differences in sanctioned behaviors among individuals of different social class or religious affiliations, and changes occur even within these over time. Also, in most developed countries there has been a remarkable change concerning the importance given the emotional experiences surrounding childbirth. Previously the aim was to deliver a healthy baby with the assistance of as much technology as possible. Professionals are now very concerned about the father's presence at birth and try to provide opportunities for much early contact between mother and baby in order to facilitate bonding with baby right after birth. Likewise, with a high number of infants having much of their primary care provided not within the family but in day care, the question of how emotional development is affected by attachment to a number of primary caregivers is also being increasingly explored. (See chapter 4.) In any event, by middle childhood children have been exposed to a number of models and to pressures from a variety of extrafamilial figures. Increasingly their influence may compete with and, during adolescence, even at times contradict and supplant that of the parents in shaping the values, behavior, and attitudes of children.

Language Development

While language development might well be considered just one of the specialized aspects of cognitive development, it will be discussed separately. This is primarily because the use of language plays a key role in the continuing emotional, social, and cognitive evolution of each child. Thus children with language problems—that is, children who have difficulties in formulating and comprehending symbolic thought and the use and understanding of verbal and nonverbal cues essential for communication—are also likely to show high rates of behavior disturbances (Cantwell, Baker, and Mattison 1979; Richman 1977).

The development of language has its precursors long before children are able to use verbal speech. For example, there is some evidence that neonates synchronize their body movements with the sound of an adult voice as early as twelve hours after birth and by three months respond differentially to friendly and hostile voices (Meltzoff and Moore 1977). In general, children understand words well before they can actually use them, although there are well-defined maturational limits to language acquisition. Thus initially words are used mainly to identify objects and people, and only during the second year can the child ask for or talk about things that are not there. During the third year children begin to play with language and in this way prepare themselves for symbolic thought (Nelson 1973). The importance of language for general development is highlighted by a number of recent findings. As an example, it has been observed that children who do not play with words are also impaired in their use of toys (Lovell, Hoyle, and Siddak 1968). In contrast, mothers usually are finely attuned to their child's language development, helping it along by talking to their children at high pitch, repeating words frequently, and using short and distinct utterances (Cross 1977; Phillips 1973). Finally, there is a close association between social class and family size in language development. Lower-class children tend to use shorter words and shorter phrases and children of larger families commonly exhibit a general delay in their language development (Rutter and Mittler 1972; Berstein 1962).

The Developmental Process

THE PERINATAL PERIOD

For each couple, the birth of their first child heralds a new developmental stage. Before they were a couple; now they are a family. Being a parent is not easy. Parenthood presents many pressures that may not be recognized, let alone reported to a physician. It may cause strain on a marriage, psychological stress for either or both parents, and resentment toward the child who has complicated their lives. The stage for the development of a new baby is often set twenty to thirty years previously, since the attitudes and patterns we employ as parents are significantly influenced by the parenting we received as children. Our own parents serve as our role models, and, even if we consciously repudiate their values and techniques in our upbringing of our own children, there is a natural tendency to revert and to repeat the type of parenting we experienced. Parenting is a major task, yet one in which we receive little formal advance preparation. For example, a new mother who has lacked the experience of feeling cared for may find it difficult to provide this experience for her infant, especially if the child proves frustrating and difficult in spite of her best efforts. A father who did not identify with his own father or father surrogate sufficiently may also find it hard to take a parental role and to assist his wife without excessively resenting the time and attention she now has to share with the newcomer. Should the baby fail to meet the parents' needs or expectations by being physically deformed or mentally handicapped, by having a congenital illness or even by not having the sex or the temperamental disposition the parents had desired, the resulting disappointment may place the child at risk.*

Events during pregnancy may have major and lasting effects not just

---

*This issue will be discussed in more detail later in this chapter.

on the condition of the infant at birth, but on the whole course of subsequent development. Maternal infections such as syphilis, gonorrhea, toxoplasmosis, and rubella during the first trimester have been clearly associated with serious congenital defects in the developing fetus (Krugman and Katz 1981). Metabolic deficiencies of genetic etiology in the mother can also have intrauterine effects on the infant (Kolodny 1972). Incompatibility of maternal and fetal blood types used to be a major source not only of intrauterine death but also of kernicterus, which was commonly complicated by cerebral palsy. Maternal drug taking during pregnancy has been implicated in a whole range of complications of handicaps; studies have been made on the effects of steroids administered early in pregnancy on the differential development of the sexual organs; the interference of thalidomide with the normal development of the limbs; the effects of barbiturates and opiates on the condition of the infant in the neonatal period; the association of maternal smoking with a lower birth weight and an increased incidence of prematurity Rush 1974). Prematurity not only results in greater biological vulnerability of the infant, but predisposes to a whole range of psychosocial problems, such as difficulties in bonding by the primary caregivers (Minde 1980).

But the newborn infant does not merely respond passively to the ministrations of the parents. Despite apparent helplessness at birth, each infant has available an innate repertoire of behaviors such as clinging, crying, sucking, and following. All these behaviors will play an important role in shaping maternal responsiveness and in eliciting caregiving behavior on the part of the mother or other primary caregiver (Brazelton, Koslowski, and Main 1974).

Some mental health workers feel that the first hour or two following birth are a special, sensitive period during which the bonding of parent to child can be actively promoted by specific manipulations (Klaus and Kennell 1982). An infant is usually in a quiet alert state during the first forty-five minutes following birth. As such a long alert state occurs only rarely during the following two to three days, Klaus and Kennell (1981) believe that close physical contact between mother, father, and the infant should be encouraged during this initial period. The general acceptance of this premise is reflected in changing birth practices, encouraging a family-oriented natural childbirth. Thus, at present, the majority of large hospitals in the developed world allow fathers into the labor and delivery room for normal births. While there is some evidence that this practice, in addition to being welcomed by both parents and to promoting a strong, more responsive mother-infant bond, actually decreases medical complications during labor and delivery, there is currently no proof that the lack of such early intimate togetherness has any adverse effect on the later development of the infant or the parent-infant relationship (Minde 1980; Rutter 1981; Sosa et al. 1980).

DEVELOPMENT DURING THE FIRST YEAR OF LIFE

Over the course of the first year, infants gradually gain control over their body. Control over the eyes is achieved in the first quarter, over the head and arms in the second quarter, over the trunk and hands in the third, and over the forefinger and thumb in the fourth. The ongoing process of biological maturation will prepare children to begin developing the motor skills that are essential for independent functioning. These include achieving the control over hands and arms that will allow them to begin exploring their world; acquiring control over their legs that will allow them to become independently mobile, thus expanding the field of exploration; and increasing elaboration of and control over cognitive apparatus and functioning.

During the first year, cognitive development proceeds from the sensorimotor level present at birth. As maturation proceeds, infants pass from a stage of reflex activity (e.g., the involuntary grasping of an object placed in the hand) through one of voluntary repetition of reflex activities (such as repeatedly thrusting the thumb or fist in the mouth, removing it, and reinserting it), to one of deliberate placing of the thumb in the mouth. True convergence of the two eyes on an object in the field of vision, essential for fixation and depth perception, first occurs at about seven or eight weeks. Some time around ten weeks of age, infants can be shown to be capable of storing the memory of a stimulus. They gradually begin to recognize that pushing an object changes its position, thus providing a different view. When they reach the point where they learn to associate these different visual perspectives with the same object, they are ready to grasp the concept of object permanence.

Object permanence is an essential prerequisite for further cognitive, emotional, and social development. Usually developed gradually some time during the first year, it becomes possible only when children can develop and retain a memory trace of an object removed from their line of vision. By this stage, if a child sees a favorite toy hidden, he or she will uncover it and regain it with delight, although if the task is complicated by first hiding and then shifting the toy without the child's knowledge, the child will continue to search for it in the original hiding place. It is not until between eighteen and twenty-four months that the child will overcome the added complexity of this maneuver to continue the search beyond the original hiding place until the toy is recovered.

The achievement of object permanence has important implications on children's relationships with their mother. By a year of age, if their mother leaves the room and the children are free to follow, they are usually not distressed; presumably they recognize that the mother still exists beyond the doorway, so that they have only to follow to find her. Toward the middle of the second year, however, children are likely to be distressed at their mother's leaving. With their increased awareness and understanding, they now seem to comprehend that their mother, though just outside the door, might at any moment move away again. Therefore they feel the need to follow her, to maintain some visual or auditory trace of her lest the mother moves to a more distant area of what the children's increasingly sophisticated memory map tells them lies beyond the door. These general developmental sequences are in no way rigid and can be drastically modified by changes in the particular situations such as interesting distractions, past experiences with other adults, and so on.

Socially we see the following changes. Anywhere from two weeks to two months infants begin to smile in response to the human voice. Soon they smile noticeably more in response to the mother (or other primary caregiver) than to others. As their visual discrimination and their ability to recognize their surroundings increase, they become noticeably more comfortable in the mother's company than in that of strangers. Yet some researchers have noted that infants as young as two months of age have shown differential patterns in relating to mothers, fathers, and strangers (Yarrow 1967). With the mother, children's movements are usually smooth and circular and their responses alternate with the mother's speaking to them. With the father, infants are more alert, sit upright, and make large and sudden limb movements. Infants also show a definite withdrawal of interest from strangers as early as four weeks of age. Some time after six months, they will begin to "make strange," hiding their face in the mother's shoulder or staring impassively when a stranger approaches.

In language development, infants of one month do little cooing or babbling. Cooing and squealing increase during the second and third months, apparently independent of environmental factors. After the third month, however, these vowel-dominated sounds occur increasingly in response either to being stimulated or to the sound of the infant's own voice. By six months, babbling consisting of an increasing number of one-syllable repetitions has replaced cooing as the dominant mode of expression. The babbling is typically interspersed with consonants, and by the end of the first year the words mama and dada have entered the vocabulary of the child who, by this stage, gives definite evidence of understanding common words and simple commands.

At age one, Bill was shorter than Krissie and had trouble standing or walking, but this did not stop him from crawling into all sorts of adventures. His parents considered his behavior a great joke. Though little involved in early care, Bill's father later enjoyed playing peek-a-boo and boisterous games with his son. Bill frequently stayed overnight with grandparents, and was excited if a visit to "Bopa's" was suggested. He could be comforted by a parent or grandparent, although he preferred his mother slightly.

Krissie, already shy, wore an eighteen-month size by his first birthday. From about eight months, he could pull himself up and move about in his walker. Krissie's father usually spent his leisure hours making home improvements, taking little part in the care of his son. Except for the odd babysitter in the evenings, Krissie's mother was the only caregiver. Krissie had two severe colds in his first year, and his mother seemed to be the only one who could comfort him.

In the area of emotional development, the crucial advance during the first year is that of the bonding that gradually develops between infant and mother, referred to as attachment. Contrary to popular belief, attachment of the child to the mother or father is by no means inevitably present at birth. It develops gradually over time as a result of ongoing exposure and mutual interaction. Anything that interferes with this ongoing interaction in the first days and weeks of life, such as prematurity or a serious illness that keeps mother or infant in the hospital and away from each other for weeks at a time, may interfere with a successful bonding, thus increasing the risk that a satisfactory attachment will not occur.

While most infants do attach, Ainsworth and associates (1978) have identified three types of attachment behavior—secure, avoidant, and anxious. In a "strange situation experiment" developed by Ainsworth and Wittig (1969), one-year-old children were observed in a playroom, first left by their mother and invited to play with a stranger, then left alone in the room, and finally in a reunion episode with the mother. Children with a "secure attachment" were able to explore their new surroundings and, being reassured by closeness of their mothers, could continue to play even in the presence of a stranger. They also greeted their mothers and were easily comforted by them when they returned. Children with an avoidant attachment tended to cry on reunion with the mother, whining and demanding her attention, but often pushing the mother away when she attempted to comfort them. Children who had developed an anxious attachment were not easily comforted by their mothers and avoided them after a separation. Some attachment theorists feel that such early manifestations of the quality of attachment predict the child's later psychological functioning (Matas, Arend, and Sroufe 1978; Phillips 1973).

If attachment is not universally present at birth, how then does it come about? In addition to the mother's usual attitudes of caring and protectiveness derived from an instinct toward the preservation of the species and from the personal pleasure that many but by no means all mothers feel at having given birth to a healthy child, through their behavior infants do much either to assist or to impede the attachment process. Many instinctual behaviors such as crying, sucking, clinging, smiling, and stroking play an active part in keeping the mother close and in encouraging maternal involvement. Bowlby (1969) describes how, over a period of time, these primary behaviors develop into goal-corrective systems that organize to maintain proximity to the attachment figures (mother, father), becoming in effect attachment behaviors.

The closeness that develops between mother and child does not become a mutual attachment until about eight months of age. At this stage cognitive development has reached the point where, concurrent with or slightly after the development of stranger anxiety, children recognize the primary caregiver, usually the mother, as more important than any other adult for their comfort and security. Once attachment has become mutual, this bond makes it difficult for mother or child to endure a separation from the other. One might equate the development of attachment with the growth of love, especially since there is some evidence that future relationships and the capacity to love may be determined to some extent by the quality of this early attachment (Matas, Arend, and Sroufe 1978). (See also p. 63.) Attachment behavior intensifies, typically reaching a peak at eighteen months, and then declines over the next two to three years to a maintenance level as children become increasingly self-reliant and independent. Although much of the early work on attachment is focused on the developmental mother-infant bond, recent research indicates that a qualitatively different but important attachment bond occurs between the infant and the father and other important adults during the same developmental phase, again dependent on the responsiveness of the father or these adults to the infant (Dixon et al 1981; Schaffer and Emerson 1964). It should be stressed, however, that there are persisting hierarchies of attachments; that is, even in institutions, children have a favorite adult to whom they will go in preference to others over prolonged periods (Stevens 1975).

Severe neglect and failure to develop a successful attachment are associated with a broad range of cognitive, emotional, and social deficits, which may include a virtual disruption of development and a blunting of the capacity for social relationships (Goldfarb 1943; Goldfarb 1955). However, most children who are removed from homes in which they are suffering severe neglect and privation and placed in families that provide adequate security and stimulation show marked developmental gains (Tizard and Hodges 1978). Though much remains to be learned in this area, it appears that the consequences of separation for a given child will depend on a number of factors, such as the degree of privation to which he or she has been exposed previously, the duration of the separation, the age at which the separation occurs (with children between the ages of one and four years being particularly vulnerable), and the adequacy and prompt availability of a suitable alternative (Rutter 1981).

AGES ONE TO THREE

Frequently called the toddler years, ages one to three are the years in which locomotor controls and skills are perfected, allowing children more freedom, greater independence, and an expanding environment. By fifteen months children can crawl, climb stairs, and frequently walk on their own. Running away from parents and other games related to this newfound mastery over the body become a source of pleasure and delight, as well as a means of reinforcing children's attachment to parents. By this age children are generally given the run of the house and by three years can run easily, jump with some control, and negotiate stairs alone with alternate feet. In addition, by this stage fine motor control has improved sufficiently so that children can hold a crayon and scribble pictures of their own, thus demonstrating the first signs of potential creativity.

Intellectually toddlers deal with their world through play, beginning by ordering and grouping objects. They may, for example, line up all their toy animals, placing them in the farmyard while the toy people are all put in or near the house. The most striking development during the second year usually occurs in the area of language. At eighteen months average children, despite a vocabulary of between three and fifty words, including a few set phrases (e.g., thank you), are not yet spontaneously combining words to form phrases. Both vocabulary and understanding progress rapidly, however, and by their second birthday children are combining words to form two-word phrases and, increasingly, using language to communicate their wants to others. Much of their vocabulary develops out of the ordering and grouping, as they use language concepts to group objects together to form categories and then to define the nature of these categories. Pigs, cows, and horses all fall into the category of animals and animals go in barns, in farmyards, or in trucks, but not in houses or cars, and so on. While constantly adding to their vocabulary, this sort of play also provides children with a way of organizing and understanding the world around them.

Toddlers also develop a sense of themselves through language. They learn their names and begin to group themselves into certain categories, each with its own specific meanings and rules. For example, a child learns that he is Johnny, and a member of the Smith family, unlike Janie next door who belongs to the Brown family. He also learns that he is a boy while she is a girl, as well as what boys are and what is expected of them. What a child learns specifically about boys will reflect the definition and attitudes of what is considered boyish in the child's particular family and its social circle. For example, a boy learns that when he grows up, he may become a daddy or husband, but will never be a mommy or wife. He learns that boys do not wear dresses (unless they are dressing up and pretending to be girls). He will learn a whole list of dos and don'ts that his particular family associates with being a boy: certain toys (e.g., dolls), activities (e.g., skipping), games (e.g., playing school) or attitudes (e.g., timidity, noncompetitiveness, sensitivity) may evoke their criticism while others (e.g., playing cars, climbing trees, "toughness," and bravery) may be encouraged. At some point, often around age three, the child will become aware that boys, like men, have penises that allow them to urinate standing up, unlike girls who, lacking them, sit down to do so. Thus a whole series of language-linked concepts help a boy develop a sense of himself. Yet this sense can only come about when cognitive and language development allow him to grasp the concept of categories and their individual characteristics.

24

Emotional development passes through three important phases during this period, well described by Margaret Mahler (Mahler, Pine, and Bergman 1975). As children's motor skills and use of language increase, they are able to venture forth and do more for themselves, thus becoming somewhat less dependent on their mother. This helps the children develop a strong sense of self as a separate person and often leads to fiercely independent behavior. Thus during the "terrible twos," it is quite normal for children to assert their independence by refusing to cooperate with parents around routines, dressing, or toilet training. But while children initially take great pleasure in asserting themselves as separate from their mother, between fifteen and eighteen months there routinely occurs a phase of rapprochement. During this stage the bond of the attachment to the parents hits a peak as children return to an intensified closeness with them. Often whiny, demanding, and more babyish, children at this stage are more vulnerable to separation anxiety if the parents leave, even to go out for the evening. Shortly thereafter, however, this anxiety recedes and again children, usually with the support and approval of the parents, begin to show signs of more independent and self-sufficient behavior (Mahler, Pine, and Bergman 1975).

At this time many parents notice their children becoming intensely attached to a special blanket or toy that seems to be essential for their ongoing security. While often dragged and taken everywhere, it seems especially necessary when the children go to sleep or face unfamiliar situations. It has been suggested that something about this object reminds the children of the safe, secure world of the early part of the first year. The blanket thus seems to serve as if the children had a part of their mother, and all the security she represents, available to them at all times. Such an object—Linus's blanket in the *Peanuts* comic strip is possibly the best-known contemporary example—is often termed a transitional object, in that it reminds children of the secure base of mother while they step forth from the safety of the relationship with her and experiment with less certain and at times anxiety-provoking relationships with other people, sometimes termed object relationships (Winnicott 1953).

The second and third year is also a time when children begin to differentiate their wants and needs from those of the parents. As the parents gradually begin to introduce limits and controls, children may struggle against them, although usually by three years of age they are prepared to submit to the will of the parents. In this, probably the earliest stage of moral development, children do as the parents say, not because they want to or in order to be good, but to avoid the loss of love or the parental anger that they fear will follow should they disobey. Toilet training is one example of the potential conflict of wills typical of this stage. Children who have reached the point where they have both the capacity for delaying evacuation and the ability to recognize and signal the imminent event sufficiently in advance are expected to hold in their stool and place it in the appropriate place at the proper time. This may make great sense to mothers, but it rarely does so for toddlers, who often experience both mild discomfort while holding in and some anxiety when placed on the toilet. If mothers, for any reason, try to force children to train before they are ready or prepared to do so, an intense power struggle may result leading to withholding, at times complicated by constipation and pain for the child and a severe strain on the mother-child relationship. Usually, however, training is completed within a few weeks when the child is ready, and in the normal child soiling rarely persists beyond age three.

Finally, this period between one and three is also the age when some children create an imaginary playmate. Often larger than life, this playmate serves to protect the children—the master—against monsters or the dark while at the same time helping the children, who may feel hemmed in by rules and adult authority, imagine that they are no longer lowest in the family pecking order. The imaginary playmate is also a good example of how play serves much more than just a recreational function, since it helps drain off energy and allows children to practice new skills and to master anxiety about feared situations. In addition, it makes it possible for children to behave like parents or other adults, thus providing them with an opportunity to practice and feel that they are like their most important role models.

> Bill didn't walk until fourteen months, and then he mostly ran. He loved emptying drawers and cupboards, and by age two his favorite word was no. At eighteen months toilet training was unsuccessful, even though Bill seemed to have the idea, but at twenty-six months he learned in a week. Bill enjoyed weekends with his grandparents, but at twenty months, when his parents left on vacation for two weeks, he became unusually quiet and withdrawn. On his parents' return he acted as if they had never been away but misbehaved for three days after. Bill was always a very involved spectator when his father played baseball on Sunday afternoons.

> Krissie was sickly in his second year and his mother was constantly phoning the doctor. An early walker, he managed stairs easily by sixteen months. He could do many things for himself but preferred his mother's help. His parents were proud of his skills with toys and crayons; his mother, a sculptor, was very involved in his play. Krissie wanted to join in his father's woodworking projects around the house, but his father felt it was too dangerous.

THE PRESCHOOL YEARS, AGES THREE TO SIX

Improved muscle coordination allows the development of further motor skills during the preschool years. Children learn to hop, skip, throw a ball, become expert in riding a tricycle and, late in the period, possibly even a small bicycle. Improved observation skills and eye-hand coordination allow them to draw first a circle and later a square. By the end of this period children are capable of drawing a person with six parts.

Meanwhile, children continue to explore their physical world, expanding their cognitive development by grouping and naming objects. Much of the learning occurs through action-linked concepts: apples are eaten, books are read, shovels are for clearing snow, and so on. Each of these objects, however, is also included in other groupings. An apple, for example, is a food and also a fruit; as it begins with the letter *A*, it is an A word, but it also has a shape and a red color that can be painted or crayoned. In this way the original action-linked concept is extended by a series of associated images, thus leading to the acquisition of new words. During this period the vocabulary, which by age three consists of about a thousand words, expands at the rate of fifty new words each month. By age three, about 80 percent of children's verbalization can be understood even by strangers. Although they still make errors, in general their grammatical constructions compare in complexity with those of colloquial adult speech, and by age four their grasp of language has advanced to the point where their speech differs from that of adults more in style than in the number of errors. By about four years children begin using complete sentences of up to eight words, sentences that are complex in their organization and notable for the increased use of relational words such as personal pronouns. By this time children have mastered vocal inflections and can use language to negotiate with the environment and to instruct themselves. Toward the end of this stage, children increasingly begin to enter the community, learning to cross roads safely and to find their own way to school and home. By now they can dress and undress themselves completely, usually become aware of their peers and spend an increasing amount of time playing with them. At first the children are not really able to play together, but rather interact with each other as they play or follow a parallel symbolic theme. By age six, however, children are capable of playing simple games by rules without adult supervision.

Until well into the preschool years, children regulate their behavior largely in response to environmental controls, but by about age five they are beginning to develop a set of internalized standards or conscience of their own. Thus their actions are increasingly controlled not by the fear or shame of getting caught, but by a growing personal sense of right and wrong. Their system of values develops as they increasingly decide what they want to be like and how they want to be seen by others. Heavily influenced by parental expectations, they take pride in activities they know that parents admire, and play out long and complicated fantasies on these themes.

Psychoanalysts refer to this as the oedipal period because they see it as characterized by the child's developing a sexual interest in the parents, particularly the parent of the opposite sex. Determined partly by the strength of innate biological drives and partly by dynamic alignments within the family environment, this attraction and the guilt and anxiety resulting from it are normally resolved by identification with the same-sex parent in favor of extrafamilial interests and activities. Failure to success-fully achieve this resolution is seen by psychoanalysts as the nuclear con-flict in psychoneurosis, and as a decisive influence in adult sexuality (Bux-baum 1959).

As children continue to align themselves with parental expectations, they begin to see themselves and to behave in a manner appropriate to their biological sex. The attitudes of one generation regarding what is sex-ually appropriate are passed on to the next. Children increasingly learn to avoid acting in ways they associate specifically with the other sex. They begin to imitate, not always consciously, the parent of the same sex who serves as a role model, while the opposite-sex parent, under typical cir-cumstances, allows and encourages this identification. During the pre-school years, children not infrequently experience severe anxiety, possibly related to what at times are stringent demands of their newly developed conscience, to increasingly demanding environmental expectations, and to the need to be like the parent of the same sex. This anxiety may lead to transitory and intense but usually normal fears that may take the form of nightmares, transient phobias, fear of the dark or of monsters, fear of bodily harm, or bed-wetting.

> Krissie made friends with a little girl down the street. Though she was sev-eral months younger, she tended to dominate their play. At first Krissie could not tolerate his mother leaving him at her house to play. He had the same reac-tion to starting nursery school at age three. Later he enjoyed all the activities, particularly the group singing, but even by age five he still had difficulty shar-ing his toys. He had a series of colds and was often absent. His mother always tried to keep him from playing with the other children if they had colds and her worries would make Krissie sullen. Krissie looked forward to the weekends when he could help his father build the new porch.

> When Bill was three and a half, a baby brother was born. Bill had wanted a brother but after a while came to resent the attention the infant received. His speech became less clear and he reverted to baby talk and bed-wetting. On a physician's advice, his father spent more time with Bill and soon the prob-lem was alleviated. Bill was always covered with bruises from falls, less from clumsiness than from being aggressive and trying everything. Bill didn't start school until age five. After two weeks he could walk the three blocks to school by himself. He enjoyed playing with boys his own age but did not always need their company.

MIDDLE CHILDHOOD: AGES SIX TO ELEVEN

This period, extending from the end of the infantile period (about six) until just prior to the resurgence of sexual and aggressive drives that initi-ates adolescence, is one in which children's attention and energies are fo-cused primarily on continuing socialization and on their adjustment to the external world, including school. Often an easier, less stressful period for both parents and children, it is one in which the strong drives and inner conflicts of the earlier years frequently seem to lose some of their urgency. Psychoanalysts have termed this the stage of latency, as they see it as providing a biologically determined breathing space between the psychological conflicts of the preceding oedipal period and the subsequent physiologically increased stresses and conflicts of preadolescence.

Others (such as Chess and associates), prefer the term middle childhood, as their observations refute the regular existence of a period of significantly reduced intrapsychic turmoil during these years. They suggest rather that with entry into school and the emphasis on continued socialization, the focus of development shifts as children increasingly begin to compare themselves to their peer group (Chess 1979). Competition with peers in every conceivable area—intelligence, appearance, strength, athletic ability, social acceptance, and material possessions—may be acute, and children's self-image, no longer merely a reflection of their parents' perception of them, increasingly takes into account the judgments of peers and teachers as well. Children, though they may at times deny it, are keenly aware of acceptance or rejection by peers and of their place in the pecking order. These inevitable social stresses lead in turn to intrapsychic conflict, as children struggle to deal with their fear of rejection. This they can do either by withdrawal or by retaliation. Should they tend toward withdrawal, they can do so physically, by not participating in activities or by avoiding volunteering answers in class to escape even the possibility of disapproval or rejection. They may rationalize this withdrawal, implying that they have no interest in being involved though they really do, or they may forget or steer entirely clear of threatening or stressful situations. Since mastering the basic academic skills being taught at this stage requires accepting the possibility of being wrong, children who are solidly committed to avoiding any risks are likely to develop learning difficulties, which in turn will further undermine their self-confidence and self-esteem.

Other children attack anxiety-rich situations head on, attempting to overcome them. If successful, their success and the resulting confidence will reinforce their pattern of direct confrontation of problems. But failure, especially repeated failure, may compound the difficulties and further undermine children's confidence in themselves and their abilities. Should they react to lack of success by clowning around or acting up in class, the reaction to their behavior may compound the damage to their self-concept and, if continued, may alienate them from school and its goals. Thus throughout middle childhood, repeated experiences in school with friends and in the home result in change and elaboration in the children's self-image and, with it, in their sense of self-esteem.

Most children look forward to beginning school, although social and cultural factors do much to influence a child's attitude and adjustment to school. While traditionally going to school was associated with furthering cognitive development, it can be seen from the preceding text that school has an impact on the child's total personality and psychological and social adjustment. While school achievement is obviously influenced by basic intelligence, other equally important determinants of academic success include motivation, work habits, creativity both innate and cultivated, cultural opportunities in and outside the home, and family encouragement and support for the value of school. Most middle- and upper-class families support education, but many lower-class children enter school lacking many of the experiences, facts, concepts, and skills possessed by their middle-class peers and valued by their middle-class teachers. Lower-class parents, who frequently mistrust the school system, often do little to motivate their children to persevere in the face of these initial disadvantages, and instead of presenting a model encouraging academic achievement frequently give at least tacit support to their children's growing alienation from school.

During these years children's thought patterns gradually shift from the concrete ordering and grouping of objects that Piaget terms the period of concrete operations, to a stage where they begin to understand concepts that allow them to start working with ideas with less need for specific objects to serve as visual props. However, true abstract reasoning, or what Piaget terms formal operations—the ability to think and to understand changes in terms of abstract concepts without the support of concrete examples to serve as props—is not achieved until well into adolescence (Piaget and Inhelder 1958).

During middle childhood the processes of moral development and gender-identity formation, begun earlier on the basis of identification, continue. The influence of the initial role models, the parents, finds increasing competition with the values and attitudes of the peer group. When, especially toward the end of these years, children begin to develop moral standards that reflect their own values, there may be much preoccupation with what is right or wrong in others' behavior. The growing ability to think in abstract terms increasingly allows children to consider moral issues in a general or abstract way (Kohlberg and Kramer 1969). This preoccupation with good and evil spills over into their fantasy life. Their imagination, continuing strong, elaborates on themes of universal good and bad, as fairy tales and monsters are replaced by police and gangsters, Kung-Fu, and so on. The search for values, and for a clearly defined sense of the self as a unique individual, will not be completed during middle childhood, but will be among the major tasks remaining for the continuing development that will occur during the adolescent years.

> Bill had no trouble starting school, but he seemed more anxious when he made the hockey team. After losing a game, he tended to be sullen and angry but he very rarely talked back to his parents. Bill's teachers thought him capable of better than average work. He didn't particularly fear success but preferred not to stand out from his pals. His father might have liked his son to be outstanding, but did admire Bill's popularity and rarely showed concern about his schoolwork. He considered that Bill's responsibility.

Krissie, who now insisted on being called Kris, was pleased by his progress in school, as were his parents. He could read and write at home before first grade. He was quick to grasp concepts, but never competed openly with other students. For him, as for his parents, learning was a personal challenge. His mother was now a well-known sculptor. Kris and his father enjoyed working together and vying with each other in such activities as skiing. Kris and Peter, friends since nursery school, had grown closer over the years and shared everything.

SUGGESTIONS FOR FURTHER READING

AINSWORTH, M.D.S., et al. 1978. *Patterns of attachment: A psychological study of the strange situation.* Hillsdale, N.J.: Lawrence Erlbaum Associates.
Provides a detailed review of issues related to attachment and its measurement.
ARIES, P. 1962. *Centuries of childhood.* New York: Alfred A. Knopf.
A good historical review of the role of children in various societies ranging from prehistoric times to the twentieth century. While this is a historical book, it is filled with sociological and cultural data of value to the person interested in child development.
BAYLEY, N. 1965. Research in child development: A longitudinal perspective. *Merrill-Palmer Quart.* 11:184–190.
A short summary of Bayley's enormous contribution to the longitudinal observation of children's physical and emotional development.
BOWLBY, J. 1969. *Attachment and loss. Vol. I: Attachment.* New York: Basic Books.
———. 1973. *Attachment and loss. Vol. II: Separation.* New York: Basic Books.
———. 1980. *Attachment and loss. Vol. III: Loss.* New York: Basic Books.
These volumes represent the most extensive exploration and analysis of children's tie to the mother, the problems of separation, the dynamics of mourning and depression, and the processes of accommodation and healing.
ERIKSON, E. H. 1959. *Identity and the life cycle,* New York: International Universities Press.
The classic volume describing Erikson's developmental theory.
FLAVELL, J. H. 1963. *The developmental psychology of Jean Piaget.* New York: D. Van Nostrand.
A very concise and still the best summary of Piaget's theoretical concepts. Fairly hard reading.
KAGAN, J., AND MOSS, H. A. 1962. *Birth to maturity.* New York: John Wiley and Sons.
A classic volume introducing modern concepts of cognitive development.
MUSSEN, P. H.; CONGER, J. J.; AND KAGAN, J. 1981. *Child development and personality.* 5th ed. New York: Harper & Row, 1981.
The latest edition of a well-organized and highly readable general textbook of child development. Presents and integrates a variety of developmental theories along with a summary of supportive research findings.
ROBERTSON, J., AND ROBERTSON, J. 1971. Young children in brief separations—A fresh look. In R. S. Eissler, et al., eds. *The Psychoanalytic Study of the Child,* vol. 26, pp. 264–315. New York: Quadrangle Books.
Looks at environmental factors that can ameliorate the stress of separation.
RUTTER, M. 1979. Maternal deprivation, 1972–1978. New findings, new concepts, new approaches. *Child Dev.* 50:–283–305.
Reviews the evidence for the effect of maternal deprivation on later development as it has accumulated during the 1970s.
———. 1980. The long-term effects of early experience. *Dev. Med. & Child Neurol.* 22:81–115.
An excellent review of how specific initial experiences at critical ages affect later psychosocial functioning.

SKEELS, H. M. 1966. *Adult status of children with contrasting early life experiences: A follow-up study.* Monographs of the Society for Research in Child Development, serial no. 105, vol. 31, no. 3. Chicago: University of Chicago Press.

A twenty-year follow-up of the effect specific interventions have on the intelligence and behavior of deprived and retarded children.

SPITZ, R. A. 1965. *The first year of life.* New York: International Universities Press.

A psychoanalytic description of the first year of life, relying on direct observation of infants.

THOMAS, A., AND CHESS, S. 1977. *Temperament and development.* New York: Brunner/Mazel. 1977.

Arising from the twenty-year New York Longitudinal Study, this book shows the significance of temperament, as it interacts with the environment, for normal and deviant psychological development.

WINNICOTT, D. W. 1953. Transitional objects and transitional phenomena. *Int. J. Psychoanal.* 34(2):89–97.

A classic paper that describes transitional phenomena as an intermediate between the infant's inner experiences of self and outer reality.

2

Harvey Golombek

Developmental Challenges of Adolescence

Introduction

Adolescence is a period of major change. Ushered in by the hormonal activity associated with the growth spurt of puberty and by changing environmental expectations, it is a stage of rapid though uneven biological, psychological, and social development. The rate at which individuals progress through adolescence varies widely. Psychological development may lag behind physical development by years. For example, a youth of sixteen may leave home, live independently, and be fully self-supporting, while a nineteen-year-old student may remain semidependent, economically and emotionally, on the family. There exists within this stage, however, a predictable sequence of physiological and psychological developments through which different adolescents pass in their own time and at their own rate (Adelson 1980). For some the developmental course is smooth and continuous (Offer 1973). For others it may be tumultuous, characterized by inner turmoil and serious behavior problems (Blos 1963), while still others demonstrate a "surgent" course (Coleman 1980; Rutter et al. 1976), characterized by spurts of progression and regression.

Normally pubescence occurs between the ages of ten and eighteen years in girls and twelve and twenty years in boys (Boutourline Young 1971). So marked is the variation in age of onset and rate of growth that one teenager may have completed biological maturation while another of the same chronological age is just beginning it. Biological maturation includes increases in height, weight, and strength and changes in body proportion as well as the development of secondary sexual characteristics and the accompanying awareness of heightened sexual urges.

Psychosocially adolescence has been defined as a period of identity transformation beginning with the youth's first asking "Who am I?" (Erikson 1968) and reaching the formal conceptualization of "This is who I am." To find this answer and attain maturity and independence, the adolescent is confronted with a series of developmental tasks. Continuing intellectual maturation increasingly allows for the development of rich abstract reasoning, which Piaget terms formal operations. This capacity allows adolescents to entertain a wide variety of complex issues simultaneously. They become able to play with ideas, strive toward a unifying philosophy, and struggle for the ultimate meanings in life.

Adolescence can be divided into three subperiods: early, mid, and late. Early adolescence includes the developmental changes initiated and indicated by the growth spurt. During this early period the adolescent remains home-centered. Behavior may temporarily show a disorganized, erratic quality along with a decreased willingness to accommodate to the expectations of parents and others, while wide mood swings and periodic bouts of feeling deprived, needy, and unloved may dominate the emotional life. Group activities with members of the same sex predominate.

Mid adolescence follows the growth spurt by about one to two years. This is the usual time of the first tentative interest and approach toward the opposite sex. This awakening of heterosexual interest often disrupts previous peer groupings and close childhood friendships. Hero worship and a tendency to idealize some adults who are used as models for identification are common. Characteristically, this is the stage when some adolescents begin to rebel markedly, where periods of irritability, wide mood swings, and rapidly changing feelings are not uncommon. Obedience to parental dictates is often replaced by conformity to peer-group standards and loyalties. Early sexual explorations begin.

Late adolescence is a period of transition as the young person consolidates his or her identity and comes to grips with the future. Late adolescents are more able to be selective and discriminating in relationships. Feeling a more complete and separate person, by this stage they are more able to form and maintain truly intimate relationships with others whose beliefs, ideals, and motives they can see and respect as clearly as they do their own. As a result, relationships are typically more varied than are those of midadolescents (Nesselroade and Baltes 1974).

Each of these subphases has its characteristic problems and demands, and each requires a different approach to counseling and treatment.

34

Developmental Tasks and Associated Sources of Potential Stress or Deviation

BIOLOGICAL MATURATION

Profound physical changes occur in every adolescent. Although individual adolescents show much variation in the rate and magnitude of these changes, little variation is evident in their sequencing or progression. Different bodily changes tend to overlap, one component beginning before others are finished. The age range for the beginning and the end of certain bodily changes varies widely. However the average adolescent female demonstrates a peak in growth at age twelve, while boys peak at age fourteen. This point in development, called the maximum growth age, is characterized by a virtual doubling of growth velocity.

It has been possible to classify the stages of pubescent development according to five levels of maturation (Tanner stages) (Boutourline Young 1971). In males progressive changes in testicular volume; axillary, pubic, and facial hair; penile length and diameter; and changes in growth rate can be accurately measured, observed, and rated according to criteria developed by Tanner (1962). Likewise, in females progressive changes in the distribution and amount of pubic and axillary hair, breast and areola development, enlargement of labia, and in menarche can all be observed and rated. It becomes possible, therefore, to accurately determine from the above observations a particular pubescent level of physical development, which can then be related to chronological age norms and assessed psychological and social maturity. For example, an adolescent boy of chronological age fifteen may show no pubescent development (Tanner stage 0) and may therefore appear very physically immature. At the same time, he may demonstrate advanced social skills that allow for successful peer relationships. Psychological assessment might reveal advanced cognitive abilities but marked immaturity in self-image and in the capacity for self-control. Thus physical development may proceed at a different rate from other lines of social, cognitive, and psychological development. Change or lack of change in one developmental line often has a great impact on the others.

All adolescents are preoccupied with adjusting to their new physical growth and developing sexuality, with the inevitable effects on body image and self-concept. Adolescents, typically, are extremely self-conscious and sensitive about their physical appearance and any deviation from "normality." Even moderate acne, unflattering nose shape, obesity, or gynecomastia can cause exquisite, though apparently quite needless, distress, as the adolescent suffers from constantly comparing the self to idealized others of the same age.

35

Early maturers generally have some advantage over late maturers (Malm-quist 1979). While they may be under stress from undue expectations placed on them because of their mature appearance, they have the strength, height, and sexual attractiveness to enforce their place in the pecking order. Later maturers, on the other hand, are forced to compete athletically and socially with peers who exceed them in size and strength. The early developers' pride in the development of their bodies only emphasizes to late maturers their own relative immaturity. Early developers' sexual interests and activities leave the late developers feeling alternately envious, inadequate, confused, and excluded. They know their day will come, but they surely wish it were here so they could feel at least part of the gang, if not the leader.

PSYCHOSOCIAL DEVELOPMENT

Adolescence may be an upsetting period, not only for adolescents but also for their families. The process of maturing and of integrating powerful but conflicting biological and social demands may generate confusion and upheaval within adolescents. Parents may respond to this confusion as if it were adolescent rebellion. The way parents respond may either assist or impede the resolution of the conflicting demands which adolescents are struggling to integrate (Friedman 1975; Ravenscroft 1974).

Mood, Drives, and Defenses

All adolescents show mood swings of some degree, but some experience these much more markedly. Mood swings may indicate an inner clash between newly intensified drives and the augmented defenses called into play against them. Such struggles may occur in any area of the adolescent's emotional life. For example, the need to be cared for and looked after is opposed by the drive to gain independence and control over one's life. Any experience or expression of normal sexual interest may be smothered in a cloak of rigid asceticism. Alternately, sexual drives may break through tenuous controls to produce a riot of indiscriminate and exploitative sexual gratification. In all such cases, the behavior reflects the exaggerated struggle, as periods of extreme constriction alternate erratically with phases of extreme impulsiveness. Such an adolescent may prolong unduly a period of crisis, actively struggling to make commitments but demonstrating great difficulties in resolving ambivalent feelings (Golombek and Garfinkel 1983).

Russell, age fourteen, was being seen because his parents were worried by what they saw as increasing depression. During his assessment, he made a number of disparaging references to his friends' sexual activities. When the examiner commented that he seemed to disapprove, he launched into a long diatribe on how disgusting their behavior was. When asked if he ever thought of himself behaving in the same way, he replied, "all the time." It quickly became clear that he was constantly preoccupied with sexual desires and fantasies. Much of his energy went into an unsuccessful struggle to suppress these, but periodically he would succumb and, almost literally in spite of himself, plunge into a sexual encounter. He would then experience relief followed almost immediately by intense guilt, a renewed determination never to slip again, and intensified disgust at his friends' normal sexual behavior.

Independence and Psychological Separation from Parents

One of the major tasks to be accomplished during adolescence is the attainment of emotional independence. This occurs through the continuing process of individuation, that process through which all adolescents achieve their own idiosyncratic synthesis of hopes, desires, attributes, skills, and defenses. Most adolescents approach independence with considerable ambivalence. They long to be self-sufficient and resent those on whom they depend. Yet they are loath to trade the security and comforts of continued dependence for the uncertainty and responsibilities of independence. They need to feel that they are gaining their independence without being overwhelmed by too much too soon. The inner struggle between these strong and antagonistic sets of needs may generate confusion and anxiety within the adolescent. These, in turn, are reflected in behavior and attitudes as intense as they are inconsistent. All too often the upheaval aggravates the parents' anxieties and precipitates ambivalent and exaggerated parental reactions that complicate the movement toward independence. The more parents perceive normal adolescent behavior as if it were pathological rebellion, the more difficulty they will have tolerating that behavior, and the harder they will make it for their adolescents to achieve mature independence without unnecessary trauma and continuing alienation.

> Joan, sixteen, had changed from a compliant and helpful child to a tempestuous adolescent, alternately demanding involvement in her affairs and complaining of being treated like a child. She objected to her mother buying clothes for her, but when told she could make her own choices, she retorted that her mother didn't care for her. Joan complained of recurrent headaches but ignored suggestions to see a doctor. Her mother finally capitulated and made the appointment for her. Joan then bitterly attacked her mother for butting into her affairs. Faced with many such situations, Joan's parents felt inadequate, confused, upset, and resentful.

Failure to progress developmentally may result from some distortion or pathological influence during childhood. Excessive rejection or deprivation, for example, may produce an adolescent who is seriously and chronically limited in the capacity to form successful relationships, to develop and maintain adequate values and beliefs, to develop appropriate self-esteem, and to establish an independent identity (see chapter 4). Such adolescents may experience identity diffusion, lacking commitment to anything or anyone (see chapter 19). On the other hand, excessively solicitous, domineering, or overprotective parents may inadvertently encourage other forms of developmental arrest. Their adolescent children may remain excessively dependent, remaining "good," submissive, and considerate throughout adolescence, showing little or no behavioral evidence of inner unrest. Although easy for parents to deal with, this type of behavior may indicate a serious delay in normal development. During childhood these adolescents established a pattern of defending excessively against their drives. The intensification of drives during adolescence is countered by an increase in their defenses crippling enough to block the normal maturation process. Such adolescents may experience an identity foreclosure in which childhood beliefs are rigidly adhered to. Burdened by strong feelings of immaturity, they are frequently unable to persevere in any activity in the face of initial difficulty or frustration. Therapeutic intervention may help remove the inner restrictions and free the path for normal development and experimentation.

> Dennis was very upset by the running battle (described in the next extract) between his father and older brother Scott, and decided, not entirely consciously, to avoid such confrontations. This meant suppressing all aggressive, hostile, or self-assertive tendencies. With few interests or ambitions, his sole aim was "getting along." His choice of a wife and career reflected his avoidance of challenge. In both areas he dealt with conflicts by placating those involved at all costs. When this failed he would become anxious, depressed, and withdrawn, the long-repressed rage surfacing only rarely. Ever pleasant and considerate, he became increasingly passive and restricted. Only his chronic pessimism and lack of energy gave any hint of the subclinical depression that lay beneath.

Adolescence frequently stirs up unresolved feelings and conflicts in parents, who may react to their child with extreme, inconsistent, or other unusual behavior. Parental stress is likely to occur as struggles to get on with psychosocial development lead to increasing demands for independence, challenges of parental authority, heightened sexual preoccupation and experimentation, provocative questioning of family beliefs and values, and critical confrontations around crucial educational and vocational choices. The ways these are handled by the adolescents and the anxiety and opposition this raises in the parents can lead to considerable tensions between the generations, tensions that may seriously test the preexisting relationship between them and the stability of the family as a whole (Ravenscroft 1974).

When the child reaches adolescence, it is appropriate that parental authority gradually recede and that the child develop greater autonomy. Parents who have precarious or incomplete control over their own aggressive or antisocial tendencies are particularly likely to be threatened by the expression of similar tendencies in their children. They may respond with rigid authoritarianism or, paralyzed by indecision, they may abdicate their parental role. Alternatively, they may belittle or plead ineffectually with their adolescents in a frequently futile and always destructive attempt to cling to the vestiges of their control (Friedman 1975).

Doug, fifteen, was the only one of five siblings to challenge his authoritarian parents, taking on his father as well as his teachers and even the law. His father responded with either hollow threats or passive disgust. Both parents would accuse Doug of being a bad influence on his siblings, or at other times plead ineffectually in a futile attempt to regain control. In response, Doug alternated between being a compliant "good boy" and a rebellious delinquent. This added to his parents' anxiety, confusion, and feeling of inadequacy, contributing to the ineffectuality and vacillation that in turn perpetuated Doug's reliance on acting-out behaviors as a way to deal with his inner anxiety.

All adolescents have mixed feelings about parental authority and are sensitive to parental anxiety and inconsistency. They may veer toward rejection of parental control at one time, while at another time use it gratefully to make decisions they cannot make themselves. As a result, adamant demands for complete autonomy may alternate with regression to childlike dependency. These vacillations in adolescents' responses to parental authority may do much to compound parental confusion, anxiety, and resentment.

Development as a Mature Sexual Individual

The hormonal changes of early and midadolescence lead not only to the development of secondary sexual characteristics but also to an accompanying increase in sexual drive. Parents have become less permissible as direct love objects, and early adolescents fill the void by becoming involved in intense friendships with, or "crushes" on, members of either sex. Early adolescents typically find and relate intensely to others who, they feel, have some quality they themselves need. The crushes of midadolescents are highly narcissistic and frequently intense, and may be so one-sided that they may exist almost entirely within the mind and fantasy of the enslaved adolescents. The object of the crush is idolized, admired, even loved, at times passively and yet passionately. This idealization temporarily keeps adolescents unaware of the erotic and frequently homosexual component of the friendship. The eventual recognition of this element often contributes to the sudden disruption of these relationships. As sexual interest and fantasy intensify, they may be accompanied by sexual explorations that are often more concerned with breaking through inhibitions and testing capacities than with any interest in intimacy. For some adolescents sexual acting-out can become a problem, but for the most part love and sex are kept quite separate. Whereas boys tend toward discussions of exaggerated sexual feats, girls are typically more taken up with romantic fantasies, to the point of preoccupation with their acceptability to members of the opposite sex. A capacity for mature heterosexual relationships and true intimacy may develop in late adolescence, as the self-preoccupation characteristic of early and midadolescence gradually recedes and a more secure and complete psychosocial identity is achieved.

39

Nancy, fifteen, made friends with her favorite disc jockey, but her interest in him soon became an infatuation. He encouraged the crush, but she became such an overbearing nuisance that he then cut her off. Nancy dealt with the abandonment by becoming increasingly dependent on her best girl friend, but the unrecognized homosexual aspect of the friendship proved too threatening for her. Still desperately needy, she became "special" friends with her history teacher and then got sexually involved with a married cousin who had wanted originally just to give her some help. When he withdrew from her, she threw herself into a series of sexual involvements with boys, trying to prove her desirability. Therapy helped her understand her underlying fears of loneliness and her need for an idealized strong protector and eventually made her capable of more appropriate involvements.

During their development, adolescents may exhibit sexual behaviors (homosexuality, fetishes, transvestism, voyeurism) that, although deviant from the norm, do not necessarily represent psychopathology. In most cases, however, the emergence of atypical sexual behaviors or strong sexual fantasies that are not socially approved may generate very disturbing feelings and forebodings. This can lead to debilitating emotional turmoil (excessive anxiety or depressive feelings) that can interfere with normal personality growth. Such adolescents are often reassured to learn that, as in other developmental areas (social and biological), changes in the sexual feelings and attractions, behavioral experimentation, and fluctuations in sexual fantasies are not unusual or ominous.

Adolescent sexual development and behavior may provoke strong sexual attitudes and feelings in parents. Repressed, ambivalently held attitudes may be activated, causing parents to respond too harshly and puritanically, or parents may be excessively permissive or overly involved in the adolescents' dating behaviors or sexual practices. In such situations adolescents frequently tune in to and comply with the parents' underlying expectations or fears, rather than their spoken admonitions, which often contradict the former.

Alice, a fifteen-year-old adoptee, was referred by her mother for increasing rebelliousness. She was defiant and abusive, both verbally and physically. She also repeatedly stayed away overnight, once attempting to be placed in a foster home. Alice was unusually attractive and physically mature, and seductive with the many older boys who knew her. Her parents fought with her, questioning her virginity and vowing to force her to have an abortion if she became pregnant.

Consultation with the mother revealed that she had grown up in a controlling family. Compliant as a girl, she had admired her rebellious older sister and now relived her adolescence through Alice, whom she envied. While she was threatened by Alice's attractiveness, she encouraged the girl's seductive behavior. Alice was indeed sexually active and was twenty-four weeks' pregnant before her parents realized it consciously. Thus she lived up to her parents' expectations and won the abortion issue at the same time.

Confronted with the burgeoning and often intense sexuality of their children, some parents may become concerned about their own (real or apparent) diminishing sexual capacity or attractiveness. This may precipitate clinical depression or attempts to seek affirmation in extramarital affairs, or even competition for the attention of the adolescents' friends.

Morals and Belief Systems

The value system of preadolescents largely imitates that of the parents. As adolescence proceeds, the increased influence of the peer group leads to experimentation and an initial identification with values that are distinctly the adolescents' own. This process usually involves modifying, giving up, and deviating from some firm parental precepts, which may cause considerable anxiety and friction within the family. Whereas previously the parents were regarded with awe and unrealistically assessed as extraordinarily powerful and wise, they are now undervalued and subject to the adolescents' inflated evaluation of their own newly formed ideas, values, and experiences.

Mid adolescents are typically intolerant of ambiguity; consequently they are attracted to moralistic and simplistic positions on highly complex issues. They thus invite polarization by their manner, which, while at best naively idealistic, is frequently arrogant and abrasive. This, combined with the adolescents' typical intolerance of shortcomings, especially in parents, creates a stage difficult for parents to weather. If these experimental dialectics are not understood as a necessary step in defining and consolidating adolescents' feelings about themselves as separate and unique individuals, the resulting polarization may lead to an irreversible weakening of the bond between parent and child.

> Scott was the only one of five children in a rigid fundamentalist family to challenge their strict authoritarian father. He observed and openly questioned the inconsistencies between his father's stated moral positions and such behaviors as speeding and tax evasion. The father, consciously aware of the contradictions, was defensive and threatening, and Scott, disillusioned and alienated by the hypocrisy, began conflicting with authorities outside the home. He became quite antisocial; when confronted with evidence of car theft or vandalism, he admitted to no wrongdoing other than getting caught.

Adolescents' changing moral, religious, educational, and vocational choices may stir up parental anxiety, criticism, and hostility, especially if parental positions are precariously or ambivalently held. Direct opposition to parental values and positions may lead to hostility and alienation, which will induce feelings of guilt and inadequacy in parent and child. Parental opposition may extend to such areas as choice of friends, recreational interests, dress, and music. Occasionally, in a misguided attempt to maintain closeness, parents may become overly involved in and identified with the adolescents' life style, thus depriving the children of the authority figure they require who can oppose and reward at appropriate times.

> Jane was a pseudomature fifteen-year-old daughter of average middle-class religious parents. Her relationship with her father had always been close, mu-

41

tually seductive, and exclusive of the mother. Jane had rejected her Roman Catholic upbringing, was sexually active, and involved in an Eastern religious movement. Her father responded by trying to "understand her." He tried marijuana with her, discussed her beliefs and the sexual mores of today's youth. Jane could deal with the hostile component of her ambivalence toward him only by escalating her dramatically unacceptable behavior. It was a shoplifting charge that led her father to seek help for the family.

The issues just cited may not always be evident in such a clear fashion but may be shifted to the usual instrumental battlegrounds of everyday family life such as cleanliness, neatness, hours of coming and going, household chores, and use of cars.

Educational and Vocational Identity

During middle and late adolescence, a number of key decisions of lifelong importance must be made. While these will be much affected by adolescents' earlier school and vocational achievement, or lack of it, they will also be influenced by pressures from parents and by pervading social and cultural values—particularly if the attitudes and aspirations of the parents conflict with those of the peer group or if the parents are seeking to live vicariously through their teenager. As a result, key decisions may be influenced more by powerful but unrecognized emotional factors than by rational evaluation.

Difficulties with Community

The task of making the transition from family to community in the 1980s is complicated by a current pervasive disenchantment with society. Adolescents are expected to find their place in a society marked by increasing social isolation, an unparalleled rate of technological change (in what Alvin Toffler has termed Future Shock), and profound economic insecurity of which they may be quite as aware as their parents. This changing world makes it difficult to anticipate, let alone plan for, adult life. Many of the traditional values around which our society has been organized—the work ethic, material success, competitiveness, the supremacy of law, concepts of sex roles, sexual morality and family life, religious beliefs—are under constant attack and, in the eyes of a well-defined and articulate minority of the adolescents' peer group, have already been discredited. Where do adolescents stand, and where is there to go in the midst of all this uncertainty? This dilemma can precipitate a crisis of psychosocial identity. If conflicts with the family have ruptured family ties and led to significant alienation, the parents will not be available—or cannot be used—to provide even minimal orientation or support during this crucial period of transition. Some adolescents, overwhelmed by demands for adaptation beyond their capacity to cope, respond by dropping out; they withdraw into a nondemanding, nonworking world, retreating to the refuge of their own fantasies for pleasure and satisfaction.

Important Tasks in Dealing with Adolescents
and Their Families

ASSESSING DEVELOPMENTAL LEVEL

The physician, counselor, or worker who recognizes that adolescents are not adults is less likely to set excessive expectations. By also recognizing that adolescents are not children, the professional avoids being patronizing or excessively authoritarian. Different circumstances call for different strengths and abilities, and consideration must be given to adolescents' ability to cope with the particular situation.

MAINTAINING OBJECTIVITY

Adolescents frequently present a problem in a dramatic fashion that may challenge the value system of the adult attempting to provide counseling. When tensions exist between parents and child, it is easy to get overinvolved in the situation and to side with one or the other. A thorough understanding of the total situation before judging or acting assists in maintaining objectivity. Information from outside the family—for example, from schools and social agencies—is essential in making an accurate and balanced assessment.

AVOIDING OVERINVOLVEMENT

Adolescents tend to involve adults in situations from which they have difficulty extricating themselves. Professionals may end up being maneuvered into doing things or negotiating concessions for adolescents who are quite capable of handling the situation themselves. Should this occur, the dependency of the adolescent is unnecessarily and inappropriately increased. For example, a therapist might be asked by a youngster to write a letter of excuse to his school explaining that recent examination failures are due to emotional problems. In this way the adolescent seeks to relieve himself of his work responsibilities hoping, but also fearing, that the adult will take charge and rescue him. Such overinvolvement or excessive closeness on the part of the professional may threaten adolescents who then frequently withdraw and become hostile. If the adult becomes hurt, responds with anger, or tries to force help on the adolescents, the situation may be aggravated by the overzealous attempt at intervention.

Parents also often invite the counselor to identify with them against their adolescent son or daughter. Overinvolvement—where one emotionally takes sides and assumes someone else's problem as one's own—runs the risk of aggravating disruptions in family life or interfering with programs of intervention already instituted by school or social agency.

DEVELOPING TRUST

Trust is built on clear and matter-of-fact communication. Counselors cannot be vague or misleading or talk down to adolescents. Arrangements regarding plans, visits, and appointments must be clear and adolescents must be notified promptly about unavoidable changes. If professionals expect respect and trust from adolescents, they must first give it.

ESTABLISHING CONFIDENCE

Adolescents must be treated as the situation demands. They will reject unnecessarily authoritarian or dogmatic attempts to direct them. On the other hand, they have no confidence in adults who allow them to behave in a manner they know is destructive, under the guise of allowing them to make their own decisions.

Adolescents expect adults to be appropriately firm and to have the courage of their convictions. Often they test adults with outrageous requests or protests, hoping to meet the strength they need to provide a sense of security. An openness and willingness to listen without preconceived judgment will bolster adolescents' sense of confidence and trust. Professionals must realize that while decision making ultimately is the responsibility of adolescents and family, the counselor may be in a position to help them recognize important factors or potential consequences that should be considered in understanding a problem and in arriving at a course of action.

Adults who counsel or treat adolescents should be prepared to share some of their own personal beliefs and values with them. They can expect to have these values met with some of the sparring typical of this developmental stage and must be able to tolerate the adolescents' right and need to choose between accepting or rejecting shared beliefs.

FACILITATING INDIVIDUATION

Psychopathology within the family may make it harder for adolescents to achieve successfully the goals of emotional independence and the formation of a separate psychological identity. If either adolescents or parents seek to avoid these conflicts by an abrupt, unilateral decision to live separately—especially if the decision is made at a point of crisis or in frustration or anger—a lasting guilt may result, which will leave both adolescents and parents with damaged self-esteem. For the professional to propose geographical separation as a solution to the difficulties of adolescent individuation would be naive. The counselor should rather attempt to help both adolescents and other family members identify and resolve the tensions they are trying to bypass. In attempting to counsel the family of an adolescent, professionals may be under major pressures, either from the family or from the adolescent, to make decisions for them. But the appropriate role for the mental health worker is that of helping the family define, as clearly as possible, the sources of conflict and of providing an opportunity to work toward a constructive resolution. Clearly the professional must be prepared to accept the family's decision if they cannot or will not use this opportunity (Steinhauer 1974).

CLARIFYING CONFIDENTIALITY

The degree of confidentiality the mental health worker should allow adolescent patients will vary with the adolescent's age, with the nature of the relationship between adolescent and family, and with the subject under discussion. Wherever possible, an adolescent's request for confidentiality should be respected. Sometimes, however, it is in the adolescent's best interests that an issue be raised with the parents. Should this be so, the matter should first be discussed with the adolescent fully and frankly, leaving no doubt that unless the teenager is prepared to raise the matter with the parents, the counselor will. For example, if an adolescent reveals serious preoccupation with self-injury and is judged to be at high risk for suicide, considerations for preserving life always supersede agreements regarding confidentiality. It can be extremely difficult to decide which issues must be shared, and this decision can reflect more the value system or anxiety of the counseling adult than the needs of the adolescent. Nevertheless, it is essential that anyone treating or counseling adolescents be aware of the need to allow each adolescent that degree—and only that degree—of confidentiality consistent with the adolescent's well-being and stage of maturity and that the counselor recognize the danger to the relationship with the patient of promising or allowing more or less.

Drug and Alcohol Use and Abuse in Adolescence

Drug use in adolescence may range from relatively harmless, transitory experimentation to persistent use with physical and psychological dependence. Depending on the pattern, the drug use may indicate a social phenomenon of no medical or psychological significance or it may be symptomatic of serious emotional disturbance. This topic is discussed in detail in chapter 19.

Principles of Management

GENERAL PRINCIPLES

There are four general principles mental health workers must keep in mind when dealing with adolescents.

1. Adolescents are often psychologically ill and not just "going through a phase."
2. Parents, family, and involved members of the community are important in assessment and treatment.
3. Any adequate assessment of an adolescent must evaluate:
    (a) Biological maturation and associated feelings (including body image and self-esteem).
    (b) Intrapsychic conflicts, in all areas listed above.
    (c) Where the adolescent stands in relation to developmental tasks.
    (d) The adolescent's relationship with the family.
    (e) Information from outside the family (e.g., schools, social agencies, etc.).
4. The goals of treatment are the attainment of psychological independence, a reduction of symptoms (including excessive anxiety or depression), and improved orientation to reality.

IMPORTANT GUIDELINES IN DEALING WITH ADOLESCENTS

1. The first contact is important. Who made it? How? How calm or upset was the person making this contact? The answers to these questions may provide clues to the resources available and to the strength and the manipulations of the people concerned.

2. Adolescents often do not present themselves or their concerns willingly. The important point is that they come. To save face, they may need to protest that help is not needed, but unless they come, nothing can be done.

3. Professionals should observe physical appearance and dress, and note any changes on future occasions.

4. A relationship of complete confidentiality should never be promised. What the mental health professional tells anyone else will depend on his or her judgment. While the adolescents' wishes in this regard must be considered, they should not bind the counselor.

5. Professionals must be prepared to inquire into all areas of the adolescents' life—school, clubs, sports and dating, and so on.

6. Manipulation should be dealt with as it arises. Adolescents may count on parents' reluctance to use existing agencies such as police and court. Adolescents may initially have trouble distinguishing in the counselor an attitude that is easygoing and relaxed from an attitude of permissiveness that derives from weakness or indifference. The easygoing atti-

46

tude is a distinct asset, while the permissive one will inevitably prove to be a liability.

7. Mental health workers must remember that teenagers may not be able to handle adult obligations and responsibilities.

8. It should be recognized that argument and challenge are part of how adolescents relate. Counselors should not be so preoccupied with the chip that they lose sight of the shoulder—and the teenager beneath it.

9. Professionals must be prepared to work with school teachers, clergy, athletic instructors, agency workers, and so forth.

10. Mental health workers must be prepared to share some of their personal values, ideas, and morals, but they should not assume that these necessarily have any special value or relevance for adolescent patients. What the professional is in dealings with the adolescent will prove more important than what he or she says.

11. In all cases, it is useful to have at least one initial family interview and probably advantageous to have intermittent total family reviews. For further treatment, the family approach seems more fitting for the young adolescent, while group or individual therapy fits later adolescents.

SUGGESTIONS FOR FURTHER READING

ADELSON, J., ed. 1980. *Handbook of adolescent psychology.* New York: Wiley-Interscience.
A comprehensive reference; contains material on values, moral development, historical and longitudinal approaches, current biological research, and gifted adolescents.

ANTHONY, E. J. 1974. "Psychotherapy of adolescence." In *American handbook of psychiatry,* 2nd ed., vol. 2, ed. G. Caplan, pp. 234–249. New York: Basic Books.
A good discussion of the general principles of psychotherapy with adolescents.

BOUTOURLINE YOUNG, J. 1971. "The physiology of adolescence (including puberty and growth)." In *Modern perspectives in adolescent psychiatry,* ed. J. G. Howells, pp. 3–27. Edinburgh: Oliver & Boyd.
Reviews physiological changes in the second decade of life to allow for a correct interpretation of variations in normal physical growth and development. Good description of Tanner ratings of pubescent stages.

COLEMAN, J. C. 1980. *The nature of adolescence.* New York: Methuen.
Outlines and reevaluates the psychoanalytic and sociological theories of adolescent development; critically discusses concepts such as "storm," "stress," "identity crises," and the "generation gap."

EASSON, W. M. 1969. *The severely disturbed adolescent.* New York: International Universities Press.
Describes inpatient, residential, and hospital treatment of severely disturbed adolescents.

ERIKSON, E. H. 1968. *Identity, youth and crisis,* 1st ed. New York: W.W. Norton.
A fundamental contribution to understanding growth and development.

FRIEDMAN, R. 1975. "The vicissitudes of adolescent development and what it activates in adults." *Adolescence* 10:520–526.
Describes typical communication patterns between adolescents and adults in the light of understanding some of the forces at work during the adolescent stage of development.

GOLOMBEK, H., AND GARFINKEL, B. D., eds. 1983. *The adolescent and mood disturbance.* New York: International Universities Press.
  A comprehensive reference integrating a broad base of investigational information. Provides clinicians with background knowledge for the effective management of mood disorders in adolescence.
HOLMES, D. J. 1964. *The adolescent in psychotherapy.* Boston: Little, Brown.
  Clearly describes therapeutic technique with adolescents, using many examples.
MALMQUIST, C. P. 1979. "Development from thirteen to sixteen years." In *Basic handbook of child psychiatry* vol. 1, ed. J. D. Noshpitz, pp. 205–213. New York: Basic Books.
  Good overview of personality development during early and middle adolescence.
MEEKS, J. E. 1971. *The fragile alliance.* Baltimore: Williams & Wilkins.
  Still a good introductory textbook in adolescent psychiatry.
OFFER, D. 1973. *The psychological world of the teenager.* New York: Basic Books.
  Study of "normal," middle-class American adolescent males.
RAVENSCROFT, K. 1974. "Normal family regression at adolescence." *Am. J. Psychiat.* 131:31–35.
  Clearly discusses the process set in motion by puberty that initiates a family development epicycle featuring a temporary regression in sibling, marital, and family functioning to earlier modes of behavior. Provides a normal framework for family members to share and to facilitate adolescent development.
RUTTER, M., et al. 1976. "Adolescent turmoil: Fact or fiction?" *Journal of Child Psychol. & Psychiat.* 17:35–56.
  Considers the concept of adolescent turmoil in the context of findings from a total population epidemiological study of fourteen- to fifteen-year-old Isle of Wight residents.
STEINHAUER, P. D. 1974. "Abruptio familiae: The premature separation of the family." In *Beyond clinic walls,* ed. A. B. Tulipan, C. L. Attneave, and E. Kingstone, pp. 204–211. University, Al.: University of Alabama Press.
  Discusses sociological and psychological factors leading many youths to leave home prematurely in a misguided attempt to solve conflicts around the establishment of independence.
WEINER, I. B.1980. Psychopathology in adolescence. In *Handbook of adolescent psychology,* ed. J. Adelson, New York: Wiley Interscience. pp.447–471.
  Focuses on frequent psychological disturbances among adolescents or those bearing special relationship to the developmental tasks of the teenage years. Reviews epidemiological data on adolescent psychopathology, indicating the limitations of both traditional diagnostic categories and problem-oriented classification within the age group.

3

Paul D. Steinhauer and Freda Martin

The Family of
the Child

Introduction—The Family

The family is the basic, universal unit that permits the survival of the human species by serving as the major functional unit for child rearing (Lidz 1963; Murdock 1960). To do so it must fulfill three fundamental tasks: (1) it must satisfy the infant's biological needs by providing a long period of physical care and dependency; (2) it must continue to provide for the physical, emotional, and financial needs of the growing child; (3) it constitutes the first and strongest influence in socializing the child as a member of a particular society. The family's ways are initially *the* ways, and all subsequent experiences are reacted to in that light. To fulfill these functions and achieve its goals, the family's structure must enable it to allow for the continued biological, psychological, and social developments of all family members (Ackerman 1958; Epstein, Levin, and Bishop 1976; Parsons and Bales 1955); provide reasonable security for all; modify usual patterns of family functioning to meet environmental or developmental demands for change; ensure sufficient cohesion to maintain the family as a unit; allow the family to function effectively and with reasonable comfort within society (Lidz 1980).

Family Structure

The family is a group, and as such it is influenced by many of the characteristic processes of other small groups (Tallman 1970; Skynner 1969). However, it is unique both in that its members share common goals without which the group would not exist and in that members depend on it for both biological and psychological survival (Boszormenyi-Nagy 1965; Epstein, Levin, and Bishop 1976; Lidz 1980). During its evolution, each family develops a definite structure—that well-defined, repetitive, and self-perpetuating set of patterns or rules (some explicit and spoken, others implicit but understood) that govern how members are expected to function and relate to each other within that particular family (Ford and Herrick 1974; Jackson 1957; Minuchin 1974). Examples would include "rules" or traditions about who speaks to whom about what, who may or may not do what, how a particular job is to be carried out and by whom.

More specifically, all families must accomplish certain tasks. The nature of these tasks will vary over the course of the family's life cycle, but their accomplishment will require the same basic skills and involve similar processes at any point in the cycle (Brody 1974; Carter and McGoldrick 1980; Glick 1955; Terkelson 1980). Thus the ultimate goal of family functioning is *task accomplishment.* Some of these tasks are determined by the culture (Minuchin 1967; Pavenstedt 1967; Pearce 1980; Rutter 1976). Others are unique to a given family. But all are influenced by that family's *values and norms.* These values and norms are derived largely from the adults' experiences growing up within their own families of origin; their internalized (i.e., psychological) derivatives of these experiences; the influences of the society in which they live; their common history and experiences since joining together to form a new nuclear family. Task accomplishment requires the family to define and perform a number of roles *(role performance).* In order to achieve its essential tasks, families use *communication* to send and receive the information needed to define and perform these roles and to accomplish the necessary tasks (Epstein 1968; Jackson, Beavin, and Watzlawick 1967; Ruesch and Bateson 1951). This includes not just the exchange of information essential for accomplishing the ongoing tasks of everyday life (i.e., *instrumental communication*) but also the expression of feeling (i.e., *affective communication*) that, depending on how it is put forth, can either assist or impede task accomplishment and successful role performance. Similarly, the quality and intensity of emotional involvement existing among family members *(affective involvement)* and how they influence each other's behavior *(control)* can either facilitate or hinder task accomplishment. Family structure is determined by the interrelationship among these dimensions of family functioning, each of which will be further defined and illustrated in this chapter.

Development of a Family Structure

TASK ACCOMPLISHMENT

A family begins when a man and woman start to live together, thus, for the first time, sharing a common existence. Immediately they are faced with a number of tasks to be accomplished. Task accomplishment is the first major dimension of family functioning and, following Epstein and Bishop (1981), can be subdivided into:

1. *Basic Tasks:*
   Tasks essential to physical survival (e.g., provision of adequate food, shelter, clothing, health care, etc.).
2. *Crisis Tasks:*
   Tasks related to the family's mobilizing to cope with stresses so severe and intense that they exceed the family's ability to deal with them successfully, thus temporarily at least threatening to disrupt the family's equilibrium (Hill 1965; see also chapter 20).
3. *Developmental Tasks:*
   Tasks that provide for the continuing development of all family members (Epstein, Rakoff, and Sigal 1968).

The decision to move from living as two individuals to functioning as part of a couple immediately presents a number of developmental tasks that will require major adjustments for both members of the couple. Habits and behavior patterns that were quite all right as long as the people lived apart will have to be modified or given up if they prove unacceptable to the partner. Alternately, the partner will have to be persuaded to develop new tolerances if these behaviors are to be retained. Thus one of the first major developmental tasks faced by the new couple is that of defining the rules under which they will live together (Jacobson 1981). The process of accomplishing this is partly conscious (i.e., direct negotiation around statements of each partner's preferences, demands, dislikes, etc.) and partly an automatic and largely unconscious accommodation to the perceived needs and preferences of the other. If successful, both partners will be satisfied that their needs are being met and the bond between them will be strengthened. If mutual accommodation is not achieved—if one or both are left feeling dissatisfied, abused, impinged upon, or unfulfilled—the bond and their ability to function successfully as a couple will be seriously undermined (Boszormenyi-Nagy and Ulrich 1981). In order to accomplish its tasks satisfactorily, the new couple will have to develop along a number of dimensions.

ROLE PERFORMANCE

The second major dimension of family functioning, one essential for successful task accomplishment, involves *role performance*. To achieve the task of mutual accommodation, the members of the couple will have to define their respective roles. This process of role definition and the willingness and ability of each to perform the roles as defined will be influenced by a number of factors.

Both partners will bring into the union their own ideas of how a husband and wife should behave and be treated. These basic expectations are based largely on their experience in the families in which they were raised. How they define their individual roles may be a carbon copy of how, when they were growing up, they saw their own parents (i.e., role modeling). Alternately, one or both partners may react against their parents' definition of marital roles by redefining roles in this new couple in a deliberate though not necessarily conscious attempt to break with their family of origin's traditional role definition (Meissner 1978), like the woman who determined not to let her husband step all over her as she felt her father had abused her mother.

Cultural influences as well as those of the family of origin may have a major influence on these role expectations (Pearce 1980). Prior to World War II, few married women worked outside the home or had separate careers. To have done so would have been interpreted widely as proof that the husband was an inadequate provider. A need for women in the labor force during World War II and later increased economic pressures and the success of the feminist movement in redefining sex roles encouraged more wives to enter the work force. At the same time, changing social attitudes defined as inadequate husbands who could not tolerate their wives working, while those who facilitated their wives' careers were termed liberated.

The more similar the couple's role expectations, the less either needs to modify or negotiate to successfully accommodate to the other's need. The more incongruent the role definitions with which they entered the union, the more each would have to change or learn to tolerate to achieve a harmonious equilibrium.

Expectations and fears remaining from past experiences may badly distort how one partner perceives the other's role performance. Such distorted perceptions, particularly in the absence of adequate communication that would allow the distortion to be identified and resolved, can seriously threaten marital harmony and effective functioning.

Mr. P had sworn that he would never let his wife dominate him as he felt his domineering mother had henpecked his father. As a result, he perceived even the most reasonable attempt by his wife to disagree or put forth an independent point of view as an attempt to dominate him. If she did not immediately capitulate when he demanded she stop controlling him, he would become enraged and accuse her of emasculating him.

> Mrs. E felt that in her family of origin, she was never taken seriously or given credit for being as capable as she was. She entered her marriage determined not to let her husband put her down as she felt her parents had for years. Whenever he questioned a position she had taken, she took this as proof that again she was not being treated as an equal and would arbitrarily announce that she had decided what the family would do. If her husband dared to question or disagree with her, she would burst into tears, insisting that he was incapable of treating her as an equal partner in the marriage.

For role performance within a couple (or family) to be successful, it must be *comprehensive* (in which case all required activities are assigned and accepted) and it must also be *complementary* (i.e., the various reciprocal roles must fit together in a way that is both efficient and acceptable to all (Berman and Lief 1975; Jackson 1957; Tharp 1963). Should these conditions be met, there will be little dissatisfaction or arguing about roles (i.e., minimal role conflict) and members will have adequate role satisfaction.

There is no single "best" or "right" way to define various family roles. What matters is not individual role definitions but that within the family there be *internal role consistency*—that is, all members see themselves as others see them and generally agree on what is expected of them (Levinger, 1965). There should also be sufficient complementarity of roles to permit successful role integration. For example, a husband who defines his role as that of the breadwinner and family decision maker may have minimal role conflict with a wife who feels fulfilled by being a housewife and mother. Should she, however, be dissatisfied with his attempt to force his definition of their reciprocal roles on her, she has five basic options: she can negotiate, submit (remaining unfulfilled and prone to depression), fight (chronic conflict), escape (alcohol, affairs), or separate.

Family role definitions should be consistent with actual role performance, since when they differ significantly confusion, disharmony, and shattering disequilibrium may result.

> Both Mr. and Mrs. C, for example, can agree intellectually upon the wife's having her own career. Should, however, Mr. C's behavior betray an unrecognized opposition to Mrs. C's working that contrasts with his stated position, the resulting inconsistency will arouse disharmony until clarified and resolved one way or another.

Ideally, role definitions will allow the psychological and other needs of each family member to be met. Members will be frustrated if they are continually expected to fit roles that neglect their own social and psychological needs even if, for a while, they appear to accept their role as defined by other family members. What matters, therefore, is that the family agree on some definition of roles that works for it, allowing enough flexibility so that each individual's needs are respected and the family is free to respond appropriately to demands for change while, at the same time, providing enough cohesion to maintain the stability of the family as a unit.

COMMUNICATION

In content, a communication can be *affective* (i.e., an expression of feeling), *instrumental* (related to the tasks of everyday life), or *neutral* (neither of these) (Epstein, Rakoff, and Sigal 1968). At the same time, any communication ranges between *clear* and *masked* (i.e., disguised and ambiguous). The more masked the message, the greater the possibility of receiver confusion, anxiety, and distortion.

Any message is either *direct* or *indirect,* depending on whether or not it is deflected from the appropriate receiver (Epstein and Bishop, 1981). To illustrate how these parameters can be used to analyze ongoing communication, consider a wife's possible responses if she were angry at her husband's failure to stop watching television to wipe their toddler's nose:

1. By a direct, clear message: "For Pete's sake, will you get up and wipe Johnny's nose!"
2. With a direct but masked message: "What the devil's the matter with you, John?"
3. With an indirect, masked message: "Why is everything left to me?" or "Suzy, turn down that radio" or slamming the door and stomping upstairs.

N. B. Epstein suggests that the more disturbed the family system, the greater the distortion of affective communication and the more likely unexpressed, accumulated feelings are to spill over and contaminate first instrumental and then even neutral communication. Thus what families term a breakdown in communication is, if it occurs frequently, usually a symptom of underlying strain or breakdown in relationships. In the well-functioning family, for example, a request for a drink of water is perceived and responded to for what it is—a direct instrumental communication. In a more dysfunctional family, that same request might be—or might be interpreted as—an attempt to dominate or manipulate (i.e., a masked, hostile communication). In families where direct expression of anger is not tolerated, anger builds up and is displaced into the control dimension. In such families parents vent their anger by finding an excuse to order children to obey while the children, rightly interpreting this as an attack, counterattack by refusing to do so. Thus "to do or not to do" becomes the battlefield on which the hostility forbidden direct expression is fought in a power struggle via masked communications. In such families an inevitable result is that the definition and resolution of problems inevitably suffers. Family therapists believe that improving communication permits the prompt identification and relief of the pressures inevitably generated in the course of family living, thus permitting and protecting more effective task accomplishment and, subsequently, family mental health (Alexander 1973).

Some families send many *paradoxical communications* (i.e., mixed messages) that simultaneously contain two mutually incompatable messages (often verbal and subverbal), as in the statement "Of course I'm not angry. I just can't be bothered discussing it" made in a voice quivering with rage. Receivers, unaware of which message they are expected to respond to but unable to respond to both, become confused and anxious. This dilemma is most marked in what Bateson termed the double bind (Bateson et al. 1956; Jackson, Beavin, and Watzlawick 1967). Here a powerless receiver is presented with a paradoxical communication by another family member too important to antagonize or alienate. Any response to either of the incompatable messages is considered wrong and attacked, and family rules forbid either clarification of the intended meaning or escape from the situation.

At one time some authors attributed schizophrenia to a defensive withdrawal by the psychotic member from the extreme anxiety generated by massive and continuous double binding within an extremely pathological family system (Bateson et al. 1956; Jackson, Beavin, and Watzlawick 1967; Lidz et al. 1957; Wynne and Singer 1963). Recently it has generally been agreed that this double-bind hypothesis of schizophrenia was originally oversold (Berger 1978; Grunebaum and Chasin 1980; Watzlawick 1963; Wynne 1976) and that the widespread use of the double bind, while not specific to any single disorder, undermines relationships, compounds confusion, and heightens anxiety in a broad range of disorders.

AFFECTIVE INVOLVEMENT

The fourth universal dimension of family functioning is affective involvement. This concerns the *degree* and *quality* of each member's interest in and concern for each other (Epstein and Bishop 1981). If a couple are meeting each other's need for affective involvement, each will provide for the other's emotional security and need to feel valued while, at the same time, tolerating the other's right to independent thought and action. The autonomy of both is assured. The satisfaction they provide and obtain will strengthen the bond between them without either demanding that the other give up the right to think, feel, or function as an individual.

CONTROL

The fifth dimension of family functioning is that of control, that process by which family members influence each other's behavior (Epstein and Bishop 1981). The reciprocal nature of role performance in families demands that those involved in reciprocal relationships constantly influence and be influenced by others. This pattern of reciprocal functioning is called *circular causality* (Jackson, Beavin, and Watzlawick 1967). Family members often try to explain their behavior in straight "A causes B" terms *(linear causality)*. Family therapists consider attempts to explain family functioning by linear causality a serious oversimplification, agreeing that circular causality with its "chicken and egg" implications is more accurate. If family transactions are viewed as a never-ending series of "A affects B who, in turn, affects A," this implies: (1) neither came first, and (2) neither is to blame.

The two systems of causality and their implications are illustrated by figure 3.1.

There are two major aspects of the control dimension: (1) *maintenance control:* the ways that members influence each other to ensure that day-to-day tasks are accomplished; and (2) *capacity for adaptation:* the ability of the family to make changes when necessary to respond to changing developmental demands or external circumstances.

To illustrate the interrelationship of these dimensions and how each must respond to a major demand for change, consider a couple's reaction to the birth of their first child (La Perriere 1980). Especially if the child is constitutionally difficult, the new mother is likely to feel overwhelmed and inadequate. These feelings will interfere with her meeting the baby's needs in a relaxed way and will leave her much in need of both practical help and psychological support from the father. He too will find the new baby unsettling. His wife, harassed and preoccupied with the baby, may have less time and may be less receptive to him. She will probably make

Linear Causality: Two Separate Interactions

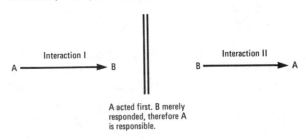

A acted first. B merely
responded, therefore A
is responsible.

Circular Causality: Single Ongoing Transaction

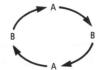

Neither came first. Neither is solely
responsible for any part of the
transaction isolated from the
context. Both share responsibility
for the ongoing transactional
patterns.

Figure 3.1 Patterns of Reciprocal Functioning

increased demands on his time and on his emotional resources (through her need for emotional support, which he may have difficulty understanding and responding to). In short, the birth of this baby is just one example of a major change that will require a significant adaptation by the couple. This will call for some reciprocal readjustment in all major dimensions of the family's functioning.

With regard to *task accomplishment,* many new tasks must be accomplished following the baby's birth. The baby will need to be fed, bathed, changed, held, taken to the doctor, and so forth. There will be multiple additional costs and possibly the loss of one source of income if the mother was previously working, or, if the mother continues to work, she will have to integrate her new role of mother with her other roles of wife, worker, and so forth. For the baby's optimal development, at least one and preferably both parents will have to bond to the baby, who will then form a secure attachment to them. This process will be facilitated by the parents meeting the infant's needs in a relaxed, competent manner. The more difficult the baby is constitutionally, the harder it will be for the parents to meet these needs.

In *role performance,* a baby's birth confronts the parents with a variety of new task demands. These require new role definitions in order to divide the new responsibilities. How this is done will be influenced by how both parents define their new roles of mother and father. Should their definitions coincide, there should be little role conflict, but if either's demands are different from what the other is prepared to provide, the potential for serious role conflict will exist.

To divide these new tasks will require that each parent state clearly his or her needs, expectations, and dissatisfactions, and explore what the other might do to meet them. This may severely test the adequacy of the couple's *communication.* Any block in adequate, clear, direct communication will lead to a damming up and displacement of frustration and resentment by one partner and a corresponding lack of understanding with subsequent anxiety, frustration, and resentment in the other. So would a tendency of either parent to withdraw, thus being unavailable to receive and understand the other's attempts to communicate.

Regarding *affective involvement,* if the partners can communicate all the essential information and if, as a result, each member perceives correctly and responds adequately to the other's needs, each will feel understood and supported by the other so that the bond between them will be strengthened. If, however, one feels misunderstood and unsupported by the other, the resulting disappointment and frustration will lead to resentment, anxiety, or guilt that, unless promptly and effectively resolved, can seriously undermine the parents' closeness and the ability of either to meet the baby's needs.

The birth of a baby presents the couple with the demand for major role adaptation in order to accomplish a variety of new tasks. The ways each partner influences the other to accept necessary role realignments to accomplish these tasks is a function of the *control* dimension. Furthermore, each major event in the child's development or the life of the family—for example, when the baby first walks, when the child starts school, when a second child is born, as the children prepare to leave home—will require further adaptations and reciprocal role realignments (Scherz 1971).

The Family as a System in Equilibrium

The family can be understood as a system in equilibrium at three interrelated levels (see figure 3.2)—the intrapsychic, the interpersonal, and the social level.

At an intrapsychic level, each person must reach a balance between biological, psychological, and social demands (for further discussion, see chapter 12). The dynamic tension between these compelling and often contradictory sets of drives, along with how each individual defends against the anxiety it generates, constitutes the intrapsychic level of equilibrium.

At an interpersonal level, all family members affect and are affected by each other. Symptomatic behavior in one person almost invariably elicits a response from other family members. For example, a child's misbehavior evokes parental discouragement, anger, and rejection, which in turn aggravate the child's feelings of deprivation and rage that contribute to the misbehavior.

At the social level of equilibrium, all members of the family—and the family as a unit—are constantly exposed to and in continual interaction with the standards and influences of the social environment.

Since these three levels of equilibrium are interrelated, stresses or

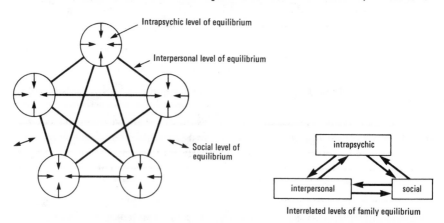

Figure 3.2 The Family as a System in Equilibrium.

events occurring at one level will inevitably reverberate through other levels of the family system. For example, a child's failure in school (event at the social level) frequently produces conflict between child and parents (effects at the interpersonal level), and these may combine to produce depression and feelings of low self-worth (effects at an intrapsychic level). In another instance, chronic marital conflict may originate from personality problems that husband and wife brought into marriage (liabilities at the intrapsychic level). These may be aggravated by the stresses and strains of living together (interpersonal level) so that neither is free to meet the children's emotional needs (interpersonal level). If the children respond to the resulting feelings of insecurity and deprivation (results at intrapsychic level) by aggressive or antisocial behavior in the community (results at the social level), neighbors, school, or police may react by bringing pressure on the family (result at the social level) that, in turn, may produce effects at all three levels of equilibrium.

Basic Principles of Family Equilibrium

Six basic principles govern family structure and the equilibrium it maintains.

1. For any family, all members assume and are assigned roles or relegate them to others in repetitive and highly characteristic ways.
2. Each family has a set of rules, explicit or implicit, that define the roles members are to assume and the ways they are to relate to each other. Examples of explicit rules could include: boys in this family must not hit girls, children are not allowed to swear at parents, you must go to bed when you are told to. Examples of implicit rules might include: we don't discuss sex at the dinner table (never stated in words, but conveyed by a frown, a change of subject, by telling the child not to yell—even though the child is talking quietly—or to sit up straight every time the subject is introduced), or "I say your bedtime is eight o'clock" (but your real bedtime is when I get angry and scream or hit, which may be at any time between eight and ten depending on how frustrated I am at the time).
3. These roles and rules govern the behavior within a given family and define the characteristic structure of that family. To say that a family has a typical structure means that given a task, be it deciding on where to go out for dinner or how to explain a given proverb, the family will approach it in a highly characteristic manner: the same members will dominate; the same ones with withdraw; the same ones will agree to anything; the same members will disrupt; and so forth.
4. Within that structure, family members are in equilibrium with one another. Thus each is constantly responding to—and being responded to by—others in a repetitive and characteristic manner. This equilibrium is not static but dynamic. A family's typical equilibrium is not defined once and accepted for all time, but is constantly being challenged and redefined by the ongoing interaction

of daily living. This is a source of much of the normal and inevitable tension of family life.

5. The family equilibrium is a self-regulating or homeostatic equilibrium (Satir 1967). Any attempt to shift a family's equilibrium from within (e.g., change in a member) or from without (e.g., input from a therapist or counselor) can be expected to evoke a reaction opposing the change and maintaining the status quo.

    This homeostatic principle operates largely beyond conscious awareness. The strength of the resistance to change may vary from family to family. In general, the better the mental health of the family, the more likely it will be to respond appropriately to demands for change. Similarly, the less adaptive the family, the greater its homeostatic resistance to change. Families may ask for help and express a desire for change while continuing to resist any measures likely to produce it. Thus parents may take a child out of treatment just as the child is beginning to improve. A husband who once complained of his wife's sexual frigidity may accuse her of being too aggressive or develop impotence as she begins to respond to or initiate sexual relations.

6. The family equilibrium is a shared coping mechanism by which the family deals with the threat of pain (e.g., anxiety, depression, rage, sexual feelings, and fantasy) or disruption. No matter how destructive or unsatisfying that equilibrium may appear to someone outside the family system, it represents that particular family's attempt to minimize the threat of pain and disruption. Thus any forcible attempt to alter it (such as when an overzealous professional tries to force a family to give up defenses prematurely) will evoke shared (i.e., group) as well as individual resistance to change.

Incomplete Boundaries: The Long-Term Effect of Incomplete Separation by the Parents

One important theoretical concept with major practical importance for family functioning is that of *boundaries.* Parents' past experiences continually influence their functioning as marital partners (Framo 1981). Particularly important is how successfully both have achieved psychological separateness (i.e., individuation) from their own parents (Lidz 1979; Meissner 1978). People who have achieved individuation have complete boundaries between themselves and the outside world. Since their boundaries are complete, they can clearly distinguish their own thoughts, feelings, needs, and motives from those of others (Bowen 1960; Boszormenyi-Nagy and Spark 1973; Lidz, Fleck, and Cornelison 1965; Meissner 1978). This makes it possible for them to tolerate differences in others without those differences becoming a threat to their own sense of self (Dicks 1967; Fogarty 1976). It is as if they are capable of saying: "I know what I think. You think differently. But there's room for both of us to have our own opinions. We need not always agree—we're two different people."

If someone else tries to make someone whose boundaries are complete responsible for that person's own behavior, they have a clear enough sense of what they are, to be able to accept responsibility when appropriate and to reject it without excessive confusion, anxiety, rage, or guilt when it is not. On the other hand, people who have not yet achieved individuation—and this includes many adults—have incomplete boundaries between themselves and others (Dicks 1967; Steinhauer, Santa-Barbara, and Skinner 1980). Never having achieved a clear and separate sense of themselves, they have difficulty tolerating independent behavior in those with whom they are closely involved, or enmeshed (Giovacchini 1976; Hoffman 1975; Karpel 1976; Minuchin 1974). The failure to develop a complete boundary around the self can lead to excessive reliance on primitive defense mechanisms such as projection, introjection, fusion, and splitting.* As they lack a clear definition of the boundary between themselves and others, differences in others become a threat to their fragile sense of self to be suppressed or avoided (Wynne, et al. 1958). It is as if they thought: "Oh, dear! You say I should think your way. But I think my way is right. At least I thought I did. Whenever someone important disagrees with me, I get all mixed up and don't know *what* to think." People with incomplete boundaries are liable to take responsibility for the inappropriate behavior of others. Therefore they are oversensitive to criticism and easily become confused, anxious, enraged, or guilty when others attack them even for behavior for which they are not to blame. Alternately, they are prone to projection, and often blame others for their own behavior (Slipp 1980). Figure 3.3 illustrates how much communication patterns (and therefore understanding) will be distorted by people whose boundaries are incomplete.

Four patterns commonly occur in families with one or both parents who have poorly defined boundaries as a result of incomplete separation from their own parents.

A tendency to blame others for one's own behavior may be exhibited. Families whose members have incomplete boundaries are particularly prone to blaming others by thinking in terms of linear as opposed to circular causality. In addition to projecting unwanted thoughts, feelings, needs, and motives onto others through gaps in their incomplete boundaries, they frequently blame others for their own behavior by implying that their actions result from or are caused by the others' behavior (Steinhauer, Santa-Barbara, and Skinner 1980).

Mother: Johnny, why did you hit Jimmy?
Johnny: Because he took my truck.

In the above, Johnny blames Jimmy for his own aggressive behavior by use of linear causality. Actually, Johnny could have dealt with Jimmy in a number of ways: (1) by allowing Jimmy to play with the truck; (2) by asking Jimmy to return it; (3) by angrily demanding that it be returned;

*See Bowen 1960; A. Freud 1946; S. Freud 1938; Mahler, Pine, and Bergman 1975; Minuchin 1974; Taylor 1975; and Winnicott 1958.

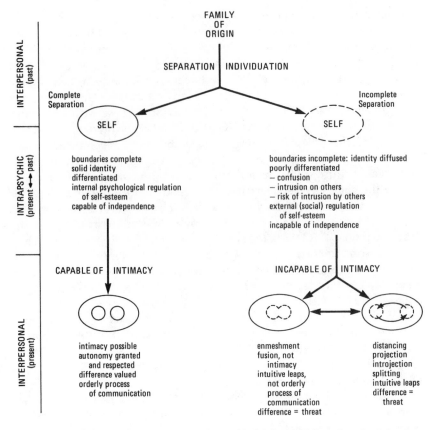

Figure 3.3 Marital Interaction as a Function of Individual and Boundary Formation.

(4) by asking a parent to make Jimmy return it; (5) by grabbing the toy from Jimmy; (6) by taking something of Jimmy's; (7) by hitting Jimmy; (8) by hitting another child smaller than he; (9) by bursting into tears. Thus Johnny's response was determined not just by Jimmy's behavior but by the way Johnny, with his particular personality and his characteristic ways of handling such situations, deals with frustration. The choice, of course, is not always conscious or deliberate.

At other times, family members whose boundaries are incomplete may reverse the process (i.e., substitute *introjection* for *projection*) and claim total responsibility for the behavior of others, another example of linear causality.

When Adam, age fourteen, failed in school, his parents were overcome with remorse. They accepted Adam's blaming them for his school failure, thus absolving him of any responsibility for his multiple episodes of truancy, failure to pay attention in class, not handing in assignments, not having studied for his exams. While it is true that Adam's upset in response to his parents' marital conflict was *one* factor contributing to his poor school performance, it is equally true that worry and disagreement over Adam's academic failure was a major source of tension and conflict between the parents. If all had recognized this and could separate out who was responsible for what (i.e., if they had complete boundaries), they would have understood the situation in terms of circular causality (e.g., we all bear some responsibility; therefore, what must each of us do to change the situation?).

In demonstrating to a family how members influence each other's behavior, one must carefully avoid unwittingly reinforcing anyone's attempts to avoid responsibility for behavior by projecting it onto others.

> A husband claimed the reason he drank excessively was his wife's intolerable nagging, which drove him to a beer parlor. She insisted it was his drinking and the accompanying abandonment of marital and parental responsibilities that made her nag. Here again we see circular causality—he drinks because she nags, she nags because he drinks. The importance of the therapist avoiding siding with either member and of not allowing either to avoid taking responsibility is underlined.

Some families may exhibit a tendency to scapegoat one or more family members (Epstein and Bishop 1981). In many dysfunctional families, one or more members are assigned and assume dysfunctional roles (Dicks 1967; Framo 1981; Skynner 1981)—assigned because other family members pressure them to accept the role; assumed because no one is trapped permanently in a dysfunctional role without some degree of collusion (Skynner, 1981). If their adjustment suffers, they are said to occupy the scapegoat role (Ackerman, 1961).

Scapegoats, who often are children, are selected because of their relatively powerless position. Their well-being is apparently sacrificed to allow the family as a whole to continue to function. (Ackerman 1961; Vogel and Bell 1960; Watzlawick et al. 1970). Epstein (1968) refers to them as being in the binder role, as they seem to bind the family together. For example, children who behave aggressively or antisocially often serve as a lightning rod drawing onto themselves the hostility of other family members who escape conflict with each other by uniting to attack the child. Sometimes the scapegoats are described as being in the discharge role, in that they discharge hostile, antisocial, and sexual drives for the entire family who then (1) derive vicarious pleasure from the scapegoat's behavior by identifying with him or her, (2) support their own defenses (repression and reaction formation) by punishing the scapegoat for badness and lack of control.

> Both Danny's parents grew up in families with authoritarian parents who allowed no expression of anger, rebellion, or misbehavior. Any aggressive or rebellious feelings were quickly repressed, since expressing them led to severe punishment. By using the defense of reaction formation, they developed into aloof but extremely successful people with extreme but conventional standards of right or wrong.
> Their son Danny, age eleven, was caught shoplifting. It became clear that for years Danny had been arriving home with expensive sports equipment that the parents knew he could not afford. With atypical naiveté, these bright, so-

phisticated parents repeatedly accepted his explanations that "a friend gave it to me." Similar blind spots occurred when Danny was found with fifty dollars when just that amount was missing from his mother's purse. Suspecting Danny was involved, they exposed him to extended and sometimes brutal interrogation but never followed through. However, when he was caught shoplifting, Danny was severely beaten, lost all privileges for three months, and had repeated sermons on how he had disgraced the family by being brought home by the police (note—not for stealing!).

The family's therapist thought Danny was serving a "discharge" role within his family. Thus his stealing could be understood (intrapsychically) as acting-out, taking the place of unrecognized but, in that family, unacceptable feelings. At the same time, by stealing, Danny was doing his parents a service that neither he nor they consciously recognized. By vicariously identifying with his behavior unconsciously, the parents found an outlet for their own deeply repressed antisocial feelings. At the same time and at a more conscious level, they reinforced their own sense of control over the powerful but disowned antisocial feelings by their response to his delinquency. Their "blind spots," the brutality of the interrogations, the statement that he had disgraced the family "by being caught," and the excessive severity of the punishment that, by its unfairness, invited rebellion unconsciously encouraged Danny to discharge their unrecognized antisocial needs, even though consciously they were sincerely appalled by his behavior.

Another scapegoat is the family martyr (usually the mother or an older sister), who constantly sacrifices her own needs to meet those of others or to keep the peace (Meissner 1978; Satir 1967). This provides some cohesiveness for the family unit, but at the expense of the martyr's becoming increasingly unsatisfied, depressed, frustrated, and resentful. All these examples demonstrate that both the scapegoated member and the family system are in collusion to maintain the complained-of symptom or behavior.

Other families may show a tendency toward enmeshment of some family members and disengagement of others. In families with one or more members with emotional, behavioral, or psychophysiological symptoms, one often finds evidence of *enmeshment.* This is a form of affective involvement in which two or more members are caught in an intense but mutually destructive bond that, though temporarily decreasing anxiety, does so at the expense of inhibiting emotional development for all involved. If a child is the identified patient, frequently one or both parents may be enmeshed with the child but minimally affectively involved with the other (Hoffman 1975; Karpel 1976; Minuchin 1974). This almost always indicates a distortion of the family system that will continue to support disturbance until the structure can be shifted so that parents can look to each other to have their emotional needs met and can work together as allies in the shared task of raising their children (Bowen 1978; Minuchin and Fishman 1981).

Such families produce individuals who remain dependent on others for regulating their self-esteem. Failure of individuation resulting in incomplete ego boundaries produces a continued reliance on external (i.e., social) approval to maintain self-esteem. Without complete ego boundaries and a well-circumscribed sense of self, the individual fails to develop the internal (psychological) mechanisms described by Winnicott (1976) and by Fogarty (1976) needed to maintain or replenish self-esteem in the face of external criticism, adverse circumstances, personal failure, or other narcissistic blows and losses. It is as if what self-esteem these people have could drain away through the gaps in the ego boundaries, unless continually resupplied by a never-ending stream of personal successes and manifestations of external approval. Such people remain, therefore, excessively dependent on the continued approval of others. The risk of alienation from those whose approval they need is so intense that they cannot bear even temporary separation from the source of the repeated transfusions of praise and approval. They are, in effect, paralyzed by their dependence on others, by their repeated questioning of their self-worth, and by their chronic vulnerability to depression.

SYMPTOMS AS AN EXPRESSION OF FAMILY DYSFUNCTION

The symptoms of an identified patient may play a key role in family members' attempts to influence one another and to maintain a dysfunctional family equilibrium. Sigmund Freud (1917) acknowledged that symptoms at times can prove useful in an individual's relationships with others. This he called secondary gain, emphasizing that while such symptoms offer the individual fringe benefits, the primary gain—the main purpose of the symptom—is to defend against neurotic anxiety. The family therapist, however, feels that neurotic symptoms, regardless of their origin, are to a major extent maintained by the responses they elicit from others. As long as symptoms pay off, not only for the individual but for the family, both child and family will rely on them to perpetuate symptomatic behavior even though consciously all express a desire for change. When symptomatic behavior no longer works for the individual and for the family, both are forced to reappraise the situation. This is often what leads families to enter treatment; the symptom is no longer working well enough or has become too frightening. Therapists do not respond directly and refuse to be manipulated by symptomatic behavior. Instead they point out what the patient is doing and reflect how the patient is using the symptom to control relationships. When the usual distortions, threats, attacks, hysterical outbursts, attempts at emotional blackmail, and so on do not succeed in manipulating or controlling the therapist, the patient is left more aware of the maneuvers and the fact that they are not working. The therapist can then help the patient recognize the degree to which similar devices are relied upon in attempts to manipulate and control others.

In certain families, for example, any attempt to discuss a certain member's behavior results in tears, accusations of being picked on, and so forth. One learns that the same thing happens at home whenever anyone tries to confront that member about undesirable behavior. The typical result is that the family members learn to put up with symptoms to avoid a scene, end up forced to justify their complaint in the face of accusations that they are unfair, or the discussion shifts to the way in which the member is defending him- or herself (i.e., the unreasonablness of the issue). In any case, the original issue has been successfully deflected—and therefore defended against—by the defensive maneuvers of the person whose behavior was discussed. But if this member is in an interpersonal situation where the typical defense will no longer work—for example, in therapy, provided the therapist avoids being intimidated, deflected, or diverted—the patient can, in time, recognize the nature of the defensive maneuvers. Only then can patients learn to achieve direct, rational, mature methods of dealing with problems. Some common uses and meanings of symptoms include:

1. The symptoms of a particular family member may have considerable communication value (Alexander 1973). For example, a statement of how miserable, lonely, hurt, or helpless one is may communicate: (a) a plea for support and/or pity; (b) an implied reproach (e.g., "look what you've done to me"); (c) an attempt to control (e.g., the martyr who uses weakness to keep the family in line).
2. Other symptoms may constitute a more direct attack. The child who vomits when angry not only demands attention but punishes parents by making them clean up. Similarly, the rituals of the obsessive-compulsive may enable a psychologically crippled wife to dominate totally a rigid and authoritarian husband. (See chapter 12 for more on obsessive neurosis.)
3. Symptomatic behavior may mask a demand that the others in the environment relax their expectations since the patient is clearly not up to them. It is as if the patient said "How can you expect me to be pleasant or to carry my weight when I'm so nervous, depressed, or crazy?"
4. Finally, some symptoms take the place of sudden, intense feeling outbursts—for example, the increased disorganization of thought in the schizophrenic in a tense, pressured situation; increased stuttering at times of tension and anger; exacerbation of psychosomatic symptoms in moments of repressed rage or grief.

THE FAMILY AS A UNIT OF TREATMENT

The viewpoint put forward in this chapter has clear-cut implications both for diagnosis and treatment. The diagnosis needs to include all levels of equilibrium (intrapsychic, interpersonal, and social) as well as the interactions among them. To those who think in this way, the unit of pathology (the patient) is no single individual but the family as a whole. The member originally referred (the identified patient) is demoted (or promoted, depending on one's point of view) to the role of "symptom bearer" for the family. Satir (1967) has referred to the identified patient as the "scab on the family sore," meaning that the symptoms are merely the obvious part of a pathological process involving the family as a unit.

If this is so, it follows that the aim of treatment becomes not merely the removal of symptoms from the identified patient, but a modification of the pathological structure and equilibrium of the family unit. Ways in which this can be done will be discussed in chapter 29.

SUGGESTIONS FOR FURTHER READING

ACKERMAN, N. W. 1958. *The psychodynamics of family life.* New York: Basic Books.
  The original textbook in psychodynamically oriented family theory.
BARTEN, H. H., AND BARTEN, S. S. 1973. *Children and their parents in brief therapy.* New York: Behavioral Publications.
  Illustrates how to "think deeply but act superficially" in dealing with the family in crisis.
BOYD, E., et al. 1974. Teaching interpersonal communication to troubled families. *Fam. Process* 13:317–336.
  Describes an approach to family intervention directed at ways in which information is exchanged in troubled families.
BOWEN, M. 1978. *Family therapy in clinical practice.* New York: Jason Aronson.
  Perhaps Bowen's most important contribution is demonstrating the significance of triangular and intergenerational relationships, particularly in poorly differentiated families.
CARTER, E. A., AND MCGOLDRICK, M., eds. 1981. *The family life cycle: A framework for family therapy.* New York: Gardner Press.
  Well-written, modern account of family organization and tasks at various stages in the family life cycle. Special attention is given to single parent and reorganized families, and to the changing role of women.
GURMAN, A. S., AND KNISKERN, D. P., eds. 1981. *Handbook of family therapy.* New York: Brunner/Mazel.
  A highly recommended, comprehensive source that enables students and practitioners to compare and assess critically current approaches to family therapy. All major schools are represented in original contributions by some of the leaders in the field. Three chapters discuss special areas: marital and family enrichment; divorce and divorce therapy; and the treatment of sexual dysfunction.
HOFFMAN, L. 1981. *Foundations of family therapy: A conceptual framework for systems change.* New York: Basic Books.
  Hoffman deals with the development of conceptual approaches since the 1950s, the issue of family typology, families producing severe psychotic disorders, theories of change, and the major schools of family therapy. Probably the best single book on the topic of strategic family therapy.
LIDZ, T. 1980. The family and the development of the individual. In *Family Evaluations and Treatment,* ed. V. K. Hofling and J. M. Lewis, pp. 45–68. New York: Brunner/Mazel.
  Concise and clearly expressed views of one of the early workers in the field of the relationship between family organization and individual personality development.
MINUCHIN, S. 1974. *Families and family therapy.* Cambridge, Mass.: Harvard University Press.
  A comprehensive description of a form of family therapy concentrating on change-producing and preventive interventions. A must for the serious student of family therapy.
————, and Fishman, C. H. 1981. *Family therapy techniques.* Cambridge, Mass.: Harvard University Press.
  A new and more sophisticated description of the structural family model and accompanying therapeutic techniques by its originator. Also contains comparisons with other major therapeutic models and numerous case examples.
MINUCHIN, S.; ROSMAN, B. L.; AND BAKER, L. 1978. *Psychosomatic families: Anorexia nervosa in context.* Cambridge, Mass.: Harvard University Press.
  Extended case studies provide a good description of the role of the structural family therapist dealing with families of anorectics by creating minor crises that are then used to shift the family's equilibrium. The rationale and conduct of the therapy have many applications in the treatment of families with other chronic illnesses.
PAPP, P., ed. 1977. *Family therapy: Full length case studies.* New York: Gardner Press.
  An excellent collection of full-length case studies by leading American family therapists. Contains direct video transcripts plus explanation by the authors.
PEARCE, J. K., AND FRIEDMAN, L. J., eds. 1980. *Family therapy: Combining psychodynamic and family systems approaches.* New York: Grune & Stratton.

The authors attempt to integrate intrapsychic and family systems theory and technique. Includes clinical examples.

RUSSELL, A. 1974. Late psychosocial consequences in concentration camp survivor families. *Am. J. Orthopsychiat.* 44:611–619.

This study of the treatment of thirty-four concentration camp survivor families in family therapy is of particular interest because of the effects of a traumatic experience on the second and third generations.

STEINHAUER, P. D.; SANTA-BARBARA, J.; AND SKINNER, H. A. 1983. The process model of family functioning. *Canad, J. Psychiat.* (in press)

A comprehensive model of family structure and functioning that defines the major parameters of universal family functioning. The model, equally applicable to functional and dysfunctional families, stresses the ongoing interaction between intrapsychic and interpersonal processes, thus integrating psychodynamic and systems theories. A self-report test of family functioning within each of these major parameters (FAM: *F*amily *A*ssessment *M*easure) has been developed.

4

Paul D. Steinhauer

Issues of Attachment and Separation: Foster Care and Adoption

This chapter will describe two groups of children separated from their natural families, those who are adopted and those raised in foster families. Even children adopted in infancy must at some point separate psychologically from their natural parents. For the increasing number of older children being adopted and for those living in foster care, memories of the natural family and of former foster families may remain prominent. It seems appropriate, therefore, to discuss Bowlby's classic description of children's reactions to separation from parental figures as background for the discussion of adoption and foster care (Bowlby 1960).

Children's Reactions to Separation

In 1960 Bowlby described three stages by which children typically react to separation from parental figures—protest, despair, and detachment—and the pathological sequelae of aborted mourning. Rutter (1972) subsequently suggested that much long-term pathology that Bowlby had attributed to separation was related more to privation suffered prior to the child's leaving the natural family. Rutter demonstrated that children from warring families that consistently failed to meet their needs did better if placed in a secure, consistent, nurturing environment than if left in the inadequate parental home.

More recently Rutter (1979) has related various long-term effects that Bowlby ascribed to deprivation to a variety of insults, each with its own psychological mechanism. Thus he attributed acute distress following separation to interference with attachment behavior; intellectual retardation to experiential deprivation; conduct and socialization disorders primarily to family discord and disturbed interpersonal relationships; affectionless psychopathy to long-term effects of abnormal early bonding. According to Rutter, separation itself, while an important stress, is less crucial an influence on ongoing development than the quality of the experience that precedes and follows it.

Individual children vary considerably in their vulnerability to separation (Rutter, 1979). The intensity of an individual child's reaction to separation may be influenced by seven factors:

1. The age of the child: Emotional distress is maximal in the child separated between six months and four years of age (Goldstein, Freud, and Solnit 1973; Quinton and Rutter 1976).
2. Previous mother-child relationship: Stayton and Ainsworth (1973) have shown there is less short-term distress following interruption of a secure attachment. This is consistent with a number of studies of separation of primate infants from their mothers (Harlow et al. 1966; Hinde, Spencer-Booth, and Bruce 1966; Mineka and Suomi, 1978). Abusive parents promote a more intense attachment, and therefore a greater response to separation, than do indifferent parents.
3. Temperament of the child: Infants respond differently to separation, probably partly because of the interacting effects of sex-linked characteristics, constitutional traits (including tendencies to withdrawal, high intensity of reaction, low adaptability), perinatal distress, and environmental influences. These factors probably affect vulnerability to separation primarily by influencing the intensity of the primary attachment.
4. Previous separation experiences: While a number of authors (Eisenberg 1962; Maas and Engler 1959; Quinton and Rutter 1976; Robertson 1970) suggest that the effect of multiple separations are cumulative, no straight-line relationship exists. Multiple placements are likely to increase vulnerability to subsequent separations. Possibly a better predictor than the exact number of separations is the quality of the child's adjustment in the longest previous placement.
5. Duration of separation: Distress is greater with a longer duration of separation (Douglas 1975; Quinton and Rutter 1979).
6. Effects of strange environment: Distress and long-term ill effects of separation are greatly reduced if the child remains in familiar surroundings, probably partly due to the continuing presence of others (including siblings) to whom the child is also attached (Heinicke and Westheimer 1965; Schwarz 1972). This suggests the potential mediating effect of multiple attachment figures and the desirability of keeping siblings together whenever possible.
7. Nature of child's situation subsequent to separation: The sooner an adequate parent substitute is available, the shorter the period in limbo and the less the

risk of serious long-term sequelae (Freud 1960). The commitment of the substitute parents to the child and their ability to tolerate the acute distress precipitated by separation also influences the nature of the child's adjustment (Raphael 1982; Tizard 1977).

Mourning is the psychological process initiated by the loss of a loved one by which a longstanding attachment (represented in figure 4.1) is gradually undone.

The aim of mourning is the giving up of the lost person. The purpose of mourning is to help mourners accept the fact that someone to whom they were attached is gone and to effect the corresponding change in the mourners' inner world—that is, the gradual withdrawal of interest, caring, and investment from the lost attachment figure. This process of detachment must be successfully completed for children to accept the finality of the loss and to be freed to reattach to a parent substitute. This process of detachment, referred to as the work of mourning, is accompanied by evidence of grief, a normal response to loss that includes signs of anger, pining, sadness, and preoccupation with memories and fantasies of the lost person.

Mourning is precipitated when children are separated from attachment figures. The more distressed the parent-child relationship, the harder it will be to complete the work of mourning (Stayton and Ainsworth 1973). Yet according to Bowlby, unless detachment occurs the child will not be free to form the new attachments needed to support ongoing development.

The crucial importance of the substitute caregiver or other significant adults (e.g., children's service worker) in actively assisting completion of the work of mourning as a prerequisite for reattachment has been stressed (Furman 1974; Palmer 1974). Yet foster parents and social workers frequently collude with children in avoiding the work of mourning and in suppressing their grief (Palmer 1974). Because of their own inability to tolerate the child's distress and the feelings of impotence evoked in them by the child's pain, they respond with a selective inattention and denial, if

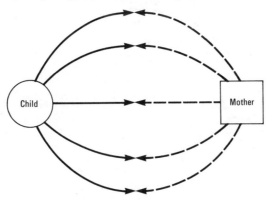

Figure 4.1 Relationship Prior to Separation.

not an active discouragement, of the child's attempts to use them to work through the mourning process.

Bowlby (1960) has described three stages of mourning: the stage of protest, of despair, and of detachment.

The *stage of protest,* shown in figure 4.2, lasts as long as the child retains hope of reunion with the lost mother (loved one or ones). The child typically cries, kicks, threatens, bargains, pleads, or behaves in any way to cause the return of the absent parent.

In the second stage, the *stage of despair* also shown in figure 4.2), the child is listless, apathetic, lethargic, and withdrawn. Adults, seeing this, often take it as proof that the child has lost interest in the lost parent(s). This is not so. Having lost hope of the mother's returning, the child accepts care from others but is not yet ready to accept a full reattachment to parent substitutes.

The stage of detachment is illustrated in figures 4.3 and 4.4.

Figure 4.3 illustrates how children respond when promptly provided with adequate parent substitutes to whom, in time, they form a secure re-

1. STAGE OF PROTEST
2. STAGE OF DESPAIR

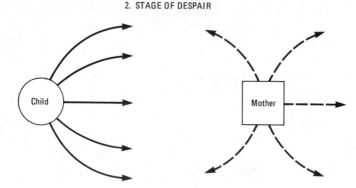

Figure 4.2 Separation.

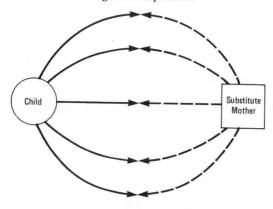

Figure 4.3 Successful Resolution.

attachment. Anna Freud (1960) has emphasized the importance of the critical period between the point of separation and that of provision of adequate parent substitutes. The longer this period in limbo, the greater the risk of permament damage. Age is also a factor here; the younger the child (once the age of six months has been reached), the shorter the limbo period that can be tolerated before psychological abandonment occurs, thus precipitating the work of mourning (Goldstein, Freud, and Solnit 1973).

Many long-term effects that Bowlby ascribes to separation Rutter (1979) attributes instead to the effects of family discord and disharmony. Most foster children experience prolonged family discord, neglect, and/or abuse prior to separation from their families. While the response of individual children varies considerably in nature and intensity, distressed and disturbed responses to separation will be intensified by the privation that preceded it. Their responses may hinder their acceptance by and their integration into their substitute families. Substitute parents committed enough to persist in spite of the children's distancing and provocative behavior can often succeed in helping them form a successful reattachment (Tizard 1977). Less committed surrogates, however, are put off by the child's persistent provocation and rejection, responding with frustration, withdrawal, neglect, or even abuse. The child then experiences at their hands a second privation that aggravates the behavior, thus increasing the likelihood of placement breakdown. Such a child, then, often shows the combined effects of privation within the natural family, one or more separations, and secondary privation within several foster families superimposed upon each other. Over the long term, children may exhibit six coping behaviors as a result of prolonged privation followed by separation.

The children may exhibit *permanent detachment.* (See figure 4.4). While Bowlby (1971) relates this to failure to complete the work of mourning, several authors relate it less to separation than to the lack of a satisfactory attachment prior to separation (Rutter 1979; Tizard and Rees 1975), especially following neglect. Other factors thought to favor persistent detachment include too long a period without adequate parental substitutes (Freud 1960), inadequate or inconsistently available parent substitutes or multiple placements (Eisenberg 1962; Maas and Engler 1959; Winnicott 1957) or a child too disturbed prior to placement to form a successful reattachment or to be tolerated in any but the most exceptional surrogate families. Should permanent detachment occur for any of these reasons, the children will reinvest the energy and love withdrawn from the original mother into themselves, which interferes with their capacity to relate to others in depth.

As toddlers, such children are overly and indiscriminately friendly (Tizard 1977; Rutter 1979), though when older they are typically described as cold and aloof, shallow, superficial, demanding, manipulative, and narcissistic in their dealings with others. Other people are used for what they can provide, valued only when they satisfy the children's needs of the moment, and discarded or turned on without guilt whenever they fail to do

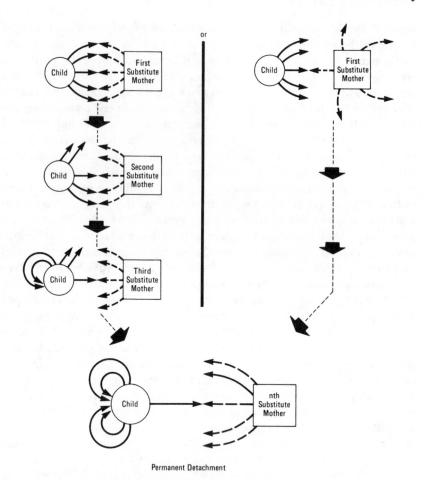

Permanent Detachment

Figure 4.4 Pathological Resolutions.

so. Alternatively, such children may combine exaggerated demands for attention and gratification with an inability to tolerate intimacy and a need to distance others. The energy withdrawn from others can be reinvested in the child's own body or in fantasy. Initially reinvestment in the child's own body results in excessive autoeroticism (thumb sucking, rocking, masturbation). Such children remain vulnerable to somatoform disorders and psychosomatic complaints later in life. (See chapter 16.) If children reinvested their energy in fantasy, the fantasy world then assumes more importance than external reality. This leads to a progressive withdrawal and an increasing turning for gratification to fantasy rather than to real experiences or other people (Freud 1960).

A second coping behavior is *persistent, diffuse rage*. Bowlby (1971) sees this as the child's response to the experienced deprivation resulting from unresolved separation, but Rutter (1979) ascribes it to disturbed family relationships primarily prior to separation. Unless worked through, this rage and the defenses developed against it may be dammed up, generalized, displaced, and diffused. This distorts the developing personality, undermines and destroys potential relationships, and dominates both mood and behavior.

Third, children suffering from the results of prolonged privation followed by separation may exhibit *chronic depression.* This depression is related to the children's need for love and security remaining unmet. While presenting at times as frank depression in the adult sense—overwhelming sadness, loneliness, hoplessness, self-destructive behavior (including drug abuse), suicidal thoughts or attempts (Adam 1982)—at other times depression presents as a continuing apathy marked by pervasive lethargy, loss of former interests, lack of drive or available energy, deteriorating school performance, inability to get started or follow through, and global, persistent pessimism. These may alternate with bouts of acting-out and frequently antisocial behavior that can be dynamically understood as depressive equivalents. (See chapters 13 and 14.)

Another coping behavior is *asocial and antisocial behavior.* This is probably related more to previously experienced family discord than to separation per se (Rutter 1972). Three sets of factors, which commonly potentiate each other, account for the frequent asocial and antisocial behavior these youngsters display. These include: (1) an inability to empathize with others, presumably derived from failure and/or disruption of attachment; (2) defects in conscience (superego) resulting primarily from disruption and discontinuity of relationships, which keep these youngsters from forming the stable identifications needed for effective conscience formation; as a result, while frequently demonstrating diffuse feelings of shame, they lack the mature conscience's capacity for experiencing appropriate guilt; (3) defects in impulse control (ego defects). These children lack the ability to bind or tolerate emotional tension, which must therefore be discharged immediately through behavior. Thus they are prone to sudden, explosive behavioral outbursts to discharge the sweeps of rage to which they are so vulnerable.

Fifth, the children may have a *low self-concept.* This results originally from the fact that the children have never felt sufficiently loved or cared about to feel valued and worthwhile. This original lack is aggravated by the compulsive though unrecognized need to set themselves up for repeated rejections, thus proving again and again that there is nothing worthwhile or lovable about them (Littner 1960).

And sixth, the children may exhibit *chronic dependency.* Many such children never become emotionally self-sufficient and autonomous. As if needing to obtain in adulthood what they missed in childhood, they transfer exaggerated demands for nurture and support from one person or agency to another, draining and alienating each source of supply and remaining emotionally, socially, and often economically dependent.

Adoption

HISTORY OF ADOPTION

Until relatively recently, those who adopted did so primarily to serve their own interests—for example, to continue the male line, to forge political alliances, to secure or protect a family's fortune—with little attention paid to the welfare of the adoptee.

Following World War II, however, adoption began to change from a service to find children for families toward one that sought to provide suitable families for children needing them. In the 1950s potential adoptees routinely were discharged from the hospital to interim foster homes for at least six months, until their freedom from serious mental or physical defects had been established. Children whose birth parents had a history of imprisonment or mental illness would never have been considered adoptable. During the late 1950s and the 1960s, an increased understanding of genetics, of attachment and bonding, and of the psychological sequelae of separation from parental figures led to babies being adopted at birth, along with less emphasis on matching of physical characteristics and the background of the biological parents. It was only in the 1960s that foster parents became the prime candidates to adopt eligible children already in their care. Previously any such suggestion on their part would have been considered evidence of excessive involvement and unsuitability for fostering.

Adoption, in marked contrast to foster care, has always been primarily a middle-class phenomenon, while foster care has remained less prestigious, with most foster parents being drawn from working-class families (Cooper 1978).

DEFINITION AND CLASSIFICATION

One must distinguish *extrafamilial* from *intrafamilial* adoptions. An extrafamilial adoption has no preexisting blood tie between the adoptee and either adoptive parent. In an intrafamilial adoption, a blood tie exists with at least one adoptive parent. Most intrafamilial adoptions consist of stepparents adopting their spouse's children from a previous marriage. A much less common and generally more problematic form of intrafamilial adoption occurs when parents or relatives of an unmarried mother adopt her baby and raise it as their own. This chapter will use the term adoption to describe extrafamilial adoptions unless otherwise indicated.

CHANGING PICTURE OF ADOPTION

Following World War II, the number of total adoptions increased rapidly, reaching a peak in the late 1960s (Hepworth 1980; Hersov 1976). Since then, although the total has remained far above pre-1960 levels, an increasing percentage—estimated in Great Britain as 70 percent and in Canada as 55 percent—of total adoptions has been intrafamilial adoptions by stepparents, thus reflecting a steep rise in rates of divorce and remarriage (Office of Population Censuses and Surveys 1976). (See chapter 26.) Thus although total adoptions have decreased slightly, both the number and percentage of extrafamilial adoptions have fallen sharply. Two factors contribute to this decline.

First, most adoptees result from illegitimate pregnancies, especially those of unmarried mothers under age twenty years (Guyatt 1980; Hepworth 1980; Hersov 1976). Second, although the number of illegitimate children remains significantly above that of the early 1960s, the number of healthy infants available for adoption has decreased sharply. Since there has been no corresponding decrease in the popularity of adoption, there are now too many applicants for too few babies. Reasons for this include: (1) new legislation permitting dissemination of birth control information and sale of contraceptives, although these may be used more effectively by older women than by those under twenty, who have traditionally been the largest source of babies for adoption (Guyatt 1980); (2) the legalization of abortion, which shortly preceded the sharp decrease in illegitimate births; and (3) the fact that significantly more unmarried mothers are now keeping their babies. This trend presumably results from changing community attitudes toward illegitimacy and increasingly available social benefits (e.g., mothers' allowance and day care) (Guyatt 1980; Hepworth 1980; Hersov 1976).

Significance of the Changing Picture of Adoption

In addition to decreasing the number of healthy infants available for adoption, these trends have other important implications.

Several studies have demonstrated that illegitimate babies raised by their mothers make less developmental progress and show more maladjustment than either legitimate children raised by their mothers or illegitimate children adopted at birth (Crellin et al. 1971; Hausknecht 1972). This may result from a number of simultaneously operative factors:

1. The children may have a genetic vulnerability to maladjustment and, in particular, to the development of conduct disorders (Cadoret 1978; Cantwell 1975; Cunningham et al. 1975; Hersov 1976).
2. Pregnant teenagers as a group are at risk for such complications of pregnancy as prematurity and prenatal and neonatal morbidity. These problems in turn are associated with a wide range of reproductive casualties in infants (Baldwin and Cain 1980; Knobloch and Pasamanick 1966; Osofsky and Osofsky 1970). Several authors (Baldwin and Cain 1980; LaBarre 1969) have related the increased risk less to maternal age than to inadequate prenatal care. Due to widespread denial of pregnancy, frequent attempts to conceal it as long as possible (Hausknecht 1972), and failure to utilize available medical and social services (Hepworth 1980), unmarried teenage mothers frequently receive less than optimal care.

3. The widespread use of alcohol and other drugs known to have deleterious effects on fetal development is common among teenage mothers.
4. Continuing high levels of psychological and social stress are reported to impair the development of the fetus and young infant (Crellin et al. 1971).
5. Those unmarried teenagers who decide to keep their babies are poorer, less advanced academically, less stable emotionally, and more immature. They have fewer resources and support systems than those who place their infants up for adoption (Guyatt 1980; Lightman and Schlesinger 1980; Vincent 1961; Yelloly 1965). This raises questions as to their parenting capacity.
6. Children of unmarried teenage mothers frequently show deficits in cognitive development (Baldwin and Cain 1980), and adopted boys have a higher incidence of clumsiness, poor coordination, and restlessness (Seglow et al. 1972). These problems are presumed to result from the social and economic consequences of early child rearing, although Fisch and associates (1976) ascribe them to a disadvantaged socioeconomic environment.

Many young unmarried mothers fail to use traditional social services (e.g., children's aid society counseling, mothers' allowance) (Crellin et al. 1971; Hepworth 1980). Yet they often remain severely economically disadvantaged and lack family and social supports, so that the potential for neglect is increased (Pozsonyi 1973; Reed 1965). Although there is a common clinical impression that their children are at risk for coming into care seriously disturbed, often after months or years of neglect or abuse (Hepworth 1980), no firm data on the frequency with which this occurs is available, and at least one study contradicts this (Sauber and Corrigan 1970).

Because of the gap between the number of adoptive applicants and babies available for adoption, and because of changing social attitudes and pressures from governments and parent groups toward adoption, many children once considered unadoptable because of age or physical, intellectual, or emotional handicaps are now aggressively promoted for adoption. Such "special needs" children currently make up approximately two thirds of all adoption placements as compared to only one third in 1961–62 (Hepworth 1980; Rowe and Lambert 1973). Many are older children with long histories of neglect and abuse, multiple placements, difficulties relating to others, and conduct disorders, all of which were long considered barriers to successful adoption.

THE UNMARRIED TEENAGE MOTHER

The literature disagrees on whether pregnancy in an unmarried teenager is symptomatic of an underlying psychological disturbance (Lewis 1971) or merely a normal extension of widespread adolescent sexual behavior (Anderson, Kenna, and Hamilton 1960). There is no single answer to this question. Unmarried teenage mothers are neither all disturbed nor all normal. Social permissiveness interacting with such psychological factors as depression, impulsivity, acting-out of unconscious wishes and conflicts, discharging the self-fulfilling prophecies of adoptive parents, or repetition compulsion can motivate illegitimacy in selected cases. The motivation, presence, and/or degree of psychopathology must be individually determined in each given case. Alternatives available to the unmarried pregnant teenager include the abortion, marriage, and intrafamilial adoption, as well as the teenager raising the child on her own as a single parent or carrying to term and placing the child up for adoption.

The number of unmarried teenagers who have *abortions* has increased markedly since the early 1960s (Guyatt 1980). Gordon (1973) has questioned whether this compromises the unmarried mother's future ability to carry to term. Abortion is often seen by unmarried teenagers and even more often by their parents as the best solution to their problem (Perez-Reyes and Falk 1973). Several authors warn against forcing abortion on unmarried teenagers, both on ethical and on practical grounds, since doing so is frequently followed by a subsequent pregnancy that is concealed until a repeat abortion is no longer possible (Gough 1966). While those who abort even despite strong family opposition may experience some guilt, depression, and anger immediately postoperatively, more frequently abortion brings almost immediate relief with little resulting evidence of lasting psychological disturbance (Perez-Reyes and Falk 1973; Report of the Committee on the Working of the Abortion Act 1974).

Marriage to the putative father, often another adolescent, has been promoted as a socially acceptable solution to the pregnant teenager's dilemma. Yet such marriages have a high rate of breakdown—in one study five times the rate of marriages contracted after age twenty—particularly if it is decided on as a solution to premarital pregnancy (Dominian 1968; Sauber and Corrigan 1970).

Another alternative, having the child reared by the mother's parents or another relative as a child of their own (i.e., *intrafamilial adoption*), frequently results in serious psychological problems as the child gets older.

ISSUES RELATED TO SUCCESS IN ADOPTION

The success of an adoptive placement depends on the nature of the relationship between the adoptive parents and the adoptee. This is determined by three sets of factors: the characteristics and needs of the adoptive parents; the characteristics (including constitution) and needs of the adoptee; and the "fit" between child and parents, that is, how much each can meet the other's needs and accept each other's limitations.

Adoptive Parents

We know less about the positive factors that make for success in adoptive parents than about negative ones in adoptive children (Rae-Grant 1978). As mentioned earlier, adoption is primarily a middle-class phenomenon (Humphrey and Ounsted 1964; Kadushin 1970; Seglow et al. 1972), though there is an increasing willingness on the part of adoption agencies to accept more working-class applicants or ones who are marginally acceptable because of their age and state of health provided they agree to adopt older, more difficult, or disabled children. Adoptive parents are generally older and, despite qualifying medical examinations, less healthy than biological parents (Bohman 1970; Grey and Blunden 1971; Maas 1960). Humphrey (1969) has suggested that positive memories of their relationships with their own parents seem the parental factor most predictive of a successful adoptive outcome. Adoptive parents whose relationship with their own parents was strained, whose self-esteem is low, or who have had trouble separating from their own families are particularly likely to have difficulty raising another's child. Extreme overindulgence and difficulty providing normal discipline may result either from guilty fantasies of having stolen someone else's child or as a reaction formation to unrecognized rejection. In either case, the resulting conduct disorder undermines the parent-child relationship, inviting further rejection and possible eventual extrusion of the child. Parental fantasies that such children, having inherited the biological taint of the natural parents, are bound to become bad, promiscuous, and so on may long precede and may unconsciously encourage the unacceptable behavior the parents consciously repudiate.

Adoption per se is rarely the single cause of psychological or family problems, though it frequently aggravates or is blamed for stresses to which the family is already vulnerable. Unfortunately, however, psychological problems of the adoptive parents, their unhappy childhood, their own bad experience as an adopted child, or even severe marital problems are frequently concealed during assessment for adoption for fear of rejection by the adoption agency. The adoptive parents' feelings about their infertility can accentuate already low self-esteem. If either parent, badly wanting a child, pushes adoption on the other or if the child is adopted to play a special role within the family (to replace a lost child, to cement a failing marriage, to help a neurotic parent feel fulfilled), that special status and the resentment and guilt evoked when the child fails to meet the unrealistic expectation will invite rejection, overindulgence, or overprotection. These or other causes of rejection (i.e., the child serving as an ongoing and unwanted reminder of infertility, especially if a natural child was conceived subsequent to the adoption; because the child they "rescued" from rejecting parents and a life of illegitimacy fails to meet an excessive need for gratitude) may interfere with the parent-child relationship and contribute to conduct and behavioral disorders.*

At a time when many potential adoptees are older and come with a history, habits, and problems of their own, several authors† favor a two-stage review process similar to that suggested for selection of foster

*See Clements 1971; Schechter 1960; Sorosky, Baran, and Pannor 1975; Tizard 1977; and Triseliotis 1973.
†Children's Services Division 1979; Cooper 1978; Freund 1976; Gross and Bussard 1970; Rae-Grant 1978; and Wolins 1963.

parents. Initially groups of potential adoptive parents hear firsthand the experiences of couples who have taken older and difficult children into their families. This weeds out some of the less suitable applicants through self-selection, leaving those who remain with a better idea of the demands and frustrations of the course they are contemplating. This is followed by one or more individual interviews with social worker(s) to deal more specifically with attitudinal and psychodynamic factors in order to complete the assessment and to assess the fit between the couple and a particular child. In spite of the difficulties involved and the significant number of breakdowns in adoptions of older and hard-to-place children, successful adoptions of such children can significantly improve their developmental prospects while providing satisfaction for the parents and a major service for the community (Jaffee and Fanshel 1970; Kadushin 1970).

The Adopted Child

Despite considerable controversy about methodological flaws, it is probably safe to conclude that adopted children are moderately overrepresented in clinical populations. Critically reviewing the evidence available from British, Canadian, American, and Swedish studies, Hersov (1976) suggests that boys are more likely to be disturbed than girls, and conduct disorders are more common than neuroses or anxiety disorders. Possible reasons for the increased incidence of disturbance in adopted children include: (1) biological inheritance (Cadoret 1978; Cunningham et al. 1975); (2) poor prenatal care of unmarried mothers (Crellin et al. 1971; Hausknecht 1972; Osofsky and Osofsky 1970); (3) neglect, abuse, lack of continuity of attachment figures prior to placement (Rutter 1972); and (4) experiences in the adoptive family (Hersov 1976; Rowe and Lambert 1973).

There remains controversy around whether there are psychological conflicts specific to the adoptive situation. Adopted children must somehow face and resolve complex identity problems arising from having had two sets of parents in their lives (Schechter et al. 1964; Sorosky, Baran, and Pannor 1975). Adopting parents are vulnerable to potential stresses unique to their special (i.e., adoptive) status, including the competition of the ghosts remaining from natural and former foster parents, the prior history and different biological inheritance of the child, and issues related to their own infertility (Kirk 1964; Sorosky, Baran, and Pannor 1975).

As mentioned, adoptive boys are significantly more likely to be disturbed than girls (Bohman 1970; Tizard 1977), and adoptive children are more likely to be hostile, insecure, and attention seeking than nonadoptive children, but less so than illegitimate children raised by their own mothers or those restored to natural families after a period in care (Tizard 1977; Tizard and Rees 1975). There is controversy around whether and how much age at placement affects placement success, but difficulties that occur are more likely to be social and educational than a need to resist reattachment or integration within the adoptive family (Eldred et al. 1976; Jaffee and Fanshel

1970; Kadushin and Seidl 1971; Tizard 1977). Identity confusion during adolescence is predictably exaggerated for many adoptees (American Academy of Pediatrics 1971; Sorosky, Baran, and Pannor 1975), partly because of the prior interference with attachment that undermines the child's own sense of identity and partly because the continued presence in fantasy, and potentially in real life, of a second set of parents, the birth parents. This favors continued reliance on the use of splitting as a defense (i.e., imagining one set of parents are good, the other bad), thus hindering the child's ability to fuse good and bad images in a single person and undermining identity closure (Schechter 1960; Sorosky, Baran, and Pannor 1975).

Both adoptee and adoptive parents know that the child's biological inheritance differs from that of other family members. This establishes the child as "special" and thus liable to scapegoating and rejection in response to extreme stress or parental or marital pathology. Inherited temperament and the long-term sequelae of privation and discontinuity in key relationships prior to adoption make many special-needs adoptees difficult to accept, let alone love. Especially if natural children were conceived after the adoption, many adoptive parents, angry, discouraged, yet guilty for feeling so rejecting, may ascribe any problems that occur to genetics, thus distancing the child while at the same time absolving themselves of any contribution to the problem (Tooley 1978).

Factors Influencing the "Fit"

Age of Adoption. The effect of the age of adoption on adoptive outcome remains controversial (Eldred et al. 1976; Jaffee and Fanshel 1970; Kadushin and Seidl 1971; Tizard 1977). Humphrey and Ounsted (1963) found a higher rate of disturbance especially in boys placed prior to six months, but Offord, Aponte, and Cross (1969) and Kadushin and Seidl (1971) demonstrated that the older the age of adoption, the greater the frequency and severity of antisocial behavior. Other studies (Eldred et al. 1976; Menlove 1965; Jaffee and Fanshel 1970) suggested that the age of adoption did not significantly affect adoptive outcome, while Kadushin (1970), in a follow-up of children adopted between ages five and twelve, found only 14 percent of adoptive parents dissatisfied, a figure used to support the claim that older child adoptions are as successful as infant adoptions. Most adoption studies suggest a parent satisfaction rate of 78 to 85 percent regardless of the age at adoption (Tizard 1977). However, since these studies rate adoptive success by parent satisfaction alone, and since adoptive parents often deny even what others report as major problems until after rejection of the child has occurred (Bohman 1970; Jaffee and Fanshel 1970; Schechter 1960; Tizard 1977), these findings may be unduly optimistic. Nevertheless, available data suggest that the risk in adoption of older children is less than was previously believed. Although it has been demonstrated that many older children can be adopted, it is generally accepted that wherever feasible, adoption should occur at the earliest possible age.

Factors associated with poor adoptive outcome include the number of previous placements, a previous diagnosis of conduct disorder, and a continuing and strong emotional attachment to the biological mother.

Assessment for Adoption. Prior to adoption potentially adoptable infants no longer undergo a prolonged period of observation in foster homes to rule out defects not obvious at birth (Illingsworth 1968). However, Rutter (1970) suggests that it is more important to assess the motivation to adopt and the personal adjustment and marital stability of the adoptive parents, factors that affect the development of any child.

More recently, the emphasis in adopting older children has shifted toward identifying and stressing potential psychological and social difficulties and presenting an accurate picture of the likely limits of the child's developmental potential. Many such children are identical to those who remain until maturity in foster homes, except that they are legally free for adoption. While it is clear that children with severe medical conditions can be adopted successfully, seriously handicapped children constitute a major strain on the parents' time and the family's stability (Franklin and Massarik 1969; Cooper 1978; Hepworth 1980). While most parents cope successfully with such children, when problems occur, these are more often in children with severe handicaps and are more likely to be behavioral than medical (Knight 1970). It is both unethical and self-defeating to withhold from potential adoptive parents any data regarding the probable nature and extent of handicaps or problems they are likely to face. Prior experience in having raised successfully their own children seems to decrease the risk of adoption breakdown.

Interaction Between Child and Parents Related to Adopted Status. Several authors note a general reluctance by adoptive parents to discuss information about their child's biological parentage and adoption openly and comfortably (Jaffee and Fanshel 1970; Sorosky, Baran, and Pannor 1976; Triseliotis 1970). Although there are exceptions (Schechter 1960), most authorities suggest discussing adoption with children when they are very young (Eldred et al. 1976; Kirk 1964; Triseliotis 1973). They do so for several reasons.

For one thing, at some point all children will learn of their adoption. It is better that they be confronted with their special status in a supportive way from trusted parents than that they remain in ignorance only to be told the truth of their origin at a time of heightened vulnerability by a nonsupportive or hostile person in a manner that is shocking for its unexpectedness and lack of preparation (Triseliotis 1973).

Failure to discuss adoption and the child's origins openly has been related to general parenting style (i.e., presence or lack of openness, marked overprotection) or to the parents' need to deny anything special about their adoptive status. (Jaffee and Fanshel 1970; Sorosky, Baran, and Pannor 1975; Triseliotis 1973). Parental shame related to infertility is probably less of a factor in this regard now than was the case twenty years ago, since the woman's movement has provided mothers with other ways of establishing their self-worth than just by childbearing. The tone and attitude during these discussions may be as important as the actual information transmitted. Children who feel that parents are comfortable discussing the subject will ask what they want to know when they want to know it.

What and when the child is told is an important issue. While there is no absolutely right way—parents must do as they see fit—a number of guidelines are suggested.

Parents should begin with a simple and concrete initial statement as soon as children begin expressing interest in where babies come from. Then the children will have at least heard and associated with themselves the word adoption, thus becoming aware of their adopted status. Beyond that, children should generally be told what they want to know, and no more or less. If children sense that the topic is an open one, they will return for more when they are ready for it.

Because of unconscious conflicts about the child's illegitimacy or adoption, adoptive parents may have trouble facing their periodic anger and disappointment with the child. All parents are, at times, angry and disappointed with their children. In adoptive families, the hostile component of this natural ambivalence is often repressed, dammed up, and eventually discharged in distorted and symptomatic ways.

Not infrequently, adopted children handle hostility to their parents by exploiting the parents' fear that the child is not securely attached and making excessive demands or blackmailing them into condoning outrageous behavior. In response, insecure parents become increasingly anxious and resentful. Guilt, in reaction to resentment and what they see as their failure, and fears that they may alienate their child forever may be handled by reaction formation. As a result, the hostile component of their ambivalence is replaced by overindulgence, overinvolvement, and an inability to limit or discipline the child, whose infantile tendencies toward omnipotence and control are thereby reinforced.

Meanwhile the adoptee must also cope with having been given up by the birth mother. But why? Because of badness? Or was it the child who was good and the mother bad? Children told early, frankly, and comfortably about the circumstances of their adoption are more likely to feel secure in their adoptive status and do well (Eldred et al. 1976). At some point all adopted children must come to grips with the fact of their illegitimacy or of being given up by the biological parents who still exist and have a history of their own, and that to some extent the child may be like one or both of them. The less freely the adoptive parents discuss the birth parents with the child, whether because of lack of information or inhibition, the greater the possibility of the child's being preoccupied with romanticized or idealized fantasies of them (Jaffee and Fanshel 1970; Sorosky, Baran, and Pannor 1975). Should the adoptive parents be critical of or attack the birth parents, children identified with them will feel that they too are being denigrated. Should this recur repeatedly, it favors the child's identifying with the birth parents, potentially undermining the sense of belonging within the adoptive family and the child's self-esteem. Thus the more adoptive parents can comfortably help adoptees accept their origins, the better the children's chance of a successful attachment to the adoptive parents that can then be used to support the child's development.

As Triseliotis (1973) points out, the fact that "disturbed" adoptees were preoccupied with what they saw as the failure of their adoptive family life is not proof that their persistent problems were indeed the result of their adoption. Nevertheless, this was how they perceived the problem, and in North America, groups of adoptees supported by some natural parents are demanding legislation to "unseal" their case records and instruct agencies to produce on request identifying information that they could use to exercise their "right" to contact with their birth mothers. This possibility has been available for some time to adoptees in Scotland and in a small minority of American states. Sorosky, who studied fifty adult adoptees following reunion with natural parents, supports opening the record on request (Sorosky, Baran, and Pannor 1976). He found 90 percent of his sample satisfied following their reunions, which, they reported, provided a sense of closure and diminished conflicts over identity. Triseliotis (1973), in a study later replicated by D'Iorio and Steinhauer (1978), is more cautious. These studies distinguished between the provision of nonidentifying information—which they supported—and the encouragement of reunions with birth parent—about which they were more guarded. Both studies found that those adoptees urgently demanding reunion differed from those seeking information only or, in the latter study, from those interested in reunion but without preoccupation or urgency. The urgent seekers were characterized by longstanding dissatisfaction with relationships within the adoptive family; low self-esteem and chronic problematic adjustment in many areas of life; nondisclosure or disclosure of only hostile background information by the adoptive parents. Their response to reunion was mixed and often involved bitter disappointment, although the adoptees claimed the meetings were helpful in their coming to grips with their situation.

These studies, and that of Jaffee and Fanshel (1970) who also found an association between longstanding dissatisfaction, problematic adjustment, and complaints of insufficient or hostile disclosure, suggest the importance of agencies routinely making background information available to adoptive parents and that they strongly suggest that this be shared freely and as naturally as possible with adopted children well before they enter adolescence.

Requests for information or reunion should be treated not as isolated events, but as stages in an ongoing process that, in themselves, may represent a crisis for the individual adoptees who are seeking to consolidate their identification. Sensitive casework at this point by an agency worker familiar with the vicissitudes of identity formation in adolescent adoptees can be extremely helpful to the adoptees themselves, the adoptive parents, and, at times, to the natural parents, all of whom are at a transition point in their lives. D'Iorio and Steinhauer, agreeing with Triseliotis, are much more cautious than Sorosky, Baran, and Pannor as to whether the advantages of reunion on request outweigh the additional anxiety and disruption that such a policy would involve for many adoptive parents. The disappointment reported by some adoptees subsequent to contact with their birth mothers is not in itself an argument against reunion, as it may be a necessary stage in the adoptee's finally coming to terms with reality, if confrontation with the natural mother as she is undermines the idealized fantasies resulting from the widespread use of splitting as a defense. The author would see no objection to reunion if all three parties involved (i.e., adoptee, adoptive parents, and natural parent) agree to it.

FACTORS CORRELATED WITH LACK OF SUCCESS IN ADOPTION

1. Children with a history of previous deprivation and multiple placements, especially within the first two years of life (Kadushin 1970; Steinhauer 1980; Rutter 1979), are at higher risk of adoption breakdown. Such children are likely to continue to show more frequent school problems and disturbed social problems especially outside the home, to have continuing difficulty with social relationships, and to place additional strain on the relationship with the adoptive parents, however accepting they may be.
2. Adoptions of children with a diagnosable conduct disorder prior to placement are at higher risk of adoption breakdown (Kadushin 1970).
3. Children suddenly removed from a successful long-term placement with foster parents who are their psychological parents are at increased risk of adoption breakdown. Currently in North America there is strong pressure toward adopting such children on the grounds of ensuring "permanence." In reality, the real sources of the pressure seem political, racial, and economic (i.e., eliminating the cost of maintaining them in foster care). The arguments that foster homes are inherently unstable, that the permanence of foster care cannot be guaranteed since some such placements break down during the child's adolescence, and that foster parents must be only minimally committed or they would proceed to adoption are all used to demand "permanency placement" (i.e., adoption). A number of authors* suggest that placements in which children have formed a stable attachment and are adjusting and developing successfully should be supported and stabilized, not undermined and disrupted by agencies and governments operating in the name of "stability."
   To accommodate such situations, a variety of alternatives such as "planned permanent" foster care, foster care with tenure, and "subsidized adoption" are being attempted increasingly for children securely attached and developing well in a long-term foster home (Derdeyn 1977). In the absence of sound evidence regarding the least detrimental alternative for this group of children, their optimal management should consist of careful planning on an individualized basis with the participation of all involved in order to find the solution most likely to provide maximal continuity for the child (Cooper 1978).
4. Adoptions involving a child who retains a strong emotional tie to a birth or foster mother are vulnerable to breakdown unless that attachment is respected

*See Cooper 1978; Derdeyn 1977; Goldstein, Freud, and Solnit 1973; Rae-Grant 1978; Steinhauer 1980; and Wiltse 1976.

and continuing access is allowed. In such cases forced separation may well favor retention and idealization of the lost mother in fantasy, thus interfering with the child's availability for successful attachment to the adoptive parents (Goldstein, Freud, and Solnit 1973; Kadushin 1970; Steinhauer 1980).

5. Adoptions in which the adoptive parent(s) have excessive expectations of the adopted child are at high risk. In such cases the child is so badly needed to meet the needs of the adoptive parents (for example, to replace a dead child; to serve as a ready-made companion for an only child; to fill an empty nest; to give their lives meaning) that the parents are unavailable to meet the needs of the child (Schechter 1960).

6. Adoptions in which the child, as a result of previous experiences, has developed a well-established personality, ways of behaving, and/or exaggerated needs that interfere with acceptability to the adoptive parents are less likely to succeed (Eldred et al. 1976).

7. The controversy as to whether or not older children are more vulnerable to adoption breakdown has yet to be satisfactorily resolved. Although the majority of those writing on the topic suggest that they are,* although not as vulnerable as had been thought previously, several studies disagree (Jaffee and Fanshel 1970; Eldred et al. 1976). Jaffee and Fanshel's data seem to indicate that the vulnerability of older children to adoption breakdown is not as great as other researchers believe. The Frequency of adoptive parents' denial of problems, the nature of Jaffee and Fanshel's sample (only those adoptions that have survived the adoption probation period) and their defining success purely in terms of adoptive parent's reported satisfaction suggest more that some older children can be successfully adopted than that the risk of adoptive breakdown in older children is not increased. Eldred's study (Eldred et al. 1976) is more difficult to evaluate since the precise criteria by which success was determined are not stated. Until the controversy is resolved by incontestible evidence, it seems wise for adoption to occur at the earliest possible age.

TEN SUGGESTED GUIDELINES FOR PLACING THE OLDER CHILD UP FOR ADOPTION

1. Placing the older child up for adoption should always be part of a carefully considered plan.

2. Older children whose adjustment is good and who are developing well with foster parents prepared to commit themselves to raise them to maturity should, generally speaking, have their placement protected, not disrupted. Foster care with tenure, subsidized adoption, or planned permanent foster care may be preferable to adoption for such children. The assurance of continued agency support should difficulties occur in adolescence may do much to help foster parents honor such a commitment.

3. Parents considering the adoption of an older child should be told clearly and directly that while most parents who adopt older children express satisfaction with their decision, they may have to face a prolonged period of excessive demands, disruptive behavior, and/or rejection.

4. Prospective adoptive parents should be told to anticipate anger, resentment, and mistrust displaced onto them from the birth parents. They should be helped to anticipate and avoid feeding into their child's use of splitting (i.e., seeing the birth parents as entirely good and them as 100 percent bad) and to

*See Bohman 1970; Eisenberg 1962; Kadushin and Seidel 1971; Offord, Aponte, and Cross 1969; Rae-Grant 1978; and Tizard 1977.

recognize that much of their child's resentment and rejection of them is displaced from the ambivalent feeling toward birth parents and previous foster parents.

5. Such adoptive parents may need continuing or periodic support, even after the adoption is made final. They should be told that the period of adoption probation may be the calm before the storm, with disturbing behavior suppressed until after the adoption has been completed.
6. Adoptive parents should be alerted to the possible flare-up in adolescence of issues and behaviors related to the adoption.
7. Prospective adoptive parents should be told that it is not unusual or abnormal during adolescence for adoptees to seek information about or to search for their birth parents.
8. Adoptive parents should be told that such searching is not necessarily a negation or rejection of them, but may be a sign of the adopted adolescents' greater difficulty consolidating their identity.
9. Prospective adoptive parents should be strongly encouraged to understand the importance to older adoptees of protecting, through letters and visits, established ties to significant figures from their past, such as siblings and foster parents.
10. Adoptive parents should be helped to see such contacts as potentially useful in helping the child form a successful reattachment within the adoptive family.

Foster Care

HISTORY OF FOSTER CARE

Around the turn of the century, foster homes gradually began to replace large institutions as the preferred placement for orphans and neglected children (Children's Services Division 1979). Foster care was grounded historically in the spirit of rescuing "good" children from "bad" parents (Maluccio et al. 1980). Early foster parents served on a voluntary basis, and were expected to meet their foster children's basic needs and to prepare them for good citizenship in exchange for the child's working in the family home, farm, and/or business. The 1930s saw the first attempt to select and approve foster homes, to provide payment to foster parents, and to match child to foster home. While foster homes continued as the placement of choice for homeless or neglected children until the 1960s, fostering, with its low financial rewards, low public profile, and low public esteem, remained a much less socially acceptable alternative than adoption (Cooper 1978). Success rates were poor, although those cases most accessible to review and research were those with multiple problems, while those foster children who did well, married, and settled down were less accessible to review. There were few guidelines on which to base decisions and much confusion regarding the role of foster parents: were they clients of the agency, substitute parents, surrogate therapists for already damaged children, members of the child welfare agency team, or all of the above (Cooper 1978; Eastman 1979; Katz 1976; Wiltse 1979)? With an increasing number of already disturbed older children and adolescents coming into care, foster care gradually and unevenly evolved into substitute family care, largely on a temporary basis. In the 1960s group homes began to rival foster homes as the preferred placement for the increasing number of teenagers in care. Originally promoted for adolescents since they demanded less intensity of relationship than foster homes, group homes were considered unlikely to arouse the same loyalty conflicts and need for distancing by the adolescents involved. (See chapter 5.) Other trends of the 1960s and 1970s included the widespread questioning of whether foster care is essentially and inevitably an unstable service (Cooper 1978; Finkelstein 1980; Prosser 1978); the intense economic, political, and racial pressures to restore or place in adoptive homes foster children who once would have been considered unadoptable because of age, mental, emotional, and physical handicaps; the growth of Foster Parent Associations, which enhanced the self-image of foster parents and provided a channel for the expression of their dissatisfaction and for demands that agencies recognize their needs and the effects of fostering on foster families as well as on their foster children.

EPIDEMIOLOGICAL TRENDS

In general, there are fewer young children coming into care, but more older children and adolescents. While the total number of children admitted to care in Canada has approximately doubled over the last twenty years, between 1966 and 1978 (Hepworth 1980), the number of children under twelve coming into care decreased by 6.2 percent, and the number of adolescents coming into care increased by 72.4 percent. This latter figure is more than double the increase in the percentage of adolescents in the general population (Children's Services Division 1979; Cooper 1978; Hepworth 1980).

Reasons for this increase include more unmarried mothers keeping their babies, changing adoption practices (i.e., fewer infants placed in foster homes for observation prior to adoption), and an unintended and paradoxical consequence of expanded protection services, which leaves some children in inadequate families longer, only to bring them into care later (Hepworth 1980).

More older, hard-to-place, behaviorally and emotionally disturbed children are coming into care (Children's Services Division 1979; Cooper 1978; Gruber 1978; Hepworth 1980). The percentage of children transferred from protection services (supervised care in their own homes) to in-care services (i.e., placements) has steadily increased (Hepworth 1980). Because placement usually occurs after a longer exposure to an inadequate family environment, it is not surprising that most foster children are more behaviorally and emotionally disturbed as well as older. Aware of their roots, with their own biography and identity and with siblings and parents with whom they often wish to maintain contact, they frequently resist rapid integration into foster families. More children enter care after having appeared before the courts, and in many jurisdictions (e.g., Ontario and Massachussetts) planned decreases in training school and residential treatment beds have shifted children who at one time would have filled these institutional placements to overflow into the foster care system (Gruber 1978). More foster children stay in care for longer periods of time, growing to maturity with little experience of living with their natural families. As a result, many of these children are profoundly disturbing to the life of the foster families in which they live (Wilkes 1979).

These factors have led to a gradual but definite shift in the nature of foster care, from traditional to specialized foster care. With the increased number of older, seriously disturbed children and adolescents entering care, traditional foster care is no longer sufficient to meet their needs. Thus to be adequate, standard care must be specialized foster care as defined in table 4.1 for many if not the majority of cases (Frank 1980).

Because of the older and more difficult children coming into care, most child welfare associations or children's aid societies, especially in large urban areas, find it increasingly difficult to obtain and maintain enough foster homes, losing in some cases as many as one in four foster homes each year (Hepworth 1980). At the same time, the number of foster homes remaining vacant because of the lack of an "appropriate" child has increased, since older, disturbed children still strongly though ambivalently attached to their natural families do not rapidly integrate, despite the wishes of traditional foster parents (Children's Services Division 1979). Because of the shortage of foster parents prepared to cope with disturbed older children, an estimated 20 percent of foster children are institutionally placed, in spite of the myth that institutional care of homeless children is a thing of the past (Hepworth 1980). Why are fewer couples willing to foster? Hepworth suggests a number of reasons, including the fact that foster care is more demanding but pays less than home day care and provides little financial incentive to compete with higher paying jobs for women in the work force. The more difficult and disturbing children coming into care, increased case loads, the generally decreased availability of backup by child psychologists and psychiatrists, the increasingly militant advocacy of children's rights, at times at the expense of children's needs, and the growing legalization of what was once the child welfare and the children's mental health field have placed both foster parents and child welfare workers under mounting pressure. This has contributed to less sensitivity and individual responsiveness within the child welfare system; intimidation and harassment of foster parents; a downgrading of the supervision of casework skills in favor of an increased emphasis on case management

Issues of Attachment and Separation: Foster Care and Adoption

TABLE 4.1

Comparison of Traditional and Specialized Foster Homes (Children's Services Division 1979)

	Traditional Foster Home	Specialized Foster Home
Role of Foster Parents	Parent surrogates: provide basic care.	Provide basic care and treatment program (i.e., parent therapists, not parent surrogates).
Types of Children	Chiefly infants and young children.	Chiefly older and "special need" children with mental, physical, emotional, and behavioral problems requiring not just care but active treatment.
Motivation	Primarily voluntary: not paid for time or service.	Primarily a career choice; paid for time and services provided.
Funding	Boarding and maintenance allowance.	Boarding and maintenance allowance *plus* increment related to special services provided (treatment, etc.).
Goal	Normalization	Remediation.
Training of Foster Parents	None required.	Ongoing training and supervision would be expected; previous professional training might not be required, depending on program.
Services Offered	Contract to provide basic care and to cooperate in plan to return child home or prepare child for adoptive placement if possible or, otherwise, to foster to maturity.	Contract to provide basic care and to cooperate with agency in implementation of management and treatment plan designed to meet the needs of the child. Might include work with biological parents toward a return home, preparation for adoption, providing a therapeutic milieu as prescribed, possibly recontracting to provide planned permanent foster or adoptive care.
Disruption of Family Life Style	Usually minimal.	Usually considerable.

(i.e., crisis intervention only) skills. The net result is a decrease in the amount and quality of casework available to support beleaguered foster parents, thus contributing to dissatisfaction and burn-out. On the other hand, programs that organize foster parents into "extended family" groupings for mutual support and relief suggest that the network model may be a potent source of support by decreasing their anxiety and increasing their sense of being listened to, understood, and included in decision making (Fein, Davies, and Knight 1979; Foster Care Committee 1972; Hazel, Cox, and Ashley-Mudie 1977; Jacobs 1980), thereby providing increased job satisfaction and less likelihood of burn-out (Children's Services Division 1979; Cooper 1978; Rosenblum 1977).

THE EFFICACY OF FOSTER CARE

An unresolved debate rages between those who consider foster care inherently damaging and those equally convinced that under satisfactory conditions foster care can effectively protect the developmental potential of children who cannot be raised in their own families. The positions staked out by those on both sides are based more often on strongly held opinions than on proven fact. Prosser (1978) has illustrated the lack of proven knowledge about the long-term effects of family placement, due largely to the dearth of adequately controlled studies comparing the long-term (i.e., adult) adjustment of children who have grown up in different types of family and institutional care. Prosser stresses the need for immediate, controlled research on the ability of various placement alternatives to meet the developmental requirements of older, special-needs children. Such research is extremely difficult in view of the large number of dissimilar children and placement alternatives to be studied; the multiplicity of variables to be controlled for; the contaminating effect of unanticipated events beyond the control of the investigators; the difficulty obtaining and maintaining the cooperation of a frequently defensive and/or antagonistic subject population; the struggle to get approval for studies that satisfy increasingly stringent human experimentation criteria; the multitude of problems involved in introducing a research protocol into large child welfare agencies with their service pressures and established ways of working; and the diffusing effect of major differences in subsequent life experience, whose influence increases with the length of time between the end of the experiment and the collection of the follow-up data. Considerable confusion has been added by the frequent failure of those reporting to specify the nature of the children studied; the children's family experiences prior to placement; the type of placement involved; the degree and nature of casework and other assistance available to help child and foster family deal with the emotional sequelae of privation, coming into care, subsequent separations, and other difficulties; and the extent of contact with the natural family following placement. Any discussion of long-term foster care that is not controlled or that fails to define clearly its position regarding all these variables may do more to confuse than to illuminate.

There is a general belief that long-term foster care is inherently unstable and generally damaging (Finkelstein 1980; Gruber 1978; Maluccio et al. 1980). Cooper (1978) suggests that while short-term fostering in preparation for adoption has a clear purpose, intermediate and long-term fostering lack a clear definition of task and their inherent instability have consistently been shown to promote insecurity for all involved. Numerous authors* have expressed concern about the number of foster children who, more from a lack of adequate planning than from any conscious decision, end up drifting into permanent foster care abandoned by parents who no longer visit and neglected by the agency that is supposedly caring for them. But it is essential to differentiate the effects of the indifferent long-term foster care that results from indecision or drift from those of planned permanent foster care. A number of authors,† while well aware of the dangers of indifferent long-term placements, maintain that planned permanent foster care, if it results from an appropriate placement and receives adequate agency support, may differ little from subsidized adoption with or without contact (i.e., visits) with the natural family and may, for selected children, be the least detrimental alternative available. These authors attribute many of the failures of foster placement to faulty matching of child and family and/or agency failure to do enough to assist and maintain placements, rather than failures of foster care per se. Rutter (1972) has pointed out how much better children develop and adjust in a secure and nurturing environment than if exposed to continuing privation, neglect, and/or abuse in their own families. Tizard (1977) and Fanshel and Shinn (1978) have warned that those children who do least well are those who are taken from foster families in which they are flourishing and restored to indecisive, rejecting, or overwhelmed natural parents. Fanshel found that children who did best in long-term foster care were those who maintained contact with their natural families. The implication is clear: allowing children to drift in care or to bounce in and out of care is more damaging developmentally than providing a planned permanent placement in an alternative family that meets developmental needs. This highlights the central dilemma of the child welfare worker: how to avoid letting children drift unnecessarily into long-term care because no one has made a permanent plan for them while, at the same time, avoiding undermining the chance of a successful reunion by giving up on parents too soon. To assist in this, Maluccio and associates (1980) call for the establishment of research-

*See Bryce and Ehlert 1971; Fanshel and Shinn 1978; Gruber 1978; Maluccio et al 1980; Sherman, Neuman, and Shyne 1973; Steinhauer 1980; and Wiltse 1976.

†See Anglim 1980; Derdeyn 1977; Fanshel and Shinn 1978; Frank 1980; Goldstein, Freud, and Solnit 1973; Madison and Shapiro 1970; Sherman, Neuman, and Shyne 1973; Steinhauer 1980; and Wiltse 1976, 1979.

able criteria for evaluating parenting capacity, an area in which, with remarkably few exceptions (Simmons et al. 1981; Steinhauer 1981) little has been written.

Maluccio and colleagues (1980) comment on the difference between what is legally a permanent placement and one that is truly permanent and is experienced as such by both the child and parents involved. He warns of the need to distinguish between making and maintaining a permanent placement. Just returning a child home or placing that child up for adoption does not guarantee permanence. In their Oregon project, Maluccio and his associates found foster homes less stable than adoptive placements, but more stable than restoring children to their own families. On the other hand, Fein, Davies, and Knight (1979) showed no difference between adoptive and natural parents in stability of permanent placements after discharge from a temporary placement.

The term permanency planning has become a catchword in North America for those who seek to save children from foster parents, as if a return home or adoption were, by definition, permanent. This is illustrated by a 1979 report of the National Commission of Children in Need of Parents, entitled "Who Knows? Who Cares? Forgotten Children in Foster Care." According to the report, "Foster care provides little love and virtually guarantees insecurity and instability for many children in its embrace."

Maluccio and associates (1980) point out that research on permanency planning is at present limited and inconclusive. They stress the need for studies of the importance of a sense of permanence to both child and foster parents; of the permanence and effects on development and adjustment of different types of placements, (e.g., foster parent adoptions, subsidized adoptions, planned permanent foster care, legal guardianship) for different types of children; of criteria for the termination of parental rights; of the role of foster parents in permanency planning; of the identification of populations at high risk for having their children come into care and the nature of services needed to prevent family breakdown; and of follow-up of planned permanency placements.

In the meantime, Pike and associates (1977) suggest that the term permanency planning has become ambiguous and is at times used synonymously with adoption planning. Pike suggests that permanency planning should mean aggressively clarifying and deciding on the intent of a given placement and, during temporary care, keeping alive a plan for permanence. Emlen and colleagues (1977), cutting through the rhetoric, define the essential criteria of permanency planning: the placement is intended to last forever, though its permanence cannot be guaranteed. The family is one in which the child has a real sense of belonging, a respected social status, and a definite legal status. The permanence consists of commitment and continuity in the child's key relationships.

What is known about factors that affect the stability of foster placements? Cautley and Aldridge (1973) have listed a number of factors commonly associated with placement breakdown. Some of these appear to have preceded placement, such as a history of behavioral problems, hyperactivity, and excessive demands by the child, as well as excessive needs and unrealistic expectations by the foster parents. Others are generated by putting together a disturbing child and an established family (e.g., discomfort with the new child; rivalry between natural and foster children; rejection by foster parents of the foster child, or vice versa; hostility between foster and biological parents; foster parents unable to tolerate and unwilling to work with the child's problems). Other factors associated with unnecessary and damaging breakdowns include avoidable emergency placements; a lack of adequate involvement of both foster parents in preplacement decision making and preparation; poor foster parent selection or matching of child to family (poor fit) (Thomas 1981); inadequate preplacement visiting as part of a competent, consistent plan; a history of previous institutional placement; rejection in the child's longest previous placement; a history of poor physical care; the presence in the home of natural children of about the same age; the absence of good placement technique due to lack of knowledge, lack of commitment at the gut level, and/or excessive case loads that make only crisis intervention rather than continuing (process) interventions possible.* Maluccio and associates warn against increasing expectations on workers in the face of limited resources. This increases their frustration, dissatisfaction, sense of failure, and the likelihood of burn-out, whereas with proper training, planning, support, and resources child welfare work can be satisfying.

Moving beyond the child and the natural and foster families, factors have been identified in the child welfare and family court systems that undermine the quality of care. These include: delays and insensitivity to developmental and psychological issues within the legal system; overloaded public agencies with excessive case loads; lack of social supports for vulnerable families; inadequate after-care services; and the short-sightedness of considering it enough to merely train workers when what is needed is to influence administrators, planners, legislators, judges, social work trainers, the community.†

WAYS OF INCREASING THE EFFICACY OF FOSTER CARE

Several authors‡ have commented on significant changes in child welfare programs resulting from increased emphasis on a careful evaluation

---

*See Aldridge and Cautley 1975; Cautley and Aldridge 1973; Fein, Davies, and Knight 1979; Gruber 1978; Littner 1960, 1974; Palmer 1979/80; Steinhauer 1980; and Wiltse 1976.

†See Anglim 1980; Children's Defense Fund 1978; Derdeyn 1977; Maluccio et al. 1980; Palmer 1974; Regional Research Institute for Human Services 1976; Steinhauer 1978, 1982; and Wiltse 1976.

‡See Derdeyn 1977; Fanshel and Shinn 1978; Littner 1974; Maluccio et al. 1980; and Steinhauer 1978.

of children's needs as seen in their family context; careful planning to maximize continuity of care and placement stability; more explicit attention and help to natural parents and foster parents, especially during the initial period in care; and a greater recognition of the importance of after-care services. Out of this, the following guidelines can be derived:

1. All those working in the child welfare area should be trained and supervised in assessing parenting capacity (Simmons et al. 1981; Steinhauer 1983). Should a child's developmental needs not be met within that child's natural family, a determined attempt should be made to assess the nature of the child's and family's problems and to help the family resolve them as much as possible, by mobilizing other available social supports that might protect the family's continued ability to function as a unit (Frank 1980).
2. Wherever possible, child and family problems should be handled without removing the child. A demand for removal indicates a crisis that may or may not be accessible to alternatives short of separation. Removal and placement should be used only as a last resource.
3. If the child's life or continued security and development remain at risk either because of the danger of imminent abuse or because of the family's inability to cooperate with or benefit from the best casework and other services available, the child may require removal from the natural family. The time to think of where a child will go *after* being placed is *before* that child is removed. In other words, children should only be removed from their families as part of an adequately formulated plan of long-term management. Agencies that operate according to the philosophy "First we'll avoid abuse by taking the child into care; then we'll start to think about what to do next" are less likely to work intensively with the family in crisis at the point of the family breakdown and are more likely to allow children to stagnate or drift into limbo.
4. Wherever possible, situations likely to deteriorate and necessitate removal should be promptly identified. A thorough assessment of child and family at an early stage may do much to clarify those factors in child and family contributing to the deterioration. The more clearly these are understood, the greater the chance of finding a satisfactory alternative to placement. Even should placement be necessary, an advance assessment and formulation will still prove invaluable in helping define the child's needs and areas of difficulty and in helping select a suitable alternative placement, thus minimizing the risk of unnecessary and damaging replacements. This is the best time for psychiatric consultation, not after things have reached the point of no return (Hampson and Tavormina 1980).
5. Emergency placements should be avoided wherever possible. They allow no time for adequate matching of child and resource, or for preparation of child and foster family for each other. Proper preparation for placement should invariably include discussing frankly with both foster parents difficulties the child is likely to present and a carefully planned series of preadmission visits for the child. Unless the risk of serious abuse is imminent, it is better for the child to remain in a known but inadequate situation a few days or weeks longer in order to allow for the development and initiation of a planned and adequately prepared alternative.
6. Intermediate placements should be avoided wherever possible, and the child should move directly into a resource suited to his or her anticipated needs as determined by a prior assessment. Intermediate placements should be reserved for children identified in advance as unable to tolerate a permanent placement

or those relatively few absolute emergencies where a planned placement simply cannot be delayed.

7. Should a separation be unavoidable, the potential risk can be minimized by:
   a. Ensuring that the move is part of an overall plan of management rather than an isolated response whose long-term implications have not been adequately considered.
   b. Preparing the child adequately for separation and placement. This involves dealing openly with the reasons for the placement and with the feelings of all involved around this. It also requires a gradual and predictable introduction to the new placement at a rate that the child can tolerate without undue anxiety.
   c. Bearing in mind that parental figures to whom the child is attached will continue to have emotional meaning despite physical separation. This implies:
      i. that separation will cause the child to mourn, either overtly or covertly. The successful resolution of this mourning, which will depend on the assistance of the foster parents and/or the caseworker, will be crucial in determining how much permanent damage the child will suffer as a result of the separation.
      ii. particularly if the separation occurred without adequate preparation, every effort should be made to see that child and parents (or surrogates) see each other following the placement so that feelings stirred up but not resolved can at least be out in the open. To avoid this on the grounds that it will prove unpleasant or traumatic is to encourage the child to repress the experience, with consequences previously outlined.

8. Skilled and committed work with foster families, despite the resistances and difficulties involved, will be crucial if the number of replacements is to be minimized. The role of the worker must be kept clearly defined, and the dangers of being drawn into competition with the foster parents or cast as a middleman (messenger) between foster parents and child recognized. The worker must be aware of the child's prior disturbance and avoid blaming foster parents for their reactions to the child's preexisting pathology. Only if they are sure that the worker clearly sees (a) the degree of the child's disturbance and (b) the fact that it existed prior to placement with them will foster parents allow examination of their reactions to the child without extreme defensiveness. The primary role of the worker is to help child and family work out their relationship with each other by learning to deal, both individually and together, with the feelings—especially hostility, anxiety, and rejection—they elicit in each other (Eastman 1979). To assume the role of an expert on child rearing, or to attempt to deal with issues purely at the instrumental level, is to invite failure. Current reality is important, but feelings left over from the past contaminate children's perceptions of the present and their behavior. They are an essential part of the child's reality.

9. Workers should learn more about child development, the psychopathology of childhood, and techniques of working with children and families. Caring is not enough. A body of knowledge is available on children's responses to separation and foster care. Through reading, in-service training, proper utilization of supervision, better use of consultants, and, above all, a critical examination of their own work, workers should continually evaluate professional strengths and learn to recognize and strengthen areas of weakness.

10. Workers need to be aware of how personal feelings influence their work. When clients make them anxious, frustrated, bored, or hostile, what happens? If they

feel love or pity for a child, how does this affect their dealings with that child and the family? How often do the quality and level of the worker's involvement reflect more his or her own needs than those of the client?

11. The difficulty that most children, foster parents, social workers, and child psychiatrists have dealing with anger openly and directly must be recognized. All of us feel rage from time to time, whether we acknowledge it or not. The more mental health workers can build a relationship with clients, supervisors, and consultants in which all feelings, both positive and negative, are dealt with in an open, direct but controlled manner, the more effective they will be. Workers must be sensitive both to their own and to the client's indirect expressions of hostility (cancellations, lateness, complaints about the agency or former workers, the derisive use of humor, attempts at manipulation, repeated requests for more money), and use these to get at the source of the underlying anger openly and directly.

12. Foster parents know more about day-to-day living with a child in their family than the worker does. Decisions affecting the child will also affect their family. Thus they should be involved in any major decisions around the child (Cooper 1978; Hampson and Tavormina 1980; Katz 1976; Wilkes 1979).

13. Issues such as the timing of the termination of parental rights and the pros, cons, and nature of visits with the natural family should be determined according to a plan based primarily on the child's needs and reviewed and updated on a regular basis. Generally speaking, those children who do best in long-term foster care are those who remain secure in their foster homes but have continuing access to natural parents to whom they remain attached but on whom they cannot depend for the caring, consistency, and guidance they need (Fanshel and Shinn 1978). Visits with the natural family should be used to make it possible for the child to maintain the continuity of important relationships; to remain in touch with—that is, to have stirred up, and therefore available to casework—the feelings and conflicts left unresolved since coming into care; to help the child see directly the reasons for coming into care. By stopping visits the relationship with the parents is not eliminated; this merely encourages the child to idealize and perpetuate in fantasy the absent parents rather than to seek solace in new and real relationships (Steinhauer 1977).

14. Decision making regarding a child in care should involve all those likely to be affected by the decision to be made. While not all will be satisfied, all—foster child, foster parents, natural parents, agency—need to feel that their position has been heard and seriously considered (Cooper 1978).

15. There needs to be greater recognition of the changing nature and demands of foster care. In view of the numbers of older, already damaged youngsters coming into care, specialized foster care has become standard, and traditional care, while less costly, is usually exploitative and inadequate.

16. More attention needs to be paid to the attraction, selection, retention, and training of a new type of foster parents, ones who are trained and prepared to act as surrogate therapists carrying out a treatment plan in their own homes. Criteria for and methods of selection have been discussed elsewhere (Children's Services Division 1979; Gross and Bussard 1970; Jacobs 1980; Wolins 1963). A number of projects have found that campaigns aimed specifically at—and prepared to pay appropriately for—specialized foster parents have less of a recruiting problem (Hazel, Cox, and Ashley-Mudie 1977). Projects involving specialized foster parents emphasize ways of routinely including foster parents within the decision-making process; clear definitions of the roles of foster

parents and social workers as colleagues and team members; patterns of service that provide support, relief when necessary, and enhance foster parent self-esteem need systematic assessment (Foster Care Committee 1972; Hazel, Cox, and Ashley-Mudie 1977; Jacobs 1980).

17. Because of the difficulties referred to earlier, there are many unanswered questions regarding foster care. Controlled studies of the permanence and criteria for the selective use of adoption, subsidized adoption, planned permanent foster care, and foster guardianship are needed, so that each of these alternatives may take its appropriate place in the care of children who cannot continue to live with their birth parents.

Conclusion

Because of the changing nature and needs of those children requiring placement outside their families, the nature of adoption and foster care is also changing and the distinction between them is, at times, less clear. Thus planned permanent foster care with guardianship may differ little from subsidized adoption or adoption with access. As foster care and adoption converge, a number of key questions face child welfare workers, clinicians, and researchers as we begin the 1980s, including:

1. What is the relationship of foster care to adoption?
2. What criteria can be used to decide which form of family placement is preferable for a given child?
3. How can one facilitate earlier but appropriate decision making, both to free children for adoption and to avoid the drift that can otherwise result from institutional inefficiency or neglect?
4. By improving the quality of foster care, can workers eliminate the damage that results from drift into long-term care, or is even optimal foster care less desirable than adoption?
5. What can be done to raise the status and satisfaction of foster parents in order to aid in recruitment and minimize burn-out?
6. Should restoration to natural families remain the primary goal for most children during their first year in care, or does an excessive push to restoration in the face of parental ambivalence or rejection increase the hazards of ongoing discontinuity or neglect?

Until more data on these topics are available, decision making for each child should be undertaken only after all those participating in the care of the child—including the child and foster parents—are involved in the planning process.

SUGGESTIONS FOR FURTHER READING

ALDRIDGE, M. J., AND CAUTLEY, P. W. 1976. The importance of worker availability in the functioning of new foster homes. *J. Child Welfare League of Am.* 54:6.
Placement success in a new foster home is highly dependent on the amount and kind of preparation the new parents get, the characteristics of the social worker, and his/her availability during placement.

BOWLBY, J. *Attachment and loss, Volume 1: Attachment.* New York: Basic Books.
A theoretical discussion of the nature and development of the child's tie to the mother (Vol. 1, 1969), of anxious attachment and separation anxiety (vol. 2, 1973); and of loss and mourning (vol. 3, 1980); using a psychoanalytic framework but drawing on the findings of ethology, control theory and cognitive psychology.

DERDEYN, A. P. 1977. A case for permanent foster placement of dependent, neglected and abused children. *Am. J. Orthopsychiat.* 47(4):604–614.
Permanent foster placement is suggested as an alternative for children who would suffer from a return to the home but whose adoption is blocked by the defense of parental rights.

FANSHELL, D., AND SHINN, E. B. 1978. *Children in foster care: A longitudinal investigation.* New York: Columbia University Press.
A comprehensive longitudinal study of the emotional and intellectual adjustment of 624 children entering foster care in 1966 and the circumstantial factors that contribute.

GOLDSTEIN, J.; FREUD, A.; AND SOLNIT, A. J. 1973. *Beyond the best interests of the child.* New York: The Free Press.
Focused attention on effect of child's age and time sense on that child's response to disruption of continuity. Popularized term psychological parent. Useful for those in the child welfare, family court, and family law fields.

MALUCCIO, A. N., et al. 1980. Beyond permanency planning. *Child Welfare* 59(9):515–530.
"Permanency planning" is receiving increasing attention from foster care workers. The authors examine the definition of permanency, the effect on practice, and the implications for service delivery.

PARKES, C. M., AND STEVENSON-HINDE, J., eds. 1982. *The place of attachment in human behavior.* New York: Basic Books.
Distinguished authors examine the influence of attachment and loss on personality development and the psychopathology of childhood and adult life. The first section (Infant-Mother Attachment) is highly recommended for all serious students of child development. Other topics dealt with include relationships between maternal depression or parental death and attachment, the contribution of attachment theory to an understanding of such diverse topics as child abuse, specific reading disabilities, neuroses, adult depression and suicide, prevention of mental disorders.

PROSSER, H. 1978. *Perspectives on foster care: An annotated bibliography.* Windsor, England. NFER Pub. Co. Ltd.
Extensive coverage of foster care literature and discussion of works on planned permanency and restoration.

RUTTER, M. 1979. Maternal deprivation, 1972–1978: New findings, new concepts, new approaches. *Child Dev.* 50:283–305.
A critical review of maternal deprivation research since 1972 is used to assess formulations proposed in 1972 and to discuss the implications of fresh findings on some new topics.

SIMMONS, J. E., et al. 1981. Parent treatability: What is it? *J. Am. Acad. Child Psychiat.* 20:792–809.
Attempts to objectify and quantify family historical data, familial factors prominent in the decision to hospitalize a child for psychiatric reasons, parental "treatability" or capacity for change, and specific professional aids needed by parents of a hospitalized child.

SOROSKY, A. D.; BARAN, A.; AND PANNOR, R. 1975. Identity conflicts in adoptees. *Am. J. Orthopsychiat.* 45(1)18–27.

Study findings indicate that such prevalent adoption practices as permanent sealing of birth records should be changed in recognition of the life-long nature of adoption.

TIZARD, B., 1977. *Adoption: A second chance.* London: Open Books.

An eight-year longitudinal study of sixty-one children institutionalized in infancy who were adopted, restored, or fostered, examining the success of the placements and the effects of early deprivation. For professionals and concerned parents.

5

Saul V. Levine

Alternative Family Styles

In contemporary North America, many children are being raised in domestic situations different from those popularly represented in the media—mother, father, 2.3 children (Masnick and Bane 1980; Reiss 1980). Along with the demise of the extended family as a common source of psychological and social support, the nuclear family itself has undergone radical transformations (Keniston 1977). Decades of rapid technological and value changes, the ethic of mobility at all costs, of narcissism, of materialism and acquisitiveness as ultimate goals, and of self-realization have manifested themselves in changes in the life styles of adults that have certainly affected their children's life circumstances and development.

Although most children are still being brought up in intact nuclear families, that majority is constantly shrinking. In today's middle-class elementary and high schools, almost every classroom contains not only children living with two married parents in traditional families but an increasing number of peers who live with one parent, more than two parents, no designated parents, or in a variety of other circumstances (Eiduson, Cohen, and Alexander 1973; Vanier 1977). Many children actually find themselves "belonging" to more than one family. As a result of the rising prevalence of separation, divorce, and common-law unions, an increasing number of children live with two parents who may not have married. They may have at least one stepparent recently introduced into the family who brought children from previous relationships. On the weekends, the stepparent's children visit their own noncustodial parent, who may live in another such nontraditional union with one or more of the children from the prior union in addition to children from the noncustodial partner's mate's previous unions. The variations on this theme, discussed in more detail in chapter 26, are almost endless.

The effects of living in different circumstances for extended periods of time have not yet been clearly defined. What is remarkable is the degree of rhetoric and rage provoked by these variations. Impugning motives and morality, lay critics have mercilessly attacked alternative living arrangements as destructive to the psyche, soma, and soul of children and adolescents, who are seen as victims. Defenders, however, have been equally hyperbolic in describing some arrangements as presaging a new millennium.

In attempting an objective analysis of alternative family styles, it is extremely difficult to tease out the variables. For example, many of the children living in altered domestic situations have ended up there through a process of sequential moves, each coming on the heels of a failed relationship or life style. As a result, ascertaining whether the current scheme of things is salutory or detrimental in the short and long term or whether it can make up for problems remaining from earlier and discarded domestic arrangements is difficult. Obviously only long-term prospective research on children and families in a variety of living arrangements will provide the kind of data necessary to draw meaningful conclusions. There appears to be only one such large-scale study in progress at the present time (Eiduson, Alexander, and Cohen 1973). This study compares the child-rearing practices of counterculture groups with those of two-parent nuclear families and studies the effect of multiple caretaking and antisexist attitudes on the psychological growth of the child.

This is not to say that there is no other information available. Nor is it to suggest that the Royal Road to Utopia is only via the intact nuclear family. There are many such physically intact units that do a disastrous job of child rearing in spite of the "ideal" structure. Thus the nuclear family is not necessarily the standard against which all other arrangements must be measured; it is just the most familiar. Comparisons will inevitably have to be made, but not with the implication of the nuclear family's inevitable superiority.

Single-Parent Families

The single-parent family is the most common alternative to the traditional nuclear family (Census of Canada 1976). Single-parent families formed 17.3 percent of all families in the United States in 1979 (U.S. Bureau of the Census 1981), and Glick and Norton (1979) have estimated that 45 percent of all infants born in 1978 will live part of their first eighteen years with only one parent. Little is known of the long-term effects of single-parent upbringing. Kulka and Weingarten (1979) showed in a twenty-year study that parental divorce in childhood does have some effect on psychological well-being in adulthood, but that correlation is weak. Research on shorter-term effects finds no significant differences in self-esteem, academic achievement, or maturity between children of one- and two-parent families (Hammond 1979; Raschke and Raschke 1979), but certain variables such as family conflict must be controlled for (Berg and Kelly 1979).

While sometimes the single-parent family results from the death of a parent or, especially in the last two decades, the choice of an unmarried mother to keep her child, the vast majority of children living in one-parent families do so as a result of a divorce or long-term separation—that is, a breakdown in the original family. When this has occurred, the child has already, prior to the separation, lived in an atmosphere of serious and prolonged domestic trouble and tensions. The effect of these tensions often lingers on after the parental split (Rutter 1979). Disagreements about divided or shared responsibilities, custody, access, finances, and approach to children, not to mention continuing interpersonal conflict between the parents who are emotionally and physically estranged yet forced to deal with each other concerning the care and upbringing of the children, often confer a degree of continuing bitterness to the home environment. There *is* evidence that children living in such circumstances are at considerable risk psychologically (Offord et al. 1979; Robson 1979). The situation of few children living with single parents is ideal (Baldwin and Cain 1980; Sugar 1976). For example, the average income of single parents is well under the national average (Census of Canada 1976; Ferri 1976). Fifty percent of these families have incomes below the official poverty line.

Economic disadvantage is the one factor consistently associated with single parenting, and it does have a negative effect (Buchler 1978). Generally speaking, such factors as social class, family size, and parental aspirations show greater influence in the lives of children than does the family situation per se. A single mother with one or more children, living on a subsistence level in crowded or dilapidated quarters and feeling absolutely overwhelmed in her family and milieu, is poorly equipped to proceed satisfactorily with her own development, let alone meet the security and developmental needs of her children (McAnarney, Roghmann, and Adams 1978; Phipps-Yonas 1980). Similarly, the growing number of unmarried teenage mothers who decide to keep their babies—adolescents who already are more likely to be psychologically disturbed and disadvantaged than those who abort (Olson 1980)—has become a major social problem (Nakashima 1977; Presser 1977; Subcommittee on Select Education 1978). Not only do their children not fare well—they are beset by higher rates of morbidity, hospitalization, and abuse (Bolton, Lauer, and Kane 1980; Kinard and Klerman 1980; Ory and Earp 1978)—but the young mothers often find themselves unsupported, out of school, ostracized, and in varying states of psychiatric disorder.* Too frequently these children end up in foster care when they are preschoolers, by which time they are already confused and disturbed (Hepworth 1980).

If the single-parent family results from a recent divorce, an extremely common contemporary phenomenon, how that process is handled will largely determine the effects on the children. If the divorce is handled relatively quickly, if continuing conflict and tension between the ex-partners are kept to a minimum, and if the parents achieve new satisfactions in their lives while continuing to parent, a sense of stability can return in time to the domestic scene, despite an inescapable period of misery for the children. (See chapter 26.) Stability in this context implies a situation meeting the same criteria one would apply to any family—a loving, happy environment; adequate nutrition, clothing, and housing; the potential for successful ongoing relationships; stimulation and teaching; consistency in discipline; and predictability of one's life (Steinhauer 1983).

The question then becomes "In a stable, loving, single-parent family, is the child at any more risk than in a similar family with two parents?" There is no evidence to suggest that this is the case. Children raised de novo by good single parents or children who, having adapted over time to a new rearing situation with one parent only, do not appear to manifest any greater incidence or prevalence of psychological disorders (LeMasters 1970; Weisner and Eiduson 1978). Further, there is no evidence that problems with sexual identity or orientation are increased among children raised mainly by a parent of the same or opposite sex (Eiduson, Cohen, and Alexander 1973; Green 1979; McLure 1976).

Reconstituted Families

Two adults living together with children from previous unions comprise the increasingly common phenomenon of newly formed or reconstituted families. Despite frequent initial stress and difficulty resulting from the attempt to blend two dissimilar and not necessarily compatible or willing nuclear families, many of these reconstituted families function in time not unlike intact nuclear families, albeit with unique features and problems. Reconstituted families are discussed further in chapter 26.

*See Cannon-Bonventre and Kahn 1979; Card and Wise 1978; Furstenberg 1976; McAnarney 1978; Menken 1972; and Moore, Hofferth, and Werthheimer 1979.

More Than Two Parents

A great deal of observation, and some clinical research, has been directed at the effects of communal living on children (Levine, Horenblas, and Carr 1973; Marcus and Robinson 1972). In particular, this has been exhaustively studied in Israeli kibbutzim and other collectives abroad (Marcus and Robinson 1972). In North America, while communes are by no means a new phenomenon—the Bruderhofs, Hutterites, and other Utopians have been here for generations—they have recently become much more common, as people have banded together for a variety of reasons.

Certainly alienation in a competitive, materialistic world has caused some people to form "intentional social systems" with built-in support, shared duties and responsibilities, and common values and goals. But even more influential for many communalists has been their shared belief system, be it political-economic (socialism), therapeutic, religious, or even anarchistic. These overriding goals have often determined the direction the communal organization pursues and have even affected the approaches to children of various members (Levine, Horenblas, and Carr 1973; Sussman 1972).

In this complex area there have been some relevant findings. Most communes in North America have continued the "proprietary" approach to children—that is, a mother (or father) knows who her children are and takes prime, sometimes sole, responsibility for their upbringing. One study reports a reversion to this model after an attempt at group upbringing (Levine, Horenblas, and Carr 1973). Interestingly, most kibbutzim are now also moving in the same direction.

To the extent that a commune works well and provides relative tranquility and support, the children appear to do very well indeed. They seem healthy, self-assured, warm, and outgoing. They go to regular schools and generally cope as well as any other children. But just as in a nuclear family under a great deal of tension, an unstable, conflicted commune engenders emotional problems in its members, including the children. Communal groups that are disorganized or full of antagonisms usually break up within a matter of months, as their members go their own separate ways. In contrast, as with successful families, communes that do well are stable, supportive, nurturant, and strong (Eiduson 1976; Levine, Horenblas, and Carr 1973).

Group Homes

In many North American cities, many children and youth, particularly in the young adolescent years, live for extended periods in officially designated group homes. The routes into these homes are many and variable, via welfare agencies (e.g., Children's Aid Societies), mental health agencies, or correctional services. Many of the homes—and youngsters—appear to be quite similar in functioning and in stated goals regardless of the designated category, official purpose, or source of funding.

Most of the residents of group homes attend regular schools in the communities in which the homes are situated. At times the homes and the children are feared, vilified, or even scapegoated by the surrounding neighbors. Amicable relations with neighbors can usually be engendered after a while, particularly if community concerns are acknowledged and treated with respect. This allows staff or representatives of the sponsoring agency to reassure anxious neighbors that many of their more fanciful and exaggerated concerns are irrational. Such person-to-person contacts are particularly effective when the adults operating the group home see to it that the youngsters in their charge eliminate provocative and outrageous behavior within the community.

It is difficult to evaluate the effect of group home living on these young people, because almost all of them have been placed in order to ameliorate or correct a previous intolerable domestic situation. Either from the results of having been raised in a destructive milieu, because of their own internalized or reactive psychopathology, or, most commonly, from a combination of the two, the group home population consists of youngsters who are, before entry, difficult and disturbed. Many have already been stigmatized and labeled "sick" or "bad" by one or more of society's major institutions. For psychological or social reasons, they have been extruded from their own often disruptive and tension-ridden families, and excluded from their communities.

Within the group homes, there is usually an attempt to provide a familylike atmosphere but usually without the demand for emotional involvement typical of most foster homes. In addition, there is often a large therapeutic thrust, both formal and informal. In some, the children are cared for by a team of child care workers and social workers with psychiatric consultation and support. Others are run by trained married couples who get similar backup. Many homes and leaders, unfortunately, lack such support but are still expected to cope with very difficult children. Within each such home, there are usually between five and ten youths who must learn to live with one another, cope with each other's behavior while sharing the responsibilities of the home and, at the same time, adapting to a new community and coming to terms with whatever emotional conflicts and behavioral difficulties led to their admission in the first place. This is no easy task. They go to neighborhood schools and, depending on how successful they are in their attempts to stabilize and adjust, develop friendships with local youngsters. Those who do well may seem no different from any of their "normal" peers. Those who do not do well frequently remain excluded and may be morbidly conscious of their unacceptability to the surrounding community, with disastrous consequences to their self-concept and self-esteem.

While it is obvious to any professional working with group homes that some children who enter these homes already seriously disturbed are immeasurably helped to go on to academic, personal, or social success, the long-term effects on the majority of group home inhabitants are not yet known. Nor are they being monitored or studied systematically. The markedly higher incidence of teenage suicide for children living apart from both parents (Garfinkel 1979) strongly suggests that premature and conflicted separation from parents prior to the satisfactory achievement of emotional separation interferes with developmental progress (Steinhauer 1974), leaving youths vulnerable to depression and suicide. We do not know about the ultimate fate of the majority of youngsters raised in group homes. There is no clear evidence that the group home experience is, in the long run, beneficial as compared to doing nothing, or to other alternatives such as remaining in their own families. Nor is it clear that children raised in group homes are at long-term psychiatric or other risk as a result of living and growing in a group-home setting. We have all seen successes and would like to believe that group homes offer an alternative for many who have been damaged by their families. But the degree of family disturbance and failure of professionals to work adequately with the family, both prior to and following the child's admission to the group home, may outweigh the group home's potential effectiveness. And if there is not an adequate social support network, there is in fact an exponential limitation on what can be accomplished by the mental health professions.

Cults

Most cults or fringe religious groups are made up largely of young (mean age 22.5), Caucasian, single, middle-class men and women who usually follow the doctrine and dictates of a living guru (e.g., the Reverend Sun Myung Moon, Maharaj Ji) and do not have a large number of young children being raised in their midst. The reasons for this are fairly clear. The cults themselves tend to support a curious kind of asexuality, so that romantic fraternization between the sexes is frowned upon (Enroth 1977). The age and marital status of the members certainly discourage the raising of children. Furthermore, in spite of all the rhetoric generated by parents confused and upset by their adolescent's leaving the family and its traditions to join a cult, most members remain in cults for less than two years (Schwartz and Kasiow 1979; Levine 1979). For the more occasional longstanding members who have married and have children while within the cult, the children are raised by their parents but are subject to the dictates of the religious leaders. For example, the children whose parents are Hare

Krishna followers attend schools that indoctrinate them while they are very young into the beliefs and dogma of that sect. They are taught and required to participate in the unique rituals—early-morning wakening, diet, showers, prayers, and so forth—from an extremely early age (Stoner and Parke 1977).

Whether this augurs well or poorly for their development and future adjustment is not known. Children of longstanding quasi-communal religious groups, such as Hutterites and Mennonites, grow up indoctrinated with the specific beliefs and values of the sect, but show no evidence of significant emotional damages. It would be fascinating to compare the children of parents who have spent their entire lives as members of such a sect with those of parents who, in late adolescence or youth, turned away from their families and their families' traditional religious identifications to enter a cult. Any attempt to draw comparisons or to make predictions on the evidence currently available would be mere conjecture. At this time, in the absence of long-term studies, there is no firm data of the effect on children of their parents' cult membership.

We do know, however, that many predominantly middle-class adolescents and young adults join cults. For those who do, the cult may serve as a substitute family, replacing the biological family from which they have become estranged. Often cult members give up family, friends, school, and other directions that they seemed to be pursuing until the cult made its appearance. They join because of feelings of alienation, demoralization, and low self-esteem, feelings they largely, though temporarily, overcome by immersing themselves in a powerful belief system and an intense group experience (S. V. Levine 1979; S. V. Levine and Salter 1976). Time spent within the cult seems to have a narrowing effect, as in a psychosocial moratorium, instead of being growth enhancing (S. V. Levine 1978). However, when members leave the cult, they tend to pick up many of their previous pursuits (S. V. Levine 1979). Some research data support the conclusion that young people who join cults are not a particularly disturbed group and that their families are no more dissonant or problematic than those in the general population (S. V. Levine 1978; S. V. Levine and Salter 1976). Many families are thrown into crisis by their son or daughter's joining a cult, and their coping resources are severely tested (Conway and Seigelman 1978; Schwartz and Kasiow 1979).

Day Care

One of the major influences on the structure of the young family in recent years has been the burgeoning of the day care movement in North America. Partly due to economic necessity and partly due to the increasing number of middle-class mothers wishing to pursue careers outside the home, more and more young children are being placed in a variety of day care services.

Family day care, also called home day care, is a service run by a private family in its own home. The vast majority of home day care services are unlicensed, unsupervised, and often "under the table" operations of variable quality. Some are clearly satisfactory and some even excellent, but in others the quality of care provided ranges from barely acceptable to grossly inadequate because of poor or overcrowded facilities, the personal qualities or inexperience of the caregivers, and the unavailability of an adequate support system with professional backup when needed (Johnson 1978). In 1980, 10 percent of the licensed available spaces in Canada were in government-supervised home care facilities.* Of the children in supervised family day care, 31 percent were infants under two years, compared to only 5 percent of the population of group day care centers (Ministry of National Health and Welfare 1980). Many authorities as well as many parents in both the United States and Canada consider family day care the preferable form of infant care (Johnson and Denine 1981; Young et al. 1973). It is certainly the less expensive form, although many agree that the cost would be comparable to community care were there an adequate support system in place and reasonable pay for the caregivers.

Some community day care is cooperative, that is, run largely by the involved parents (usually mothers). Other centers have sophisticated programs, run mainly by a professional or trained staff. Still others are operated in a family home by an untrained but usually well-motivated mother who is in the same position as those women whose children she cares for. Within each of these categories, a broad range in the quality of day care exists, ranging all the way from superb substitute parenting to day care that is inadequately staffed, overcrowded, and, in essence, exploitative of desperate parents and potentially damaging to their children.

The effects of long-term day care on children placed in it from an early age are not yet known. Evidence now available suggests that day care neither assists nor impairs intellectual development (Belsky and Steinberg 1979), except for children from socially disadvantaged families, who show less than the usual decline in IQ after eighteen months of age when exposed to day care (Caldwell 1972; Golden et al. 1978; Ramey and Smith 1977). There are no data on how generalizable to real-life functioning any such relative gains are, or even whether they persist through the school years. As to effects on emotional development, the bulk of the evidence suggests that the child's attachment to the mother is not disrupted, even when day care is begun during the first year of life (Belsky and Steinberg 1979; Clifford 1973). Several studies suggest that the mother remains the

*Of the more than five million children in home day care in the United States, 94 percent were in totally unregulated, unsupervised situation (Devine-Hawkins, 1981).

110

preferred adult over the day caregiver (Farran and Ramey 1977; Kagan, Kearsley, and Zelazo 1978; Riciuti 1974). With the exception of a single study (Blehar 1974) whose findings have not been replicated by other more rigorously controlled ones, the bulk of the evidence suggests that given excellent day care, significant disruption of the parent-child bond is unlikely. The National Day Care Study (*Children at the Center* 1979) has demonstrated that in small groups, especially if supervised by trained personnel, there is less hostility and conflict, less aimless wandering and apathy, and more involvement and warmth between caregivers and children. Except in the case of day care for infants or toddlers, the staff–child ratio seems to have a less important effect on the quality of the experience than the total size of the group or the training of the supervisors. In the area of social development, day care children interact with peers more, both positively and negatively, than home-reared children. Some early evidence suggests, however, that long-term involvement in day care is associated with increased apprehension and decreased cooperation with adults, as well as with decreased educational involvement after school entry (Belsky and Steinberg 1979). In summary, much of the data quoted above is suggestive, and while one cannot yet predict with certainty the results of a long-term day care experience, it is probably appropriate to endorse Belsky and Steinberg's conclusion that the effects of day care are mediated by children's experiences at home, so that when day care supports good parenting it is beneficial, while when it encourages the parents to abandon their parenting responsibilities or when it attempts to compensate for what a child is not receiving from disinterested, rejecting, or overwhelmed parents, the net effect is probably detrimental.

Low-cost, readily available day care is being seen more and more as a right rather than a privilege. Leaving aside the philosophical question of whether this is desirable, mounting economic pressures will result in an increasing number of children being placed in day care in the coming decades. Some day care centers will operate where the parents work or study, in order to encourage easier access. There is evidence from other countries that absence of the child from the family need not be deleterious in any way, if the agency or center is regularly able to meet the child's developmental needs and if the parents made up for a reduced amount of time spent with the child by a high-quality, mutually rewarding relationship when they are together (Belsky and Steinberg 1979). If these ideal "ifs" cannot be approached, inadequate day care, through its chronic failure to meet the developmental needs of those children entrusted to it, is likely to predispose vulnerable children to such long-term ill effects as inability to trust adults, social insecurity, poor object relations, and frank psychopathology. It is incumbent, therefore, upon North American communities to define and legislate stringent criteria for quality day care and to see that these are properly enforced as an important step in prevention of emotional disorders. (See chapter 27.)

Variations on a Theme

In addition to young people who come from families with the alternate living styles already discussed, there are others who come from yet different circumstances. For example, one child might be living with two divorced mothers who have moved in together to share expenses and child rearing. Another might be raised by a homosexual couple, male or female. A third might be living with his father as the "househusband." These and other variations are seen from time to time in most western cities. Furthermore, some of these changes are sequential. For example, a child may have lived in a traditional nuclear family for some years, then in a commune, and finally with a single parent. He or she will obviously be the product of all these major influences as well as others: constitution, personality, peer influence.

As long as certain basics of child rearing are supplied, it can be assumed that most children will demonstrate remarkable resilience and resourcefulness while continuing to proceed toward the increased social competence and capacity for mastering tasks of greater complexity that represent the long-term goals of successful development.

Thomas, in a recent review (1981) of current trends in developmental theory, has stressed that adaptive functioning and optimal development are more likely to occur (Thomas, 1981) when there is consonance—a "good fit"—between the properties, demands, and expectations of the child-caring environment and the child's own capacities, motivations, and styles of behaving. Similarly, dissonance—a "poor fit"—between the child's needs and capacities and the qualities, demands, and expectations of the environment is likely to produce excessive (i.e., intolerable) stress that, in turn, predisposes to disturbances of behavioral functioning and developmental blocks or distortions. These in turn aggravate the dissonance, further undermining the likelihood of a supportive and helpful environmental response. Thus it is not just the parenting capacity of the biological parents but the capacity of the child's total environment to perceive accurately and respond appropriately to that child's basic developmental needs that will favor optimal continuing developmental progress. The necessary combination of love, attention, stimulation, teaching, expectations, stability, consistency, and limits may be supplied by parents, parental surrogates, or other suitable environments. Parents or surrogates who are themselves conflicted, neurotic, rejecting, insensitive, and psychologically or socially overburdened will not be able to meet these needs consistently, either in an intact nuclear family, a single-parent family, or any of the alternatives cited earlier. What matters most is the capacity of the environment to meet the child's needs on a continuing basis. This, rather than who meets them or the domestic alignment of the key adults in the child's life, will determine whether or not the child achieves his or her genetically determined potential.

SUGGESTIONS FOR FURTHER READING

BELSKY, J., AND STEINBERG, L. D., 1919. What does research teach us about day care: A follow-up report. *Children Today* 8(4):21–26.
The effect of day care on the intellectual, emotional, and social development of children ranges from neutral to positive. Children's experience improves with a decrease in group size. This is a summary of the 1976 report by Bronfenbrenner et al. to the Department of Health, Education, and Welfare.
EIDUSON, B. T., AND ALEXANDER, J. W. 1978. The role of children in alternative family styles. In *J. Soc. Iss.* ed. N. Feschbach and S. Feschbach, 34:147–167.
An examination of parents and children in alternative family styles points to changing attitudes toward achievement, future planning, and authority. These changes have implications for child-rearing practices.
EDUSON, B. T.; COHEN, J.; AND ALEXANDER, J. 1973. Alternatives in child rearing. *Am. J. Orthopsychiat.* 43:720–731.
A comparison of the child-rearing practices of counterculture groups with those of two-parent nuclear families. The effect of multiple caretaking and antisexist attitudes on the psychological growth of the child is discussed.
FARRAN, D., AND RAMEY, C. 1977. Infant day care and attachment behaviour towards mothers and teachers. *Child Dev.* 48(3):1112.
The growing trend toward placing infants in group day care at very early ages may have serious effects on the development of the mother-child attachment bond.
HEPWORTH, H. P. 1980 *Foster care and adoption in Canada.* Ottawa: Canadian Council on Social Development.
A comprehensive nationwide overview of Canadian child welfare services, studying long-term trends in their development from 1959 to 1979.
KINARD, E. M., AND KLERMAN, L. V. 1980. Teenage parenting and child abuse: Are they related? *Am. J. Orthopsychiat.* 50(3):481–488.
The methodological difficulties of examining this relationship are described. The hypothesized association may be compounded by the association of each variable with social class.
LEVINE, S. V. 1979. The role of psychiatry in the phenomenon of cults. *Can. J. Psychiat.* 24:593–603.
A variety of theoretical and practical issues, both clinical and social, are derived from the author's extensive work with cult members and their parents.
MCANARNEY, E. R. 1978. Adolescent pregnancy: A national priority. *Amer. J. Dis. Child.* 132(2):125–126.
A brief report on the scope and severity of a problem that urgently needs to be addressed by government. Prevention of adolescent pregnancy is stressed as a priority. Areas needing research are discussed.
REISS, I. L. 1980. *Family systems in America.* 3rd ed. New York: Holt, Reinhart and Winston.
An attempt to understand the trends in family styles and the social factors shaping them. This revision takes advantage of major advances in research and available data of the last five years.
RUTTER, M. 1979. Maternal deprivation, 1972–1978: New findings, new concepts, new approaches. *Child Dev.* 50(2):283–305.

A critical review of new findings in such topics as the bonding process, critical periods of development, links between childhood experience and parenting behavior, and children's resilience in the face of deprivation.

Schwartz, L. L., and Kaslow, F. W. 1979. Religious cults, the individual and the family. *J. Mar. & Fam. Therap.* April:15–26.

A description of the recruitment and conversion techniques of cults, the kinds of youths vulnerable to them, the dynamics of the recruit's family, and the most effective modes of therapeutic intervention.

PART II

Classification and Assessment in Child Psychiatry

6

D. R. Offord

Classification and Epidemiology in Child Psychiatry: Status and Unresolved Problems

Classification

An adequate classification system in child psychiatry would serve clinical, research, and administrative and planning purposes. The psychiatrist would have a shorthand way of communicating with other psychiatrists about patients. Ideally when a psychiatrist carefully and accurately classified a patient in a particular category, that classification would dictate the most effective type of treatment for that patient. In the research area, a well-developed classification system would enable investigators to compare results on, for instance, etiologic factors or treatment outcomes on groups of patients who have been defined in the same way. Last, in the administration and planning area, an appropriate classification system would make it possible to collect meaningful statistics on the types of patients seen in clinical settings and to match resource allocations to the frequency and distribution of particular types of disorders in the child population. Thus an adequate classification system is a prerequisite for advancement in almost all facets of child psychiatry.

117

The criteria for an acceptable classification system have been outlined by Rutter (1977*b*). They include the requirements that the classification system must: (1) be based on facts, not concepts; (2) provide adequate coverage of patients seen in clinical settings; (3) enable mental health professionals to differentiate adequately between various disorders; (4) be reliable (precise) due to the fact that two psychiatrists must be able to show a high level of agreement on a patient's diagnosis, given the same data on which to base their diagnosis. The system also must: (5) be valid (accurate). The most important aspect of validity is that the categories in the diagnostic system must differ in predictable ways on some variable or variables other than the symptoms that define them (Rutter 1978). These variables could include ones associated with etiology, course, response to treatment, or some other aspect of the disorder. Finally, the system must: (6) be seen by psychiatrists as being both manageable and useful.

Until recently there was widespread dissatisfaction with the two major classification systems in use, the *Diagnostic and Statistical Manual of Mental Disorders, Second Edition,* (DSM-II) (American Psychiatric Association 1968) and the *International Statistical Classification of Diseases, Injuries and Causes of Death (Eighth Revision)* (ICD-8) (World Health Organization 1965), primarily because the disorders were not defined with sufficient precision and the categories were too broad.

In the mid-1960s, dissatisfaction with these two systems resulted in a third classification introduced by the Group for the Advancement of Psychiatry (1966). This new system divided childhood psychopathological disorders into ten major categories with multiple subcategories. While somewhat more precise than the other two systems, its categories remained broadly defined and no attempt was made to operationalize them.

In addition to these clinically derived categorization efforts, empirically derived systems have been developed that use multivariate statistical techniques such as factor and cluster analyses to identify syndromes (Achenback 1980; Achenbach and Edelbrock 1978). Achenbach (1980) notes that most child psychiatric disorders have not received widely accepted operational definitions, due partly to limited knowledge but also because many of them lack the sufficiently cohesive symptom picture needed to define with precision discrete clinical entities. This approach sees child psychiatric disorders as lying at the extreme ends of a behavioral continuum, rather than consisting of clearly circumscribed clinical disorders that a child either has or does not have. Achenbach suggests that at this stage a classification system should include both clinically and statistically defined syndromes or clusters. Then the degree of overlap among syndromes or categories derived by both approaches could be determined, depending on the acceptability of syndromes as already defined above, in order to work toward deciding which syndromes merit inclusion in a further classification system.

More recently, two new classifications have been introduced. *The Diag-*

nostic and Statistical Manual of Mental Disorders (Third Edition) (DSM-III) has been launched by the American Psychiatric Association (1980), while the *International Statistical Classification of Diseases, Injuries and Causes of Death (Ninth Revision)* (ICD-9) an international classification of disease, is endorsed by the World Health Organization (1979). Containing a new diagnostic system for mental disorders for children and adults, ICD-9 is an outgrowth of seminars and task forces extending back into the mid-1960s (Rutter et al. 1969; Rutter, Shaffer, and Shepherd al, 1975; Tarjan et al. 1972).

A COMPARISON OF DSM-III AND ICD-9

A comparison of the two systems in the area of childhood and adolescent psychiatric disorders brings to light both important similarities and differences.

Both systems attempt to be more precise in the description of each diagnostic entity. DSM-III has taken this a step further by employing precise operational diagnostic criteria with specific inclusion and exclusion criteria for each entity.

Both systems employ a multiaxial classification. Each disorder is classified along several independent dimensions, but as table 6.1 illustrates, the axes used in the two systems are not identical. In both DSM-III and ICD-9 Axis I refers to clinical psychiatric syndromes. Axis II in both systems includes specific delays in development in areas such as learning and language, but in DSM-III Axis II also includes personality disorders, a diagnosis rarely used in childhood. In ICD-9 personality disorders are covered under Axis 1. Axis III in DSM-III is identical to Axis IV in ICD-9 as both refer to coexisting medical or physical disorders. Mental retardation is covered under different axes in the two systems—Axis 1 in DSM-III and on its own separate axis, III, in ICD-9. Axes IV and V differ in the two

TABLE 6.1

Axes Used in the Diagnoses of Psychiatric Disorders in Children and Adolescence

Axes	DSM-III	ICD-9
I.	Clinical Syndromes	Clinical Psychiatric Syndromes
II.	Personality Disorders and Specific Developmental Disorders	Specific Delays in Development
III.	Physical Disorders and Conditions	Intellectual Level
IV.	Severity of Psychosocial Stressors	Medical Conditions
V.	Highest Level of Adaptive Functioning in Past Year	Abnormal Psychosocial Situations

schemes. In DSM-III they refer respectively to severity of psychosocial stressors and highest level of adaptive functioning in the past year, while in ICD-9 Axis IV refers to coexisting medical conditions and Axis V to abnormal psychosocial situations.

The number of separately named child and adolescent psychiatric disorders has increased significantly in both DSM-III and ICD-9 compared to their predecessors. This proliferation of disorders is particularly marked in DSM-III; there has been criticism that the number of disorders listed is excessive in relation to our knowledge of validated child psychiatric syndromes (Rutter and Shaffer 1980).

Field studies have been carried out to discover the strengths and problem areas of both systems and to establish the reproducibility of the disorders primarily through obtaining estimates of interrater reliability. Little or no work has been done on test-retest reliability. These studies on ICD-9 (Rutter, Shaffer, and Shepherd 1975) and DSM-III (Cantwell et al. 1979*a,* 1979*b;* Mattison et al. 1979; Russell et al. 1979) report remarkably similar results (Rutter and Shaffer 1980). The better coverage of disorders in childhood and adolescence and the multiaxial approach in both systems have met with approval and were seen as advances over the previous systems. Interrater reliability was good for the broad groupings of syndromes but poor for finer subdivisions and in complex cases. For instance, the average interrater agreement for Axis I on DSM-III was 54 percent but dropped as low as 20 percent for complex cases (Mattison et al. 1979). It should be noted that these percentages are inflated because of agreements due to chance. Psychometric studies of DSM-II and ICD-8 were not carried out when those classifications were introduced. However, Freeman (1971) did carry out a reliability study on the GAP classification scheme.

While DSM-III and ICD-9 are separate classification systems, DSM-III has been designed and the coding categories organized in such a way that in most cases a diagnosis in one system can be made comparable to a diagnostic category in the other system.

DSM-III

Since DSM-III is the classification system most widely used in North America, a summary of it will be given. Table 6.2 provides an outline of the disorders usually first evident in infancy, childhood, or adolescence. These are covered on Axis I. Within these broad categories, the disorders themselves have many subdivisions. These have been described in detail in the DSM-III (American Psychiatric Association 1980) and have also been summarized by Spitzer and Cantwell (1980).

Table 6.3 outlines the disorders usually first evident in infancy, childhood, or adolescence that are covered under Axis II in DSM-III. "Specific developmental disorders" refer to delays in circumscribed areas of devel-

TABLE 6.2

Disorders Usually First Evident in Infance, Childhood, or Adolescence (Covered on Axis I in DSM-III)

1. Intellectual:
    Mental Retardation

2. Behavioral (Overt):
    Attention Deficit Disorder
    Conduct Disorder

3. Emotional:
    Anxiety Disorders of Childhood or Adolescence
    Other Disorders of Infancy, Childhood, or Adolescence

4. Physical:
    Eating Disorders
    Stereotyped Movement Disorders, Including Involuntory Motor Movements (Tics)
    Other Disorders with Physical Manifestations.

5. Pervasive Developmental Disorders

opment that are not due to some other disorder. Examples include delays in reading or arithmetic.

In diagnosing psychiatric disorders in children and adolescents using DSM-III, clinicians and researchers are not limited to the disorders described for Axes I and II. Many disorders from the adult section of the classification, such as affective disorder and schizophrenia, are often appropriate for children and adolescents.

Axis III, "physical disorders and conditions," allows the psychiatrist to identify any current physical disorder or condition that has potential relevance to the understanding or management of the patient. Axis IV, "severity of psychosocial stressors," is scored on a seven-point scale. Examples for children and adolescents of the different points on the scale are provided in DSM-III (American Psychiatric Association 1980, p. 27). Similarly, Axis V, "highest level of adaptive functioning in the past year," is scored on a nominal five-point scale; examples of applying the scale are available in DSM-III (American Psychiatric Association 1980, p. 29).

Various chapters in this book provide further details of the subcategories in DSM-III and the major classes and subclasses of disorders.

TABLE 6.3

Disorders Usually First Evident in Infancy, Childhood, or Adolescence
(on Axis II in DSM III)

Developmental

Specific Developmental Disorders

121

FUTURE DIRECTIONS

The development of a satisfactory classification system for the psychiatric disorders of childhood and adolescence is an ongoing process. As more information becomes available about etiology, course, and response to treatment of various disorders, this will provide the basis for a more valid categorization of childhood disorders. Conversely, it is hoped that DSM-III and ICD-9 will stimulate further work on etiology, response to treatment, and so forth, of children with different disorders. Immediately needed are further studies of the reproducibility—that is, interrater and test-retest reliability—of the different diagnostic categories. Acceptable levels of reproducibility for a particular category must be established before the validity of that category can be studied—that is, before the ways in which that category differs from others in terms of etiology, course, response to treatment, or other variables can be determined (Rutter 1978).

The degree to which reliability and validity can be established for different proposed categories, whether they originate from empirical work, DSM-III, ICD-9, or some other diagnostic scheme, will determine whether particular categories should be preserved in a classification system or dropped from it.

Epidemiology

Child psychiatric epidemiology is concerned with the distribution in a population of the psychiatric disorders of children. Information derived from studies in this area has two major uses: scientific and administrative.

Scientific uses of epidemiological data center on discovering the causes of these disorders. The data can identify what factors in the environment are associated with the presence of a condition. From this information causal chains leading to disorders can be hypothesized, and the accuracy of these chains can be tested by mounting and rigorously evaluating intervention programs aimed at breaking the chains at some point. Undertakings of this type have been termed experimental epidemiology (Robins 1978).

An administrator of a child mental health facility can use epidemiological data to allocate more rationally scarce child psychiatric diagnostic and treatment services. Geographic areas that are relatively over- or underserviced can be readily identified. In addition, if a relationship can be demonstrated between demographic characteristics and the distribution of child psychiatric morbidity and if accurate predictions of population trends are available, this will allow more effective planning for future child mental health needs.

PREVALENCE OF CHILDHOOD PSYCHIATRIC DISORDERS

Our knowledge about the occurrence of child psychiatric disorders in a population has been based almost exclusively on prevalence studies. These studies provide data on the number of cases existing in a population at a given moment or period of time. Studies aimed at the determination of incidence—that is, the number of new cases defined in a population over a given interval of time—are almost nonexistent in child psychiatry because of the difficulty in ascertaining precisely the onset and duration of childhood disorders (Earls 1980*a*).

The determination of the prevalence of childhood psychiatric disorders has been hampered by a number of problems, some of which have been highlighted in the section on classification. They include difficulties with definition of disorder, instrumentation, sampling, source of information, ages examined, and location of studies.

The definition of disorder in child community surveys has been approached in four ways (Links 1982). Some studies have arbitrarily chosen individual behaviors as signifying deviance. Others have used symptom loading, that is, a score of equally weighted symptoms, as indicating psychiatric disturbance. Still other investigators have employed statistical means to denote deviance, deciding, for example, that any behaviors that occur in fewer than 10 percent of the children studied would be considered deviant. Last, a few investigators have employed a clinical assessment of parent or child interview data in order to arrive at what would be considered to be abnormal. Obviously each of these methods of defining disorder can be expected to lead to different prevalence rates.

The development of suitable instruments for community surveys has been difficult, time consuming, and expensive. In addition, unfortunately most investigators have attempted to develop their own instruments, which has made the comparison of results across studies impossible. The instruments can be divided into direct and indirect measures. Direct measures obtain data from the children themselves, as by established achievement tests or child questionnaires. Indirect measures collect data from important people in the children's life such as parents or teachers. The psychometric properties of the various instruments, including measures of reliability and validity, have not always been established. The validity of the instruments has been tested in one of several ways—through their ability to discriminate children in the general population from those seen in child mental health centers; their capacity to replicate the results of direct clinical assessments; their success in matching an indirect clinical appraisal based on data from parents, teachers, or the children themselves;

and last, the strength of their association with other instruments in the field. All of these procedures to establish validity have certain weaknesses (Earls 1980; Links 1982).

Most instruments have not gathered data on specific disorders but have obtained information that provides an estimate of general childhood maladjustment or, at best, of childhood disorders characterized by aggressive or rule-breaking symptoms such as fighting or stealing (conduct disorder) and those identified by nonaggressive internalized symptoms such as worry and anxiety (emotional disorder) (Rutter, Tizard, and Whitmore 1970).

An accurate estimate of prevalence of a disorder in a population requires that a representative and sufficiently large sample be examined. Community child psychiatric studies have not met these criteria. Little attention has been paid to calculating the appropriate nature and size of the sample needed to make prevalence estimates of a certain precision. In several studies, for example, the sample frame has been public school listings, which, of course, exclude from the sample those children attending private schools and those in institutional settings (Links 1982).

The estimates of prevalence of child maladjustment vary depending on the sources of data used. In a major child epidemiological study using both parent and teacher data, Rutter, Tizard, and Whitmore (1970) observed that for each data source, 50 percent of the children identified as being deviant on screening procedures were eventually designated as having psychiatric disorder. However, these two sources, parents and teachers, identified the same children as being maladjusted in only 7 percent of the cases (Gould, Wunsch-Hitzig, and Dohrenwend 1981). It is not known which source of data or which combination of sources is most valid in identifying disturbed children, but it is clear that studies that use only one data source will almost certainly underestimate the actual prevalence of childhood psychiatric disorders.

Most studies have focused on a particular age group. As a result, we do not know much about the distribution of maladjustment over the age span of childhood and adolescence.

Last, because many of the best surveys have been done in unique settings—for example, the Isle of Wight, (Rutter, Tizard and Whitmore 1970), Martha's Vineyard (Earls 1980*b*), and Kauai, Hawaii (Werner and Smith 1979)—the opportunity to generalize results has been greatly reduced (Links 1982). Given all these problems and limitations, Gould, Wunsch-Hitzig, and Dohrenwend (1981) concluded in a critical review of twenty-five United States prevalence studies of childhood disorders that the prevalence of clinical maladjustment of American children was probably no lower than 11.8 percent.

THE RELATIONSHIP BETWEEN CHILDHOOD DISORDERS
AND UTILIZATION OF SERVICES

Two studies, one in the United States and one in Britain, address the problems of the adequacy of the delivery of child mental health services (Langner et al. 1970; Rutter, Tizard, and Whitmore 1970). Langner's study, carried out in New York City, reported that less than half the children with marked or severe impairment from middle- or upper-class families had had any therapeutic contacts. In low-income families, this proportion dropped to about one third. If a more meaningful measure of a therapeutic contact was employed—that is, a contact of two months or longer—the proportion dropped to one third and one quarter respectively. In their study of ten- and eleven-year-old children on the Isle of Wight, a semirural setting off the coast of England, Michael Rutter and his colleagues found that nine out of ten children with psychiatric disorder had not been expertly diagnosed or assessed, let alone treated. In both the Isle of Wight and New York studies, the better educated sections of the community made better use of services than the poorer sections, which, as will be discussed, needed them the most.

There is no reason to believe that the findings of these two studies do not apply more widely. They bring into focus a major problem in the delivery of child psychiatric services: the services reach only a minority of children who need them, and those who receive services are not necessarily the ones with the most serious psychiatric illness.

CORRELATES OF DISORDERS

In the literature, several factors associated with the occurrence of child psychiatric disorders have been termed correlates or risk factors of disorders. Again, the correlates are usually to child maladjustment in general rather than to specific diagnostic entities. Some of the factors are peculiar to the children themselves and others to their environment.

Sex

Most studies report higher rates of maladjustment for boys than girls (Links 1982). This difference was found in twenty-two of the twenty-five community studies that published rates according to sex (Gould, Wunsch-Hitzig, and Dohrenwend 1981). The sex ratio varies by general type of disorder. Conduct disorders are two to three times more common in boys than in girls. On the other hand, emotional disorders occur equally in the two sexes. During adolescence and thereafter the rate for emotional disorder is greater for females.

Age

The limited available evidence indicates a slight rise in the rate of psychiatric disorder between late childhood (9–12) and early adolescence (13–16) (Rutter et al. 1976). In addition, depression and school refusal are much more common in adolescence. These same data point out that some disorders are more persistent than others. For instance, three quarters of the children with conduct disorder at age ten still had a psychiatric disorder at fourteen. This was a significantly worse outcome than that demonstrated in children with an emotional disorder at age ten.

Other Correlates

A number of other factors originating in the child have been demonstrated to place children at increased risk either for psychiatric disturbance in general or for the development of a particular disorder. For example, children with mental retardation or brain damage are at significantly increased risk for psychiatric disturbance in general (Rutter, 1977a; Rutter, Tizard, and Whitmore 1970). On the other hand, reading disorder (where the child's reading level is significantly below his or her IQ score) places a child at increased risk for conduct disorder but not for emotional disorder (Rutter, Tizard, and Whitmore 1970).

In addition to these child-related factors, factors within the environment also put some children at risk for psychiatric disorder.

Social Class

Michael Rutter and his colleagues (1975) used similar techniques to establish prevalence rates of childhood psychiatric disorders in a middle-class area, the Isle of Wight, and a poor inner-London borough. Both conduct and emotional disorders were found to be twice as common in the poor areas. The greatest difference between poor and middle-class populations appears to be the excess in the former of childhood problems beginning in the early school years and running a chronic course (Rutter 1981). Only a small difference in the rate of disorders arising for the first time in adolescence was found. Other findings support the idea that within a population, the rates of disorder increase as one descends the social class ladder (Langner et al., 1970; Rutter, Tizard, and Whitmore 1970). For example, Langner and his group reported that in their New York City study, the percentages of children with impairment from high-, middle-, and low-income groups were eight, twelve, and twenty-one respectively. The evidence, as far as we have it, consistently suggests a strong link between low social class and increased prevalence rates of childhood psychiatric disorder.

Family Factors

Several family factors are strongly associated with children with conduct disorder. They include broken homes, marital discord, parental deviance (including psychiatric illness and criminality), and large number of siblings (Offord and Waters 1983). While parental deviance, especially recurring psychiatric illness, is a risk factor for childhood psychiatric disturbance in general, broken homes, marital discord, and large number of siblings are correlates of conduct disorder but not emotional disorder (Rutter 1978; Offord and Waters 1982).

Many of the same methodological problems that plague the definition of child psychiatric disorders also hinder work in the correlate area. The definitions of the correlates must lead to reproducible measures, and, of course, any success in learning the extent to which these risk factors are associated with specific psychiatric disorders depends on the degree to which these disorders can be defined satisfactorily. Although a number of risk factors have been identified, it is not yet clear precisely how they interact with each other and the degree to which individual, family, and demographic correlates operate independently or produce their effect through interaction with other variables. In addition, we know little about the variables that intervene between the occurrence of risk factors and the increased prevalence of disorder (Offord and Waters 1982). Such data are urgently needed if information about risk factors is to be converted into a form that can aid prevention and treatment endeavors.

School Influences

Recent work (Rutter 1980) has confirmed earlier studies that found marked differences in both academic achievement and rate of psychiatric disturbance in children attending different schools. However, this latest study has ruled out more convincingly than before the possibility that the differences in pupil outcome in various schools could be accounted for by the characteristics pupils possessed before they entered these schools. In Rutter's study, the children had been tested extensively at age ten, before beginning secondary school. The results found during their secondary school careers could not be explained by the pupils' academic or behavioral characteristics on entering high school. Two points should be emphasized about Rutter's work. In his study, the differences between the worst and best schools in academic and behavioral indices were marked. And it was not one or two isolated factors but many acting together that appeared to contribute to this difference. These factors, discussed in more detail in chapter 27, make it clear that schools can be an effective, health-producing factor in a child's life. What is not yet known is how to change a "bad" school into a "good" one.

A detailed review of the evidence regarding the relationship between these and other risk factors specific to each child psychiatric disorder is covered in the chapters describing that condition.

FORMATION OF CAUSAL CHAINS

Knowledge of the existence of possible causal chains can provide direction to and a rationale for intervention programs aimed at the prevention of particular psychiatric disorders. Figure 6.1 provides an outline of one such possible causal chain. The evidence for the validity of this chain is mixed (Offord 1982), but the chain may account for a significant proportion of antisocial behavior.

(a) Learning Disorders ⟶ (b) School Failure ⟶ (c) Low Self-Esteem ⟶ (d) Antisocial Behavior

Figure 6.1 Possible Causal Chain

As can be seen from the figure, breaking the chain at any of the points (a), (b), (c), or (d) could be expected to reduce the incidence of antisocial behavior. The limited data available in the literature support the hypothesis that the major childhood psychiatric disorders to some extent share common causal chains; therefore, breaking one causal chain may have widespread payoff in reducing the incidence of several types of childhood morbidity (Robins 1979). More work in this area needs to be done.

FUTURE DIRECTIONS

Child psychiatric epidemiology is in its formative stages, and many lines of investigation merit pursuit. Community surveys are needed in which the discrete disorders and the potential correlates are defined reliably, where adequate sampling procedures are carried out, and where the population studied covers a wide age span.

Data from such surveys can form the basis for further work. For example, prospective studies could be launched to determine the natural history of individual symptoms or disorders. This lack of detailed natural history studies makes it impossible to distinguish symptoms that are ominous from those that are transient (Robins 1974). In addition, studying the natural history of conditions would enable mental health professionals to determine those factors that can be used to predict the duration of a disorder. Up to now workers have spent most of their energy determining the predictors of the occurrence of the disorder rather than the predictors of its duration. The latter data are needed particularly to plan treatment more effectively (Robins 1979). Further, as information accumulates about causal chains, it can provide a background against which true experiments can be carried out and innovative prevention or treatment programs rigorously evaluated.

Finally, it is important to note that a sizable proportion of children reared in families with many or all of the known correlates of psychiatric maladjustment remain free of disorders and develop and adjust well (Offord and Waters 1983). Further epidemiological work should focus on what factors protect these children and how these protective factors operate to support children's development and adjustment even in adverse circumstances (see Rutter 1979 and chapter 27 herein).

SUGGESTIONS FOR FURTHER READING

ACHENBACH, T. M., AND EDELBROCK, C. S. 1978. The classification of child psychopathology: A review and analysis of empirical efforts. *Psychol. Bull.* 6:1275–1301.
Reviews the rationale and efforts of the empirical approach to the classification of childhood psychiatric disorders.

EARLS, F. 1980. Epidemiologic methods for research in child psychiatry. In *Studies of children,* pp. 1–33. New York: Prodist.
Covers some basic points about epidemiology in general and summarizes the current state of child psychiatric epidemiology.

GOULD, M. S.; WINSCH-HITZIG, R.; AND DOHRENWEND, B. 1981. Estimating prevalence of childhood psychopathology: A critical review. *J. Amer. Acad. Child Psychiat.* 20:462–476.
Provides a critical review of the prevalence studies of childhood maladjustment carried out on U.S. populations.

LINKS, P. S. 1982. Community surveys of the prevalence of childhood psychiatric disorders: A review. *Child Dev.* in press.
Is a critical review of community surveys aimed at determining the prevalence of childhood emotional and behavioral disorders. Future directions of work in this field are outlined.

ROBINS, L. N. 1978. Psychiatric epidemiology. *Arch. Gen. Psychiat.* 35:697–702.
Outlines the current state of development, research issues, and future directions of psychiatric epidemiology.

———. 1979. Longitudinal methods in the study of normal and pathological development. In *Grundlagen und Methoden der Psychiatrie,* vol. 1, ed. K. P. Kisker et al., pp. 627–684. Heidelberg: Springer-Verlag.
Gives a thorough review of the issues in carrying out and evaluating longitudinal studies; an annotated bibliography of the major longitudinal studies of childhood psychopathology is provided.

RUTTER, M. 1977. Classification. In *Child psychiatry: Modern approaches,* ed. M. Rutter and L. Hersov, pp. 359–384. Oxford: Blackwell Scientific Publications.
Covers the basic requirements of a classification system for children's emotional and behavioral disorders.

RUTTER, M., AND SHAFFER, D. 1980. DSM-III: A step forward or back in terms of the classification of child psychiatric disorders? *J Amer. Acad. Child Psychiat.* 19:374-394.
Provides a critical review of the DSM-III classification of the psychiatric disorders of childhood and adolescence.

RUTTER, M., ET AL. 1976 Isle of Wight studies, 1964–1974. *Psychol. Med.* 6:313–32.
Provides a concise summary of the extensive child psychiatric epidemiologic investigations carried out by Michael Rutter and his colleagues in Great Britain.

SPITZER, R. L., AND CANTWELL, D. P. 1980. The DSM-III classification of the psychiatric disorders of infancy, childhood, and adolescence. *J. Amer. Acad. Child Psychiat.* 19:356-370.
Provides details about the DSM-III classification as it applies to the psychiatric disorders of childhood and adolescence.

7

Elsa A. Broder and Eric Hood

A Guide to the Assessment of Child and Family

A thorough assessment of the child and family forms the foundation on which adequate diagnosis and effective intervention are based. Without this foundation, therapy proceeds blindly. In this chapter the goals, techniques, and common problems of assessment are examined. An outline for organizing data collected in the course of an assessment is included along with a discussion of how to present findings to the family and aspects of report writing.

In assessment, there is a series of questions to be answered that define the problem and the ways it can be resolved. Keeping these in mind helps the process to become more goal-directed and in itself more therapeutic. How the examiner approaches the task can, for healthier families, provide a model that they can use to define and solve problems on their own. Thus, for some, assessment may also be treatment. The questions are:

1. What is the nature of the problem (diagnosis)?
2. Is it a problem that requires action?
3. What are the factors causing and maintaining the problem (formulation)?
4. What action, if any, is needed and by which members of the family system? (treatment plan)
5. Who can best carry out the treatment? Is referral necessary?
6. Will the family accept the treatment plan (contract)?

130

Children are individuals in their own right. They are also immature organisms dependent on parents and others. Hence it is essential to investigate not only the children but their ecology (Hobbs 1975). A complete assessment must include inquiry into the following areas:

1. The development of the individual child in comparison with norms of physical and emotional development.
2. The internal dynamics and personality of the child, including cognitive and emotional adequacy, conflicts, and ways of defending against anxiety.
3. The interactive aspects that include consideration of how the child fits into the family, how the child helps to maintain the family homeostasis (see chapter 3), and how the family fits into the larger society.
4. The development of the family as it faces, at different ages with changing capabilities, the different tasks that are required (Erikson 1963; McGoldrick and Carter 1982; Stierlin and Ravenscroft 1972).

Initial Anxieties

Parents often approach their child's psychiatric assessment feeling anxious, guilty, and afraid of being blamed and criticized. These fears are made worse by the common expectation that blame will be laid particularly on the mother. In addition, parents may be concerned that they did not seek help earlier, even though caregivers or physicians advised that the child would grow out of the problem in time. On the other hand, some parents approach assessment with relief that their concerns are respected, taken seriously, and will be fully investigated.

Sometimes evaluation has been obtained under pressure from outside agencies such as the school or the court. Parents' motivation to seek help and to participate enthusiastically is diminished by their resentment at this intrusion into personal lives. A child's difficulties and unhappiness are more likely to be expressed in behavior than in words, with disturbing behavior the most common presenting complaint. With the emphasis on bad behavior or poor achievement, the child is likely to feel criticized and belittled. It is no wonder that all may be concerned that the assessment will be a repetition of previous unhappy experiences.

The First Encounter

The first encounter, be it over the telephone or face to face, is very important for establishing rapport and setting expectations. Identifying data, including who makes up the family and introduction to the major parental concerns, can be obtained by telephone (Mackinnon and Michels 1970). Some examiners use a questionnaire and/or behavioral checklists, the purpose of which is explained to the family at this time. By supplying basic information, such forms allow a more economical use of interview time, requiring the examiner to spend less time in data collection and enabling him or her to focus more on the interaction between child and family. A number of questionnaires and checklists have been rigorously tested for reliability and validity (Quay 1977; Rutter and Graham 1968; Spivack and Swift 1977). Some are completed by the parents, others by schoolteachers or workers who have intimate contact with the child.* Having some data before the first appointment allows the examiner to anticipate the nature of the problem and, where indicated, to obtain written consents in order to collect reports from other agencies, therapists, or schools. In addition, it allows for thought about the problems, the development of initial hypotheses, and the planning of appropriate strategies for clarification and verification.

The clinician should determine in advance how the parents are planning to prepare the child and the family for the forthcoming interview. Many parents will need help to tell the child frankly why the assessment has been requested and what they hope to achieve through the assessment. It may be necessary to explain why it is important that the father and siblings be involved. Both parents and children should have a rough idea of what to expect. The appointment times, the duration of the interview, the number of possible contacts, and whom they will meet should all be mentioned in advance. Financial arrangements should also be made. If audiovisual recording or direct observation are planned the family should be advised and, for recording, give prior written consent.

Surroundings and Equipment

Although assessment can be carried out almost anywhere, some surroundings are more conducive to the task than others. Freedom from interuption is essential, as is sufficient time.

The interviewing room should be comfortable, quiet, and with a relaxed atmosphere, large enough to seat a whole family while allowing a child some freedom of movement. Furniture should be free of sharp pointed edges and easy to keep clean so that parents and examiner need not be concerned if children climb or make a mess.

*See Conners 1969; Rutter 1967; Sonis and Costello 1981; Spivack and Swift 1977; and Werry, Sprague, and Cohen 1975.

For examination of the child, fancy toys in great variety are not necessary. Relatively nonstructured materials that can serve as a stimulus for expression of fantasy are best. Basic equipment should include pencils, crayons, paper, several puppet families, plasticine, a ball, and a target game such as bean bags. It is useful to have graded books to test reading ability and mathematics. Little other equipment is needed to complete an adequate assessment unless a neurological or physical examination is indicated. Then standard medical equipment should suffice.

While it is most comfortable for clinicians to carry out interviews in their own familiar settings, it may be necessary to see children and families at home, in the offices of other agencies, within an institution, or at school. Assessment procedures may be adapted so that the necessary information can be gained. An on-site visit can reveal a great deal about the child or family, allowing for more spontaneous expression of feelings, behavior, and interaction. When the child has behavior problems in school, direct observation in the classroom, gymnasium, and schoolyard may be of great value, as may be direct discussion with the teacher.

Theoretical Perspective

Some authorities contend that an adequate assessment needs only to ascertain how children are currently functioning in the major areas of their lives, arguing that the here and now is what one uses in therapy and not the past.* Others belive that one cannot fully understand the immediate problems without knowing what has gone before.†

Theories of change can be grouped into those models based on insight, those based on concepts of learning, and those based on paradox (Feldman 1976; Schwitzgebel and Klob 1974; Watzlawick, Weakland, and Fisch 1974). An examiner working from an insight model will collect data about the past, centering on areas of conflict and defense mechanisms. At the other extreme, those using a paradox model will want to know the current operation of the system, the function of the symptomatology, and those mechanisms blocking information exchange. Our contention is that one must know about all—the factors leading to the development of the problem (predisposing and precipitating determinants) as well as those currently contributing to the difficulty (perpetuating determinants). Without information about all of these, the clinician lacks the understanding needed to devise a strategy for effective treatment (Broder 1975; Hood and Anglin 1979).

*See Haley 1978; Minuchin 1974; Palazzoli et al. 1978; Patterson 1977; and Stuart 1971.
†See Cohen 1979*b*; Freud 1962; Guerin 1976; McDonald 1965; and Rich 1968.

Structure of an Interview

Whether it is with an individual or family, every interview has a basic structure. In the *beginning* the clinician makes contact with the person or persons to be interviewed. The clinician identifies his or her professional background and establishes a cooperative working relationship. This is what Haley (1978) calls the social phase. During this time the tone and direction of the interview are established. Anxieties need to be calmed and people made comfortable enough so that they can take an accommodative and active role in the process.

In the *middle* phase the work of the interview is accomplished. Information needs to be collected from each person present about those factors that have contributed to the development and maintenance of problems. The examiner should be clear about the task, accomplishing this goal as efficiently as is possible, not digressing to pleasantries.

Finally there is the *ending* phase. This is the part of the interview most commonly ignored. It is important to draw the interview to a close, making sure that no participant is so troubled that he or she might act out feelings in an impulsive, destructive way. What has been covered should be summarized and plans regarding what will happen next made clear. The clinician should attempt to ensure that, however stormy the interview has been, people feel they have been treated respectfully, that their concerns have been given an adequate hearing, and that no one has been scapegoated, battered, or abused in the process.

All interviews, whether for assessment or treatment, should be planned and goal-directed. It is not helpful to allow people to ramble irrelevantly or to avoid coming to grips with issues because there might be discomfort. However, a light touch is required in exploring areas of weakness or difficulty to prevent having the family become unduly ashamed and defensive. It is important to avoid becoming entrapped in an alliance with one or the other parent or child. The clinician must try to see how ready the family is to consider alternative explanations for what has been happening and to make productive use of what is suggested. Parents must be helped to realize that their cooperation and involvement are essential if a solution is to be found.

Sources of Data

Within the assessment interview there are two main sources of data: the *content* (what people say) and the *process* (what people do). The *content* includes not only the information shared about the history, current problems, and events but also what is omitted or avoided. It includes the family's interpretation of what has been said or what has occurred. The *process* is the manner in which people behave, their ways of relating to one another, and the nonverbal metacommunications, or "communication about communication" (Watzlawick, Beavin, and Jackson 1967), about behavior.

Another source of information is the examiner's reactions to the family or child. These may be unrelated to the verbal content and may accurately reflect covert or nonverbal messages being passed to the examiner. However, at times they are part of the countertransference that is the professional's "partly unconscious or conscious emotional reactions to his patient" (American Psychiatric Association 1975, p. 38). Professionals cannot work equally well with all types of people and problems, but they should know themselves well to recognize personal sensitivities and prevent them from interfering.

Assessment Format

Various formats for conducting an assessment are possible. Each provides a particular type of information. The child identified as the patient can be seen alone, with the parents, or with the whole family, or any subgroups of its members can be interviewed.

A *family diagnostic interview* is considered by many to be a good way to start. Such an interview helps the examiner to understand the family environment and, by focusing on family interaction, may help to relieve tension and anxiety by making the child feel less singled out. It may also give children an opportunity to relax and feel out the examiner while still receiving the support of their parents. This can be helpful where there are difficulties around separation. Adolescents, in particular, respond well to this form of interviewing, seeing it as an opportunity not only to hear what is being said about them but also to define themselves and share information about other family members. Fisher (1976) has reviewed the many formats family diagnostic interviews can take.

Seeing the parents independently allows for exploration of material that they may be reluctant to discuss in front of their children, such as their sexual relationship, marital problems, differences of opinion, financial difficulties, thoughts of placement outside the family, and secrets such as adoption or common-law marriage. With very omnipotent children it may be therapeutic to begin to differentiate the members of the family by introducing hierarchy, supporting the parents as the most powerful (Kantor and Lehr 1975; Minuchin 1974; Westley and Epstein 1970).

In *interviewing children,* the younger they are the more likely the clinician will utilize play rather than talk as a vehicle for communication. In child interviews a variety of play materials are made available, and children are allowed some freedom to explore, play, and communicate spontaneously. Rapport is established, and what the children talk of, play with, and the way they relate to the interviewer are observed. Toys and drawings may be used to explore how the children feel about the problems that have led to the assessment and their roles and relationships within their family. Some examiners feel that a more valid and reliable examination is obtained by structuring the interaction. Others allow it to flow freely (Hodges et al. 1982; Rutter and Graham 1968).

Should novice examiners feel unsure of themselves and their skills at conducting an assessment of young children, a less active, observational stance will be helpful, allowing the children freedom to use the play materials and come to the therapist when ready. In contrast to examination of adults, much of the mental status examination of children can be performed through observation alone.

There is no single right way to conduct a play interview.* Those preferring to use a more structured format for at least part of the interview can employ a number of techniques to tap the child's inner thoughts and to elicit main areas of conflict.

FREE PLAY

In free play the child is allowed to move around the room exploring the play materials and activities of choice. How the child moves, physical development, fine and gross coordination, laterality, relation to examiner, and age appropriateness of activity can all be assessed.

DISCUSSION WITH CHILD

As the child plays or draws, the examiner can begin to explore the various areas of the child's life, beginning with more objective concrete questions about school, teacher, recreational activities, friends, and home life. Children may be surprisingly candid in telling what they do to annoy parents and teachers. As trust and cooperation are obtained, the more emotionally laden topics related to problems can be explored.

PROJECTIVE METHODS

Various projective methods may be used to explore the inner life of the child. These include:

*See Allen 1942; Chess and Hassibi 1978; Cohen 1979*b;* Gaensbauer and Harmon 1981; Goodman and Sours 1967; Lawrence 1976; Looff 1976; Pruyser 1979; Simmons 1974; Werkman 1965; and Winnicott 1971.

1. Puppet play.
2. Drawings and the stories the child tells about what has been drawn. Spontaneous drawings can come first, then the examiner may ask the child to draw the family doing something together. "Children may speak to us more clearly and openly through their drawings than they are willing or able to do verbally" (Di Leo 1977).
3. Three wishes, with a discussion of what the child would do with each wish if granted.

> Mr. and Mrs. A requested an assessment of their ten-year-old daughter, Joanne, to determine which of them should receive custody. When asked directly with whom she would rather live, Joanne refused to commit herself. Her three wishes, however, included a trip to England, one thousand dollars, and a new house. Asked what she would do with these, she said that she wanted the trip to have a holiday with her grandparents and the money to spend on the trip. When asked about the new house, she replied that she and her siblings would live there with their mother, far away so that her daddy would not be able to visit.

4. Animal questions, such as, If you were to turned into an animal, but could choose what kind of animal you would be, which would you choose, and why? Give three choices.
5. Squiggle game. In this game the children and the examiner alternately turn a meaningless set of lines, or "squiggles," into a picture and then tell a story (Winnicott 1971).
6. Desert island. The examiner asks something like: Of all the people in the world, which three would you choose to take to live on a desert island? A variation of this is which three people would be taken in a lifeboat.
7. Tree-house-person test. The child is given a blank piece of paper and told only to draw a house, tree, and person. Given good dexterity and cooperation, this test is thought to reveal something about how children view themselves (self-concept), their bodies, and their relationships with others (Buros 1972). Some examiners approach this more directly by asking children to draw a picture of themselves.

While all of these methods can help the examiner tap the inner life of the child, they also reveal other aspects of the child's functioning, such as thought processes, feelings about the family, fine motor coordination, laterality, and ability to concentrate. They also serve as a vehicle to open up communication, particularly with constricted youngsters.

Adolescents are usually able to verbalize in a way similar to adults. They may or may not be particularly cooperative, and initial surliness may be a cover for shyness, resentment at being assessed, fear that some grave secret will be revealed or that they may be found crazy. It takes time, patience, and skill to create an atmosphere sufficiently free and uncritical to allow a troubled adolescent to feel safe enough to confide about emotionally painful and conflicted areas (Golombek 1969; Holmes 1964; Meeks 1971; Oldham et al. 1980; see also chapter 2).

Sometimes questions arise as to the physical and neurological functioning of the child. For those who feel competent, a complete *physical and neurological examination* can be performed. This is better done at the end of the interview and with a parent present. If the examiner cannot perform the examination, appropriate referrals can be made to a pediatrician, neurologist, or family doctor. It is wise to explain to the parents and the child what procedures may be done and the rationale for requesting them.

PSYCHOLOGICAL TESTING

Psychological testing can be especially helpful if there are questions about the child's level of intelligence or the presence of specific learning disabilities, organically based dysfunction, thought disorder, or psychotic ideation.

Additional Technical Points

The immediate use of first names for either examiner or parents blurs roles, detracts from the professional nature of the relationship, and may be resented as an intrusion. The same applies to calling the parent "Mom" or "Dad." Requesting the use of first names may have a variety of meanings, including an unconscious resistance to the process—"Let's pretend that this is a social rather than a professional visit"—or an attempt to make the situation less frightening. Unless the meaning of the request is clear and the examiner is sure that the change will be salutary, the more traditional modes of address should be employed. Children should be asked what they wish to be called, and diminutives like "dear" or "son" should be avoided, as should the use of nicknames without the child's consent.

As no one can accurately remember all the information revealed, notes should be made during the assessment interview. Under some conditions—for example, if court involvement is possible—almost verbatim recording is essential. Most families do not object to the examiner taking notes and many even appreciate it as indicative of a thorough approach. A seating plan, similar to the one in figure 7.1, detailing where everyone sits and who interacts with whom can be helpful and may graphically illustrate when someone is being left out or if there is little or no communication between any of the family members.

During the interview the examiner must pay careful attention to the level of anxiety. It is inevitable that discomforts and apprehension will arise. Some tension can be helpful, but too much can lead to an inability to relate constructively and to take an active role in the assessment process.

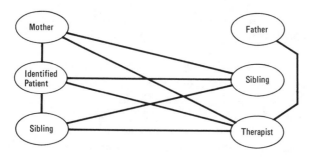

Figure 7.1 Seating Chart.

Examiners will find that structuring the interview is often helpful in allaying anxiety, as is demystifying the process by describing fully the procedures that will be followed.

Problems in Assessment

On occasion, one parent or sibling may refuse to be involved. Some facilities will not do an assessment in this circumstance. When this occurs, it seems unfair and perhaps poor practice to punish those who are willing to come by withholding intervention. Yet the absence of an important family member is an issue that requires examination, and it might well be considered unproductive to begin therapy without that individual's involvement.

Some adolescents may request that their parents not take any part in the assessment. Although in some instances this wish can be respected, the reason for the request should always be explored carefully. Where there is concern about issues of safety of the adolescent or others, professional responsibility demands that the parents be informed about the seriousness of the adolescent's condition and their involvement be sought. In such situations the adolescents should be encouraged to speak to their parents first. Should they refuse, they should be informed of the examiner's intention of involving the family, preferably before contact is made. While an explanation of what will be kept confidential and what will be revealed may be in order, it is a mistake to promise total confidentiality.

Some children may refuse to leave their parents. In these cases the clinician can invite the parents into the playroom to help the child settle. How the family deals with such happenings can be quite instructive. Reassurance about where the parents are waiting, even for a short visit, may be necessary for the very anxious, dependent child.

If after several visits the examiner is not clear about the nature of the problems and the child is showing disturbed behavior, admission to a hospital with continuous observation may be another way to achieve clarification.

Possibly the most difficult, but least obvious, problem occurs when the examiner's own feelings are touched in such a way that they interfere with the assessment process. In families when there has been separation or divorce, or when there are divided loyalties, considerable pressure may be exerted on the clinician to join in an alliance with one side or the other. Any such alliance must be scrupulously avoided, as should the tendency to side with the children and ignore the parents' positions. Children can be very difficult, can have a major impact on parents and families, and are not always the victims.

Organization of Material

An outline for the organization and recording of the data collected follows. It begins with identifying data and moves through history of present and past difficulties, the history of the family and development of the identified patient, to reporting of interview impressions. It ends with formulation, diagnosis, and proposed plan of treatment.

In preparing a written record, the clinician should make clear the sources of the data, indicating which come from direct observation and which from inference or hearsay. Too often, inaccurate or highly speculative material are recorded and, by virtue of having been written in a record, become accepted as hard fact.

Written records should be clear and easily understandable to both the lay and professional reader. Professional jargon is largely unnecessary and may block rather than assist communication. The fact that there is an increasing expectation that patients have a right to view their own records should be kept in mind—records should be clear and objective with unpleasant facts or observations presented with compassion and justice.

OUTLINE OF ASSESSMENT DATA

Identifying Data

Name, age, address, telephone number, legal status (natural child, adopted, foster) school, grade.

Referral Source

Persons or agencies involved in the referral process.

Chief Complaint(s).

A concise list of issues of concern: usually behavioral observations.

Sources of Information

A list of persons interviewed, the types of interviews, reports obtained, and telephone contacts.

History of Current Difficulties

Description of problems; duration; how they were noticed; by whom; way in which they create difficulty; what precipitates them; where, when, what makes them better or worse; child and family's explanation of the causes; what attempts have been made to help? What are the goals in seeking help now?

History of Previous Difficulties

A review of earlier problems of the family and its members; description of the problems, duration, what help was obtained, the results, the feelings about the help received.

Family History and Development

1. Constitution of family—Age, education, occupation, elucidating separations, deaths, moves away as relevant.
2. Parents' early life experiences—A brief review of their families of origin; style; quality of relationships; management of discipline and conflict; sharing of affection and feelings; attitudes toward work, school, sex, money, the law, relevant life events.
3. Courtship and marriage—How the couple met; what attracted them; expectations of marriage or union; significant factors in early adjustment (sexual, social, and economic); description of previous liaisons and marriages.
4. Arrival of children—Planning for children; pregnancies; births; abortions or miscarriages; effect of each child's arrival; personalities and achievement of children; adoptions, fostering, placements, hospitalization.
5. Current marital and family functioning—Style of marriage, ability to cope with developmental changes, responsibilities; sexual relationship. Daily routines—meals, recreation, role functioning, employment. Economic factors, living conditions, cultural and ethnic factors, legal issues. Significant illnesses, deaths, losses, changes, separations, divorces, and their consequences. Relationship to extended family, community, school, church, courts, police, children's aid society and other services.

Development of Child

1. Pregnancy, delivery, neonatal period (including parental reactions), early physical and temperamental style (see table 1.1, p. 8–11), developmental milestones, establishment of feeding, sleeping, toilet routines.
2. Activity level, reaction to stimuli, general responsiveness.

3. Quality of early relationships, bonding and attachments.
4. Stresses: emotional, physical; illnesses and injuries.
5. Preschool development and personality.
6. Response to discipline.
7. Introduction to school; emotional reaction; progress at school, behavior with teachers and classmates.
8. Hobbies, interests, sports, chores, work history.
9. Physical development: age at puberty and reaction to it, interest in sexual matters, sexual relationships, feelings about sexual matters.
10. Development of conscience and morality.
11. Degree of individuation from family—involvement with peers, activities in community.
12. Contact with police and other community agencies.

Examination of the Family

Who Participated. General description of each individual and the family as a whole.

Structure and Organization of the Family. Repetitive patterns of interaction; alliances, coalitions, subsystems; power hierarchy; separation of generations; boundaries between individuals; degree of individuality; cohesiveness, interdependency; enmeshment. Clarity of roles and functions. Rigidity and flexibility of system; openness to information; homeostatic mechanisms.

Communication. Clarity, ambiguity; directness, indirectness; displacement. Consequence of verbal and nonverbal communication. Metacommunication (rules about what can be said, by whom, to whom, how) content, themes, preoccupations, avoidances, quantity.

Affect. Emotional tone, expression, intensity, variation, rules about expression. Comfort level with feelings, responsiveness.

Control and Decision Making. Leadership style, flexibility, consistency, form of reinforcement, cooperation, resistance, attitude to feedback.

Conflict Resolution. Method and style. Management of differences and disagreement; areas of difficulty.

Developmental Parameters. Age-appropriateness of expectations, roles, intergenerational issues. Management of autonomy and individuation. Fit between developmental task of adults and those of children.

Examination of the Child

Mental status (compared with developmental norms) consists of:

Appearance. General appearance, physical development, gender attributes, dress, grooming, posture, gait, voice, manner of speaking, articulation defects, facial expression, coordination, laterality, presence of odors, contusions, lacerations, scars, needle tracks, and so forth.

Relationship to Examiner. Nature of relationship formed; working alliance, social manner, eye contact, involvement in activities, appeal of child.

Behavior and Activity. Description of main activities, themes. Activity level, goal-directedness, persistence, concentration, reaction to stimuli, age-appropriateness. Impulsiveness, compulsiveness, messiness. Habits, tics, involuntary movements.

Perception, Sensorium. Consciousness, alertness. Orientation in time, space, and person. Memory for recent and remote events. Auditory, visual, and recognition skills; accuracy. Hallucinations, illusions.

Thinking Processes. Content—main themes, general knowledge; dreams, fantasies, daydreams, wishes, obsessions, delusions. Function—organization, coherence, disturbance in flow, ability to use abstract reasoning; estimate of intelligence; defense mechanisms. Language—comprehension, fluency, expressiveness, specific disorders. Insight and judgment—of own problems, of consequences, objectivity, concepts of morality.

Affect. Emotional tone of interview, range, variation, intensity, appropriateness to content; awareness and control over feelings.

Attitude Toward Self and Others. View of self, ideals, aspirations, goals, sense of responsibility. Body image; sexual identity. Self-esteem, feelings of belonging vs. alienation and of being loved. Trust in self and others; feelings about others.

Other Observations

Other observations include tests, evaluations, reports, and earlier assessments, such as psychological tests, electroencephalograms, education assessments, and so forth.

Formulation

Formulation is the process by which historical information, clinical observations, and other data are synthesized to reach a diagnosis and to suggest a plan of treatment. It is a speculative and subjective attempt to combine facts and observations with generally accepted theories and knowledge of biological, psychological, familial, and social functioning in order to explain the patient's level of achievement, blocks or distortions of development, adaptive and defensive mechanisms, and symptom formation. Although formulation may appear to be a procedure that can be carried out only after all available data have been collected, it actually begins as soon as the clinician acquires any information about the case. Initial theories and presumptions about the patient's difficulties are continuously modified as more information becomes available.*

Significant factors in the patient's development and difficulties are grouped in four major areas—biological/constitutional, familial, sociocultural, and psychological. The contributing factors can also be grouped according to whether they are seen as predisposing, precipitating, perpetuating, or protecting. By using the grid shown in table 7.1, it is possible to examine the interactions of the various contributing factors.

The following case history illustrates how a case might be formulated.

*See Cameron et al. 1978; Cohen 1979a; Goldberg, Lessers and Schulman 1966; Group for the Advancement of Psychiatry 1966, 1973; Kline and Cameron 1978.

Linda is a fourteen-year-old girl, adopted at birth, who has been increasingly rebellious since age eleven. Truancy, running away, use of drugs, and a recent suicide attempt are major concerns. She has been closely involved with an anti-social subculture. Her middle-class parents have had little marital satisfaction, and each has had serious psychiatric difficulties. Father repeatedly fails at his work and is highly critical of his wife and daughter, while mother suffers psy-chotic depressions and episodes of alcohol abuse. The parents unite to criticize Linda, who contains her feelings but runs away for relief. She was a pleasing child in early years and did well in school. She seems bright and articulate and has been able to maintain a fairly positive relationship with the guidance teacher at her school.

TABLE 7.1

Contributing Factors to Patient's Development Formulation

	Biological Constitutional	Familial	Sociocultural	Psychological
Predisposing	None identified. No information on nutrition of biological mother during pregnancy or delivery.	Adopted at one month. Father's ambivalence about adoption. Chronic marital conflict. Guilt-inducing style of parents. Repeated failures of father. Mother models avoidance through alcohol abuse and psychotic illnesses.	Lack of siblings. Adult-orientated household. Finances precarious.	Maternal illness and hospitalization may have affected bonding and development of basic trust. Differentiation not valued.
Precipitating	Early maturation. Use of nonprescription drugs.	Shame and criticism about tattoo and behavior in general. Parents' lack of acceptance of differentiated thought and behavior. Need to individuate.	Discomfort with schooll and peers. Involvement with antisocial groups. Rejection by "in crowd."	Severe suicide attempt. Onset of puberty with increased sexual drives, questioning of adult values and need to differentiate. Fantasies about lost natural parents.

TABLE 7.1 *(continued)*
Contributing Factors to Patient's Development Formulation

	Biological Constitutional	Familial	Sociocultural	Psychological
Perpetuating	Mature appearance elicits inappropriate expectations. Impulsive tattoo.	Parents only united by scapegoating of child. Poor communication skills. Model of avoidance of expression of feelings. Father's repeated failures. Mother's repeated absences in alcohol and psychosis.	Social isolation of family. Support of delinquent subculture. Increased expectations at school.	Anger at parents turned on self. Guilt about feelings and behavior. Lack of acceptable outlet for feelings. Parental rejection evokes fantasies of rejection by birth parents.
Protecting	Temperamentally an easy child. Good physical health. Good intelligence. Attractive.	Financial support from extended family. Positive aspects of work ethic and upward striving.	Provision of camps, dance lessons, adding to skills. Friendship and concern of guidance teacher.	Well-developed ego skills. Capacity to relate positively.

The examiner then interweaves these factors and presents them in paragraph form.

Linda, a fourteen-year-old girl, presented at emergency after having taken a serious overdose of her mother's tranquilizers. She also gave a history of rebelliousness, running away from home, involvement in a delinquent group, and use of drugs.

Linda was adopted at one month. Although she was temperamentally an easy child, it is questionable whether bonding was complete and basic security achieved, as her adoptive father was ambivalent about the adoption and her mother had repeated hospitalizations for psychiatric problems. The persistent parental conflict required Linda to stabilize the marriage, with parental inadequacies and dissatisfactions being displaced onto the child. She was saddled with the responsibility of her mother's illness and made to feel responsible even though she strove to be a pleasing child. Since the family was unable to tolerate expressions of negative feelings, anger was internalized, causing her to withdraw into herself, leading to feelings of loneliness and isolation.

This isolation and lack of siblings made peer relationships difficult to achieve. Early maturation and her adoptive status increased Linda's sense of being an outsider. She relieved this by escaping to an "outsider" subculture in which she may have unconsciously sought her fantasied natural parents. Mother's depression and dysfunction and the hostile criticism of both parents intensified feelings of guilt and alienation that Linda repeatedly tried to escape by running away, using drugs, tattooing, and then finally attempting suicide.

The difficulties are perpetuated by interacting patterns of scapegoating, mutual rejection, and projection of feelings of guilt among family members across unstable ego boundaries. Linda's involvement in an antisocial subculture provides an illusion of intimacy and support based on collusion against external authority. Fortunately Linda is able to use her intellectual strengths in her own interest and to capitalize on a degree of trust and warmth provided by her guidance teacher. Her mastery of numerous skills suggests a good capacity for healthy development beyond the current crisis.

Differential Diagnosis

The differential diagnosis consists of a list of conditions to be considered in arriving at a diagnosis. The consideration of other possibilities prevents the examiner from falling into the trap of premature closure by thinking that the most apparent difficulty is the only or even the basic problem.

Provisional Diagnosis

The examiner reaches a provisional diagnosis based on the data available from the differential diagnosis. A standard recognized nomenclature is used (most likely from DSM-III or ICD-9).

Treatment Plan

Any treatment plan should arise out of the formulation. It must be feasible and acceptable to the family and should specify the type of treatment, by whom, and the goals.

Prognosis

The prognosis is the natural history of the disorder and the examiner's estimate of what can be achieved if treatment is instituted.

Contract Making and the End of the Assessment

Once all the data have been collected and analyzed, the clinician must present the findings to the family in simple, explicit terms, illustrated if possible by examples that occurred or were discussed in the course of the assessment. At this time the family may experience considerable anxiety, which may impede their ability to hear what the examiner is telling them. For this reason more than one session may be required for the findings to be heard and assimilated. This is particularly true when a diagnosis such as mental subnormality, genetic disorder, or psychosis must be communicated to the family, or when hospitalization is recommended.

If the clinician is planning to undertake the treatment, general objectives, methods of treatment, time, attendance, and fees must be negotiated. When referral is recommended, the rationale must be explained and feelings of disappointment, sadness, anger, and of being blamed worked through. The referred family should be prepared to have some aspects of the assessment repeated, as most settings like to do their own evaluations. The examiner should be familiar with the facilities available in the community, so that whatever suggestions are made are feasible. It is better to set realistic but limited and obtainable goals than to attempt the impossible and succeed only in frustrating everyone involved.

Reports to Other Agencies

Upon completion of an assessment, a clinician may be asked by a variety of agencies to provide a report. No information can be released without written consent. Before a report is sent, it should be clear why the report is being requested and the response should address only the questions being asked. Although labels are useful for research and treatment consideration, in the wrong hands they can have serious repercussions (Hobbs 1975). A report mentioning the possibility of schizophrenia and brain damage could lead to undue pessimism, intensifying the child's difficulties. Once prepared, the contents should be reviewed with the family, if possible. Even if the clinician must be critical or makes recommendations contrary to the wishes of the family, a relationship can be maintained if the rationale is explained.

In time, children grow up and may request to see their files or to have information sent to another setting. Clinicians must remember that such requests do not permit the release of information about the patient's parents or siblings unless they too have signed a consent.

Conclusion

An adequate assessment is an essential step toward effective treatment. It must take into account the nature of the problem, the desires and capabilities of the family and child, and the style of the therapist. At its completion, it should provide enough data to lead to a clear understanding of the problem and to suggest realistic plans for future management.

SUGGESTIONS FOR FURTHER READING

BANDLER, R.; GRINDER, J.; AND SATIR, V. 1976. *Changing with families: A book about further education for being human,* Palo Alto, Calif., Science and Behaviour Books.
  The principles of neurolinguists are applied in this book which contains many valuable points to demystify assessment and therapeutic work with families.
CHESS, S., AND HASSIBI, M. 1978. *Principles and practice of child psychiatry.* New York: Plenum Press.
  An excellent basic text demonstrating how concepts of nature and nurture can be used productively to understand the psychopathology of children.
FISHER, L. 1976. Dimensions of family assessment: A critical review. *J. Marr. & Fam. Counsel* 2:367–382.
  A very complete review and integration of various schemata for the assessment of the family.
GOLDSTEIN, J., FREUD, A. AND SOLNIT, A. J. 1973. *Beyond the best interests of the child.* New York: Free Press.
———— 1979. *Before the best interests of the child.* New York: Free Press.
  Classics of particular value to anyone doing assessments in the child welfare or custody and access areas.
GOODMAN, J., AND SOURS, J., 1967. *The child mental status examination.* New York: Basic Books.
  A basic book reviewing various aspects of the child mental status examination.
GRAHAM, P., AND RUTTER, M. 1968. The reliability and validity of the psychiatry assessment of the child. II: Interview with the parent. *Brit. J. Psychiat.* 114: 581–592.
  A series of articles studying the reliability and validity of information obtained in structured interviews with mothers and with children in the psychiatric assessment of children.
HALEY, J. 1978. *Problem solving therapy.* San Francisco: Jossey-Bass.
  A classic book illustrating strategic work with families. The first chapter is a particularly valuable discussion of the first interview with the family.
HOOD, E., AND ANGLIN, J. 1979. *Clinical assessment in children's services.* Ontario: Ontario Ministry of Community and Social Services, Children's Services Division.
  A thorough, practical, basic discussion of the process of assessment.
LEWIS, M. 1978. *Clinical aspects of child development.* Philadelphia: Lea and Febiger.
  A review of aspects of child development and its applications in clinical practice.
MINUCHIN, S., AND FISHMAN, C., 1981. *Family therapy techniques.* Cambridge, Mass: Harvard University Press.
  This and Minuchin's other book, *Families and Family Therapy,* give a complete and thorough account of the author's structural approach to family assessment and therapy in a form that is easily understood and can be applied.
MOUSTAKAS, C. E. 1973. *Psychotherapy with children.* New York: Ballantine Books.
  A complete review of the ways of doing psychotherapy from a nondirected, client-centered, theoretical orientation. Basic principles are equally relevant to process of assessment.
PATTERSON, G. R. 1968. *Living with children.* Champaign, Ill., Research Press.
————. 1975. *Families.* Champaign, Ill.: Research Press.
  Both are do-it-yourself, fill-in-the-blanks books teaching basic principles of child management with a social learning theory orientation. Useful as an introduction to a behavioral approach to treatment planning.

Schwitzgebel, R. K., and Klob, D. A. 1974. *Changing human behavior.* New York: McGraw-Hill.
A complete discussion of how human behavior may be changed using a social learning theory paradigm. One useful approach to treatment planning.

Simmons, J. E. 1981. *Psychiatric examination of children,* 3rd ed. Philadelphia: Lea and Febiger.
A detailed description of the ways in which the psychiatric examination of children can be carried out.

Sonis, W. A., and Costello, A. 1981. Evaluation of differential data sources. *J. Am. Acad. Child Psychiat.* 20:3, 597–610.
A review of different sources of data collection and discussion of ways of evaluating these sources.

Watzlawick, P., Weakland, J. H., and Fisch, R. 1974. *Change: Principles of problem formation and problem resolution.* New York: Norton.
A still provocative book that challenges old notions of how change comes about and provides much valuable information about new ways to think about and organize data to help patients change how they are behaving and what they are doing. Useful in considering treatment planning.

Winnicott, D. W. 1971. *Therapeutic consultations in child psychiatry.* New York: Basic Books.
A delightful book in which Winnicott describes his consultations with children, including a discussion of his use of the squiggle game.

PART III

Common Syndromes in Child Psychiatry

8 *Klaus Minde and Susan Goldberg*

Infant Psychiatry

History of Infant Psychiatry

Eva, a seven-month-old girl, was referred to a child psychiatrist by a geneticist. Her mother complained that Eva never smiled at anyone, and the pediatrician thought she suffered from a specific genetic abnormality. On examination, it became clear that Eva's father rarely smiled and had never shown any gentleness toward his wife. Mother had waited desperately for a smile from this, her first child, but when none occurred by six weeks had "given up" and administered to Eva only perfunctorily. During examination, mother clearly failed to notice the obvious though not exuberant smiles and pleasure Eva showed in her presence.

John, aged three months, was referred to a child psychiatrist because he "screamed more than twelve hours a day." His mother needed to go back to work and did not know how to leave the infant. Further exploration revealed that John had been delivered by a different physician from the one mother had seen all along. This delivery had involved much technology and left mother "enraged" during her hospital stay. John began to cry almost continuously after hospital discharge, and as a result, fed about forty times a day. On examination, John was restless, very precocious in his motor development and seemed unable to relax and cuddle.

It may surprise the reader that children so young are evaluated and treated by psychiatrists. Yet public awareness of potential psychological problems of infancy and the number of psychiatrists working with infants have grown rapidly in the last decade.

Although psychiatric tradition has theoretically always recognized the psychological importance of infancy, several historical trends have recently combined to translate this theoretical interest into a more direct and pragmatic one.

153

THEORETICAL WORK BY PSYCHIATRISTS WHO OBSERVED INFANTS

Much of traditional psychoanalytic theory has been concerned with reconstructing from the analyses of adults the inner experience of babies. For a long time this reconstruction depended exclusively on retrospective recall of early experiences by adults because the infant, as a nonverbal organism, rendered traditional psychoanalytic methods inapplicable. More recently, however, psychoanalysts have found in behavioral studies of infants an additional source of information that could be verified, and some, including Spitz and Cobliner (1965), Mahler (1965), Escalona and her colleagues (Escalona et al. 1952), and Sander (1964), have carried out empirical studies of infants themselves or of mother-infant interaction. Bowlby's landmark volumes on attachment and loss (1969, 1973*a*, 1973*b*) integrated much of this work with studies of development in animals and humans. The resulting impact has contributed to major studies, particularly in developmental psychology, of the early parent-infant relationship.

INCREASED "PSYCHOLOGIZING" IN PEDIATRICS

With the rapid and widespread success of Benjamin Spock's *Baby and Child Care* in 1946, it became clear that parents were interested in and receptive to advice about the emotional and social development of their children. Pediatricians have, therefore, become increasingly aware of the child psychiatry and developmental literature. Lately developmental and behavioral pediatrics have emerged as important subspecialties, and numerous pediatricians have engaged in empirical studies of infant behavior and development.

EMPIRICAL RESEARCH ON INFANTS BY DEVELOPMENTAL PSYCHOLOGISTS

Beginning in the late 1950s with Robert Fantz's demonstration (1956) that infant visual behavior could provide information about perception and cognition, innovative methodology for studying the psychological experiences of behaviors developed rapidly. That these technological advances coincided with the translation of Piaget's books on infancy (1951, 1952, 1954) provided further impetus to the enterprise, and infancy has since become a major research area in child development.

TRENDS IN EDUCATION AND EARLY INTERVENTION

Educational institutions, originally designed to serve children from the age of five to seven onward, have gradually been augmented by a variety of structured experiences first for preschoolers and now for infants. In part the trend has been a response to the increasing number of mothers with children under five who enter the work force and to the increasing expecta-

154

tions after World War II that "everybody deserves an equal chance in life." Thus many of these programs have been generated by efforts to provide better preparation for formal schooling among children in otherwise disadvantaged circumstances (e.g., Head Start). In addition, governments and courts have increasingly ruled that public education must be extended to children with special needs. This has given rise to efforts to implement early detection of those who fall into this category.

These various movements cross-fertilized each other, resulting in the channeling of a vast amount of energy and enthusiasm into clinical and research programs focused on infants. As our understanding of infancy has grown, we have also become aware of the needs of infants and parents, including those who may require psychiatric consultation or treatment.

The Role of Psychiatry in Infancy

In spite of the common belief that early experiences play a major formative role in the child's development, empirical studies, most of them admittedly focused on cognitive skills and using IQ scores as outcome measures, have failed to find consistent relationships between early experiences or characteristics of infants and later individual differences (McCall 1979). For example, studies of breast versus bottle feeding have shown few personality differences at later ages (Caldwell 1964). Cognitive style in infancy did not predict cognitive style at age ten (Kagan, Lapidus, and Moore 1979), and comparisons of children spending a large amount of time in day care with those spending their entire infancy at home show few resulting differences in cognitive, social, or personality measures (Belsky and Steinberg 1979). This has led some child developmental theorists (Kagan, Kearsley, and Zelazo 1978) to argue that development is discontinuous and that infancy is no more or less formative than any other period of life. Others (Sameroff 1975; Sroufe 1979) have argued that previous approaches to such studies have been overly simplistic and that we must think in a more complex fashion to disentangle the thread of continuity from infancy through later developmental periods. The authors' view is consistent with the latter position. (See chapter 1.)

Because the infant and environment engage in mutually regulating transactions, any single experience or infant characteristic is unlikely to be traceable to a specific later outcome. Rather, such features will influence subsequent steps in the chain of transactions that lead to emergence of a particular trait, ability, or behavior pattern. Features of the child or the environment that remain stable over a long period (e.g., a child's physical handicap, family socioeconomic status) are more likely to have direct traceable effects on development.

155

At the same time, infancy is the period in which the behavioral foundations are laid for subsequent cognitive, emotional, and social skills. If these foundations are well established, the child is equipped with resources that will assist in negotiating later developmental changes. To the extent that development in infancy is hampered, extra efforts will be required at a later time to compensate for these deficiencies.

Thus psychiatric treatment of infants can be a powerful preventive measure (Fraiberg 1971). Therefore, the role of the infant psychiatrist is not limited to treating specific disorders of infancy, but includes promoting mental health through advising those concerned with normal development. Since poverty of emotional experience and lack of cognitive stimulation will set the stage for subsequent developmental compromise, the professional's role includes aiding parents whose knowledge of infants' needs is meager, whose resources for child rearing are limited, or whose infants present them with normally stressful conditions (e.g., developmental handicap or acute illness) and consulting with those outside the family concerned with infants (e.g., day care centers). Although in some communities there now exist some support systems, such as infant stimulation programs for parents (Huntington 1979), these have primarily stressed cognitive aspects of infant development. While cognitive skills are important, they represent only one part of the child's life space. The child psychiatrist is uniquely equipped to emphasize and address the socioemotional aspects of normal development.

Yet traditionally child psychiatrists have relied either on some production or comprehension of language or play, and are therefore poorly suited to direct work with infants. There is also little bona fide knowledge available on the prevalence or treatability of infant mental health problems. Furthermore, there are special problems in defining psychopathology in such a young child. For example, infants are even less able than older children to request help when in emotional distress. Since their parents often feel guilty and inadequate, they are often not inclined to talk about their concerns to mental health professionals, hoping that the rapid developmental changes characteristic of infancy will allow the child to "outgrow" problems. Since both normal and psychopathological functioning change quickly in infancy, all too often physicians agree with parents to wait things out and fail to notice maladaptive behaviors that do not disappear but simply change into a new form.

Disorders of Infancy

Despite this rather limited data base and the caution we must exercise in labeling any infant as disturbed, the most recent nomenclature for psychiatric disorder (DSM-III) cites three conditions specific to this age group: reactive attachment disorder of infancy, disorders of eating, and developmental disorders. This chapter will discuss each of these disorders in some detail and also offer a brief review of other psychiatric conditions that can be diagnosed during infancy and that may be amenable to treatment at that time. Some of these will be cross-referenced to other chapters in which the condition is discussed more fully.

REACTIVE ATTACHMENT DISORDERS (313.89)

An attachment disorder in infancy is characterized by the absence or distortion of normally occurring developments in the relationship of infants and their caregivers. As outlined in chapter 1, there is a normal sequence of attachment behaviors. Within the first month of life, infants show anticipatory approach behaviors at feeding (e.g., turn their head and open their mouth when put in the feeding position), smile preferentially to the mother's voice, and use differentiated cries to signal specific needs. Within the next three months, infants can be soothed by the mother's voice and will increasingly cling to her when faced with strangers. During the second part of the first year, protest or distress at separations, wariness of strangers, and accompanying delight at reunions with the mother become evident. Later on, imitation of mother's or other caregiver's gestures or vocal inflections and a frequent "checking" with mother when playing away from her are important social behaviors. In the second year, enrichment and elaboration of these behaviors, use of a "transitional object" (e.g., an old blanket or other special object), and an increasing tolerance for separation from the primary attachment figures develop.

A disorder in this normal process can occur at various times (Kolvin et al. 1971), leaving some clinicians (Call 1982) to subdivide the disorder into primary attachment failure of early infancy, anaclitic attachment disorder of infancy, and symbiotic attachment disorder.

Primary Attachment Failure

Symptoms associated with primary attachment failure vary according to onset, but include poor weight gain, excessive sleep and/or crying, and difficulties in feeding. In particular, in primary attachment failure the infant avoids visual tracking of the mother, is apathetic, and shows none or few of the normally occurring active social behaviors such as mutual smiling.

Anaclitic and Symbiotic Attachment Disorders

Children suffering from anaclitic and symbiotic attachment disorders have made a normal attachment to the primary caregiver but show a general regression after six to fifteen months. Symptomatology in the anaclitic type of disorder may include rocking, head banging, or other automatic behaviors, as well as poverty of play, poor language or toilet functioning, and predilection toward minor physical illnesses and/or self injury. Problems observed in the symbiotic attachment disorder center around the failure of infants above eighteen months of age to separate from their mother and are often coupled with hypersensitivity to the mother's behaviors and moods. Finally, infants usually show an inability to involve themselves with people outside the immediate family.

The predisposing factors of any attachment disorder can be quite varied. First and foremost, there are environmental events that can hinder the formation of normal attachment, such as an extensive early hospitalization of the infant or mother. Disruption of the mother-infant bond can also occur through maternal death or desertion, with consequent multiple and/or insensitive caregiving. The infant may also be born with a cognitive impairment or a difficult temperament and thus may respond in unusual ways to normal caregiving procedures. Mentally retarded and physically abnormal infants (e.g., those who are deaf, blind, or have other handicaps) present the ordinary parent with extreme caregiving challenges. Finally, factors within the parents, ranging from inexperience to deep-seated feelings of ambivalence toward the infant or difficulties in establishing a relationship with any other human being are often found in families of infants with attachment disorders. Most often, however, a combination of environmental, child, and parental factors makes up the matrix within which such difficulties and conflicts arise (Mahler 1965). Severe forms of reactive attachment disorder are responsible for the "failure to thrive" syndrome, an eating disorder characterized by the infant's refusal to eat in response to parental insensitivity to the infant's needs, abrupt weaning, or general tension between parent and infant.

Since some forms of attachment disorder are very serious and may, without intervention, lead to death, treatment must be started promptly. Its exact form obviously depends on the individual case. It is preceded by a detailed observation of both parents and the infant together as well as an examination of the infant alone, and aims to create a developmentally appropriate support system for both parties. Such a system may include the provision of outside social support for the parents, a therapeutic nursery experience for the infant, or the therapeutic engagement of the parents with someone who can provide the kind of interpersonal experience that will facilitate their ability to meet the infant's day-to-day needs with more competence and sensitivity. Such treatment is often difficult and may require long and intensive involvement (Mahler, Levinson, and Fine 1976).

EATING DISORDERS

Both pica (307.52) and rumination disorder of infancy (307.53) are characterized by gross disturbances in eating behaviors (Bentovim 1970). The essential feature in pica is the infant's persistent eating of nonnutritive substances such as paint or plaster, hair, sand, or clothing. The disorder begins at twelve or twenty-four months and usually remits in early childhood. The infant does not show any aversion to food but is most often either poorly cared for or mentally retarded. Complications may follow the ingestion of paint or the formation of hairballs. (See also chapter 9.)

Rumination of infancy, which commences between three and twelve months, features the repeated regurgitation of food and weight loss or failure of normal weight gain. Infants are normally observed to spit out and/or rechew food following a feeding, and while they may arch their back during this process, there is no facial evidence of visible discomfort. In contrast to pica, infants are often hungry and irritable between episodes of regurgitation and are difficult to feed. The latter characteristic, as well as the odor of half-digested food, often discourages the primary relationship. As the mortality rate from malnutrition in this disorder may be as high as 25 percent, remediation must be implemented rapidly. Treatment may include hospitalization of the infant to safeguard nutritional status, followed by a closely supervised feeding regime during which a competent nurse or other health professional observes and assists the reestablishment of a mutually satisfying parent-infant relationship.

Eating is obviously of essential importance to an infant, and consequently conflicts with caregivers are often expressed in feeding disturbances. The most extreme example of such conflict or incompatibility is the infant with the "failure to thrive" syndrome. This condition is characterized by weight and growth below the third percentile following an initially normal growth development, despite normal physical functioning and availability of food. It often requires long-term treatment for the parent-infant dyad, as parents may be overtly or covertly rejecting the infant or may show strong conflicts in the caregiving role.

DEVELOPMENTAL DISORDERS

The practicing clinician will encounter two distinct types of developmental disorders: mental retardation and infantile autism.

Mental Retardation (317.0x; 318.0X; 318.1X; 318.2X)

The essential feature of mental retardation, according to DSM-III, is a significantly subaverage general intellectual functioning that results in or is associated with deficits or impairment in adaptive behavior.

Mental retardation is usually divided into four subtypes, reflecting the degree of impairment (mild [317.0X], moderate [318.0X], severe [318.1X], profound [318.2X]) as measured by specific intelligence tests. In infancy these tests have little predictive validity—they predict poorly the future intellectual functioning of child. The reason for this is that "intellectual" development during infancy is primarily measured by assessing a child's motor behavior. Later intellectual skills have very different components that cannot be assessed in infancy. A child's early motor skills show little correlation with the later acquisition of social, verbal, or other interactional skills. For this reason, it is only for severely (IQ between 20 and 34) and profoundly (IQ between 0 and 19) retarded infants that the diagnosis of mental retardation can be made with confidence during the first year of life, and for infants with moderate retardation (IQ between 35 and 49) during the following year. Mild retardation (IQ between 50 and 70) cannot be reliably diagnosed until the child reaches school age.

Profound, severe, and moderate retardation are almost exclusively due to damage of the central nervous system and often associated with other physical defects, such as epilepsy. In contrast, mild retardation (317.0X) is often the result of lack of cognitive stimulation, interpersonal deprivation, or other stressful environmental factors, such as poor nutrition. This condition is, therefore, much more frequent among the poor. Treatment will obviously vary with the specific condition, ranging from the use of major tranquilizers to the counseling of parents and the institution of specific infant stimulation programs. It is important to realize that the care of a retarded infant is very stressful to most affected families and calls for great sensitivity on the part of the diagnosing physician. (See chapters 18 and 22.)

When transmitted to the family in an impersonal way, detailed information about such a child will not usually be retained initially but must be presented on a number of occasions in a supportive way.

Infantile Autism(299.0X)

Distortions of the development of all basic psychological functions important for the acquisition of social skills and language are seen in infantile autism (Eisenberg and Kanner 1956; Kolvin et al. 1971; Rutter 1976). The essential features are lack of responsiveness to people, gross impairment of communicative skills, and bizarre responses to various aspects of the environment, all developing within the first thirty months of life.

The failure to develop interpersonal relationships is characterized by the lack of responsiveness to and interest in people. Thus these infants may refuse to cuddle, avoid eye contact, have no social smile, and are often suspected of being deaf. There is usually no language present until the later preschool years. However, even nonverbal communication skills are severely compromised. Finally, the bizarre responses to the environment may take several forms. There may be a great deal of anxiety expressed in response to minor changes in the environment; such as when chairs are moved to different places in the home or doors are left open instead of being shut. There may also be ritualistic behaviors such as repeated hand clapping, touching of specific objects, or whirling movements when the head is slightly turned by the examiner. Sometimes the children stare into the sun without blinking much and may not respond to any type of physical pain.

Many of the symptoms characterizing infantile autism can be present in children with known organic conditions and/or associated mental retardation. This suggests that the condition results from disturbances within the central nervous system. Although difficult to test accurately, 40 percent of all affected children have IQs estimated below 50, and only 25 to 30 percent perform at an IQ of 70 or above. Infantile autism is discussed in greater detail in chapter 15.

OTHER DISORDERS

Physiological Problems of Psychological Origin

In addition to the specific disorders described earlier, infants can show a wide range of psysiological symptoms of primarily psychological origin. While these have not yet found their way into the official *Diagnostic and Statistical Manual of Mental Disorders,* they are nevertheless of clinical importance and should be recognized and treated by the practicing psychiatrist.

The most frequently encountered symptoms are various types of sleep disorders. Some 10 percent of infants fail to develop regular sleeping patterns by three to six months. These same infants often also have difficulties in their interaction with others (Anders 1982; Bernal 1973). They cry more during standard play observations, are less clear in their behavioral cues, and, as a consequence, are often perceived by their caregivers as relatively difficult and unrewarding. Anders (1978, 1982), who has done extensive studies on children with troublesome sleep patterns, suggests that irregular sleep is a reflection of these infants' generally poor behavioral integration. This implies that at least some behavioral difficulties in infancy can be a function of extreme biological variations. On the other hand, sleep disorders can also reflect infants' excessive anxiety or fear, caused by acute or repeated traumatic events. (For further discussion of sleep disorder, see chapter 9.)

Other symptoms denoting conflicts between the infant and the environment are problems in bowel and bladder function; frequent constipation; stool withholdings; resistance to toilet training or excessive toilet rituals, which reflect either an undue power struggle between the infant and the outside world or serious regressive tendencies within the infant.

Regressive behaviors in turn are usually seen when the environment actively discourages or inhibits the infant's growth and development. Excessive masturbation or general apathy combined with unduly long sleeping periods are other symptoms of regression. They frequently signify that the infant lives in a nonstimulating or emotionally depriving milieu and is attempting to cope with the ensuing depression by withdrawal, stereotypic activities, or regression to developmentally earlier behavior.

It is clear that all the abovementioned symptoms must be evaluated carefully. Their intensity and duration, as well as any accompanying stresses and deficiencies in the milieu of the infant, must be assessed thoroughly in order to form a basis on which useful remedial action can be planned and executed. They are discussed further in chapter 9.

Psychological Disturbances with Physical Origin

Other disorders of infancy include psychological disturbances with physical origin. Normal psychological development in infancy depends on the infant's ability to communicate internal physical states (e.g., hunger), affects (e.g., pleasure), and cognitions (e.g., recognition of familiar people) nonverbally and on the ability of adult caregivers to read and respond to these signals. Any physical impairment of the infant typically disrupts this normal communication system, placing extra demands on the caregiver. Thus physical impairments are potential sources of psychological disturbance. Three types of physical problems will be considered: those that are evident at birth, those that become evident later in infancy, and chronic or life-threatening illness.

Conditions Evident at Birth. Birth is, in and of itself, a highly charged emotional experience for parents. When the birth produces an obviously impaired infant (e.g., one with spina bifida, cleft palate, Down's syndrome), all of the parents' joyful expectations and plans are thwarted, and it is necessary for parents to reconcile these expectations with their shock and grief. Often parents experience severe guilt over such births, blaming themselves for not following the obstetrician's recommendations more stringently. Klaus and Kennell (1982) have written with great sensitivity about caring for parents who must confront these problems so that they can realistically accept the infant they will care for and learn to meet his or her special needs. (See chapter 22 for a more extensive discussion of parental reactions to the handicapped child.)

Throughout the infant's development, these parents are typically required to provide extra physical care, have less opportunity to see the rewards of normal development, and interact with a baby whose communications may be qualitatively different from those of normal infants.

The largest group of babies with physical problems at birth are those born prematurely. Although most of these babies eventually develop normally, initially they require special medical care and are known to be at risk for subsequent developmental problems. In addition to disappointment and grief over their failure to produce a normal baby, parents in this group have been presented with their infants before they are psychologically ready for the birth. Highly trained medical and nursing personnel "take over" the care of the infant, and parents, at first, have few opportunities to become involved with their offspring. In recent years concern has been expressed over the possibly detrimental psychological effects of experiencing neonatal intensive care, as few neonatal intensive care units can give much attention to the psychosocial needs of infants or parents. Psychiatrists and other health professionals have responded to this concern with efforts to use highly sophisticated medical technology while providing a comfortable psychological environment for infants and parents, particularly when the infant is able to move into transitional care. Once these infants go home, their development must be compared to postconception rather than postnatal agemates, which means that parents have to wait a longer time for developmental milestones. These babies may also be temperamentally more difficult to care for (Goldberg 1978), and parents may require some continuing support (Minde 1982).

Conditions That Emerge in Later Infancy. Many permanently handicapping conditions are difficult to identify at birth or in early infancy and only become evident as one or more aspect of the infant's development does not progress normally. Such conditions include blindness, hearing impairment, and cerebral palsy. Fraiberg's work with blind infants provides many examples of potential psychological difficulties in such cases (Fraiberg 1977). Often the parents' first suspicion that something is different or unusual about the baby is just an intuition, without any clear delineation of the problem. Later it may become clear that the infant does not make eye contact, is not developing normal facial expressions, does not respond to sounds, or is not progressing in motor skills. Until a diagnosis can be established, parents are confronted with distorted communications from their baby and, because they have no explanation for them, often feel that they themselves must be failing as parents. The family pediatrician, who is usually the first medical professional to see these infants, can usually only tell parents that it is "too early to tell. We just have to wait and see." An extended period of frustration as well as communication difficulties between parents and infant may then lead to psychological problems as parents withdraw, feel rejected by their baby, or become overprotective and anxious. Such families will need not only an explanation of their infant's problems, but support in moving beyond the disturbed interactions that have developed before they can undertake the new task of meeting their infant's special needs. (See also chapter 22.)

Chronic or Life-threatening Illness. Serious illness is psychologically stressful for the child and family at any point in development. During infancy there are two additional complications. Because of limited cognitive and language skills, the infant cannot be adequately informed about what is happening or prepared for frightening or painful experiences. Therefore, serious illness and hospitalization may be considerably more traumatic for infants than for older children. This is especially frustrating for parents who can do nothing verbally to help or reassure the infant. Second, instead of impinging on a parent-child relationship that has previously been a source of comfort and reassurance for the child, illness in infancy affects the parent-child relationship while it is still in the process of being established. Thus formation of the bond between parent and child may be disrupted. When the infant recovers, patterns established during the illness may persist even though they are no longer adaptive. For example, mothers

163

whose infants were seriously ill for a long time as neonates continue to be inactive with their babies several months after the infants have recovered, while mothers whose babies were ill for a shorter time changed their behavior as the infants' behavior changed (Whitelaw et al. 1981).

If the infant is chronically ill, potentially disruptive stresses will continue to affect the parent-child relationship and the infant's development. (See also chapter 21.) In those cases where the death of an infant is likely or imminent, most families can benefit from professional support to prepare for this possibility and later to work through the process of grieving in a way that does not interfere with the adequate care of other children at home or of a new infant, should one subsequently be born. (See also chapter 24.)

Diagnosis

More than any other group of children, infants are dependent on those who care for them. The assessment of psychological disorders in this age group, therefore, is not complete without a detailed examination of the infant and the parents and/or other important caregivers. While such an examination initially follows the usual format (e.g., including a thorough history of the parents' personal, educational, and medical history, as well as surveying their own caregiving and other interpersonal experiences), an assessment of an infant should also include a period during which the clinician observes the mother or father in action with the child. The type of interactions to be studied may vary. For example, an infant who has trouble eating may be observed during a feed, while an unresponsive baby may best be evaluated during a play session. Despite the different settings, the clinician records similar types of data. These can be divided into those relating to the infant and to the caregiver.

INFANT VARIABLES

These include capacities or sensitivities in each of the following areas:

1. *Gross motor development:* the ability to roll, sit, stand, and so on.
2. *Fine motor development:* coordination in manipulative skills such as holding a toy, working a pegboard, and so on.
3. *Sensory development:* responsiveness to visual, auditory, kinesthetic, or vestibular stimuli and the coordination of these responses.
4. *Interactional development:* communicative and language skills, the ability and style of expressing needs and wishes, and method of relating to familiar and unfamiliar people.

5. *Affective development:* the ability to express emotions through facial and vocal expression and gestures.

Some of these functions can be reliably assessed by formal tests such as the Bayley Developmental Scale (Bayley 1969). An evaluation of interpersonal skills and affect, however, has to be primarily based on clinical knowledge and sensitivity.

PARENTAL VARIABLES

These include the following areas.

1. *Sensitivity to the infant's present state.* Does the caregiver identify the infant's present state and needs? How does the caregiver introduce the infant to the interviewer? Does the caregiver notice if the infant is tired or hungry, or wants a toy out of reach?
2. *Ability to meet the infant's needs.* Once a need is identified, how does the caregiver respond? Does he or she try to soothe the baby if fussy, feed if hungry, help the baby to get the toy? Are these interventions intrusive, or do they follow the infant's cues?
3. *Willingness to engage with the infant.* Is the caregiver interested in the baby? Does he or she try to learn more about the infant and show pleasure, pride, worry at appropriate times? Does the caregiver feel an important part of the child's life space and see a role in facilitating the child's development?

Such an observational period can also be used as a preliminary test of the treatment potential of both infant and caregiver. Thus a guiding remark by the clinician to the parent that is taken up and leads to a change in the infant's behavior may well be of prognostic value. Likewise, the response of the infant to the interaction of the examiner may identify specific strengths or shortcomings in either the infant or the caregiver.

In addition, each evaluation of an infant requires a thorough assessment of the family support system. For example, are there neighbors or friends who talk to or otherwise support mother? Are sensitive public health facilities accessible to the parents? How much does the spouse or extended family help in the baby's care?

Finally, the clinician must always be aware of the rapid developmental changes that normally occur during this period of life. Diagnoses of specific psychopathological states should be arrived at with caution and only after an extended evaluation of both child and the milieu over time. This approach helps the clinician assess clearly the capacity of the infant to compensate for potential caregiver deficits and guides him or her in later treatment.

Treatment

Brief summaries of potentially effective treatment strategies for individual psychiatric conditions in infancy have already been given. While these summaries provide the reader and student with some guidance, it seems important to outline some important treatment approaches used for infants, since many general treatment modalities used by child psychiatrists are most effective in young children.

Two basic forms of treatment, direct and indirect, have been employed with infants (Johnson, Dowling, and Wesner, 1980, Mahler, Levinson, and Fine 1976).

Clinicians providing *direct treatment* believe that the best way to assist infant development is by working directly with the infant. Some have done so by using psychoanalytic models, while others have relied primarily on behavioral approaches. (See chapter 28.) It is of interest that most accounts describing the direct treatment of infants by professionals appeared in the literature over thirty years ago, while in more recent publications the specially trained mother or substitute caregiver is frequently reported to be the infant's direct therapist.

Indirect treatment, that is, treatment of the mother or other caregiver, is based on the assumption that mothers still regard infants as part of themselves and consequently will automatically transmit changes within themselves to their infants. Advocates of indirect treatment also believe that the most effective way of providing a disturbed infant with the required stimulation and care is through the caregivers' better understanding of an infant's developmental needs. The counseling given the caregivers can be of dynamic or reflective nature, emphasizing dealing with the mother's conflicts, which allegedly are interfering with her effective mothering. They can also, however, be based on a more behavioral model, resulting in straightforward advice to mothers about infant management.

While control studies comparing the clinical value of specific intervention techniques have not yet been done, it seems that disturbances in feeding, sleeping, toilet training, as well as those following short separations or other environmental stresses, can be modified with good results. It is also clear that an infant's psychological care can never be separated from his or her physical well-being, and much of our treatment effort must be directed at preventing disadvantages and strengthening the parenting skill of the infant's caregivers. In addition, we must harness those characteristics that make some infants less vulnerable to environmental stresses and strengthen their natural coping mechanisms. Such an approach usually requires the involvement of various professionals, such as pediatricians, educators, or other special support groups. The child psychiatrist, however, with comprehensive training in early development and familiarity with medical and nonmedical treatment models, is potentially well suited to take a leading role in the coordination and integration of such treatment endeavors.

SUGGESTIONS FOR FURTHER READING

ANDERS, T. F. 1982. A longitudinal study of nighttime sleep-wake patterns in infants from birth to one year. In *Frontiers of infant psychiatry,* ed. J. D. Call and E. Galenson, pp. 150–170. New York: Basic Books.
An excellent summary of the significance of sleep disorders in early infancy.

CALL, J. D. 1982. Toward a nosology of psychiatric disorders in infancy. In *Frontiers of infant psychiatry,* ed. J. D. Call and E. Galenson, pp. 117–128. New York: Basic Books.
An interesting attempt to conceptualize disorders of infancy.

GOLDBERG, S. In press. Some biological aspects of early parent-infant interactions. In *The young child: Reviews of research,* ed. S. G. Moore and C. R. Cooper. Washington, D.C.: National Association for the Education of Young Children.
A discussion of parent-infant interaction and the way it is affected by conditions that handicap the child.

KLAUS, M. H., AND KENNELL, J. H. 1982. *Parent-infant bonding.* 2nd ed. St. Louis: C. V. Mosby.
An updated version of the earlier (now classic) book that covers family relationships during pregnancy, labor, and delivery. Separate chapters cover the birth and care of premature infants and of those with congenital malformations, stillbirth, and infant death.

MAHLER, M. S., PINE, F.; AND BERGMAN, A. 1975. *The psychological birth of the human infant.* New York: Basic Books.
Summarizes most of the important insights and achievements that Mahler and her colleagues have brought to child development. While clearly based on psychoanalytic theory, it is a must for anyone interested in child development.

MINDE, K., AND MINDE, R. 1981. Psychiatric intervention in infancy: A review. *Journal of the American Academy of Child Psychiatry,* 217–238.
A recent review examining the value of specific psychiatric treatment for infants and young children.

OSOFSKY, J. 1979. *Handbook of infant development.* New York: John Wiley & Sons.
A collection of review chapters on infant development covering cognitive, social, and affective development as well as theoretical and practical issues, including clinical applications and interventions.

SPITZ, R. A. 1946. Anaclitic depression: An inquiry into the genesis of psychiatric conditions in early childhood, II In *The psychoanalytic study of the child,* vol. 2, ed. R. S. Eissler and A. Freud, pp. 313–342. New York: International Universities Press.
A classic study examining psychologically determined conditions in infancy.

9

Quentin Rae-Grant, Robert P. Carr,
and Graham Berman

Childhood Developmental Disorders

Phenomenology and Management

This chapter will discuss a number of problems that children often encounter during development. These symptom complexes are a major cause of concern for parents or guardians and are among the main reasons for their bringing their children for professional assessment and treatment. Specific syndromes, that is, clusters of associated symptoms and signs, will be defined and described, along with their known or postulated etiology, their frequency, associated factors such as the likely prognosis without treatment, and preferred modes of intervention.

DEFINITION

The symptoms of childhood developmental disorders illustrate the problem of classification discussed in chapter 6. Following the increasingly favored phenomenological approach to diagnosis, one must recognize that the same symptom may occur in the normal child, the child with a developmental disorder, the neurotic child, and the psychotic child.

For example, most preschoolers have occasional temper tantrums. If these are frequent and persist into middle childhood, they are likely to be features of a developmental disorder. But psychotic children also show frequent tantrums when frustrated, as do children with conduct disorders and epileptics with a temporal lobe focus.

168

The differentiation among these various conditions, any one of which may show the given symptom, is made on the basis of: (1) the frequency of the symptom, (2) the severity, (3) the age-appropriateness (that is, whether normal children show the symptom at that particular age), (4) the degree to which the symptoms interfere with functioning, and (5) the presence or absence of other associated symptoms, such as autism, obsessionality, and so on. Thus a comprehensive assessment is required to establish a diagnosis and to move from the manifest symptom and behavior to identify the underlying process and its degree of severity.

The symptoms discussed herein have been studied as to their usual ages of onset and of maximum frequency and have been related to the developmental tasks occurring at these ages. In general, the interaction of genetic (i.e., constitutional) factors, ongoing maturation, and environmental factors determines the "goodness of fit" between child and parenting figures. This in turn determines whether or not normal or excessive stress will disturb behavioral functioning and interfere with ongoing development (Thomas 1981).

In *normal* children, these symptoms occur frequently but are short-lived. They do not interfere significantly with overall competence or merit concern and intervention. If the parents realize this and avoid overreacting to them, the symptoms resolve, usually without attention or intervention, and do not interfere with ongoing development. Some parents, however, not realizing their innocuous nature, become concerned or upset by the symptoms, particularly in response to exaggerations of their significance by grandparents and physicians. If parents and environment respond to such symptoms with excessive anxiety or by allowing children to use them to manipulate the environment to their advantage, the symptoms are positively reinforced and thus become an increasingly prominent part of the child's behavioral repertoire. At this stage a diagnosis of developmental disorder would be made. For such a diagnosis one would take into account the severity and duration of the symptoms and the degree to which they were interfering with the child's overall functioning. It is the degree of developmental interference that should determine whether or not professional intervention is required. The differences in the characteristics of symptoms in the normal child, the child with a developmental disorder, and the child with a serious psychiatric illness are summarized in table 9.1.

ETIOLOGY AND PATHOGENESIS

In general, developmental problems occur when new developmental tasks are being faced. The problems are usually amenable to parental guidance. Many will disappear with time, but minimal prompt intervention, particularly using the parents as therapists, can help accelerate the resolution and decrease complications.

TABLE 9.1

*Comparison of the Normal Child, The Child with a Developmental Disorder,
and the Chronically Disturbed Child**

Normal Child	Child with Developmental Disorder	Chronically Disturbed Child
May show signs and symptoms of moderate degree and/or of transient duration.	Signs and symptoms are excessive and prolonged.	Some signs and symptoms may be identical to those of the child with a developmental problem, from whom they can be differentiated only by the history and examination.
Onset of symptoms is related to accentuation of stresses of ongoing development.	Onset of symptoms is related to accentuation of stresses of ongoing development.	Symptoms do not seem related to a developmental stage.
Symptoms are transient.	Symptoms are time-limited and should recede in response to parental guidance and the passage of time.	Symptoms are persistent and relatively independent of external events.
No intervention indicated.	Assessment is indicated; minimal if any treatment will be required.	Following an adequate assessment, treatment is indicated.†

*The chronically disturbed category includes children with psychoneuroses or personality disorders (see chapter 12), attention deficit disorders (see chapter 10), conduct disorders (see chapter 13), or psychoses (see chapter 15).
†For further discussion of methods of treatment, see chapter 28.

Why should some children respond in an abnormal way to the stresses of normal development that most children their age mediate without problems? Four main sets of factors appear important.

First, some children exhibit *unusually strong biological drives and/or other constitutional factors.* Those children whose biological drives are unusually intense, especially if these are reinforced by other constitutional factors that interfere with their yielding to environmental demands (e.g., high persistence, low adaptability), are more vulnerable to exaggerated conflict in response even to parental demands that are neither premature nor exaggerated. Thus the child constitutionally primed to struggle tenaciously against even reasonable parent requests for toilet training may, given susceptible parents, provoke an exaggerated and prolonged struggle. The additional stress that this can generate may not be confined to the battle around toilet training and, in extreme cases, can undermine the relationship between parent and child or produce an excessive reliance on fixed attitudes and pathological defenses that may seriously distort many aspects of future development and adjustment.

170

A second factor that may provoke abnormal responses is *a sudden increase in demands of the external environment upon a basically normal child.* Consider a child's response to premature parental demands for toilet training or parental insistence, in spite of the child's cues, on expecting too much too soon and with too little allowance for occasional mishaps. Such parents are demanding that the child delay the relief afforded by elimination and put up with the resulting physical discomfort until a parentally approved time and place are available in exchange for parental satisfaction and praise. Most families mediate this task without major upset, though it can precipitate major battles eliciting conflict, anger at those on whom the child depends for survival, and anxiety should the parental expectations exceed the capacity of this or any other child of that age to deliver.

Third, *abnormal or excessive responses of the environment to demonstrated behavior may elicit abnormal responses.* Most developmental disorders evoke a response from parents. That response can be natural; it can be supportive even though not approving; or it can be one of exaggerated rage, rejection, condemnation, or punishment that is both unreasonable and destructive. For example, most parents avoid overreacting when coping with bed-wetting and train their child to take appropriate responsibility for cleaning up after an accident. Other parents, however, react to enuresis or, even more so to soiling (encopresis) with an extreme reaction to the "dirty" behavior that evokes in them excessive disgust. This exaggerated response may become a major factor in perpetuating the symptom, a continuing source of excessive hostility or concern, and the reason for the family's seeking help.

And, fourth, *the basically normal child's difficulty coping with rapid biological changes may cause him or her to respond abnormally.* At times, a child's biochemical, endocrine, and developmental changes can disrupt a previously stable homeostasis between that child and the environment. The upheavals of adolescence, in particular, illustrate this point. Neither the adolescent nor, in many cases, the environment knows how to cope with the rapid mood fluctuations, the dogmatic statements, the insecurities, and the criticisms as the adolescent seeks to stabilize the hormonally induced disequilibrium and come to a new integration within the self and with the world. Most youngsters pass through this stage with relatively little of the *sturm und drang* commonly but erroneously considered typical of adolescnece. Those who have trouble tend to fall into two main groups. Children who before puberty had difficulties controlling their own behavior or managing relationships with others may, under the disorganization of the hormonal upsurge, respond in a chaotic and uncontrolled manner that precipitates multiple crises for them and their families. On the other hand, those who have been required to restrict their normal curiosity and exploratory behavior and who have been denied experimentation with new ways of coping by a rigid and punitive environment often have trouble containing this upsurge of pressure and activity within the emotional straitjacket that has been imposed upon them. They may have only two alternatives: to resort to an excessive reliance on phobic, obsessive, or other neurotic defenses in an attempt to contain their biologically increased drives; or to deny these and reinforce their repression by espousing the ascetic, doctrinaire, authoritarian answers provided by a hierarchically organized religion or cult (Kutty, Froese, and Rae-Grant 1979; Levine 1979). (See chapter 5.)

Developmental disorders are not confined to childhood and adolescence. Leaving home, courtship, engagement, marriage, promotion at work, achievement of milestones such as turning forty or fifty, and retirement can constitute periods of temporarily heightened stress at which developmental problems in adult life frequently occur. Thus developmental problems can occur in people of any age, although they are more frequent in the young simply because these are the years during which more change and more learning of new cognitive and social skills occur.

The more commonly occurring developmental disorders will be discussed within the framework of the major functional area affected, the age of appearance, and the frequency. All conditions pertaining to each functional area will be discussed in the age sequence in which they normally appear.

Specific Developmental Disorders

FEEDING DISORDERS

The initial establishment of feeding patterns depends on a close interaction between child and caregiver. Abnormalities of the child's neurological, muscular, or alimentary system or a constitutional irregularity of biological rhythmicity may cause difficulty establishing a satisfactory feeding pattern. So can problems the caregiver has in understanding or responding to the child's signals of hunger or satiety. Usually satisfactory feeding patterns are established when the parent feeds the child in an empathic and appropriate way, recognizing when the child is hungry and has had enough, thus establishing a pattern of regularity and reliability. But in many families and cultures eating has acquired complex meanings. Past personal experiences of privation lead some parents to place great importance on food. Furthermore, parents with some psychiatric disorders or those who themselves have felt deprived as children often have great difficulty recognizing and responding to the feelings and needs of others. This may interfere with their ability to recognize when their child is hungry or has eaten enough. As a result, children may be starved, fed irregularly, or overfed, thus interfering with their development of an appropriate sense of hunger or satiety. In childhood the rituals and conventions around eating and mealtimes may become quite oppressive in such families. When this occurs, food may become the focus for battles deflected from a number of other areas (e.g., control, autonomy, conflict between the parents, etc.).

Feeding Disorder with Colic (307.50)

"Good mothers have good babies," says an old adage equally applicable to all child caregivers. One of the first measures used to validate parenting competence is whether the baby is gaining weight and feeding properly. Mothers who are anxious and uncertain, especially with their first child, often watch their child's feeding and weight gain with considerable anxiety. If this maternal anxiety is communicated to the child, it interferes with both comfort and feeding, frequently resulting in the "three-month colic" (Spitz and Cobliner 1965). To diagnose colic initially requires a full physical examination to rule out conditions such as obstruction or enteritis. The contrast between colicky children in the hands of an inexperienced mother and those of a trained nurse is graphic. One observes, in the mother's attempts, the tension with which she holds the baby, often at an awkward, propped-up angle, lacking molding and contact with her body as she feeds. This tension most frequently stems from inexperience, particularly a failure to transfer parenting skills from grandmother to mother. It can also reflect the mother's comfort in her personal life and particularly in her relationship with her marital partner (Lakin 1957). A minority of mothers, particularly those who have had an unsatisfactory infancy and childhood, find the demands of an infant too intrusive on their own limited emotional resources. These mothers have considerably more difficulty meeting their children's needs, even though they may wish to do so. For their infant feeding becomes a tense, anxious, frustrating experience, instead of providing the relaxed satisfaction that normally accompanies the relief of hunger. Three-month colic, which in itself may have little long-term significance, may be the first indicator of a long series of problems (Wessel et al. 1954). These may stem from maternal anxiety, from a child's difficult constitution, or from a mismatch of a child's temperament and mother's ability to respond, as in the "poor fit" referred to by Thomas (1981). Thus the child's characteristics play a part in determining the maternal response (Levy 1943). Levy first noted that mothers who later become overconcerned and overprotective are often those whose infants suffered earlier from colic and failure to gain. These are most frequently oldest children or ones who have special meaning because of their sex, their birth order, or their having been conceived and delivered after a number of miscarriages (Spitz and Cobliner 1965).

Most feeding disorders are self-limited, particularly when those people supporting the family can reassure the mother as to her competence and that of the baby. The mother should be helped to get close to and enjoy rocking her infant. She will then find that this soothes the child and places her in a participant and parenting role, instead of in the role of an anxious, self-critical observer who repeatedly rushes to the scales to see whether the infant and she are passing or failing in their mother-child interaction. If the required reassurances succeed in bolstering the competence and confidence of the mother, the symptoms are often graphically relieved.

Rumination Disorder of Infancy (307.53)

This rather rare disorder, much more serious than colic, usually appears at a somewhat later age. It consists of repeated regurgitation of partly digested food after a period of normal eating. The food is brought up into the mouth without nausea, retching, or associated gastrointestinal disorder to be chewed, reswallowed, or ejected from the mouth. Along with this there is arching of the back and straining with the head held back. These children, who progressed normally until the rumination began, start to lose weight or fail to gain as expected (Bakwin and Bakwin 1972). The potential mortality from malnutrition is reported as high as 25 percent, particularly when the regurgitation immediately follows feeding (Halmi 1980). The condition is often associated with retardation, in which case the onset is frequently delayed until beyond three to twelve months, the usual age at which the rumination begins. Rumination alarms and discourages the parents, who are often alienated by their physical revulsion at the constantly regurgitated food. Rumination disorder should be distinguished from pyloric stenosis and from infections of the gastrointestinal tract. Both of these can cause regurgitation but are associated with physical abnormalities and require medical intervention.

Recent reports have suggested a lack of environmental stimulation as a major causative factor. Sheagren and associates (1980) report on three premature children who developed this syndrome in the neonatal period but who responded dramatically to environmental enrichment and stimulation.

Pica (307.52)

Pica is the persistent eating of nonnutritive substances. Most children, at some time, ingest inedible materials such as eggshells, but this usually decreases after age twelve to fourteen months. Its persistence beyond two years merits concern and investigation. Pica is not usually associated with any physical impairment, but where the material ingested contains lead the possibility of lead encephalopathy and other complications exist (Bakwin and Bakwin 1972). This is particularly likely in poor families or in areas in which lead-based paint is still found in old houses. Where pica accompanies an adequate diet, the condition generally subsides without intervention, although occasionally the ingestion of hair and the formation of hairballs complicating trichotillomania (hair pulling) may cause intestinal obstruction, requiring surgical intervention (Halmi 1980).

Persistent pica has been associated with mental retardation or with emotional and social deprivation, at times accompanied by child neglect and poor supervision. Attempts to explain pica on the basis of the child's automatic and primitive attempt to remedy some particular nutritional deficiency have had only tentative support (Lourie, Layman, and Millican 1963; Ronaghy and Halsted 1975).

The appearance of the clearly developed picture of pica suggests intervention at two levels. Primary prevention includes improving inadequate social conditions and overcrowding. Most families of a child with pica require extensive social agency assistance to cope with the disadvantaged conditions in which they live, their inadequate finances, and the emotional emptiness and neediness the parents frequently show. Pica can also be associated with infantile autism, schizophrenia, and such rare physical disorders as the Kleine-Levin syndrome, which is discussed later in this chapter.

Anorexia nervosa and bulimia are two major eating disorders whose incidence seems to be increasing in recent years. Since they commonly begin during adolescence, they will be discussed in chapter 19.

SLEEP DISORDERS

Nocturnal Fears: Nightmares

Children vary in the ease with which, as infants, they establish predictable and rhythmic sleep patterns. Infants sleep up to as much as sixteen hours a day, but some wake frequently during the night. Others are soon able to sleep through, allowing the parents more rest and relaxation. There are good indications that the factors determining sleep patterns are at least partly related to temperament.

In the preschool years, sleep can be a problem for many children. Some of these difficulties are probably related to anxieties aroused by children's passage through the stage of separation and individuation. During these years children depend on stable surroundings and the availability of the parents to maintain a sense of "self" as distinct from "other." This is very much related to their feeling of security. At night, not only are the parents visually absent, but the decrease in familiar sounds removes the reminders of their availability. Some deaf children have particular difficulty at this time because of their inability to perceive the usual audible signs that parents are still available. The child who repeatedly gets out of bed to seek reassurance but is met with hostility and parental inability to understand finds it even harder to keep an internalized image of supportive parents. A vicious cycle develops in which the child needs increasing reassurance but uses methods to obtain it that arouse even more parental hostility and rejection, becoming, as a result, still more anxious. Since preschoolers have little capacity for abstract conceptualization, they often handle this conflict by projecting the unwanted aggression and "badness" outward onto imaginery monsters and bogeymen, who further augment their anxiety (Bauer 1976). Some children's anxiety may stem from a fear of reexperiencing frightening nightmares or concerns originating in folklore and stimulated by nursery rhymes. Younger children often seek to handle these fears by trying to sleep in the parents' bed. Should this become a habit, it can cause problems later. The practice is probably best discouraged immediately, since the implications and the difficulty of breaking the habit increase as the child grows older.

Most children at some point, but especially in the preschool and early school years, experience occasional nightmares that may or may not be related to events of the day. Usually these resolve spontaneously. In addition, most children, particularly in early adolescence, experience periods of insomnia secondary to rapid changes or frightening events in their lives. Like adults, children tend to exaggerate how long they stay awake; their anxiety about not sleeping is in itself one of the major factors perpetuating full wakefulness. Sometimes just encouraging a child to rest quietly even if sleep is impossible is enough to neutralize this secondary anxiety. Frequently children at this stage sleep better if the lights and sounds of household activities are not shielded from them. Should something more be needed, small doses of medication, particularly chloral hydrate, can reestablish a regular sleep pattern and undermine the expectation of insomnia that interferes with sleep.

Over the last fifteen years, attempts to understand the sleep disorders have centered basically around electroencephalogram (EEG) studies of sleep patterns. As the stages of sleep deepen, EEG activity changes from the regular alpha wave to the delta wave through to the deepest stage, Stage Four, characterized by low-amplitude slow waves and sleep spindles. This stage is more frequent in the early hours of sleeping. REM (rapid eye movement) sleep is the early and light stage during which most dreaming and the accentuation of nightmares occur. Each night the level of sleep changes through several cycles, so that the child experiences several periods both of REM and of deep sleep (Broughton 1968).

The main sleep disorders that cause concern include nightmares, sleepwalking, and night terrors. Several authors (Anders and Weinstein 1972; Kales and Kales 1974) include enuresis in this category, but while it has EEG patterns similar to sleep disorders in children, it will be discussed separately as an elimination disorder.

Nightmares are fairly commonly reported. They should cause concern only when they are so frightening and persistent that they interrupt or make the child fight against sleep, or where the pattern of repeated nightmares requires investigation because of possible links to disturbing events in the child's life. Most children report their dreams pleasantly and rather concretely, with the sophistication of the description of content increasing with age. However, two sleep disorders are considerably more frightening to those who observe them: sleepwalking (somnambulism) and night terrors (pavor nocturnus). Both are considered manifestations of rapid arousal from deep sleep instead of the usual more gradual movement back through the stages (Broughton 1968; Kales and Kales 1974). There is a distinct relationship between sleepwalking and night terrors, as the presence of one makes the other ten times as likely (A. Kales et al. 1980).

Sleepwalking (307.46)

A typical sleepwalking attack starts with the individual sitting up quietly, generally an hour or two after falling asleep, getting out of bed, and moving about in a confused and clumsy manner. As time goes on, the behavior becomes more coordinated and complex, so that the child navigates around the house and performs apparently purposeful activities. The eyes are open, exhibiting a glassy stare. The sleeper is very hard to arouse (Broughton 1968). For parents the most unnerving feature is the zombie-like or robotlike appearance presented. The typical attack lasts from one to twenty minutes, during which the person can talk, dress, or go to the toilet, all quite appropriately. The attack generally subsides with the sleeper returning to bed. The child, when awakened, presents a disoriented, confused, and rather fearful appearance. There is no memory of the behavior the next morning.

Sleepwalking usually starts in the preschool years but can continue into adolescence, at which point it usually subsides. It is more common in children with a family history of sleepwalking or night terrors and in boys than girls. There are, however, well-documented cases of sleepwalking persisting throughout life, particularly if the symptoms remain after age thirteen. A. Kales and associates (1980) report that those who sleepwalk as adults had their first attacks at a later age than those who experienced spontaneous remission.

Investigation of sleepwalking should include consideration of the frequency and duration of the attacks as well as whether there is an associated illness. Frequent and continuing attacks have been associated with fairly major environmental disruption or with more serious psychological disorders (Keith 1975). A brief episode, on the other hand, is more likely the result of such factors as a febrile illness or some acute dislocation in the child's life (e.g., a move) (Kales et al. 1979) and has little inherent significance.

Sleep Terror Disorder (Night Terrors) (307.49)

While night terrors share with somnambulism the same pathogenesis and implications, they present a remarkably different clinical picture. They are characterized by an abrupt sitting up in bed with a blood-curdling scream, the eyes open and apparently fixed. There are also physiological changes typical of those occurring in an acute anxiety attack (i.e., heart rate of up to 180 beats per minute, profuse perspiration, and increased respiratory rate and depth). Seventy percent of the children have little immediate recall, if awakened, of the source of the anxiety (Fisher et al. 1973). Most typically, they remember only an intense fear, although a few can give more detailed dream content. Like sleepwalking, the attack typically occurs in the early hours of sleep, but night terrors usually begin and remit spontaneously earlier than sleepwalking. Broughton, in an early but definitive article (1968), attributes both night terrors and somnambulism to abrupt waking without the intervening patterns of gradual arousal that usually occur from very deep (Stage Four) sleep. This also helps account for the confusion and lack of memory, since it is known that in Stage Four, imagery is very much less than it is in REM (Stage One) sleep.

Because of the concern that such terrors engender, children suffering from them are good candidates for short-term psychiatric intervention. An isolated episode should not cause alarm or immediate intervention, as the occasional episode occurs in as much as 15 percent of the population (Broughton 1968). For the child whose terrors are occasional and who lacks other obvious psychological or familial problems, reassurance and follow-up for several months are probably sufficient. When the terrors are frequent, one should inquire about external stresses such as the death of a parent, injury, trauma, proposed or past hospitalization, assessing the child's personal and social life to delineate and resolve as many stresses as possible. To relieve parental anxiety should the attacks continue, a trial of diazepam, to which the attacks often respond well, is certainly justified. Imipramine, which alters the distribution of stages of sleep, has also been reported to have some success (J. D. Kales et al. 1980; Pesikoff and Davis 1971). In severe and prolonged cases, however, medication alone is only one part of adequate treatment and should be accompanied by psychological intervention and counseling to ensure resolution of the conflicts generating the terrors.

Other disorders affecting sleep include narcolepsy, cataplexy, sleep apnea, and the Kleine-Levin syndrome.

The presenting and key component of *narcolepsy* is the occurrence of compelling periods of sleep during the day from which the patient awakes refreshed. A second manifestation is cataplexy, a sudden paralysis in the antigravity muscles, frequently brought on by emotion such as laughter or rage and leading to sudden collapse with clear consciousness. Also present in about 50 percent of cases is sleep paralysis, which occurs as the patient is falling asleep or awakening and, in full alertness, is unable to move. This can be particularly distressing when it is accompanied by hypnagogic hallucinations often associated with fear and apprehension.

Sleep apnea is the sudden cessation of breathing during sleep, repeated several times each night and resulting in fatigue during the day. Most sufferers are also loud snorers, and increasingly loud snoring often presages an attack in which there are also involuntary flailing movements.

The *Kleine-Levin syndrome* consists of periods of hypersomnia accompanied by irritability, social isolation, and binge eating. It should be distinguished from anorexia nervosa (bulimic type), but occurs in males more than females and is accompanied by bizarre sexual behavior, disorientation, and incoherence. (Lavie et al. 1979; Reynolds et al. 1980; Vardi et al. 1978).

The understanding of all these conditions is increasing rapidly with the development of sleep laboratories, the direct observation of sleep and EEG patterns, and the correlation of these with various physiological changes.

ELIMINATION DISORDERS

Toilet training, Functional Constipation

Toilet training is the regimen by which parents teach children voluntary control of their excretions. Successful bowel and bladder control, like the establishment of a regular feeding pattern, depends on cooperation between parent and child. Any factor in either parent or child that disrupts this ongoing interaction or presents or exaggerates difficulties around toilet training may predispose to the development of bowel or bladder disorders.

In our society the importance of cleanliness and the general adult reaction of disgust with bowel contents make this a particularly difficult task for many parents. Many adults cannot empathize with children who lack bowel control or cannot comprehend that they cannot control themselves. Their children, in turn, feeling helpless and misunderstood, often deny the problem. They pretend not to notice, ignore it, and hide "the evidence," thus merely increasing the parents' discomfort and disgust.

Teaching a child to assume voluntary control of bladder and bowel is usually accomplished by age three, with bowel control preceding that of the bladder. Most families complete toilet training without significant problems by gradually increasing their expectations, encouraging cooperation, praising appropriate behavior, and avoiding disparaging reactions to failures. A few parents, however, are excessively harsh and rigid, inappropriately permissive, or vacillate inconsistently between the extremes. In spite of this most children, even in these families, are successfully toilet trained.

The occasional child who has difficulties in bowel control may develop them as the result of a constitutional vulnerability, such as a tendency toward constipation, biological irregularity, or extreme negativism. Many encopretic children show deficiencies in their body image. They have unusual difficulty describing the sensations of bowel fullness and emptiness or of pelvic muscular contraction and relaxation. Their human figure drawings tend to be quite primitive, suggesting a failure to define body shape.

Rigid and perfectionistic tendencies in insensitive parents can make toilet training a battleground in which the giving or withholding of feces or urine causes a major struggle that leads ultimately to a breakdown in the parent-child relationship. Toilet training is a task in which children, almost for the first time, can assert their own individuality. They can choose immediate evacuation in response to discomfort or can temporarily resist the impulse and endure the resulting discomfort in order to please and protect their relationship with the parents. Should the pressure to relieve themselves overpower the desire to please, there may result a clash of wills that may be the first sign either of a primarily oppositional character or of what may become the predominant mode of parent-child interaction (Anthony 1957). Thus for a few individuals, toilet training is strongly linked with the later development of aggressive or passive-aggressive personality styles. In such cases the style results not from the toilet training per se; rather the training problems are symptomatic of the basic clash of personalities and the innate inflexibility that undermine the child's development, thus contributing to the mounting oppositionality that increasingly becomes deeply rooted in the child's character and personality.

There are two main developmental disorders related to elimination, *enuresis* and *encopresis*.

Enuresis (307.60)

Definition and Classification. Enuresis is the involuntary voiding of urine sufficiently frequently to cause concern after the age at which voluntary control is usually established, arbitrarily set at age three in North America. Thus enuresis has been defined as involuntary voiding at least twice a month for children age five to seven or once a month for older children. The term is reserved for cases with no associated physical disorders such as diabetes, seizures, or genitourinary malfunction. The voiding may occur during the day (diurnally), at night only (nocturnally), or both.

Enuresis is further classified as *primary* (or continuous) when voluntary bladder control has never been established or *secondary* (or discontinuous) when there has been a dry period of at least a year. Secondary enuresis is much more likely to have a psychogenic cause than primary enuresis, where a developmental delay or sleep disturbance is more likely responsible.

The symptom itself is less important than its effect on the child's social activities and self-esteem. Frequently parents seek help to enable the child to go to camp or to stay over with friends. Such situations provide the motivation needed to persuade the child to cooperate with a regimen to help become dry. Enuretic children away from home—at camp, for example—may remain dry only to resume bed-wetting on return home. This may be because at camp enuretics are frequently identified, segregated, and subject to ridicule and teasing by their peers. This pattern of doing better away from home may in itself cause much discomfort for the family (Burke and Stickler 1980).

Prevalence. Enuresis occurs only at night in about 80 percent of all enuretic children, both night and day in 15 percent, while approximately 5 percent are enuretic during the day only. In this latter group, enuresis is much more likely to result from associated physical and physiological factors. As children become older, the proportion of enuretics continues to decline: for example, about 16 percent of children are enuretic some time after age five; only 7 percent after age seven; and by age eighteen the number of enuretics has dropped to about 2 percent (Starfield 1972). By adulthood, somewhat under 1 percent remain enuretic.

Epidemiology. Enuresis occurs in all populations without discrimination as to race, social class, or country. Nevertheless, it has some important associations. Boys are much more frequently affected than girls and are more likely to continue into adult life (Marshall, Marshall, and Lyon 1973). Enuresis is much more frequent in the delinquent population. There is often an associated history of sleepwalking and a family history of generally poorer care, as evidenced by dental neglect. The family history is positive in 75 percent. Enuresis, as mentioned earlier, has been implicated in the development of the oppositional personality (Pierce 1980b).

Etiology. Four sets of factors have been implicated in causing enuresis: developmental, urological, psychological, and neurophysiological. Those who see enuresis as a *developmental* phenomenon underline the age factor, the spontaneous remission rate, the value of persuasion and reassurance, and the lack of other differences between groups of enuretics and nonenuretics. A few enuretics show distinct *genitourinary abnormalities* although, curiously, correction of these abnormalities eliminates the enuresis in only a rather small percentage of cases (Esman 1977; Shaffer 1976). *Psychological* formulations suggest that enuresis may be an act of rebellion or regression, a bid for attention, an expression of resentment of parents or siblings, a clinging to infancy, or an anger equivalent. The timing of the onset of enuresis in discontinuous cases—for example, after the birth of a sibling or following a separation—seems to add weight to this hypothesis (Umphress et al. 1970). Several interesting studies have related nocturnal enuresis to *sleep disturbance,* producing reasonable evidence that it is a disorder of arousal from deep sleep that precipitates the voiding (Broughton 1968; Kales and Kales 1974; Ritvo et al. 1969). Especially if voiding occurs early in the night, the enuretic usually wakes with no memory of having urinated. Enuretics rarely report dreams accompanying the voiding, although signs of automatic dysrhythmia, including alterations of heart and respiratory rate, may occur. Some children do report dreaming of fires, accidents, gun fights, waterfalls, or lakes, but these are at least as likely to result from the incorporation of the wetness into dream content as to be occurring simultaneously with the voiding. When enuresis persists into adolescence, there is usually an associated history of chronic family discord and erratic, irregular, and unpredictable parental expectations. Despite this, the assumption that enuretic children are generally unhappy has not been proven. The enuresis is often simply accepted as part of the family's life. This certainly is true of the 1 percent that persist into adulthood. Occasional

enuresis is not incompatible with marriage and an otherwise normal life.
Management. Despite the frequency with which enuresis is part of a developmental delay, it is important to identify and treat separately the minority of cases in which the problem is symptomatic of a physical condition. Children with spina bifida or with neurological or other organic causes for a neurogenic bladder may be unable to regulate bladder function. Other physical conditions that may first present with enuresis, particularly of sudden onset, include: epilepsy, diabetes mellitus, spinal cord disorders, sickle-cell anemia, diabetes insipidus, and regional genitourinary problems such as calculus, infection, or intestinal parasites (Shaffer 1976).

There is a dazzling array of physical and pharmacological treatments used for enuresis, most of which do no better than a placebo. Stimulants have been used to arouse the level of sleep, as have sedatives to reorganize the sleep pattern. Atropine, belladonna, and numerous other drugs such as caffeine have also been tried. For the large majority of enuretics who do not suffer from the previously mentioned physical conditions, the following measures in sequence should be considered:

1. After a thorough assessment and examination has ruled out significant findings, reassurance and counseling the parents to try a program of home management should be tried. The parent who brings the child can usually document whether the enuresis is primary or secondary, sources of stress or disruption within the family, and, in particular, the patterns by which toilet training have been attempted (Starfield 1972). This person can also supply a baseline of the frequency of the enuresis and describe factors that increase or decrease its frequency.
2. Since nocturnal enuretics tend to excrete a larger than usual volume of urine of low specific gravity, restricting fluid intake prior to bedtime should be recommended.
3. It should next be suggested that the parents wake the child to go to the bathroom before they go to bed.
4. Establishing a system of token rewards for dry nights using a chart or calendar may prove helpful, especially in younger children. This method emphasizes successes while ignoring failures. As children become older, however, they should be expected to take responsibility for removing and putting wet sheets in the laundry as an important symbolic step toward establishing control over the enuresis (Esman 1977).
5. If the preceding measures prove unsuccessful, the use of conditioning techniques such as the "bell and pad," in which the first few drops of urine activate an electrical circuit that rings an alarm that wakes the child, should be considered. This is highly successful with well-motivated children and families, and often results in improvements in the child's self-esteem, the family's comfort, and the child's status in the family (Burke and Stickler 1980). If the conditioning apparatus is not working, one should check on the state of the batteries or, even, whether they have been included or the apparatus plugged in, since some families, despite their expressed desire for a cure, handle their ambivalence about the use of the device by "inadvertently" defeating the apparatus. When successful, this method is rarely followed by the substitution of another symptom as an alternate expression of the suspected psychological conflict, as had previously been hypothesized (Denckla, Bemporad, and MacKay 1976).

Other instruments on the market directly apply a "small" shock to the child's genitals. As they can lead to quite severe shocks and even genital burns, particularly if improperly adjusted or if turned up more than recommended, these should not be used.

6. The one medication that has consistently shown strikingly better success than placebo is imipramine. The dosage recommended is between 25 and 75 milligrams in a single dose (i.e., 25 mg a day for ages ten and under, 50 or 75 mg for those older). This is given in midafternoon if the wetting occurs early in the night or much later should the enuresis occur closer to morning. If successful, the drug should be continued for two months, after which it should be discontinued at least temporarily (Rapaport et al. 1980; Werry et al. 1975–76). The success rate is 80 percent.

7. Many other methods and medications have been recommended, but with no more success than can be accounted for by chance.

8. In cases of secondary or discontinuous enuresis, particularly where obvious associated stress exists, enuresis is likely to be reactive. Here psychotherapy should be part of the management. Indeed, even when medication is the primary intervention, at least part of its success stems from the parental involvement with the child and from the parents' increased feeling of competence in helping to eliminate the symptom (Umphress 1970).

Encopresis and Functional Constipation (307.70)

Description and Definition. Much less frequent than enuresis, encopresis consists of fecal soiling after the age when bowel control is usually physiologically possible and after toilet training should have been accomplished—between the ages of two and three years. Anthony (1957) defines encopresis as the passage of stool of normal consistency at culturally inappropriate times and places in the absence of any organic cause. The children soil their clothing but vehemently deny it, despite the evidence or the discomfort of bystanders. Some children try to conceal their soiling by hiding their dirty clothes and the excrement, often in places seemingly selected to elicit the maximum revulsion, for example in a drawer of clean clothing or in the mother's purse. Some children soil at school, acquiring unflattering though descriptive nicknames, while others reserve their soiling for home.

Epidemiology, Course, and Differential Diagnosis. Soiling is four to five times more common in boys than in girls (Hoag et al. 1971). Its incidence is difficult to measure, as most estimates come from child guidance clinics. Even in that selected population, the proportion of encopretics is small. Encopresis usually subsides, with or without treatment, by adolescence, although there may be reports of continuing staining, and encopretics show an increased risk of delinquent behavior in later years.

Associated Conditions. Encopresis is associated with abdominal pain, constipation, and, about one third of the time, fecal impaction (Hersov 1976). Because of the possible association of chronic constipation with an enlarged colon, an adequate assessment of these children should include a complete physical, barium enema, and rectal examination.

Constipation, by itself, is not cause for concern. It is generally intermittent, self-limiting, and nonnoxious, despite common myths to the contrary. It becomes a problem, however, if children retain so much feces that they become bloated and uncomfortable or complain of colicky abdominal pain. Such cases may have a lower colon loaded with feces, leading to an overflow diarrhea (fecal incontinence) occurring around the impacted fecal mass. Parents usually complain about the soiling, not the constipation, which may be discovered only on examination. This "functional megacolon" must be distinguished from Hirschsprung's disease (aganglionic megacolon), in which a grossly dilated lower bowel shows a characteristic picture on X-ray examination. This disease results in gross loading of the abdomen with fecal masses, associated neither with incontinence nor with the psychological and family problems typical of functional constipation. Where the X-ray is equivocal, the diagnosis can be confirmed by bowel biopsy (Pierce 1980a).

Other problems of elimination control include fecal play and coprophagia (the eating of filth or feces). Both may accompany encopresis, but particularly coprophagia is associated significantly with maternal depression and psychological unavailability verging on the deprivation syndrome discussed in chapter 4.

Etiology. The basic problem appears to be a developmental one, with psychological factors seeming to contribute to, exacerbate, or perpetuate its course. Encopresis often produces disproportionate disgust in parents. While normally parents react less intensely to their own child's feces, the mothers of many encopretics experience such anger and depression that they may reject or punish to the point of abuse, particularly in response to what they see as deliberate, hostile, aggressive soiling. Encopretic children are often as verbally and emotionally "constipated" as they are physically retentive; as a result, they evoke little spontaneous warmth, even from noninvolved adults (Bemporad et al. 1971).

Management. There are three main approaches to treatment, surgical, psychotherapeutic, and behavioral. Since none can claim consistent success, a combination of all three may be required for successful management of a symptom highly troublesome to child, family, and environment.

1. *Surgical treatment:* A surgical technique is reported to produce dramatic results when used in constipated children with colonic dilatation. The colon is vigorously evacuated by repeated enemas. The children are given continuing doses of stool softeners and told that with any further soiling they will be returned to the hospital for more energetic investigation and treatment. Proponents report that very few patients return. While undoubtedly some cases can be handled this way, whenever possible the overly vigorous use of laxatives and enemas should be discouraged to avoid potentially serious psychological complications. The exception is when the colon is impacted, in which case rapid evacuation of the bowel and small doses of stool softeners are a major part of total management (Pierce 1980a).
2. *Psychotherapeutic treatment:* Psychotherapy of encopretics must involve both child and family, either separately or together. The aim is to improve communication

between parents and child, to allow ventilation of hostility and guilt, and to mediate aggression and struggles for control. The child's therapist must attempt to help the child find alternative ways of expressing natural but blocked feelings of rage and desires for independence by establishing a working partnership between child and parents. And the parents' therapist attempts to help the parents examine their frequent overreactions and develop reasonable and dispassionate alternatives in dealing with the encopretic child.

3. *Behavioral methods:* As with enuresis, a behavioral reward system that reinforces times when the child has not soiled may assist in eliminating encopresis.

SPEECH DISORDERS

Speech Delay

While wide variations exist, most children say a few words by their first birthday and a number of phrases by age two, though many normal children may still say only the odd word by their second birthday. It is important to distinguish accurately and as early as possible those children whose late speech signifies a significant problem from those normal youngsters who just happen to develop speech late. This distinction cannot be made from the quality of the speech alone, but rather must be based on an assessment of the characteristics of the babble, the nature of the child's play, the child's social responsiveness, the response to sound, and the child's understanding of language.

Epidemiology. About 1 percent of children are seriously delayed in developing speech. About 5 percent begin school still unable to be understood by strangers (Morley 1965). The causes of speech delay include: (1) mental retardation, in which all other developmental functions are uniformly retarded (see chapter 18); (2) infantile autism (see chapter 15); (3) lack of environmental stimulation and negative psychosocial factors, for example, the deprivation syndrome (see chapter 4); (4) emotional or behavioral disturbance.

Differential Diagnosis. Many children with delayed speech are referred to psychiatric clinics because the parents are anxious and dissatisfied with casual—and often incorrect—reassurance that their child is quite normal and that speech will develop in time. The child who cannot speak is in danger of losing out on early and important types of learning. Early, accurate diagnosis of delayed speech is important to avoid missing conditions that can be helped. The parents may be so anxious because of the language delay that they undertake secondary measures that further interfere with healthy speech development. From a thorough evaluation, parents need to know the cause of the delay and whether their child is developing normally though slowly, aphasic, or retarded. They must also learn how to encourage the child without excessive pressuring that causes further discouragement. It is important to identify the deaf child who cannot receive the auditory stimuli needed to develop speech and the child with cerebral palsy whose problem is in the expressive area.

185

Developmental Articulation Disorder (315.39)

Developmental articulation disorders constitute a specific failure to develop and to articulate consistently the sibilants *(s, z, sh, zh, ch, ji)*. These are among the last sounds to be mastered, and lisping is defined as a persistence of this mispronunciation past age seven. Like baby-talk, lisping is at times considered cute and reinforced by adult encouragement and amusement. In younger children, lisping requires no intervention since spontaneous mastery of the sounds usually occurs, making speech therapy unnecessary. The incidence and social significance of lisping varies from culture to culture. Especially in adolescent boys, it tends to be associated with effeminacy, so that a short course in pronunciation may help avoid much teasing and rejection.

By definition, this disorder has no neurological or structural basis. The rest of language and other development is normal. The diagnosis, therefore, is made both from the circumscribed articulation deficit and by ruling out such other conditions as mental retardation, infantile autism, child psychosis, and hearing or visual defects.

Stuttering (307.00)

The term stuttering is usually used synonymously with stammering, although some authors (Barber 1954) reserve *stuttering* to describe repetitious speech, while using *stammering* to indicate speech with unusual hesitancy and pauses that disrupt the usual word flow. Both of these should be distinguished from *cluttering,* characteristically rapid, nervous speech in which the last part of the words or certain sounds or syllables are omitted in the pressure to produce the thought.

Epidemiology. About 1 percent of the population are stutterers, with the incidence somewhat higher in Europe (Silver 1980). In western cultures, stuttering is more common in ambitious, upwardly mobile families (Ingram 1959). Males are two to five times as frequently affected as females (Bloodstein 1969; West 1958), and there is often a family history in one or other parent or in a sibling (Ingram 1959). Though not uncommon in normal three-year-olds, stuttering at this age may cause disproportionate parental concern. Children who stutter often have associated reading and writing problems.

Description. Stuttering consists of interruptions of the flow of speech with blocking, repetition, and hesitations followed by explosive utterances and scanning. Confirmed stutters may grimace as they try to force speech or may utilize a number of mechanisms such as stamping the foot. Some of these may have been learned in speech therapy as alternatives and modifiers of the condition. Stuttering is made worse by pressure and by having to speak in public. Not infrequently, stutterers can carry on individual conversations but are unable to talk in front of a class. Four out of five stutterers recover spontaneously if free from pressure, but if the condition persists, stuttering deserves intensive systematic training to desensitize the stutterer to the anxiety-provoking situations that precipitate and perpetuate it (Shames 1968).

An important side effect of stuttering is the discomfort it arouses in those who hear it. Stuttering has, therefore, been considered a hostile, controlling, and aggressive maneuver to challenge the hearer to produce the word at a stage when the empathy originally evoked by the difficulty has turned to discomfort, frustration, or even rejection. During the school year, mocking peers and classmates may produce considerable stigmatization, undermining self-confidence and socialization (Shames 1968).

Etiology. Various theories have been advanced as to the cause of stuttering. Earlier it was ascribed to mixed laterality and cerebral dominance, or even to a miniature epileptic seizure (West 1958), although the evidence for the latter is tenuous. Psychogenic theories have related stuttering to obsessive-compulsive mechanisms and battles for family control, while psychoanalysts have implicated the oral-sadistic and anal-sadistic stages of development.

Management. Since no form of therapy has produced convincing results, multiple methods have been used, including various forms of speech therapy (distraction, teaching sing-song intonation and repetition of monotone syllables, delayed playback of speech), suggestion (hypnosis), and relaxation therapies. All have produced some temporary remissions, but the results are often short-lived. Classical psychotherapy or psychoanalysis have also been used with, at best, indifferent results. The psychotherapies are more helpful in diminishing secondary social and emotional consequences than in modifying the stuttering itself. More modern treatments are based on learning theory. They attempt, through desensitizing the patient to the stuttering, to modify both the stutter and the associated behaviors by teaching the stutterer to monitor and control the air flow. Supportive intervention to diminish secondary social consequences can be a useful adjunct (Shames 1968).

4. Elective Mutism (313.23)

Elective mutism is a persistent refusal to speak in certain social situations despite a clearly demonstrated ability to comprehend and talk in others. Typically the child refuses to talk—for example, at school—while continuing to talk freely at home, or the converse. Electively mute children have normal language skills, though speech development and articulation may be somewhat delayed. Elective mutism, however, is not related to these delays, as is shown by the clear contrast between child's ability to speak in one situation and the refusal to do so in another.

Epidemiology, Course, and Associated Conditions. This is a relatively rare condition with no associated family history, apparently more frequent in girls than boys. One study (Bradley and Sloman 1975) found elective mutism appeared predominantly in children of immigrant families, being diagnosed during the first year of school. Associated psychological or developmental problems such as enuresis, excessive shyness, school refusal, temper tantrums—in other words, controlling or oppositional behavior—are common (Hayden 1980). In general, the mutism is of brief duration and self-limiting, but it can lead to scapegoating and labeling in school. The diagnosis is used only when other causes of speech problems and major psychiatric disorders have been excluded.

Management. Treatments attempted have included a variety of psychotherapies aimed at decreasing the child's need to struggle for control with adults and at improving the child's self-esteem. Combined with speech therapy, this yields mixed results. Not frequently, the mutism may be the last remnant of a major disturbance, most of which has responded to treatment. Rarely, in such cases, the induction of speech under hypnosis in the situation in which it is normally avoided may allow the child to give up this at least partially self-imposed ban on communication.

STEREOTYPED MOVEMENT DISORDERS

In DSM-III, a number of disorders featuring a dysregulation of gross motor movement were grouped together under the rubric of stereotyped movement disorders. They include acute and chronic tic disorders, Gilles de la Tourette syndrome, and other stereotyped movement behaviors such as head banging and rocking.

Tic Disorders (307.21; 307.22; 307.20)

Tic disorders have been divided into *transient* and *chronic,* but both groups are very similar except for duration. Tics are recurrent, repetitive, rapid, apparently purposeless movements affecting primarily the head and face and, in decreasing frequency and descending anatomical order, the arms, body, respiratory and alimentary systems. By concentrating on controlling them, the sufferer may be able to voluntarily suppress them for a while, but inevitably the concentration lapses and the tic returns. Arbitrarily, any tic disorder lasting for at least one month is defined as acute, while those persisting beyond one year are reclassified as chronic (according to DSM-III).

Epidemiology. Many normal children experience transient ticlike movements, which commonly appear between the ages of seven to ten. Some studies have suggested a prevalence as high as 23 percent of the total child population (Kanner 1972), but Rutter, in his studies on the Isle of Wight, found an incidence of less than 1 percent (Rutter, Tizard, and Whitmore 1970). Tic disorders are approximately three times as common in boys (Silver 1980), and there is often a family history (Golden 1978).

Etiology. The etiology of tic disorders has shifted away from earlier, basically psychogenic formulations following substantial evidence that tics may be secondary to organic difficulties. Their frequency and severity are exaggerated in response to anxiety and excitement, and they decrease when the child is distracted or involved and disappear during sleep. This led to the theory that tics discharge diffuse anxiety or are remnants of specific, once-meaningful actions whose original purpose has over time been lost leaving only the tics, now disassociated from their original stimulus and meaning. Recent reports of tics as a side effect of methylphenidate and of relatively low dosages of dopaminergic agents (Esman 1977) support an organic or biochemical origin (Denckla, Bemporad, and MacKay 1976). (See chapter 29.)

Differential Diagnosis. A number of conditions should be ruled out before diagnosing a tic disorder. The principal differentiation is from Gilles de la Tourette's syndrome (see below), which is characterized primarily by the presence of vocal tics and coprolalia. Various forms of chorea also feature purposeless activities, but careful observation easily distinguishes these from tics. Sydenham's chorea, a neurological sequel to rheumatic fever, produces writhing or choreiform movements of the muscles of the extremities, face, and trunk, along with lowered muscle tone and emotional lability. Huntington's chorea is a progressive, genetically transmitted, familial, neurological degeneration with an eventually fatal outcome that affects only males but is transmitted by females. Myoclonic seizures are sudden, twitching movements of various muscle groups and are distinguishable from tics by electromyography (Silver 1980).

Management. Management has varied with the postulated etiology and has shifted from psychotherapeutically oriented to psychopharmacological treatments as evidence of the major neurological component to the etiology has accumulated. Some psychological intervention with child and family is still justified in motivated cases, however, to minimize the disruption of the child's normal development and to moderate the disproportionate concern, resentment, hostility, and intervention of other family members. Various family and behavioral interventions have been used to demonstrate to the patient the effect of the tic on relationships with others and its relationship to intrapsychic conflicts. One form of behavior therapy, using the principle of negative practice, has the child deliberately repeat the tic as fast as possible for brief periods of time, interspersing these with rest periods. This is in order to help the child gain control over what once was automatic behavior (Yates 1958). Work with the family is directed toward minimizing pressures on the child and reducing other sources of family tension that aggravate the tic.

Chronic motor tic disorders are much less common than the acute disorder and probably less frequent than Gilles de la Tourette's disease, though the actual incidence is unclear. Follow-up studies suggest that only approximately 5 percent continue to have significant, though not disabling, tics while the majority are either symptom free or show only very minor residual tics by midadolescence. Psychotherapy for children with chronic tics probably helps most by bolstering the child's self-esteem and decreasing family pressure and rejection in the face of a troublesome symptom until natural remission occurs. In both transient and chronic tic disorders, some children are helped by haloperidol (Barker 1975).

Gilles de la Tourette's Disorder (307.23)

The principal features of this syndrome are the presence of multiple tics, at least initially somewhat progressive and including, in 60 percent of those affected, the pathognomonic but not essential feature of vocal tics and coprolalia (Eisenberg, Ascher, and Kanner 1959).

Epidemiology. The frequency of this syndrome, regarded as a rarity until the last fifteen years, cannot be accurately assessed. With increasing attention, however, the number of cases diagnosed has increased so markedly that several large studies are currently under way. The diagnosis should be made with great care, as the syndrome implies an irreversible and lifelong illness. If untreated, the symptoms persist, undermining self-esteem and causing alienation from family and peers as common complications. Despite earlier reports suggesting intellectual deterioration, more recent studies indicate that, if anything, those affected have above average intelligence (Eisenberg, Ascher, and Kanner 1959).

As with the other stereotyped movement disorders, there is continuing disagreement between psychological and somatic theories of causation of Gilles de la Tourette's disorder. Recently there is an increased weighting of neurological factors as the primary condition, while much of the reported psychological and family pathology is considered reactive to the organic syndrome. Although individual case studies have reported underlying psychotic processes or severe neurotic character traits, recent large-scale surveys fail to confirm a significant association with major mental illness, and there has been no recent evidence of a specific personality type associated with the disorder (Golden 1979; Silver 1980). A higher than normal frequency of hard or soft neurological signs (Golden 1979), abnormal electroencephalogram findings, scores on the Bender Gestalt Test in the organic range (Silver 1980), and a greater proportion of left-handedness all indicate the role of organic factors. The clear response to haloperidol is evidence that the defect lies in the dopaminergic pathways (Brunn et al. 1976; Feinberg and Carroll 1979; Golden 1978).

The differential diagnosis includes the other stereotyped movement disorders. Assessment requires a careful history and a thorough neurological examination to rule out possible associated brain dysfunction.

Like many chronic conditions in which traditional approaches seemed equally limited, many treatments have been tried for Tourette's disease without significant effect. At present, the treatment of choice is the administration of haloperidol, with pimozide as an almost equally effective alternative (Brunn et al. 1976; Feinberg and Carroll 1979). This may be augmented by psychotherapy to help the patient maintain or rebuild self-esteem and to increase family acceptance. A self-help group of families of patients with Tourette's disease does exist and can be very supportive to families prepared to meet with others struggling to overcome the social stigma imposed by the condition. The dosage and side effects of haloperidol are discussed in chapter 29.

Head Banging (307.30)

Head banging may occur in normal children but can also be associated with various serious conditions. Beginning early, at about the time when voluntary movement of the head and trunk becomes possible, it may persist throughout the preschool years as repetitive, rhythmic banging of the head against the sides of the crib or other objects by a child who usually does not otherwise appear distressed. Silberstein has tried to distinguish between head banging of an autoerotic nature and that which occurs during temper tantrums (Silberstein, Blackman, and Mandell 1966). In autoerotic head banging, the child persists in a vigorous, noisy, and at times alarming fashion until exhaustion and sleep terminate the behavior. Such head banging occurs more frequently in severely deprived children, particularly those suffering from hospitalism, and is often accompanied by other self-stimulating habits such as rocking, trichotillomania, (hair pulling), pica, or thumb sucking. On the other hand, temper-tantrum head banging typically begins later as part of the diffuse and violent explosion of rage characteristic of tantrum behavior. More frequent in retarded children, head banging has been related to their delay in motor development and their ability to adjust. One should consider mental retardation or other severe developmental disorders in the differential diagnosis, being careful to rule out infantile autism and schizophrenia.

Management. There are basically two treatment approaches. One, addressed to the hypothesized lack of maternal stimulation, attempts to encourage the mother or caregiver to be more responsive to the child, although the factors causing the original deprivation may make this difficult to achieve (Silberstein, Blackman, and Mandell 1966). Alternative interventions geared toward protecting the child during episodes of head banging include cushioning the crib bars or having the child wear a helmet for protection until the symptom disappears, which it usually does. Where the head banging complicates severe mental retardation, behavior modification may help minimize this often potentially self-destructive behavior.

Rocking

Rocking, which appears somewhat later than head banging, consists of a rhythmic back-and-forth swaying of the trunk, usually with the child in a sitting position, particularly at night. It may be sufficiently violent to move the crib across the room. While rocking can occur in normal children, marked rocking is more common in those who are retarded, severely deprived, or developmentally delayed. Frequently rocking follows or occurs simultaneously with head banging (Broughton 1968). It is postulated that these activities are pleasurable and tension relieving, and they may accompany autoerotic activities.

Rocking rarely requires treatment. Intervention, if indicated, is more for an underlying disorder of which rocking is but a symptom. However, in 1949 Lourie postulated that the rhythm of both rocking and head banging was determined by that of the heart and with some success introduced an alternative metronomic stimulus. Others have tried to provide an alternative source of rhythmic satisfaction such as a rocking horse, swings, and so on.

MISCELLANEOUS DEVELOPMENTAL DISORDERS

Nail Biting, Thumb Sucking, and Finger Sucking

These symptoms are so common that many, if not most children, show them at some point in their development. Their consequences are entirely innocuous, although thumb sucking has been implicated as potentially damaging to proper dental alignment.

Thumb sucking is basically a comfort mechanism that usually disappears either before, or just after, school entry. Painting the thumb with noxious substances rarely helps, as children learn to like even something as bitter as aloes. Usually, when they have outgrown the need for it, they gradually give up the habit, although even up to age ten to twelve it may recur during television watching or just before or early in sleep.

Some *nail biting* occurs in up to 40 percent of children between ages five and eighteen. While sometimes seen as early as one year of age, the incidence peaks in boys at age twelve to thirteen and in girls at age nine (Malone and Massler 1952). Nail biting is usually a simple tension-associated mechanism occurring in anxious and fidgety children. Only severe cases require investigation, and for parents who remain concerned, intervention with child and family is directed toward relieving the underlying tension (MacFarlane, Allen, and Honzik 1962). The amount of nail biting itself is an inaccurate indicator either of the need for, or of the progress of, therapy. A program of systematic, positive reinforcement for controlling the habit proves successful in some children. A significant number of high-pressure, achievement-oriented adults continue to bite their nails.

Breath-Holding Spells

These extremely alarming attacks can occur in children as young as six months, though they are more usual between the ages of one and five. A typical attack follows some precipitating event such as an injury, prohibition, or punishment that sets off brief but intense crying, followed by breath holding. The child may appear cyanotic, with generalized rigidity or opisthotonos and impaired consciousness, with or without tetanic convulsive movements. Because of the similarity to epileptic seizures, epilepsy is the main condition to be ruled out in the diagnosis. (See chapter 11.) Clinical features that may distinguish between the two include the facts that: breath-holding attacks have an obvious precipitant that is absent in epileptic seizures; crying precedes breath holding but rarely precedes a seizure; and opisthotonos and cyanosis appear *during* the breath holding rather than after, as in epileptic seizures (Livingstone, Pauli, and Pruce 1980). The diagnosis can be confirmed by the presence, in epileptics, of significant abnormalities in the EEG that are usually absent in breath holders.

Breath-holding attacks, fortunately, are self-limiting, as the breathing automatically resumes after loss of consciousness, leading to rapid recovery. The importance of breath-holding spells lies in their power to evoke such alarm in parents that they can become extremely overindulgent to avoid any conflict that might precipitate an attack. This rewards the breath holding, making it a potent form of emotional blackmail (Bakwin and Bakwin 1972).

Temper Tantrums

Tantrums are even more frequent in young children than breath holding, although the two are often associated. In response to frustration, limits, or controls the child shouts, screams, and lies kicking and thrashing on the ground. Tantrums can occur at home or in public, where they are even more embarrassing to parents. Tantrums are frequently attempts by children to force parents to give them what they want, though, if frequent, they may also indicate a stubbornly persistent temperament in a constitutionally strong-willed and demanding child. In later life the same persistence that frequently leads to tantrums when frustrated as a child can, if constructively redirected, contribute greatly to competence and successful achievement.

While, like breath-holding spells, tantrums themselves are unimportant, they may prove an effective weapon in the battle for control of the family. Punishing a screaming child who is out of control is more likely to provoke than to shock the child out of a well-established temper tantrum. Argument or discussion at the height of a tantrum are similarly useless (Bakwin and Bakwin 1972). If necessary, the child should be held to avoid injury to self, others, or the surroundings and should be bodily removed from the situation with minimal interaction. Systematic periods of "time out" where the child is isolated in response to a misdemeanor can prove particularly effective by depriving the child of the reinforcing attention, anxiety, or other reaction that the tantrums produce. Parents should be reassured that by being firm and taking charge early in the tantrum they are providing the control and security of which the child, at the moment, is incapable. Discussions of issues should occur after, rather than during, a tantrum. Ideally, tantrums should get neither a positive nor a negative reaction, since either can reinforce the behavior. Specific causes or precipitants should be identified and avoided wherever possible, as long as in doing so the parents are not being blackmailed into making inappropriate "special" provisions for the child. The management, then, is to discourage the disruptive component without breaking the spirit and persistence that lie beneath it.

Masturbation

Masturbation is frequent even in young children, some of whom may even experience orgasm. In itself, masturbation is almost universal, at least in adolescent boys, has no clinical significance, and is not correlated with any pathology or aberrant sexual behavior in later life, traditional myths to the contrary. It has no effect on health, growth, or later development. For that reason parents should be advised to ignore it or, at the most, induce gradually in the child a sense of where to conduct it without incurring negative reactions. Masturbation only becomes a concern when child or parents are preoccupied with it, or if the child fails to develop a normal sense of sexual privacy (Bakwin and Bakwin 1972). On these occasions, when a major part of the time is spent in public masturbation and other autoerotic activities, an investigation to rule out the possibility of a pervasive developmental disorder or serious environmental deprivation is indicated. Failure to develop a normal sense of privacy may lead one to investigate why modesty, which usually increases during middle childhood, is not present. Parents' preoccupation with their child's masturbation, except under the rare, potentially pathological conditions just described, is more likely to result from a problem in the parents than one in the child, though continued exposure to excessive parental involvement in what should remain the child's business may secondarily cause excessive guilt or overstimulation. Other exploratory sexual activities, such as inspection of each other's genitals and mutual exhibition and sex play, either heterosexual or homosexual, with peers or siblings, are common in children and early adolescents. Again, like masturbation, they represent normal curiosity and responses to stimulation. They require no outside intervention unless they become a major preoccupation, or unless the child is obsessed by guilt because of them. For all these activities, reassurance and some instruction on the normality of exploratory behavior may be much needed by parents who become disproportionately concerned because of their own sexual concerns or family or religious beliefs. In such cases it is the compulsivity of the parental overinvolvement or the associated guilt in the child, not the sexual activity per se, that is significant enough to merit investigation.

Atypical Gender Role Behavior

As early as age three, some children begin to show behavior and interests more typical of the opposite sex. If of brief duration or limited extent, these behaviors may be insignificant and are usually discouraged by most parents. However, persistent cross-sex behaviors, including toy and clothing choice and peer preference, when accompanied by wishes to belong to the opposite sex, may presage a later homosexual orientation or even a transsexual outcome (Green 1980).

Despite the fact that gender-disordered children often manifest cross-sex behaviors as early as parents can recall, such children tend to be referred only sometime after starting school. The motivation to seek help may result from teacher pressure, name calling from peers—effeminate boys suffer more intense peer rejection than do tomboyish girls—or from the parents' growing realization that the child is not outgrowing the behavior.

In addition to preferring female peers, effeminate boys are frequently frightened by the rough and tumble that they associate with male peer activities. This difficulty in establishing relationships with male peers, if persistent, may lead to further social ostracism, as with time these children tend to be isolated from the female peer group as well. Although the overt feminine behaviors may decline with age, if untreated, these boys tend to retain some female mannerisms that feed into their being labeled "faggots" by their peers.

Tomboyish behavior in girls usually has a more benign course. Most tomboys outgrow their intense cross-sex behaviors as they move into adolescence. In addition, they seldom experience peer rejection. These two factors may account for the lower incidence of either a transsexual or homosexual outcome as compared to effeminate boys. Discriminating factors that may point to a less normative outcome are not well understood, but possibly consist of a more intense, longstanding cross-sex orientation with more marked cross-sex wishes.

Etiological factors are not well understood. Currently, despite efforts to uncover biological factors, such as hormonal and neuroendocrine differences, psychological factors in early childhood are still hypothesized as most important.

Treatment of the gender-identity disorders includes a combination of individual psychotherapy for the child with accompanying parental involvement. Therapy attempts to help the child identify with and adopt the features of the biological sex, particularly through encouraging more successful involvement with and modeling on the same-sex parent (Rekers et al. 1977). Behavior modification has been used to extinguish effeminate mannerisms in boys or masculine mannerisms in girls in order to decrease their rejection by the same-sex peer group. The aim of these efforts is to reduce the child's alienation and social distress while improving the child's self-esteem. The long-range effects of such intervention on the subsequent orientation remain to be determined (Green 1979).

SUGGESTIONS FOR FURTHER READING

ANTHONY, E. J. 1957. An experimental approach to the psychopathology of childhood: Encopresis. *Brit. Med. J.* 30:146–175.
A classic article in the field outlining the difference between the three types of encopretic children in his clinical experience. Toilet training, maternal attitude, and environmental effects are all discussed, along with recommendations for treatment.

BROUGHTON, R. J. 1968. Sleep disorders: Disorders of arousal? *Science* 159:1070–1078.
The first in-depth electroencephalogram study of sleep disorders, examining the disruption of sleep patterns now associated with nocturnal enuresis, nightmares, night terrors, and somnambulism. Broughton also gives a detailed description of a typical attack of each of those disorders.

EISENBERG, L.; ASCHER E.; AND KANNER L. 1959. A clinical study of Gilles de la Tourette's disease in children. *Am. J. Psychiat.* 115:715–723.
A well-written article that contains seven extremely well documented case reports. Birth history, childhood events, milestones, disease history, and family environment are all examined.

GOLDEN, G. S. 1979. Tics and Tourette syndrome. *Hosp. Prac.* November 14, pp. 91–100.
A very good article that gives a useful basic insight into the nature of the stereotyped movement disorders. Phenomenology is reported in detail, and through examination of several factors, Golden concludes that some organic cause is always present.

GREEN, R. 1975. The significance of feminine behavior in boys. *J. Child Psychol. & Psychiat.* 16:341–344.
The most general of Green's recent articles, which examines previous studies of feminine boys and the treatments tried in an effort to determine the effectiveness of current treatment procedures in changing the sexual orientation of these boys. Green states that the problem may be in the direction of the treatment and not in the difficulty of the problem.

KALES, A., AND KALES, J. D. 1974. Sleep disorders: Recent findings in the diagnosis and treatment of disturbed sleep." *N. E. J. Med.* 290:487–497.
In this definitive overview article, Kales and Kales not only concern themselves with the usual sleep disorders (somnambulism, night terrors, enuresis) but also with narcolepsy, hypersomnia, insomnia, pregnancy, drug withdrawal, duodenal ulcer, coronary artery disease, asthma, and hyper/hypothyroidism).

LEBOVITZ, P. S. 1972. Feminine behavior in boys: Aspects of its outcome. *Am. J. Psychiat.* 123:1283–1289.
A study of fifteen men who were formerly judged to be "feminine" as boys. The average age of the study was 21.5 years. Subjects were questioned with respect to history of the problem, current sexual orientation, and attitude toward parents. One of the better studies of this kind.

RAPOPORT, J. L., ET AL. 1980. Childhood enuresis. *Arch. Gen. Psychiat.* 37:1146–1152.
A double-blind crossover study designed to measure the effectiveness of imipremine hydrochloride, desipramine hydrochloride, and methscopolamine on enuresis. All subjects were tried on placebo in order to ascertain presence/absence of placebo effect. Out of forty, twenty-three boys were successfully treated using the results of the study.

SHAMES, G. H. 1968. Dysfluency and stuttering. *Pediatr. Clin. N. Am.* 15:691–704.
A fairly standard but comprehensive treatment of the most common speech disorders. Shames outlines the boundaries of normal development and stresses the importance of assessing the effect of environmental factors before proceeding with treatment.

10

Klaus Minde

Disorders of Attention

Introduction

During the past two decades, hyperactivity, or attention deficit disorder (ADD) as it has been named in DSM-III, has become probably the most commonly diagnosed disorder in childhood (Freeman 1976), with 5 to 12 percent of all school-aged boys in the United States so considered (Miller, Palkes, and Stewart 1973). While initially described in North America, more recent studies have shown it occurring commonly in such diverse countries as Germany, New Zealand, and Uganda (Minde and Cohen 1978; Sprague, Cohen, and Eichlseder 1977). Investigators of attention deficit disorder have produced hundreds of scientific papers about the syndrome and done much to describe its phenomenology, natural history, and treatment. This chapter will examine primarily those clinical aspects of hyperactivity relevant to the practicing health professional. It will discuss definitions of the term, describe the clinical picture and its outcome, and present current approaches to etiology and treatment.

DEFINITION AND COMPARISON OF TERMINOLOGIES

During the past ten to fifteen years the diagnostic labels "hyperactive" or "hyperkinetic" have been applied to an increasing number of children whose behavior is characterized by developmentally inappropriate excessive motor movements, attentional problems, poor impulse control, and a decreased ability to inhibit emotional responses. At the same time, a variety of other labels such as minimal brain damage (MBD), minimal brain dysfunction, and minimal cerebral dysfunction have been widely used in the diagnosis of this complex of symptoms. The latter terms suggest that

197

hyperkinesis is associated with damage, albeit minimal, to the brain. This has not yet been documented (Werry and Sprague 1972), and since many children who are called hyperactive do, in fact, exhibit other behavioral difficulties in addition to the motor restlessness and poor concentration, the whole entity of the hyperkinetic syndrome or ADD has been questioned by a number of experienced clinicians and researchers (Sandberg, Rutter, and Taylor 1978; Schachar, Rutter, and Smith 1981). In addition, the great variation in children labeled hyperactive by different authors has made the comparison of research findings difficult. Because of these difficulties of definition and the increasing evidence that the term hyperactive may subsume a number of clinically similar yet distinct entities, this chapter will use the term attention deficit disorder. Many of the studies reviewed, however, have been based on samples whose clinical manifestations were diverse and inadequately defined.

HISTORICAL PERSPECTIVE

A description compatible with our current knowledge of ADD appears in the German physician Heinrich Hoffmann's children's story, "Der Struwwelpeter," published in 1854, one of whose main characters, der Zappelphilip, could not sit still at the table and showed many other features characteristic of a youngster with ADD.

Children described as "restless ... irritable ... disobedient ... emotionally quite unstable" were next reported by Hohman (1922), who examined children after recovery from the acute phase of von Economo's encephalitis. Other authors (Blau 1936; Kasanin 1929; Strecker and Ebaugh 1924) described a similar picture in children following recovery from head injuries.

The autonomy of ADD as a syndrome was not suggested until 1937, when C. Bradley accidentally discovered the therapeutic usefulness of dextroamphetamine in calming children. Bradley had originally used the drug for its sympathomimetic effects to ease the headaches of children who had undergone what were then routine pneumoencephalograms performed on almost all patients entering his hospital. To his surprise, the drug also calmed the behavior of a great many children who displayed those symptoms currently associated with ADD, thus focusing attention on a possible common etiology of the disorder. However, follow-up studies of these same children (Bradley 1957; Laufer and Denhoff 1957) suggested that the syndrome constituted a separate clinical entity, leading to a more detailed investigation of its etiology, course, and treatment.

Apart from these trends in medical research, a number of social changes focused attention on the ADD child. Beginning in the late 1950s, public education services for children with behavior and learning difficulties began in earnest in North America and Europe (Dunn 1973). In addition, newly developed psychotropic drugs such as the phenothiazines seemed to help substantially many severely emotionally and educationally handicapped children and adults, thus promising for many an equal chance to grow and develop according to their basic abilities (Minde and Cohen 1977).

The initial enthusiasm for treating ADD with drugs has been followed by a more sober reassessment of pediatric psychopharmacology because of the apparently excessive use of stimulants in children (Sprague and Sleator 1973; Walker 1975). Such a reassessment was also prompted by follow-up studies that failed to demonstrate any long-term benefit of medication on the behavior and educational achievement of emotionally disturbed and specifically on ADD children (Gittelman-Klein and Klein 1976; Menkes, Rowe, and Menkes 1967; Rie et al. 1976; Weiss et al. 1975).

CLINICAL PICTURE

It is convenient to divide the manifestations of ADD into essential or primary symptoms and associated or secondary symptoms. Primary symptoms are those that must be present to make the diagnosis, while secondary symptoms are commonly associated features.

Essential (Primary) Symptoms

The first essential feature of ADD is the child's *inability to maintain attention.* In school these children are described as having a short attention span, as being distractible, disorganized, and inattentive. At home attentional problems are characterized by a failure to follow through on parental requests and instructions or by the inability to engage in activities, including play, for periods of time appropriate for the child's age. Clinically inattention to appropriate stimuli both at home and at school may at times be labeled "daydreaming."

However, it is important to realize that the behavior of ADD children is quite variable. Typically symptoms fluctuate from time to time and from situation to situation, and variable and inconsistent functioning is a common characteristic. Thus a child's behavior may be well organized and appropriate on a one-to-one basis or in specific tasks or activities but disorganized when in a group or at school. Likewise, difficulties may emerge only in school, while home adjustment is generally satisfactory.

The other essential feature of children with ADD is their *poor ability to inhibit both motor and emotional impulses.* In practical terms, this results in a low frustration tolerance. They seem unable or unwilling to delay gratification; they give up quickly and rapidly become upset when things or people fail

199

to behave as they wish (Wender 1971). Their school work is performed sloppily and impulsively, with frequent, careless errors.

More recent work has understood this impulsivity somewhat more generally by suggesting that the major difficulty is the ADD child's inability to restrict behavior as the situation demands. This implies a general failure to develop self-control, so that both adults and peers see these children as disobedient and oppositional (Barkley 1978; Whalen and Henker 1976). For example, they are more likely than others to run off in several directions at once rather than to plan and organize their actions with foresight and judgment. This, in turn, is often interpreted by the environment as typical of a younger child and labeled "immature."

Another common feature of ADD is the *higher level of aimless activity* these children display. The overactivity is expressed both by gross motor (e.g., jumping, running, climbing) and minor motor (e.g., fidgeting) behavior. At home these children are often described as "always on the go" and as having difficulty sitting still. In school they are reported as fidgety, restless, overactive, and disruptive of others at play and at work. In young children hyperactivity shows an excessive gross motor activity such as running and climbing. In older children and adolescents the hyperactivity may express itself in general restlessness and fidgeting. The overactivity seems haphazard, poorly organized, and lacking a clear goal orientation. In situations where high levels of motor activity are expected and appropriate, such as during free play or in competitive sports, hyperactive children are indistinguishable from the average child.

A minority of children with ADD do not show excessive motor activity. Reliable statistics on the extent of this group are not currently available, but Anderson (1956) and Wender (1971) as well as the most recent classifications (DSM-III in the United States and the ninth revision of *International Statistical Classification of Diseases, Injuries and Causes of Death* in Britain [Rutter, Shaffer, and Shepherd 1975]) subdivide children with attention deficits into those with and those without excessive motor activity.

Associated (Secondary) Symptoms

About 50 percent of all children with ADD have *significant learning impairment* (Conners 1967; Langhorne et al. 1976; Minde et al. 1971; Safer and Allen, 1976). They do not achieve adequately in some or all school subjects despite adequate general intelligence. The reasons for this academic failure are considered related to two problems.

One reason for academic failure may be the difficulty all ADD children have in paying attention to the material presented by the teacher (Freibergs and Douglas 1969; Swanson and Kinsbourne 1976). Their lack of attention was initially thought to make them distractible, making it hard for them to shut out extraneous activity in the classroom and concentrate on the academic task at hand. More controlled studies of the psychophysiology of ADD and normal children (Hastings and Barkley 1978; Laufer and Denhoff 1957), however, found that in contrast to the formulations of clinical investigators, the ADD children are not overstimulated by their environment and/or deficient in inhibitory mechanisms. In contrast, these studies suggest that some ADD children are underaroused and attempt to optimize their level of stimulation by their excessive behavior and interactions with the environment (Rosenthal 1973; Satterfield and Dawson 1971; Zentall 1975). For example, studies comparing overstimulating environments to less stimulating ones have generally found that with increased stimulation, typical ADD behavior decreases (Gardner, Cromwell, and Foshie 1959; Zentall and Zentall 1976).

The definition of ADD, however, is not sufficiently clear cut to allow safe generalizations about this population. Hence one subgroup of these children may indeed show specific psychophysiological abnormalities characterized by underarousal, while others may not.

Another associated phenomenon of these youngsters' attention deficit is their particular learning style. Douglas and her students (1976) have documented that ADD children respond less to intermittent reinforcement and, at least in the laboratory, show more improvement in behavior and task performance in response to punishment than when given no feedback or positive reinforcement (Worland 1976). This knowledge cannot be applied within most schools, however, as reinforcement for appropriate behavior will always be irregular. Class size demands that a child remember good behavior as well as the academic material for some time without immediate reward.

Another reason for academic failure may be the fact that a relatively high number of ADD children (about 15 percent) also have a specific learning disability (Minde et al. 1971). In practice this means that the affected child can adequately perceive the learning material presented—there is no problem hearing, seeing, or touching—but the child has a problem processing information appropriately. The difficulty may be in retaining spoken words, sentences, or letters (auditory memory); deciphering sounds (auditory discrimination); or duplicating designs (visual motor integration). The child may also lack the visual memory needed to sequence letters to create specific words or to decode letters or words. (See chapter 17.)

This suggests that learning-disordered children should have more difficulty with subjects requiring abstract reasoning (e.g., history, literature, geography) than in mastering more concrete academic tasks, such as multiplication or rote reading. This has been confirmed by various studies (Minde et al. 1971; Prinz and Loney 1974). Prinz and Loney also documented that the tested IQs of ADD children did not differ from those of normal controls in grades 1 and 2 but was substantially lower by grade 6, suggesting that failure to learn and retain the academic material increasingly penalized these youngsters during their later school years.

It is obvious from the preceding text that the child with ADD has to cope with multiple handicaps. Some of these, such as the excessive motor movements, will be expressed directly as *behavioral difficulties*. Others, such as the attentional deficit, may occur primarily in specific situations, thus influencing key interpersonal relationships. These in turn will shape the child's later reactions to the world at large. Hence a particular child's behavioral difficulties may vary greatly depending, among other things, on the child's age and interaction with the surrounding milieu.

To understand the multiplicity of behavior difficulties associated with ADD, it helps to consider the behavior problems of such a child as resulting from a "poor fit" between the child and the important properties of his or her environment. This concept of the "goodness of fit" as a way to understand maladjustment, first elaborated by Henderson (1913) and further developed by Thomas and Chess (1977), holds that optimal development will occur if there is "consonance" between an individual's temperament, motivational patterns and abilities, and the expectations, demands, and opportunities of the environment. The "goodness of fit" model is particularly helpful in understanding behavior problems associated with ADD since it is not a homeostatic but a homeodynamic model—it has as its end result developmental change rather than the maintenance of an equilibrium. (See also chapter 1.)

In order to illustrate the relationship between various behavioral difficulties in ADD children and environmental influences at critical points in the developmental process, we will examine these difficulties in a developmental sequence, keeping in mind that the reaction or tolerance of the environment determines the child's response and even whether the diagnosis is ever considered.

Attention Deficit Disorder at Different Ages

INFANCY

About 60 percent of children diagnosed as having ADD in middle childhood have a history of extreme restlessness in early infancy (Stewart et al. 1966; Werry, Weiss, and Douglas 1964). They are often also described as colicky (Stewart et al. 1966) and averse to being cuddled (Brazelton 1961). Their motor development is typically somewhat accelerated, but both bowel and sphincter training and speech acquisition are delayed

(Schain and Reynard 1975). Despite the high percentage of young ADD children who have general developmental irregularities, only a few are referred to health professionals by their parents, presumably because of our society's belief that children have a right to run around and have fun without responsibilities. Also, parents of small unruly children are often made to feel responsible for their children's behavior by friends as well as professionals, so that they tend to blame themselves rather than examining the potentially deviant transactions between the child and the environment.

PRESCHOOL AGE

Preschool ADD children usually present far more serious management problems than infants because they are much more mobile, fearless, and seemingly unable to learn from experience (Stewart and Olds 1973). Parental complaints during this stage center on their children's incessant and aimless activity, now complicated by their ability to climb. They consequently have more accidents and poisonings than normal children (Stewart, Thach, and Freidin 1970) and need very intensive supervision (Ross and Ross 1976). They often need less sleep than their agemates and are prone to severe temper tantrums when frustrated or angry. Generally showing little concern for the feelings of others, they are often genuinely unaware when they have hurt another child. This may lead to their being shunned by other, calmer children, and it is during these preschool years that they often experience their first rejection by being excluded from nursery school or asked not to visit a neighbor's child. Nevertheless, the difficulties at this point still appear quite specific. For example, Schleifer and colleagues (1975) compared twenty-eight preschoolers with ADD to sixteen matched control children in a special nursery. During free play, the ADD children were socially and motorically indistinguishable from their normal peers. During structured periods in which the children were required to remain seated and participate in activities introduced by the teacher, however, the hyperactive children were more aggressive and spent more time out of their chairs doing irrelevant things. This lack of difference during free play between ADD and normal children has been confirmed by recent, more detailed observations by Cohen and associates (1981).

MIDDLE CHILDHOOD

Clinical descriptions and research on the school-age ADD child have shown that many children who fit the criteria of ADD during their preschool years continue to show attentional difficulties during their school years and that the disorder may now increasingly affect major aspects of the child's life (Campbell, Schleifer, and Weiss 1978; Cantwell, 1975*b*).

At home and in school, the children remain overactive, although at this age increasing opportunities for participation in sports and other organized activities can sometimes provide socially acceptable outlets for them. Other facets of the syndrome, however, make life more difficult at home. ADD children have rapid mood changes. They frequently rebel against any type of discipline and hence often precipitate arguments among and general unhappiness of family members. These struggles in turn often leave the children feeling guilty and wondering whether anyone can really like them despite their bad habits. They find it hard to talk about these feelings to anyone, since talk means reflecting on past events, which is not an easy task for them. They often become more stubborn, more antagonistic, and consequently more isolated and lonely. While some parents have the ability to understand their child's difficulty and to remain caring and sympathetic, both school authorities and peers often see only the nonperforming bully. Thus with ever-increasing academic difficulties, and ostracized by their peers and adults, many ADD school children are left socially isolated, often with a reputation for being a quitter or a poor sport (Stewart and Olds 1973). Others become more aggressive and the leaders of groups of younger peers (Minde 1976). In school, performance gradually drops because of the previously outlined lack of attention, impulsivity, and the need for consistent reinforcement, conditions usually not possible in the average school setting.

ADOLESCENCE

Early investigators considered ADD a time-limited condition that disappeared as the child grew older (Bakwin and Bakwin 1966; Eisenberg 1966). While the symptoms of hyperactivity do, indeed, diminish with age (Mendelson, Johnson, and Stewart 1971; Minde, Weiss, and Mendelson, 1972; Weiss et al. 1971), adolescent ADD children remain more active and impulsive than controls and can be identified by observers in the classroom (Minde et al. 1971). Behaviorally, too, things remain difficult. In the most detailed follow-up to date (Weiss et al. 1971), 70 percent of the mothers of sixty-four children with a mean age of thirteen years and average intelligence complained about their children's aggressivity, emotional immaturity, and poor academic functioning. Eighty percent of the children had repeated at least one school grade, 10 percent were in special classes, and only 5 percent were doing above average work. Thirty percent had no close friends, and 25 percent showed some antisocial behavior. Similar data were reported in several similar studies (Denhoff 1973; Huessy, Metoyer, and Townsend 1974; Mendelson, Johnson, and Stewart 1971), in which the parents described their ADD children as rebellious and disobedient, and 40 percent had seriously considered having them live away from home. These clinical studies all suggested that underneath their outward rebelliousness, these youngsters often feel terrible about themselves and that much of their acting-out is their attempt to cover up their underlying misery and depression. Recent experimental studies have confirmed that the self-esteem of ADD youngsters is significantly lower than that of peers (Hoy et al. 1978).

ADULTHOOD

There is suggestive evidence (Cantwell 1975a; Menkes, Rowe, and Menkes 1967) that links ADD in children with specific psychopathological conditions in adulthood, such as alcoholism in men and conversion disorders in women.

Etiology

There is still considerable controversy around the extent to which ADD is an autonomous child psychiatric diagnostic entity (Minde 1980; Schachar, Rutter, and Smith 1981). A number of studies using complex multivariate analyses have failed to find significant correlations between the symptoms of the presumed ADD syndrome (Langhorne et al. 1976; Routh and Roberts 1972; Werry 1968). Additionally, some researchers argue that no valid distinctions exist between ADD children and other children referred for treatment of conduct disorders. For example, Sandberg, Rutter, and Taylor (1978) demonstrated that children identified as ADD by the Conners Scale of Hyperactivity (1973) did not differ from a general sample of children referred to a child psychiatric clinic on symptoms denoting general aggressivity or other conduct problems. Thus despite much recent research emphasis, the specific etiology of ADD remains unclear.

ORGANIC FACTORS

The possible contribution of organic factors to ADD has been sought in brain lesions, genetic defects, biochemical imbalances, infections, poisoning, and minor neurological abnormalities. Historically, hyperactivity was first noted in children after brain injury or infection (Blau 1936; Strauss and Lehtinen 1947). This "organic" hypothesis of the etiology of ADD was supported by other studies associating it with a variety of viral infections (e.g., pertussis) and poisonings, especially of lead (David et al. 1977; Thurston, Middlekamp, and Mason 1955). Lately Cantwell (1972) has also examined adults with past histories of hyperactivity and claimed that ADD does not disappear in adulthood but simply changes its symptomatology. In contrast to Cantwell, whose data are based on retrospective accounts of disturbed adults, Weiss and her colleagues are continuing to examine the long-term outcome of this condition by following seventy-five children previously diagnosed as ADD for at least ten years through intensive interviews and psychological tests (Hechtman et al. 1976; Hopkins et al. 1979; Weiss, Hechtman, and Perlman 1978; Weiss et al. 1979). While not all their data have yet been analyzed, the following findings are becoming apparent. Few ADD young adults aged seventeen to twenty-four are seriously emotionally disturbed or chronic lawbreakers (Weiss et al. 1979). In fact, only 10 percent of the adults previously diagnosed as having ADD exhibited moderate or severe psychopathology. The clinic group had no more contacts with the police than the controls except for stealing and showed no difference in the nonmedical use of drugs (Hechtman et al. 1976). However, psychological test data confirmed that the cognitive style of these young adults was still more impulsive than reflective, and they perceived themselves as less able to relate to others, less happy, more tense, and more hyperactive than did their normal peers. They had also, on average, significantly more car accidents (1.3 vs. 0.5). Academically they continued to do less well up to the point of graduation and were less well liked and trusted by their teachers. However, the thirty-nine youngsters with full-time jobs at the time of the interview were rated by their employers as equally reliable and hard working as the controls. Whether the apparently good occupational functioning of these young adults primarily reflects the low demands of the jobs they held at that time in their lives and whether marital or parental role demands can be met adequately later will be determined only by future studies.

These data suggest that ADD loses much of its social stigma once formal education has stopped and real adult life has begun. They also show, however, that some form of attentional deficit continues and that the many social and academic failures of their early years have left their mark, in a damaged self-esteem (Hoy et al. 1978; Weiss et al. 1979) and unhappy memories of their childhood.

Other studies have tried to establish retrospectively an association between prematurity, prenatal and perinatal medical complications, and a variety of psychological behavioral and neurological abnormalities in children (Knobloch and Pasamanick 1966). While these studies indeed documented some statistical association between a compromised neonatal history and later behavioral disturbances, the absolute difference between the experimental and control groups was small (32 percent of the normal and 38 percent of the compromised births showed behavioral difficulties) and the samples were poorly matched for socioeconomic class. In a subsequent similar study carefully controlled for socioeconomic factors, no differences in the rate of birth complications were found (Minde, Webb, and Sykes 1968). While more recent follow-up studies of premature infants have also demonstrated that both learning disorders and hyperactivity are statistically somewhat more common in infants who at birth weigh significantly less than expected by their gestation (Fitzhardinge and Ramsey 1973), most such infants escape later pathology in spite of this increased risk.

Studies of neurologically heterogeneous groups of ADD children (Werry 1968; Werry et al. 1972) have repeatedly found that these children exhibit a higher number of so-called soft neurological signs. However, these soft signs, which include differences in lateral dexterity, fine motor coordination, and lateral thresholds to touch, have also been found in children with behavior disorders (Prechtl and Stemmer 1962), with learning difficulties (Hertzig, Bortner, and Birch 1969), and even in adult schizophrenics who showed premorbid asocial behavior (Quitkin, Rifkin, and Klein 1976). Moreover, there is as yet no clear-cut evidence that the soft signs are valid indicators of brain damage (Shaffer 1978).

Various researchers have reported an increased incidence of minor physical anomalies (MPA) in ADD children and have seen this as a possible pointer to organic problems (Rapoport and Quinn 1975; Waldrop and Goering 1971). Minor physical anomalies include such things as malformed ears, hypertelorism, variations in the lengths of fingers and toes, a high palate, or increased head circumference. More recent studies, however, showed that nonaffected siblings and parents of ADD and retarded children also had an abnormally high number of minor physical anomalies (Firestone et al. 1978; Quinn and Rapoport 1974). High anomaly scores have also been found in children with speech and hearing difficulties (Waldrop and Halverson 1971) and in those with learning difficulties (Rosenberg and Weller 1973). The nonspecificity of these findings makes the possible usefulness of an increase in MPA "markers" in the early detection of problem children extremely questionable.

The most specific formulation of a relationship between brain dysfunction and ADD comes from the work of Wender (1971), whose model is based partly on the quieting effect of amphetamines on ADD children. Wender suggests that various neurotransmitter systems within the brain, such as the dopamine system, may mature at different rates, thus causing an imbalance of excitative and inhibitory systems in the nervous system that, in turn, is responsible for the abnormal activity. While others have tried to confirm Wender's hypothesis using sophisticated studies (Satterfield and Braley 1977), no empirical support for his theory has so far been documented.

GENETIC FACTORS

The recognition that brain damage was not the major cause of most cases of ADD has stimulated research into other etiological factors. The high ratio of nine males to each female (Safer and Allen 1976) as well as the frequent history of other relatives who appeared to have been overactive during their early years suggested some genetic factor operative in the hyperkinetic syndrome.

Two controlled psychiatric studies of the biological parents of ADD children have been reported (Cantwell 1972; Morrison and Stewart 1971).

Both showed that more parents of ADD children reported symptoms compatible with ADD in their own childhood (16 percent for fathers, 5 percent for mothers respectively) than did the parents of the controls (2 percent for fathers, none for mothers). Thirteen percent of all male relatives combined showed the diagnosis. Furthermore, both studies revealed a higher than expected incidence of alcoholism (10 percent and 30 percent) and sociopathy (5 percent and 16 percent) in the fathers and of hysterical symptoms in the mothers (12 percent).

Two adoption studies by the same authors (Cantwell 1975a; Morrison and Stewart 1973) confirmed ADD much more frequently in the biological first- and second-degree relatives of ADD children than in those of adopted children. Similar data were reported in a study of the full and half siblings of seventeen hyperactive children that found ten of the full but only two of the twenty-two half siblings to show symptoms of ADD.

Twin studies, the traditional method for evaluating the role of genetic factors in any illness, have been limited in this condition. Lopez (1965) found that all four monozygotic twin pairs, but only one out of the six dizygotic pairs studied, were concordant for ADD. Since both same-sex and other-sex pairs were used in the dizygotic group, differences may be related to sex rather than zygocity. In another study (Willerman 1973), mothers of ninety-three sets of same-sex twins rated their children in the Werry-Weiss-Peters Activity Scale (Werry et al. 1970). By arbitrarily defining children scoring in the top 10 percent as hyperactive, Willerman derived a heritability estimate of 0.82 for boys and 0.58 for girls.

While the preceding data suggest that there is some evidence for genetic factors in ADD, it is important to recognize that the studies are suspect because the authors knew the group to which the children belonged while they conducted the investigation. In addition, as Cantwell (1976) points out in his review of genetic factors in ADD, one cannot generalize from one twin study to the general population, especially in a disorder that most likely includes a heterogeneous group of children.

ALLERGIES

Recently it has been suggested that artificial colors, flavors, or preservatives in food cause ADD-type behaviors (Feingold 1975). While few physicians have followed this idea, some uncontrolled studies have confirmed Feingold's thesis of ADD children's hypersensitivity to colors or additives (Crooke 1975). Feingold claims that food additives and salicylates may cross-react with each other to cause colic in infants and, later on, irritability, emotional liability, hyperactivity, and poor attention span. Even among those who believe that diet can cause ADD, differences of opinion are strong. For example, Crooke (1975) has blamed sensitivity primarily to common foods such as wheat, milk, corn, and eggs, while Levin (1978) considers sugar the most disturbing agent. While the dietary theory of hyperactivity has not been clearly proven so far (Conners et al. 1976), it is currently being investigated by a number of respected researchers (Swanson and Kinsbourne 1980; Williams et al. 1978).

Treatment

Children with ADD are multiply handicapped. They thus require a multi-focused treatment approach that may include pharmacological, educational, as well as psychological, remediation at different stages of development. While each form of treatment will be discussed separately, a combination of interventions may have to be developed to meet the needs of each individual child.

PHARMACOTHERAPY

Drug treatment is the easiest, least time-consuming, and most frequent intervention used in the treatment of ADD children. As pharmacotherapy in children is described at length in chapter 29, this aspect of the treatment will be discussed here only briefly. Drugs used to treat children with ADD have included the major tranquilizers (chlorpromazine, thioridazine), antidepressants (imipramine, amitriptyline), minor tranquilizers (diazepam), and lithium carbonate as well as the psychostimulants (dextroamphetamine and methylphenidate). Reviews of the voluminous literature on the subject are available (Barkley 1977; Gittelman-Klein 1975; Schain and Reynard 1975; Sroufe 1975; Whalen and Henker 1976).

While the placebo-controlled double-blind studies vary in methodology and results, they agree on the following points:

1. Psychostimulants are more effective than other pharmacological agents for ADD children.
2. Psychostimulants appear to influence two major aspects of behavior:
    (a) Cognitive behavior, especially selected measures of attention such as vigilance, choice reaction time, cognitive style, and concept learning (Baxley and Leblanc 1976; Douglas et al. 1976).
    (b) Social adaptive behavior, as measured by parent or teacher questionnaires (Sleator and Von Neumann 1974) or during direct behavioral observations.*
3. The effect of stimulants on the ADD child's test performance is very short-lived, peaking between one and two hours after administration and disappearing after four hours (Swanson et al. 1978). Changes in behavior follow a similar pattern (Rapoport et al. 1978).

*See Barkley and Cunningham 1979; Campbell 1975; Cohen et al. 1981; Humphries, Kinsbourne, and Swanson 1978; and Whalen et al. 1979.

4. Improvements in both cognitive tasks and on behavioural measures do not carry over once the drug is withdrawn (Swanson and Kinsbourne 1976). This is not surprising considering other studies of drug-dependent learning (Overton 1964), but it raises the issue of the long-term efficacy of stimulant therapy. While Swanson and Kinsbourne's theory of state-dependent learning in ADD children has not been confirmed in later studies (Steinhausen and Kreuzer 1981), Rapoport and associates (1978) have demonstrated that even optimally medicated children are not different in academic achievement and social acceptance from a group of dropouts from drug treatment. Weiss and her group, comparing sixty-six children—some treated with amphetamines, some with phenothiazines, and some untreated controls after five years on a number of academic and social variables—reported virtually identical results (Weiss et al. 1975; Weiss 1981). On the other hand, Sleator, Von Neumann, and Sprague (1974) found that 26 percent of their sample of methylphenidate-treated children functioned adequately when the stimulant was exchanged for placebo after two years.

5. There is dose specificity to the therapeutic benefit of psychostimulants. While some prescribe enormous doses of methylphenidate (e.g., up to 200 mg per day) (Millichap 1973), several authors (Sprague and Sleator 1973; Werry and Sprague 1974) found does of 0.5 milligrams per kilogram consistently superior to higher doses. These investigators contend that if the psychostimulant dosage is increased until improvement in social behavior is maximized, cognitive performance may actually deteriorate to levels below those obtained when children are given placebos. Swanson and colleagues (1978) also demonstrated that five patients receiving an average of 19 milligrams methylphenidate did worse on a paired associate learning task than when they received only 10 milligrams. Similar observations have been made by Barkley (1979), who observed that children receiving 1.0 milligrams per kilogram became increasingly withdrawn and preferred solitary to group play.

    The side effects experienced by some children taking stimulant medication encompass sleep and appetite disturbances (Conners 1971), sadness and withdrawal (Katz et al. 1975), an increase in heart rate and blood pressure (Aman and Werry 1975), as well as reversible growth retardation (Puig-Antich et al. 1978; Satterfield et al. 1979).

PSYCHOLOGICAL TREATMENT

Since drug treatment has not proven as beneficial as some have claimed in the past, the development of alternative treatment methods has been of interest to many clinicians. Individual psychotherapy as the sole method of treatment has been tried with ADD children but has not been successful (Cytryn, Gilbert, and Eisenberg 1960).

BEHAVIOR MODIFICATION

Operant conditioning has been evaluated in a number of well-designed studies on small numbers of hyperactive children. Jacob, O'Leary, and Price (1973) reported improvement following a three-month study of eight hyperactive children treated in ordinary classrooms by daily evaluations of problem behaviors by the teacher. Other studies using a similar design of rewarding specific behaviors such as "on-task" behavior and academic performance with sweets or money have also reported significant decreases in scores on the Conners Scale of Hyperactivity and in abnormal behavior (Ayllon, Layman, and Kandel 1975; O'Leary et al. 1976; Rosenbaum, O'Leary, and Jacob 1975).

Another approach to the treatment of ADD children has been directed toward modification of their impulsivity. The aim was to provide inattentive children with alternative strategies of problem solving by teaching them to slow down and think before they acted. Theoretical justification for this approach comes from the work of Meichenbaum and his colleague (Meichenbaum 1977; Meichenbaum and Goodman 1971), who used younger children's tendency toward self-verbalization as a technique by which older children might learn to curb their impulsivity and poor attention. Several studies using this method on school-age children have reported impressive changes in cognitive style (Douglas et al. 1976; Nelson and Birkimer 1978), although long-term follow-up data are not yet available. The technique is less useful in preschoolers (Cohen et al. 1981).

Investigations combining behavioral treatment with pharmacotherapy (Hohman 1922) have shown that the behavioral approach affects primarily academic performance while medication more clearly influences social behavior (Wolraich et al., 1978). More recently Mash and Delby (1979) have reported promising results in attempting to evaluate the effects of parent training programs on child management of ADD children.

The findings from behavior modification studies to date appear to suggest that: hyperactive children do show improved behavior during behavior modification treatment; these improvements are not associated with changes in academic performance unless the programs specifically focus on academic performance (Cunningham and Barkley 1978); and behavioral improvements, as a rule, do not generalize to nontreatment settings and are not maintained beyond termination unless parental counseling allows for a continuation of behavioral reinforcement at home.

DIETARY TREATMENT

Dietary treatment based on the hypothesis that ADD may be caused by food allergies has created much controversy among the public as well as within the scientific community. While many testimonials support Feingold's specifically designed K-P diet (Feingold 1975), the available scientific literature seems to indicate two main points.

First, most hyperactive children do not show dramatic improvement when placed on a diet free of additives. Improvements, when they occur, are more frequently seen by teachers than by parents (Conners et al. 1976; Williams et al. 1978).

Second, scientifically sound studies of additives are extremely difficult to carry out because of the uncertain adherence to the recommended diets and problems with the specificity of instruments measuring changes associated with the diet. The first difficulty is highlighted in a study in which all foods eaten by all family members of the forty-six children investigated were provided by the investigators for a ten-week period (Harley et al. 1978). This included the snacks for the entire school classes of the children involved. The second problem is highlighted by the results of Williams and associates (1978) and Levy and colleagues (1978), who failed to find behavioral changes after challenging their patients with food additives prepared by the Food and Drug Administration, while Swanson and Kinsbourne (1980) found clear-cut changes on a learning task following the same dietary manipulations. In the latter study, however, the children's learning deteriorated only when they were given 100 milligrams of the color blend, rather than the 26 milligrams initially suggested by the Nutrition Foundation (Lipton 1975) and administered by the groups of Williamson and Levy.

It appears that food additives are not inert substances and can impair learning. There is, however, currently no evidence that they "cause" ADD or that dietary restriction can "cure" it.

Summary and Conclusions

It is clear from the preceding text that ADD remains a syndrome whose clinical symptomatology, treatment, and final outcome still cause much controversy among both clinicians and researchers. The reasons for this continuing ambiguity seem clear. ADD, like many other syndromes associated with behavioral abnormalities, is determined by a complex transaction of numerous variables and thus defies any univariate model of a traditional medical disease. For this reason, future research in ADD, as in other areas of child psychiatry, will focus increasingly on delineating factors that will predict a positive response to drugs or to different types of behavioral management. For example, in their study of the 240 children, Loney and associates (1978) have suggested three predictors of response to medication. These were age at the time of referral, the retrospective maternal recollection of perinatal complications, and hyperactivity. Even in this large sample, only 25 percent of the variation in the children's responses to methylphenidate was predictable from their age at referral, degree of perinatal complications, and their score on a hyperactivity factor. In later work, Loney (1979) pointed out that aggressivity alone is the best predictor of later functioning in ADD children. Yet aggressivity often precedes ADD and results from specific ecological antecedents in the children's families. These may or may not coincide with those of ADD, again implying that much of the later behavior of ADD children may be related to early environmental factors (Loney 1979; Milich and Loney 1979).

Whalen and Henker (1980), writing on the social ecology of psychostimulant medication, have suggested that much of the poor predictability of outcome in these children may result from the way they were introduced to medication and to society's tolerance for medicating its members. While this introduces a far bigger sociological variable, at the same time it highlights some of the concerns expressed in criticisms of DSM-III and the decision of its authors to include in the classification conditions whose basic epidemiology is still largely unknown (Minde 1980; Rutter and Shaffer 1980).

In conclusion, it appears that ADD, while it has stimulated a great number of excellent investigations, has also illustrated the continuing tenuous knowledge base in the field and the complexity of human nature and development.

SUGGESTIONS FOR FURTHER READING

Barkley, R. A. 1981. *Hyperactive children: A handbook for diagnosis and treatment.* New York: Guilford Press.
A practical and up-to-date text to aid clinicians in diagnosing and treating hyperactivity. Stress and medication as well as behavior modification techniques are dealt with.

Cantwell, D. P. 1976. Genetic factors in the hyperkinetic syndrome. *J. Acad. Child Psychiat.* 15:214–223.
Clearly delineates the evidence for and against specific genetic factors operating in hyperkinetic children.

Douglas, V. I., et al. 1976. Assessment of a cognitive training program for hyperactive children. *J. Abnorm. Child Psychol.* 4:389–410.
A very well written article documenting the usefulness of cognitive training methods for some hyperactive school-aged children.

Loney, J., et al. 1978. Hyperkietic/aggressive boys in treatment: Predictors of clinical response to methylphenidate. *Am. J. Psychiat.* 135:1487–1491.
The most comprehensive article available, which attempts to assess what specific behavioral parameter will predict outcome at adolescence for hyperactive children.

Schleifer, M., et al. 1975. Hyperactivity in preschoolers and the effect of methylphenidate. *Am. J. Orthopsychiat.* 45:38–50.
The original article that demonstrates the diversity of the hyperactive syndrome. It documents that hyperactivity can be clearly diagnosed in preschool children and that hyperactive children vary a great deal, with some showing their behavior only in specific situations and others in almost every setting.

Stewart, M. A., and Olds, S. W. 1973. *Raising a hyperactive child.* New York: Harper & Row.
Provides an academically stimulating and humane description of scientific data and the clinical realities of raising a hyperactive child. It can be useful for both professionals and selected parents.

Rapoport, J. L., and Ferguson, H. B. 1981. Biological validation of the hyperkinetic syndrome. *Dev. Med. & Child Neurol.* 23:667–682.
Reviews all the evidence for and against the validity of this concept of attention deficit disorder. The authors conclude that there is currently no good evidence for the existence of the syndrome.

WEISS, G., et al. 1979. Hyperactives as young adults: A controlled prospective 10-year follow-up of the psychiatric status of 75 hyperactive children. *Arch. Gen. Psychiat.* 36:675–681.

The classic ten-year follow-up study of researchers in Montreal, following up hyperactive children to young adulthood.

WHALEN, C. K., AND HENKER, B. 1980. The social ecology of psychostimulant treatment: A model for conceptual and empirical analysis. In *Hyperactive children: The social ecology of identification and treatment,* ed. C. K. Whalen and B. Henker, pp. 3–51. New York: Academic Press.

Presents the best summary of ecological factors associated with hyperactivity. It examines the response of society to the syndrome and our attitude toward psychostimulant medication, and in that way provides a very cautionary note about the effects a new syndrome can have on medicine and society in general.

WOLRAICH, M., et al. 1978. Effects of methylphenidate alone and in combination with behavior modification procedures on the behavior and academic performance of hyperactive children. *J. Abnorm. Child Psychol.* 6:149–161.

Provides the best available evidence on how particular treatment methods such as behavior modification or psychostimulants affect specific areas of functioning of children with attention deficit disorder.

11

William Hawke and Douglas McGreal

Convulsive Disorders and Other Neurological Conditions Commonly Associated or Confused with Psychiatric Illness

Introduction

This chapter contains information about common neurological conditions frequently associated with emotional problems, neurological conditions that originally present as functional disorders, and common functional conditions that simulate organic disease.

The questions to be answered when assessing a child for a possible neurological problem are "Is there a lesion, and, if so, where and what is it?" The answer to the first part of the question is not always clear, and the interpretation of physical findings can be difficult. Much has been written about so-called soft neurological signs (Rutter 1977). The ones commonly seen include awkwardness and poor coordination, surplus movements of athetoid or choreic type, difficulty in rapid alternating movements of the hands, and poor finger localization. Psychiatrists and other professionals not trained in neurology often consider these soft signs as indicative of organic disease, but the trained observer can usually distinguish between the incoordination of the youngster who is merely clumsy and the early signs of a cerebellar tumor, the sensory inaccuracies stemming from lack of attention or delayed development and the learning problems based on an underlying organic process. Many children referred for psychiatric or educational assessment operate at the lower end of the normal range of neurological functioning. They often demonstrate mixed laterality, have delayed maturation patterns, or give a history of similar developmental characteristics in other family members. Recognition that these patterns do not indicate organic cerebral disease often clarifies the clinical picture and saves a great deal of unnecessary investigation (Livingston, Pauli, and Pruce 1980; Rutter 1977; Shapiro et al. 1978; Wender 1973).

Another area requiring care in interpretation is that of electroencephalography. There are considerable variations in the "normal" electroencephalogram (EEG) at different ages and under different physiological conditions, such as hunger and drowsiness. The response to hyperventilation may be considerable, depending on the enthusiasm with which the child breathes or the metabolic state, leading the unwary observer to class the response as unstable, epileptiform, or suggestive of an epileptic diathesis when, in fact, it is within the broad range of normal. If possible, it is wise to have the record read by an electroencephalographer who has wide experience reading children's EEGs in order to obtain an accurate diagnosis. (Bosaeus and Sellden 1979; Stevens, Sachdev, and Milstein 1968).

Neurological Disorders Commonly Associated with Emotional Problems

CONVULSIVE DISORDERS[*]

Changes in the state of consciousness, slight or significant, reflect changes in cerebral function and are a common reason for neurological assessment. Seizures are more common in children than in adults, and the clinical pattern determines the diagnosis.

One of the first questions asked is "Is this epilepsy?" The term epilepsy is reserved for paroxysmal, inappropriate discharges of impulse from some neurones, recurring at intervals and producing certain motor, sensory, or other changes in the child. Several clinical patterns are recognized. Howev-

[*]A comprehensive discussion of the neurological aspects of epilepsy can be found in O'Donohoe (1979) and Robb (1981).

er, not all "fits" or "seizures" are due to epilepsy. To be so diagnosed, they must be recurrent. Many children have seizures that disappear spontaneously with age. They are not considered epileptic, though the relationship of these seizures, usually associated with fever, to epilepsy is under active investigation. The term convulsive disorder is more appropriate for these cases, since it implies neither etiology nor prognosis.

Major seizures, or grand mal, are those in which the patient loses consciousness, falls to the floor, and may either be stiff or show rhythmic movements of the limbs. The eyes roll backward, and there may be cyanosis, vomiting, or incontinence. After a variable period of time, consciousness returns; the patient may be confused, have no memory of the seizure, have a headache, or fall into a deep sleep.

Partial seizures affect more restricted areas of function. They may or may not be associated with loss of consciousness or may develop into a major seizure. Movements observed may be simple, as in the face or limbs on one side, or complex, as when the patient shows organized movements that are uncontrolled and inappropriate. Speech and thought processes may be involved, and the patient may or may not retain some awareness of the events.

Minor seizures are more common in infants and children. The term includes seizures that consist of whole or partial body jerks, brief loss of muscle tone of the head or trunk, and other brief seizures that are not major or partial.

Absence attacks, or petit mal, are a separate form of minor seizure in which there is brief loss of awareness without loss of limb tone. The patient does not fall. The eyes may flicker, and there may be small movements of the hands or slight, jerking of the upper limbs. Petit mal attacks rarely last longer than twenty to thirty seconds, after which the patient resumes the previous activity, usually unaware that an attack has occurred. There may be urinary incontinence. Petit mal commonly develops at five to seven years of age and may be interpreted as daydreaming. It is associated with a particular abnormality on EEG and does not respond to the drugs usually used to treat other forms of epilepsy (O'Donohoe 1979).

Diagnosis of seizures, while usually depending on information available from the patient and eyewitnesses since doctors rarely see an attack, is usually not difficult. However, problems may arise particularly with the partial or minor types of seizure. The neuronal discharge that starts the focal seizure arises in an area of the brain that may have other functions—motor, sensory, or psychic. For example, a seizure originating in the motor strip will cause movements in the associated area of the opposite side of the body as the first sign; in the sensory area there will be numbness or tingling in the appropriate area; and the onset in other parts of the brain may cause loss of speech, inappropriate speech or behavior activity, visual or auditory hallucinations, or combinations of these.

Partial seizures arising from the temporal lobe often produce the behavior pattern known as a *psychomotor attack.* These are characteristically sudden in onset without any precipitating cause, involve complex motor activities often presenting the same pattern in each episode, and cease as suddenly as they began, often without the patient being aware that the attack has occurred. The classic example often quoted is the boy in school who suddenly rises from his desk, walks to the corner of the room, urinates in the wastepaper basket, and then returns to his seat—all without conscious knowledge of these activities. If these symptoms are not followed by an overt seizure, it may be difficult to decide whether the problem is primarily organic or psychological. EEG findings while the child is awake or asleep may be useful if they are abnormal, but they must always be correlated with the clinical symptoms. A normal EEG will by no means exclude an organic disorder. An even more confusing situation exists when the patient with a known seizure disorder has, in addition, episodes of apparently altered consciousness that are functional. Even the skilled observer assessing an EEG done during an attack may not provide a definite diagnosis. Patients with temporal lobe (psychomotor) seizures are more likely to display behavioral abnormalities in addition to true psychomotor attacks (Bear, 1979; Blumer 1979).

EMOTIONAL PROBLEMS COMMONLY FOUND IN CHILDREN WITH CONVULSIVE DISORDERS

In addition to those problems associated with any chronic disabling disease (see chapter 21), some specific problems accompany convulsive disorders (Ward and Bower 1978).

Problems Resulting Directly from the Disease Itself

Children suffering from convulsive disorders may exhibit episodes of peculiar behavior, spells of confusion associated with transient episodes of petit mal, or longer periods of confusion and abnormal behavior that can accompany petit mal status or temporal lobe seizures.

These children may show behavior commonly associated with organic brain damage, such as hyperactivity, impulsive and uncontrolled behavior, labile mood swings, and various educational difficulties due either to general limitation of ability or to specific learning disabilities (Rutter 1982; Stores 1978; Wender 1973).

In addition, epileptics may show behavioral syndromes resulting from focal damage to specific areas of the brain, as in the frontal lobe or temporal lobe syndromes. Children with frontal lobe syndromes behave much like lobotomized or senile patients, generally lacking concern about their environment or their personal appearance. They show diminished drive, poor judgment, impulsivity, and, often, disturbances in recently acquired cognitive function, as well as failure to appreciate the effect of their behavior on others. Children with a temporal lobe syndrome show patterns more like those of children prone to psychomotor attacks along with labile mood swings with impulsive, uncontrolled, and often extremely explosive behavior on minimal provocation. Impaired cognitive functioning is frequently evident in short- and long-term memory disturbances (Lindsay, Ounsted, and Richards 1979).

A number of children show behavior similar to that of a mentally retarded child. In some cases the retardation is considered primary, in that both the intellectual deficits and the behavior result from congenital or perinatal factors, while in others the retardation is secondary to the convulsive disturbance. Repeated severe convulsions can cause minute areas of cerebral hemorrhage and gliosis, which can cause intellectual deterioration. Another pattern, often called pseudoretardation, occurs when the child, though not retarded, appears so because of excessive medication.

Occasionally children with repeated, almost intractable temporal lobe seizures later develop behavior that can mimic psychotic disturbances such as schizophrenia (Kanner 1944; Kolvin et al. 1971; Miller 1975; Rutter 1981).

Problems Resulting from the Child's Reaction to the Disease

Children with convulsive disorders show many of the reactions to chronic handicap described in chapter 22. Those particularly common in these children include:

1. Anxiety over the possibility of an attack in school or on the street and worry about the future (e.g., marriage, work, etc.).
2. Feelings of being different from the other children in the neighborhood or family who do not have the limitations resulting from the convulsive disturbances.
3. Resentment, especially when they compare themselves to nonaffected siblings who are free both from the convulsions and from associated limitations.
4. In later years, increasing isolation and withdrawal from the community because of the attacks and the associated feelings of alienation.

Problems Resulting from the Family's Reaction to the Disease

While the general patterns of family responses to chronic illness are discussed in chapter 21, convulsive disorders commonly evoke anxiety over the future of the child, particularly concerning: education, marriage, and the possibility of employment; shame and embarrassment because their child has convulsive disturbances that are evident to friends and neighbors; guilt, if there is a family history of convulsive disturbances.

In addition, some extremely permissive and overprotective parents, are unable to provide the child with a convulsive disorder a suitable environment in which to develop. For example, some parents sleep even with the older child or adolescent. Others forbid children with convulsions to cross the street by themselves, while still others are unable to set and consistently follow through on limits, thus creating a behavioral Frankenstein.

Problems Resulting from the Medical Program

Problems resulting from the medical program are usually secondary to the amount of medication prescribed and the regimen on which the child is placed. Not infrequently, in order to control the convulsions the child's medication is increased to the point that the child becomes dull, slow in school, and lacks normal drive and initiative. This is particularly true if the convulsions are extremely difficult to control, as physicians may repeatedly increase dosages in order to achieve seizure control. Fortunately, the current technique of assessing anticonvulsant blood levels reduces the likelihood of such overdosage.

Children with convulsions are often placed on a fairly rigid regimen, forbidden to do many activities typical of their age group. In fact, however, probably only three restrictions need be applied: the child should not swim alone, should not ride a bicycle on a busy road, and, in all probability, should limit climbing (Robb 1981).

The Effect of Emotions on the Frequency of the Convulsions

Every type of convulsion—petit mal, temporal lobe, grand mal, and so forth—can be affected by emotional tension and environmental situations. There have been numerous instances where formerly well-controlled attacks suddenly increase in frequency just at the point where an adequate history reveals precipitating emotional factors in the environment. In addition, it can often be predicted when there will be increased frequency of convulsions—for example, at examination time.

While much is being written about pseudoconvulsions, it is most unlikely that any child will have a true convulsive episode based purely on psychogenic factors unless there is an underlying convulsive diathesis.

PSEUDOSEIZURES

The term pseudoseizures is used to discuss various conditions that appear to be due to convulsive disorders but that, in fact, are not. The common conditions under pseudoseizures are syncope, narcolepsy, and functional (psychogenic) seizures (Riley and Roy 1982)

Syncope

A common cause of loss of awareness is vasomotor syncope, the common "fainting spell." Several mechanisms may be involved, but it is generally agreed that the initial problem is one of peripheral vasodilitation resulting in inadequate venous return to the heart. As a result, the lack of oxygen reaching the child's brain causes partial or complete loss of consciousness. This usually occurs when the child has been standing for some time or suddenly stands up, and then experiences blurred vision, lightheadedness, stomach sensations, clammy sweatiness, and loss of consciousness. Gravity plays a part, and there may be vagal influences that slow the heart rate. There is pallor and a thready pulse, but the period of unconsciousness is brief. With full return of consciousness, the child is usually aware of what has occurred and may have a headache, vomiting, or tiredness. If the hypoxia lasts longer, there may be stiffness or twitching of the limbs with rolling of the eyes and, in some children, loss of consciousness with very little warning. Frequently there is a family history of similar episodes. Syncope may be very similar to a seizure, and the diagnosis is made on a full assessment and the history. While syncope can occur in small children, it is much more common in adolescents.

Breath-holding attacks, described in chapter 9, are in response to pain or frustration. They constitute a particular variety of cerebral hypoxia affecting children from the age of about six months up to six to seven years.

Loss of consciousness may also occur with *migraine,* especially the basilar type that occurs more in teenagers but is still uncommon. The attack may be preceded by vertigo, double vision, weakness or paresthesias, nausea and vomiting, visual disturbances, and ataxia as well as the headache. If there is loss of consciousness, it is usually brief (Brown 1977).

Narcolepsy and cataplexy, two other forms of pseudoseizure, are discussed with the sleep disorders in chapter 9.

Psychogenic Causes of Loss of Consciousness

Full or partial loss of consciousness can result from psychological factors generally associated with unpleasant visual experiences (sight of blood, accidents, etc.). Both vagal and peripheral factors are thought to be involved. Sometimes a conditioned response can result in a particular set of circumstances precipitating a loss of consciousness through syncope, anxiety being a potent factor. Hyperventilation, if excessive, will result in peripheral vasodilatation and cerebral vasoconstriction and may cause syncope (Riley and Roy 1982).

COMA

The ultimate loss of awareness is coma, which is occasionally precipitated by or simulated in psychological states. The situation and surroundings of the unconscious patient often provide clues. The physician or mental health worker should consider drug overdose, coma secondary to seizures or head injury, metabolic comas (diabetic, hypoglycemic, uremic, or hepatic), encephalopathy (including Reye's syndrome), intracranial vascular lesions (including expanding lesions), or endocrine abnormalities. A rapid examination for neck stiffness, signs of head injury, smelling of the breath, pupil reactions, blurring of optic discs, eye movements, patterns of respiration, and skin coloration may provide clues as to etiology. The EEG can be helpful if there is drug intoxication or if the cause is psychogenic.

CEREBRAL PALSY

One chronic condition, cerebral palsy, is becoming less common because of improved obstetrical and perinatal care. The term implies that the underlying cerebral dysfunction is nonprogressive. The condition may result from damage occurring at about the time of birth, usually from hypoxia or hemorrhage, or may occur during the formative years (acquired cerebral palsy) as the result of trauma, infection, or metabolic insults. Clinical descriptions include three main types: the spastic child, the athetotic child, and the ataxic child. Psychological complications affecting all three forms are described in chapter 22 (Gardner 1968).

The spastic child may have spasticity affecting the arm and leg of the same side (i.e., hemiplegic); both legs in a symmetrical fashion, perhaps with lesser involvement of the arms (i.e., diplegic); or all four limbs in varying degrees (i.e., quadriplegic). These children show increased muscle tone with a clasp-knife rigidity noted in movement of the limbs, increased deep reflexes, and extensor responses. The spastic form is much more likely than the other types to be associated with such complications as mental retardation, disturbances in vision or convulsions, and so forth.

The athetotic child has a marked awkwardness in any attempted movement, with associated overflow movements involving various body parts. These children's speech articulation is usually disturbed and they also show: unsteady gait or lack of balance; a false increase in tone, which, under relaxation, eventually appears normal; and normal or slightly decreased deep tendon reflexes and flexor plantar responses. This condition usually results from hypoxia affecting the basal ganglia, whereas the spastic form is usually caused by hypoxic effects in the motor cortex.

The ataxic child is relatively rare. The condition results from a disturbance affecting the cerebellum or the cerebellar system. It is associated with decreased muscle tone, reduced deep tendon reflexes, normal plantar responses, nystagmus and intention tremor, with marked general incoordination of fine movements.

The emotional problems associated with cerebral palsy, as described in chapter 22, may be those due to cerebral palsy itself but often result from the complications that accompany the condition.

DISTURBANCES IN MOVEMENT

Besides cerebral palsy, a number of different conditions can affect normal movement patterns—fatigue, weakness, incoordination, involuntary movements, changes in tone, seizures, and the like—and assessment requires a full history and physical examination. Fatigue and tiredness often appear as psychological symptoms, but it is important to be sure that an organic origin is not being overlooked. Weakness may be associated with fatigue as in *myasthenia gravis,* a condition frequently still undiagnosed in the early stages during which the presenting symptoms are considered psychogenic. Confusion is more likely when the symptoms are generalized and less so when they are bulbar. Demonstration of fatigability of the eyelids and a Tensilon test are diagnostic.

In the early stages, weakness due to *polymyositis* or *dermatomyositis* may be misdiagnosed and considered functional, particularly if dysphagia is an early symptom. Later diagnosis of this condition is usually made through muscle tenderness and recognition of the skin lesions, supported by biopsy and an electromyogram.

Lack of coordination and involuntary movements are characteristic of *lesions of the basal ganglia and cerebellum* and in the early stages may not be easy to recognize. *Dystonia musculorum,* though rare, is very frequently thought to be psychogenic because of the absence of abnormal signs when the patient is examined lying down. The subtle differences in tone and posture that occur when the patient is upright are often initially thought to be functional in origin.

Another condition that, though rare, is important to diagnose since treatment is available and effective is *Wilson's disease.* In this condition copper is deposited in various organs, causing damage to the liver and the basal ganglia that produces various abnormalities of movement. However, in some children psychiatric symptoms that precede the motor disability may be the first indication, and unless the physician thinks of the condition, takes a careful family history, and looks for the diagnostic Kayser-Fleischer ring in the cornea, the correct diagnosis may be delayed.

Tremors, not uncommon in children, usually represent an exaggeration of the normal physiological tremor seen in many individuals and are often familial. An intention tremor most evident when reaching for an object is not benign and usually indicates cerebellar dysfunction.

Tics or habit spasm are particularly common in boys, have a good prognosis, and often have a very strong familial history. Including repetitive, organized movements such as blinking, sniffing, head shaking, neck stretching, coughing, grunting, and so forth, occurring alone or as multiple movements, they are discussed further in chapter 9.

Gait abnormalities may be readily recognized—the hemiplegic or diplegic gait of cerebral palsy; the ataxic gait of cerebellar disease; the waddle of muscular weakness; the drop-foot gait of peripheral nerve damage; and the reeling, drunken pattern of intoxication—but some are less obvious, such as that of the early stages of musculorum deformans. Hysterical gaits may be quite bizarre, but the absence of any abnormal neurological findings consistent with the observed pattern of the gait makes this condition suspect. A full and detailed psychiatric history should show a psychogenic reason for such a gait and confirm the diagnosis (Rose 1979).

Neurological Conditions That Originally Present as Functional Disorders

HEADACHE

Headache is common in children but is rarely of serious significance. First it must be determined how much the headache interferes with normal activity and whether or not there are objective physical findings. Concern increases with (1) a short history, (2) associated vomiting, especially in the morning, (3) loss of balance or altered physical ability, and (4) definite physical findings on examination, such as a skull bruit, choking of the optic fundi, and increased blood pressure.

Headaches may occur at any age. Even in infants, it may be possible to recognize, often in retrospect, the abrupt occurrence of pallor, quietness, vomiting, and sleep that are due to migraine. In the older child, leading questions may be needed to extract the details of the symptomatology that are essential to accurate diagnosis since, in most cases, the physical findings are unremarkable. The most common cause of headache in young children is not tension but *migraine,* although the classical migraine pattern of the older child and adult is uncommon (Rees 1971). The pain is frontal, occipital, or in the region of the temples, and usually bilateral. The character is usually throbbing or aching, the latter becoming throbbing with exertion. Blurring of vision and "dizziness" may be associated, and stomach sensations—pain or nausea—are also present. Vomiting followed by sleep frequently ends severe attacks. A specific trigger for the child's migraine can rarely be identified, but inquiries about food sensitivity should be made. In the migraine patient, any problems involving the head or neck—sinus, teeth, ears, throat—may make the migraine more frequent or more severe. There is usually positive family history, although the headaches occuring in other family members may be dismissed by many as tension, eye strain, sinus infection, or allergy. A full description by the individual is often necessary to provide substantiation. Nonspecific vascular type headaches of the type associated with fever, hot rooms, or hot days may be seen. Some children are more susceptible to them than others. In general, eye trouble and allergies rarely cause headaches, but since infection causes a recognizable pattern of headache, the teeth and temporomandibular joint should be considered if the pain is atypical.

Tension headaches usually occur in the older child or adolescent and are fairly easily recognized by the typical description of a band around the head or pain at the back of the head with extension to the neck and shoulders, combined with a history suggesting tension. Tension and migraine may be closely associated. In some instances tension triggers the onset of the migraine, while in others the headache is actually the combination of a tension and a migraine headache. It may not be profitable to attempt to separate the two components in some cases. In the migrainous adolescent, the headaches may at times become constant with exacerbations, a kind of status migrainous. This may generate anxiety that complicates management.

A number of symptoms sometimes called migraine equivalents and described well by Brown (1977) may occur in children without either the typical or even an atypical headache. The most common are episodes of cyclic vomiting lasting a few days without any precipitating cause or demonstrable pathology in the gastrointestinal tract. Episodic attacks of vertigo, usually of short duration with no demonstrable abnormalities in the vestibular system, are often migrainous equivalents. A sensitivity to motion sickness—for example, a tendency to go to sleep or become nauseated while being driven in a car—are typical of these children. In such cases the diagnosis can be made only through a detailed family history and the absence of other findings to account for the symptoms. In some but not all of these children, migrainous headaches develop in later life.

Migraine may, in some children, be extremely resistant to treatment, even though some newer and specific drugs have been developed to treat the actual attack and others to prevent or limit the occurrence of the episodes. In view of this, the treatment of migrainous headaches is probably best left to the internist or the neurologist.

PROGRESSIVE DETERIORATIVE DISEASES

These uncommon conditions can cause deterioration in intellectual function alone or, more commonly, in motor, sensory, and mental faculties. Only those that might be referred to a child psychiatrist if the organic basis has been missed will be discussed.

Until recently, the most common of these conditions has been *subacute sclerosing panencephalitis (SSPE)* due to the chronic measles virus. With more intensive inoculation against measles, the condition has become rare. It often presents initially with dementia, but later brief myoclonic-type seizures develop. The diagnosis can be confirmed by the very characteristic EEG and cerebrospinal fluid findings. There is as yet no satisfactory treatment.

Huntington's chorea occasionally presents as deterioration in a child, before the characteristic movement disorders occur. More commonly, seizures are the initial symptom. A positive family history allows one to diagnose these changes in intellectual function and behavior at an early stage, but occasionally the adults in the family may not have developed symptoms until after the child is affected. There is no satisfactory treatment, but genetic counseling is important.

Ataxia telangiectasia occasionally presents with intellectual deterioration, but this is usually preceded by problems in coordination. The diagnosis is made by the characteristic telangiectasias developing in the sclera of the eyes.

In *tuberous sclerosis* there is a wide spectrum of involvement; lesions of the skin, seizures, intracranial calcification, mental retardation, and dementia all occur. This condition should be considered in an infant with retarded development and myoclonic seizures.

Disorders of gray matter due to *storage diseases* occur most frequently in infancy, presenting usually as failure in development, and are discussed in more detail in chapter 18.

The child who has a *specific learning disability* and/or a *specific language disability* is usually unable to progress at a normal rate in the school system. Since most intelligence tests are based on children who have followed the normal educational stream, the results are obviously affected by repeated school failure. In such children repeated intelligence tests over the years often show gradually decreasing scores secondary to their educational limitations (Lickorish 1971). In the past this was not recognized, and so many of these children, suspected of having a deteriorative process, were admitted to hospitals for a neurological examination, a lumbar puncture, and even an air encephalogram. Today this condition is recognized and, fortunately for the children, such investigation is no longer carried out.

SLEEP DISTURBANCES

Although this subject is discussed in chapter 9, there are several areas of interest from the neurological point of view. *Temporal lobe seizures* often occur in sleep and may not be recognized readily unless there is overt seizure activity. The pattern may be that of a nightmare or night terror that, if recurrent, usually recurs at the same stage of consciousness—shortly after falling asleep or just before waking. Breathing problems, cyanosis, focal movements, or incontinence are signs suggesting a seizure problem.

Migraine may be associated with what appear to be night terrors, with the behavior presumably reflecting changes in local blood flow within the cerebral cortex. A full family history should be obtained. The symptom responds well to chlorpromazine given at bedtime.

Sleep apnea is being increasingly recognized as a cause of nocturnal as well as waking problems, though so far few children have been implicated. Evidence of airway obstruction is important and the child may snore or wake frequently, briefly, with a startle. In the morning, after waking, the child may be unduly tired or confused and may complain of headache. Drowsiness during the day may occur, and the true diagnosis may be missed unless the possibility of sleep apnea is considered.

It is common for infants to cry out at night and for older children to wet the bed. Less common, but still normal, are such activities as talking in sleep, nightmares, grinding the teeth, and limb or body jerks occurring as the child falls asleep. Even less common are night terrors and sleepwalking, both of which are discussed in chapter 9. A family history of migraine occasionally occurs, but most children with night terrors or sleepwalking have a family history of a similar sleep disorder, especially those children who do not reveal enough emotional problems to account for the symptoms. They often respond well to chlorpromazine or dilantin given at bedtime.

Another interesting problem is that of *sleep paralysis,* usually described in the older teenager and young adult. The frequency is uncertain, since most patients do not seek medical attention. The person is aware but neither fully awake nor asleep, and any movements other than respiratory ones seem impossible. This may cause panic, but the ability to move suddenly returns. If attacks are frequent, considerable reassurance may be needed, and a trial with methylphenidate is justified.

Emotional Disturbances Simulating Organic Disease

Many if not most emotional disturbances simulating organic disease are considered under the discussion of the dissociative disorders (see chapter 12). However, as far as the neurological system is concerned, disorders of apparent consciousness, movement, or sensation may often be classified broadly as "hysterical." Many or most children lack the typical *belle indifference* that results from repression and the subsequent lack of knowledge of the conflict situation responsible for the symptomatology. Such typical reaction patterns are more common in the older adolescent or adult than in the younger child, who seems to be aware of the problems producing the symptoms and to be using the symptoms in a conscious, deliberate way to obtain increased attention from the environment or to avoid an unpleasant situation. If attention is sought, the symptoms may arouse anxiety in the parents, who respond by increased attention and affection. The escape sought is frequently from a difficult situation at school. For example, the child may suddenly develop visual problems that interfere with seeing the chalkboard or the print in books, or may develop weakness or paralysis, almost invariably of the dominant hand, which makes it impossible to write. In most cases the diagnosis and the origin of the symptom become apparent after an adequate psychiatric history. A common problem in management is the difficulty convincing the parents that the child does not have organic disease but may be deliberately using the symptoms for attention or escape.

Conclusion

A number of conditions that straddle the border between neurology and psychiatry have been described, along with others that, while clearly falling within one or the other area, have symptoms that can confuse the diagnosis. Although ongoing research will undoubtedly further clarify the neurological and psychological components contributing to these conditions, it will probably always be important for physicians and neurologists to remain alert to the psychological sequelae of neurological illness and for psychiatrists and psychologists to be careful to rule out neurological causes, especially where there is a sudden, unexplained onset of marked personality or behavioral change or any suggestion of the conditions described herein.

SUGGESTIONS FOR FURTHER READING

BOSAEUS, E., AND SELLDEN, U. 1979. Psychiatric assessment of healthy children with various EEG patterns. *Act. Psychiat. Scand.* 59:180–210.
Significant relationships are showing up between clinical variables in psychiatric assessment and EEG patterns.

BROWN, J. K. 1977 Migraine and migraine equivalents in children. *Dev. Med. & Child Neurol.* 19:683–692.
A review article dealing with definition, classification, etiology, precipitating factors, pathology, the clinical picture, the relationship to school failure, and management.

GARDNER, R. A. 1968. Psychogenic problems of brain-injured children and their parents. *J. Am. Acad. of Child Psychiat.* 7:471–491.
The manifestations, psychodynamics, and therapy of some of the more common psychogenic problems. The discussion is divided into sections dealing with the problems that stem from the parents and those that stem from the child. The complex interplay of factors is kept sight of.

KESSLER, J. W. 1972. Neurosis in childhood, in *Manual of child psychopathology,* ed. B. B. Wolmar, pp. 387–435. New York: McGraw-Hill.
Chapter is concerned with those emotional problems that are included in the diagnostic categories of phobia, hysteria, and obsessive-compulsive neurosis.

LINDSAY, J., OUNSTED, C., AND RICHARDS, P. 1979. Long-term outcome in children with temporal lobe seizures. I: Social outcome and childhood factors. *Dev. Med. & Child Neurol.* 21:285–298. II: Marriage, parenthood and sexual indifference. *Dev. Med. & Child Neurol.* 21:433–440. III: Psychiatric aspects in childhood and adult life. *Dev. Med. & Child Neurol.* 21:630–636.
This study of 100 subjects shows a low occurrence of overt psychiatric disorder in adulthood. Those disorders that do occur (schizophreniform psychosis and conduct disorders) are related to various childhood profiles.

LIVINGSTON, S.; PAULI, L.L.; AND PRUCE, I. 1980. Neurological evaluations of the child. In *Comprehensive textbook of psychiatry,* vol. 3, ed. H. I. Kaplan, A. M. Freedman, and B. J. Sadock, pp. 2461–2473. Baltimore: Williams & Wilkins.

A readily available discussion on differentiating between recurrent spells of neurological or psychogenic origin and the diagnostic techniques (e.g., clinical history and laboratory procedures) used when physical or neurological deficits are not detectable.

KANNER, L. 1944. Early infantile autism. *J. Pediat.* 25:211–217.
The original description of early infantile autism as a clinical syndrome.

KNOBLOCH, H., AND PASAMANICK, B. 1975. Some etiologic and prognostic factors in early infantile autism and psychosis. *Pediatr.* 55(2):182–191.
Describes a group of autistic children examined in infancy and the early preschool period and considers the relationship of "autism" and "infantile psychosis" to perinatal complications and associated disorders. Findings are compared with those of two studies of older children.

REES, W. L. 1971. Psychiatric and psychological factors in migraine. In *Background to migraine: Fourth migraine symposium, September 11th, 1970,* ed. J. N. Cumings, pp. 45–54. London: Heineman.
An overview of research. The author points out a need for research studies using random, representative samples rather than clinical populations.

RILEY, T. L., AND ROY, A. 1982. *Pseudoseizures.* Baltimore: Williams & Wilkins.
Discusses diagnosis and treatment of neurological, cardiovascular, and psychological (i.e. hysterical) conditions which may cause sudden loss of consciousness and which may be confused with epilepsy. The use of EEG in arriving at the correct diagnosis is dealt with.

ROSE, F. C., ed. 1979. *Paediatric neurology.* Oxford: Blackwell Scientific Publications.
A good general textbook covering the neurological disorders of childhood.

RUTTER, M. 1977. Brain damage syndromes in childhood: Concepts and findings. *J. Child Psychol. & Psychiat.* 18:1–21.
Includes a clear discussion of the confusion existing around the interpretation of soft neurological signs and on the relationship of brain damage to psychiatric disorder.

———. 1981. Psychological sequelae of brain damage in children. *Am. J. Psychiat.* 138:1533–1544.
Brain injury causes increased risk of both intellectual impairment and nonspecific psychological sequelae. The risk is related to the severity of the lesion. Psychiatric sequelae are related to abnormal neurophysiological activity, preinjury behavior, cognitive level, and psychosocial circumstances.

———. 1982. Syndromes attributed to minimal brain dysfunction in childhood. *Am. J. Psychiat.* 139(1):21–33.
Considers two main concepts of MBD: a continuum notion and a syndrome notion. While subclinical damage can occur, it must be substantial and does not cause a single syndrome. The syndrome possibility remains an alternative, but the claims exceed the proof as yet available.

STORES, G. 1978. School children with epilepsy at risk for learning and behavior problems. *Dev. Med. & Child Neurol.* 20(4):502–508.
Data from four preliminary studies designed to identify vulnerable school-age epileptics suggest that a persistent left temporal spike, especially in boys, is associated with reading problems, inattentiveness, dependency, and other disturbed behaviors. The drug phenytoin may adversely affect cognitive functioning.

WARD, F., AND BOWER, B. D. 1978. A study of certain social aspects of epilepsy in childhood. *Dev. Med. & Child Neurol.* 20(1) Supplement 39.
Parental attitudes evoked by epilepsy, especially at an early stage, are significant to the child's later adjustment. This study illustrates the social and personal factors that condition parental response. The approach taken is individual and anecdotal rather than quantitative.

WENDER, P. H. 1973. Minimal brain dysfunction in children: Diagnosis and management. *Pediatr. Clin. N. Am.* 20(1):187–202.
The most common cause of chronic behavioral problems in children, minimal brain dysfunction responds well to minimal intervention but is often unrecognized or inadequately treated. A practical guide to diagnosis and management.

12 *Paul D. Steinhauer and Graham Berman*

Anxiety, Neurotic, and Personality Disorders in Children

This chapter will discuss those conditions labeled anxiety disorders in DSM-III, as well as other disorders appearing elsewhere in that classification sharing a common etiology, for example, some somatoform disorders. Most of what traditionally were termed neurotic and personality disorders will be covered.

Definition

All people experience anxiety in the presence or anticipation of new and potentially threatening situations such as examinations, athletic competitions, stage and speaking performances, job interviews, visits to doctors or dentists, and so forth. Anxiety has two main components: an *affective* component, that is, a subjective discomfort consisting of a sense of apprehension, restlessness, accelerated thinking, erratic concentration, and a mild though often undefined sense of foreboding; and a *somatic* component, that is, increased heart rate, raised blood pressure, sweating, coldness and clamminess of the extremities, palpitations, breathlessness, abdominal distress with or without increased urinary frequency, and/or diarrhea.

Both the affective and subjective responses are mediated by the activation of the norepinephrine system, a hormonal altering response of the autonomic nervous system to anticipated danger. Most people learn to tolerate these symptoms or find ways such as denial, activity, or diversion to allow themselves to continue functioning successfully. Others, however, suffer incapacitating anxiety even without any real or impending danger, or rely so extensively on the maladaptive use of defenses to neutralize anxiety that they may develop a psychoneurotic disorder. Although they are unaware of the reasons for their anxiety or their symptoms, a careful history and observation of their behavior will demonstrate that they are responding to situations considered innocuous by others as if they were dangerous and, therefore, anxiety provoking. These situations appear to have special meaning for them, either because the trigger situation is unconsciously and symbolically linked to past experiences and repressed psychological conflicts, or because their symptoms serve an important though unrecognized role in their relationships with others.

David, age fourteen, was referred for behavior problems at home, severe underachievement in school, and lack of friends. Unknown to his mother and stepfather, David had been stealing compulsively for two years without being caught. He was distressed about his stealing but unable to stop. He had no idea why he stole; he just knew that he would suddenly feel desperately unhappy and could feel relieved only if he stole. In therapy it became clear that the episodes of distress and the stealing that masked and replaced them were triggered by stimuli that reactivated the grief David had repressed following his father's death when the boy was nine.

On the other hand Jan, at fifteen, had shown no emotional or behavioral symptoms until the recent deterioration of her parents' marriage. She then began to experience periods of intense anxiety, at the height of which she would steal. Each such episode occurred after a battle between the parents or whenever separation seemed particularly imminent. Her stealing stopped soon after the parents sought marital counseling, which they used successfully. Thus Jan's behavior appeared related not to psychological conflict but to the family stress with which she was forced to cope.

Prevalence

In their Isle of Wight study, Rutter and associates (1970), studying ten- and eleven-year-olds in a largely small-town population, found the prevalence of psychoneurosis to be approximately 2.5 percent in the general population and 34.1 percent in a clinical population. In their 1973 study, Rutter and colleagues found that the prevalence of psychoneurosis in a large metropolitan area was approximately twice that of the Isle of Wight, while that of emotional disorders in adolescence was higher still (Rutter et al. 1976). Whereas more girls than boys were psychoneurotic during early and middle childhood, there were almost as many neurotic boys as girls during adolescence. Leslie (1974), studying an inner-city population, found twice Rutter and associates' number of severe disorders (neurotic) and triple the number of total disorders. She considered this more the result of the urban environment than of the age of the children, who were about two years older than those studied by Rutter and associates. In the United States, Cantwell (1974), studying the dependents of military families, found 10 percent of them neurotic, with twice as many girls in the neurotic sample. Rosen and colleagues (1968), studying a psychiatric outpatient clinic population, found 6.1 percent of the boys and 8.4 percent of the girls had diagnoses of psychoneurosis but that 20.7 percent of those hospitalized in a general hospital psychiatric ward were considered psychoneurotic.

Classification

The number of different theoretical viewpoints in psychiatry is paralleled by a number of different classifications, none entirely satisfactory. Recent classifications (e.g., DSM-III in North America, ICD-9 in Europe) have emphasized observation, description, and phenomenology rather than postulated cause. Both ICD-9 and DSM-III use a multiaxial format to permit more precise diagnosis and to convey more information about the biological, psychological, and social dimensions of the patient's condition. On DSM-III, most psychiatric diagnoses are listed on Axis 1, while personality and developmental disorders are listed on Axis 2.

For any diagnosis, the severity of a given patient's illness may vary greatly. One patient may be thoroughly incapacitated by a phobic disorder, for example, while another with a milder phobia may show minimal functional impairment. As a result of this variability, there is considerable overlap. No single diagnostic category is, by definition, more severe than any other. Thus diagnoses refer to the nature, not the extent, of the psychological disturbance.

Development of Anxiety (Neurotic) Disorders

How does the development of a child with a neurotic (anxiety) disorder differ from that of the normal child described in chapter 1?

CONSTITUTION AND TEMPERAMENT:

Children constitutionally low in adaptability, who show an intense physiological response to minimal stimulation (Thomas and Chess 1977), will experience more than usual anxiety in the course of normal living. While extreme temperamental differences (e.g., the "difficult" child) may interfere with bonding and attachment (see chapter 1), major bonding and attachment difficulties are usually associated with more serious psychiatric conditions (e.g., personality disorders) rather than with anxiety disorders. It is probable, though not proven, that less extreme constitutional and temperamental deviations contribute to the development of anxiety disorders. Many aspects of temperamental style, cognitive ability, appearance, and body build affect a given child's adaptability and the ongoing transactions between the child and others, thus influencing the probability of later difficulties.

PARENT–CHILD INTERACTION:

Parent-child interaction is important at all stages of development. Ongoing transactions between child and parents—and, later, with the broader social environment—have long-lasting effects on all participants (Thomas 1981). Children learn to react to people as essentially comforting or non-comforting, reliable or nonreliable, while parents view children as rewarding or frustrating, demanding or easy, cuddly or distancing. Some parents are more able than others to perceive and respond successfully to the highly specific needs of their child. The more sensitively and appropriately they can respond to their particular child's needs, the more satisfying the relationship will be (the better the fit between parents and child). On the other hand, where parents are unable to perceive or respond appropriately to their child's needs, the resulting dissonance will lead to excessive stress, disturbed behavioral functioning, and interference with optimal development. In addition, parents model behavior for their children and by action and attitude influence their emotional set to life and its events. From the depressed parent children learn to be pessimistic and expect the worst. With the anxious parent they do not know what to expect but learn to worry about many possibilities. The phobias of parents are passed on to their children through excessive empathy and encouragement of children's normal fears. The paranoid parent sets the child on a course of mistrustfulness of the world. Prejudice is equally available to modeling and learning. Obviously two parents present very different models so that children, depending on the degree of closeness or affiliation with each, selectively learn behavior sets that fashion their way of facing tasks, stress, and setbacks of life. Thus the mutual interaction between constitution (i.e., continuing genetic influences), maturation, and learning through modeling and selec-

233

tive reinforcement will shape the emergence of new and more complex psychological attributes as development proceeds (Thomas 1981).

SEPARATION AND INDIVIDUATION

From about nine months until two and one-half to three years of age, children become increasingly aware of themselves as individuals living in a family of other individuals. In doing so they develop their own mental picture of themselves and others (Mahler, Pine, and Bergman 1975).

At about eight months of age, children recognize that things have a permanent existence of their own. This recognition, referred to in chapter 1 as object permanence, is followed by a stage of marked curiosity about the nature of things in general and themselves in particular. It is characterized by the cognitive process of ordering and grouping described on pages 20–22. During this period of intense curiosity, children develop an acute interest in their body, exploring and naming body parts. In due course they compare and contrast their body with those of others. This may lead to a period of particular interest and curiosity about the genitals, which are recognizably different from those of parents and some other children, as well as to a preoccupation with the processes of elimination, which they soon realize are very important to the parents although they, the children, alone can control them. As these individual recognitions coalesce, an increasingly coherent picture of themselves as separate persons with their own unique characteristics begins to take shape. Normally these curiosities and preoccupations are associated with little, if any, anxiety, although for children who have experienced major surgery, prolonged, painful, or repeated immobilization, a great deal of nude body contact with the parents (Galenson et al. 1975), or the loss of a sibling or parents, the curiosity may be associated with severe and/or lasting anxiety (Galenson and Roiphe 1971; Roiphe and Galenson 1973).

Up to this point children have been influenced primarily by responses to their biological drives and by the ways that others, especially parents and siblings, respond to them. Some conflict is inevitable between biological drives that demand immediate release and parental and—increasingly with age—extrafamilial demands for behavioral and emotional control or modification in order to retain the approval and avoid the displeasure of others. Thus the child increasingly learns to control biological drives and emotions in order to behave in what the environment defines as an acceptable manner.

At about this stage children recognize and begin to use the stimulation and relaxing potential of masturbation to comfort themselves when the parents are unavailable. There is some, though not yet conclusive, clinical evidence that the fantasy which accompanies masturbation is very much colored by the nature of the parent-child relationship (Greenacre 1971).

When there is a good fit between children's needs and parents' ability to meet those needs, progress toward the developmental goals of task mastery and social competence is enhanced. For these children masturbation is typically associated with pleasant and loving fantasies. However, where a poor fit between children and parents exists, either because children's needs are excessive or because parents are unavailable or psychologically unable to meet them, task mastery and social competence are likely to be impaired and masturbation is more likely to be associated with themes of loss, disappointment, and deprivation. These fantasies, often sadistic or masochistic in nature, combine with the parents' attitudes and direct responses to the child's early sexual behavior to shape children's sexual attitudes, feelings, behavior, and involvements (Greenacre 1971; Parens 1968; Sarnoff 1976). These, in turn, evoke secondary responses from parents and others, so that ultimately sexual attitudes and behavior result from the interaction of genetic, maturational, and environmental factors (Thomas 1981).

THE DEVELOPMENT OF AMBIVALENCE

As children achieve stable inner pictures of themselves and others, they develop an increased ability to see themselves as others see them. This, in turn, allows them to think of themselves as more or less like others in a world of similar people. Then they can actively imagine taking the role of another family member, while assigning a parent or doll to represent them in fantasy and play. This allows them an increased awareness of the power structure of the family and of the advantages of being a parent. This creates a new kind of conflict for children. At times they feel hostile and resentful of the authority of the same parents to whom, much of the time, they feel affection. In response to the tension between these affectionate and hostile feelings, they develop a variety of defenses, mental mechanisms used to decrease discomfort at unacceptable wishes or feelings. For example, a child might be unusually solicitous toward a parent to convince herself that she was not jealous or resentful. This oversolicitousness, an example of reaction formation, would be a defense against the emergence of resentment and hostility that, if recognized, might cause the child to be punished or at least temporarily cut off from the parents on whom she depends for her continued security. Psychoanalysts have termed this struggle to learn to tolerate ambivalence the Oedipal struggle and called this stage the Oedipal stage.

LEARNING TO LIVE WITH AMBIVALENCE: CONSCIENCE FORMATION

Children's affection for their parents and their wish to avoid displeasing them helps them resolve their resentment of the parents. They do this by developing a conscience, or superego. Whereas before they needed the parents to enforce family rules, now they begin to police themselves even in the absence of the parents. Previously children's feeling of being good or bad depended on whether they were pleasing the parents. Now they increasingly begin to regulate their own self-esteem and to define goodness or badness by whether they obey or transgress these newly internalized concepts of right or wrong. The resulting inner tension allows them to control their own behavior for longer periods, even in the absence of parents. Because many family rules are directed against sexual and aggressive behavior, most children develop adequate control over their fantasy and excitement and become reasonably conforming and socially agreeable by middle childhood (ages six to ten).

THE RESULT OF LIVING WITH AMBIVALENCE

Even by middle childhood, most children have not yet achieved a stable mental picture of themselves and others. When excited or anxious, their capacity for thinking and behaving realistically is impaired. At these times they may fear loss of control over their sexual feelings or over the hostile component of their ambivalence to the parents. This potential danger serves as a source of anxiety. Should they lose control, the parents might retaliate by becoming angry or rejecting. Should they transgress the dictates of their conscience, they would feel guilty or ashamed. The more intense this anxiety, the more strenuously and rigidly they defend against their sexual and aggressive feelings. The reason for their particular choice of defense is not always clear, but children tend to model themselves on their parents and to use the same defenses they see their parents using to cope with anxiety. This form of learning—role modeling—plays a major part in defense selection and, therefore, in symptom formation. Most children successfully defend against conflicts and anxieties by pushing them out of awareness (i.e., by repressing them). This leaves them comfortable and sufficiently free of anxiety to function and develop satisfactorily. If the child's defenses are adequate, frightening wishes or fantasies, along with the defenses opposing them, are successfully repressed. They remain, according to analytic theory, in the unconscious portion of the child's mind, a potential but not an actual source of anxiety.

If at some later stage the child encounters a situation sufficiently close to an unconscious conflict that has been repressed, the existing defenses may prove insufficient. The child then experiences a sudden breakthrough into consciousness of the reinforced conflict along with the anxiety accompanying it. This in turn calls for the urgent development of new defenses to contain the now out-of-control anxiety and to repress once again the unwanted conflict, restoring the more comfortable status quo. When such a breakthrough occurs, the resulting symptoms, some of which result from the anxiety itself and others from the unsuccessful, excessive, or overly rigid use of auxiliary defenses called into play against the anxiety, are known as neurotic symptoms (Tolpin 1970).

236

Sometimes instead of experiencing a dramatic breakthrough (i.e., neurotic symptoms) a child gradually develops a personal style that, while reasonably adaptive, shows continuing distortion due to the excessively rigid and automatic overuse of defenses. In such cases the pattern of defenses originally called forth to neutralize conflicted impulses has become such an integral part of the child's personality structure that it no longer appears to be anything out of the ordinary and is accepted as part of the child's makeup. When this occurs, it is known as a personality disorder or neurotic personality disorder.

The Childhood Neuroses: Anxiety Disorders

A childhood neurosis may be precipitated in any child predisposed to one by the existence of a repressed conflict between intense but unacceptable feelings and the defenses against them. The precipitating cause may be anything that reactivates repressed conflicts and stirs up anxiety against which the available defenses can no longer defend. The resultant neurosis represents the most successful compromise that the child can find, given that child's particular personality resources and the responses of the family and larger social environment. The family reaction frequently, though inadvertently, perpetuates the child's illness. Parents, for example, may reinforce neurotic defenses by allowing the child extra protection, attention, or freedom from responsibility because of the symptoms. Doing so makes the symptoms pay off for the child (secondary gain), thus making it worthwhile to perpetuate them. Childhood neurosis, then, represents a complex interaction between intrapsychic and interpersonal factors joining in an unsuccessful attempt at adaptation. Through the neurotic symptoms, the patient is trying to reestablish a comfortable control over unwanted fantasies and fears while, at the same time, using the neurotic symptoms to maneuver others into providing protection or compensations.

Children with an anxiety (neurotic) disorder are not usually aware of the intense inner conflict between opposing tendencies and the defenses against them. Often they are conscious only of their symptoms and distress, which they see as unrelated to conflict or only to conflict that is exclusively interpersonal. Many of these concepts are illustrated in the following case example.

Jane, a pubescent twelve-year-old, eldest of four in a devoutly religious family, was referred for psychiatric consultation a month after being hit in the eye with an icy snowball. Severe hemorrhage, intense pain, and the loss of vision in that eye required her to be hospitalized with both eyes bandaged, under orders to lie perfectly still to avoid further bleeding. A month later, full recovery of sight was still not certain, but she was discharged from the hospital on strictly limited activity.

Jane was referred for a number of uncharacteristic behaviors that had developed since the accident. She showed extreme sensitivity and was easily upset if treated in what she considered "the wrong way." She had recurrent nightmares, repeating the accident. In one dream, however, she was berating the boy who threw the snowball when her father came to his defense. Shocked and enraged, she killed her father and was instantly overcome with remorse. She was sobbing when she awoke. She was obsessed with hearing the latest weather report, becoming unreasonably fearful at any mention of snow. Her parents and doctors were concerned by her unnaturally "saintly" endurance of all the pain and discomfort she had suffered. She showed no anger. Instead she constantly expressed exaggerated concern for the guilt and emotional suffering of the boy who hurt her. Yet the one time he tried to visit, she flew into a rage and refused to see him. Within half an hour she resumed her extreme concern for his welfare.

Certain aspects of Jane's background are significant. Both her parents were intelligent and deeply concerned. The father was described as a kind man whose only flaw was an explosive temper. The mother, upwardly mobile and better educated than her husband, frequently experienced frustration but preferred to withdraw when angry, even though this frequently resulted in headaches that she would suffer in silence.

Before the accident Jane's parents had never considered psychiatric help for her but, in retrospect, they recognized her as the most oppositional and easily upset of their children. She passed grades easily, but school teachers thought she was underachieving. Jane often remarked that she was stupid.

Jane had been repeatedly sexually molested by a male babysitter over a period of years from the age of six and had long shown distrust and hostility toward boys. This had receded in the few years before the accident but returned in strength after it.

PREDISPOSING FACTORS

Let us examine those factors that Jane's psychiatrist saw as contributing to the development and maintenance of her symptoms. Prior to her injury Jane had been considered asymptomatic, although there was some behavioral evidence of ongoing inner struggles against the environment. The babysitter's seduction had been followed by several years of distrust and hostility toward males, but that seemed to have been repressed successfully some time prior to the injury.

Prior to the accident, Jane seemed to have been undergoing a similar internal struggle to control her hostile and aggressive feelings. The most stubbornly determined of her siblings, she fought harder against parental demands for conformity and achievement before eventually submitting, partly to protect her relationship with her parents and partly because the family's values defined anger as something "unworthy," to be controlled (like the mother), not expressed (like the father). She eventually established a precarious control over her anger. After she did so the intensity of the struggle diminished and the conflict was again repressed.

This repression allowed her to avoid chronic battling and constant resentment of pressures placed on her by the parents she loved. It allowed her to function relatively comfortably and productively. Evidence that her defenses were barely sufficient to the task were her stubbornness, the exaggerated sensitivity, and the underachievement. All these factors discussed contributed by predisposing Jane to the development of a neurotic or anxiety disorder given a sufficient precipitant.

PRECIPITATING FACTORS

In Jane's case the precipitating factor was the injury and the pain, immobilization, and anxiety it produced. These greatly increased the amount of anxiety and rage she had to deal with, while at the same time separating her from the parents on whose support she had always depended in difficult situations. Jane knew that outbursts of rage were unacceptable in her family. She experienced intense anxiety that her rage might erupt, alienating her parents and evoking intense guilt. In a desperate attempt to contain it, she developed a number of auxiliary defenses (e.g., the obsession with weather reports, the extreme oversolicitousness for the boy who threw the snowball [i.e., reaction formation], barely masking the hostility that lay beneath it), but these were not enough to keep the anxiety from breaking through in her dreams (i.e., when her defenses were down). The single nightmare in which she killed her father suggests a reactivation of resentment against her father (or the parents) whose demand for such tight control over her anger led to her extreme ambivalence in the first place. At the same time, the fact that the snowball thrower was a boy reactivated the conflict around males as untrustworthy aggressors that had originated in the seduction by the babysitter but had, since its repression several years before, lain dormant. Thus the injury precipitated a posttraumatic neurosis by recharging a latent set of repressed but potential conflicts that, once activated, produced an overt neurotic disorder.

PERPETUATING FACTORS

In Jane's case there were no perpetuating factors, either intrapsychic or interpersonal. If her earlier development had been less satisfactory so that she had not developed the generally satisfactory impulse control and the ability to mediate internally conflicting biological and social drives, the resulting psychological weakness might have perpetuated her disturbance. Alternately, if the parental reaction had been less supportive—had they been unable to provide the support and security she needed; had they been so overindulgent as to encourage excessive and prolonged regression; had her symptoms been incorporated into a chronic struggle between husband and wife as, for example, if one had harshly condemned the "crazy behavior" while the other had insisted that the behavior needed love and understanding, not criticism; if the mother, because of a deep mistrust of men, had needed to reinforce her daughter's mistrust and hatred of males; or if the father, because of his discomfort with his own rage, had needed to insist that Jane's anger was intolerable; if either or both parents had needed to deny the existence of a problem, because of embarrassment at their child's needing to see a psychiatrist—then what began as an inner conflict (i.e., a neurotic problem) might well have been reinforced and perpetuated by the family's ongoing response to it. It is not unusual for children with neurotic or anxiety disorders to have what was originally a psychological disorder perpetuated by the family's reaction to the child's symptoms or by the mobilizing or focusing of latent or chronic family tensions on the neurotic child's symptoms, which distract from other sources of family tension. In any such case, Jane, who was extremely sensitive to tension between her parents, might have responded with an exacerbation of symptoms whenever marital conflict seemed imminent.

Fortunately, in Jane's case none of these occurred. The parents were appropriately concerned, sought help promptly, and cooperated well with Jane's therapist. They understood the meaning of Jane's symptoms and helped her realize that her anger at the snowball thrower was not only acceptable but understandable. With their help Jane's conscience allowed her to begin expressing the anger she had previously repressed. Concurrently her anxiety over the hostile and sexual feelings she was struggling to contain decreased so that she could recognize and discuss them. Her therapist, not content with mere ventilation, made Jane and her parents aware of how the family taboo against anger had predisposed her to react excessively to her injury. The parents were able to help Jane develop a more tolerant attitude toward both her anger and her sexual feelings. This allowed her to experience aggressive and sexual feelings as normal rather than "bad" or "sinful." Thanks to the family's preexisting strengths, this was achieved over the course of twelve twice-weekly psychotherapy sessions. A follow-up three months later showed Jane functioning productively and, in several areas, more comfortably than before the accident.

GENERAL DISCUSSION OF THE CASE STUDY

This case has been described as resulting from the interaction of two separate regulatory systems:

1. The psychological structure or internal regulatory system, which could alternately be described as one individual subsystem (i.e., Jane's) within the family system. This was Jane's way of balancing the conflicting pressures of her wishes, fears, and demands that she adapt to meet the needs of others in order to protect her place within the family.
2. The family system, within which a repetitive set of interactions governs the regulation of tensions generated in the course of living. (See Henderson 1982; Steinhauer 1983; also chapter 3.)

All people and all families have such regulatory systems. The families of children with anxiety disorders (psychoneuroses as opposed to post-traumatic neuroses) have family systems that are chronically maladaptive in that they encourage the production of anxiety disorders in their members and interfere with the efficient resolution of the inevitable stresses of daily living.

Types of Anxiety and Personality Disorders of Childhood and Adolescence

GROUP I.

Group I disorders consist of those in which the child's available defenses are insufficient to contain the anxiety that results from repressed (i.e., unconscious) conflict. In figure 12.1, it is represented diagrammatically by a model that shows anxiety bursting through the available defenses.

Posttraumatic Stress Disorder (Traumatic Neurosis) (308.30—Acute; 309.81—Chronic or Delayed)

In a posttraumatic stress disorder, symptoms appear suddenly, precipitated by an exposure to unusual stress. Following the triggering event, the child remains preoccupied with the stress, reexperiencing the trauma in thoughts and/or dreams, remaining relatively uninvolved in the external world. An example would be the case of Jane.

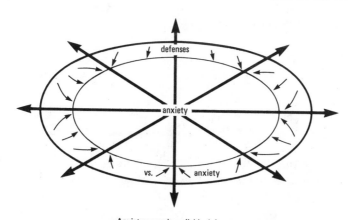

Anxiety exceeds available defenses

Figure 12.1 The Neurotic Child: Group I—Defenses Insufficient.

241

Anxiety Neurosis (or Anxiety States) (300.01—Panic Disorder; 300.02—Generalized Anxiety Disorder)

Anxiety states are characterized by acute, generalized anxiety and worry, either persistent (300.02) or episodic (300.01). As the anxiety is generated by unconscious conflict, there is no valid external reason for it, and it is not related to the child being separated from parental figures. In children, generalized anxiety and panic disorders are of relatively short duration, as children rapidly succeed in developing defenses that structure the difficulties into a more circumscribed symptom.

> When Ann was three, her father left home to live with his secretary. As her mother came to terms with the situation Ann soon got over her upset and visited her father each weekend, but when she was four and one-half and she developed intense generalized anxiety, fearing that her mother would disappear or that she herself would die. She had no defenses sufficient to ward off her anxiety, but like most anxiety disorders in children, her problem did not last long. Instead it developed into a different and more structured disorder, in this case a phobic disorder.

Phobic Disorders (Phobic Neuroses) (300.23)

A phobic disorder is a persistent, irrational, excessive fear of a specific object or situation. Feelings that the child is too guilty or too fearful to accept are projected onto some external object or situation (e.g., dogs, horses, subways, school). As long as this external threat is then avoided, the child can remain anxiety free. The phobia may bring secondary rewards, such as additional concern and care from the parents or permission to avoid unwanted activities. The following history of Ann, the girl introduced in the preceding case study, illustrates this mechanism.

> Ann became afraid that a kidnapper would come and get her during the night. Her generalized anxiety diminished as she structured her neurosis and her life around this phobia. She protected herself by moving into her mother's bed. In therapy sessions Ann repeatedly enacted the same fantasy with a doll family. The girl would go away with her father. A robber would kill the mother. Then the girl, who was also a doctor, would revive the mother and look after her.

When her parents had separated just before she turned four, Ann was at the height of her struggle with her ambivalence toward them. She was competitive with her mother for her father's affection but, at the same time, angry at her father for deserting them both. This was very upsetting for Ann since, at the same time, she loved them both too. Her original anxiety disorder had resulted from her inability to handle this ambivalence toward her parents. By organizing her diffuse anxiety into the more structured phobia, she could confine it to one part of her life (bedtime), functioning more comfortably the rest of the time. Ann wanted to be with her father but could not give up the tremendous rage she felt toward him for deserting them. She handled this unacceptable rage by putting it outside herself (i.e., by projecting it onto the kidnapper). Then, to neutralize her fear of the kidnapper, she took to sleeping with her mother, which not only protected her from the kidnapper but at the same time reassured her that her anger and competitiveness would not hurt the mother she loved and depended on. We can also see the phobic mechanism in Ann's play, when she projected her angry feelings onto the robber who then killed the mother while Ann, represented by the girl, was aware only of protective feelings toward her mother.

Separation Anxiety Disorder (309.21)

The child with a separation anxiety disorder is afraid of any separation from the principal attachment figures and/or from familiar surroundings. These children may suffer extreme anxiety at any attempt or threat of separation. They often refuse to sleep over with friends or to take school trips or go on errands outside the home, preferring to shadow or even cling to the parents than to experience panic or somatic symptoms at the slightest threat of disruption. The onset of the disorder may be preceded by a loss or a change of environment.

School refusal (school phobia) is a disorder that frequently combines features of a phobia with those of a separation anxiety disorder. In this condition the child refuses to attend school because of an intense but irrational fear expressed through a combination of frank anxiety and somatic symptoms. Technically it differs from a true phobia in that the disturbance is often deeply rooted in a pathological parent-child relationship, in which the parent's intense need to maintain a continuing attachment is blocking the normal development of independence. The child typically is symptom free as long as there is no pressure to leave home or parents, since school is the phobic situation onto which the conflict has been projected. Sometimes a minor physical illness serves as a precipitant. Most children with school phobia are better than average students and reasonably well adapted socially but show a number of psychoneurotic features. A smaller but still substantial number suffer from a personality disorder. This chronic form, which may result if the acute stage is not adequately treated or may develop gradually following a long period of repeated absenteeism for questionable illnesses, is more common in older children. Here the process is more insidious and difficult to interrupt as the children are so much more dependent on their mothers and more immature in their social adaptation. An even smaller group of older children or adolescents shows this behavior as the manifestation of an underlying psychosis.

Management consists of returning and maintaining the child in school. The sooner this is achieved, the better the prognosis. Persistent inattendance aggravates and fixes the pathology. Instead of the anxiety that was a feature of the acute stage, the chronic stage is dominated by evidence of passive aggressiveness (oppositionality) and hostile dependence. Secondary gain (additional advantages obtained from the phobic behavior) such as time alone with mother, treats, bribes, and so forth, may also be prominent in the chronic stage, especially within the neurotic group of children (Coolidge et al. 1960).

The first stage of treatment involves getting the child back to school as soon as possible. Child and family must be assessed adequately to ensure that the child is capable of returning to school (which is almost invariably the case) and to study factors within child and family that are perpetuating the problem, as well as those strengths that can be utilized to support the child's return. When this is done, parents and child must be informed that, while the inability to attend school is symptomatic of an emotional disturbance requiring treatment, an essential part of that treatment is getting the child back to school immediately and school attendance is nonnegotiable. From this point on, the treatment may vary. Some therapists merely inform the parents that it is up to them to derive a workable method of returning the child to school. Psychotherapy sessions several times a week are then used to help parents and child identify and resolve difficulties occurring as they attempt to implement their chosen plan.

> Kenneth, referred to a psychiatrist at age fourteen, had been away from school and in home-bound teaching since developing diabetes just over a year earlier. His mother, frightened by the diagnosis, became even more overprotective than she already was. Kenneth was assessed as being capable of returning to school, although he insisted he was too panicky to tolerate it. The therapist reiterated to the parents the primary importance of their getting Kenneth back to school in spite of his objections. They reluctantly agreed, and twice-weekly sessions were set up with all three so that the therapist could assist in the process.
>
> By the next session, Kenneth's parents were still letting him stay at home. He had complained of a stomachache, and though they doubted that he was ill, they were afraid to upset him. The therapist repeated that the parents must overcome their anxieties in order for Kenneth to overcome his and return to school. They had let themselves be manipulated into undermining the treatment.
>
> In the following session, an incident was recounted in which Kenneth had refused to dress for school. His father threatened that he would dress him, but his attempt to do so turned into a physical battle that ended with the father slapping Kenneth. The mother came to her son's defense, the father capitulated, and Kenneth stayed home. The therapist outlined the role of all three. Kenneth's refusal to dress had provoked his father's physical intervention. The father was supported in his attempt to take a firm stand, and the mother was shown that she had colluded in Kenneth's avoidance of school. Fortunately she was able to acknowledge this, and she subsequently told Kenneth that thenceforth he could dress himself or be dressed, but he alone was responsible for the consequences of his obstinacy.
>
> The next day Kenneth went to school and basically continued to attend despite frequent short absences in which his mother colluded. The therapy sessions, soon reduced to one a week, continued for over a year concurrent with individual therapy for Kenneth and the mother. Kenneth was, by this time, attending school regularly and without anxiety, and there was some increase

in family harmony. However, neither family nor individual psychotherapy succeeded in modifying the excessively close bond between mother and son that contributed to an obvious but unacknowledged effeminacy. The parents eventually left therapy to avoid handling this.

An alternate plan of management is illustrated by the case of Alice, age eleven, who had been out of school for a much shorter period of time.

An emergency assessment had established that while Alice was capable of returning to school in spite of her anxiety, her parents seemed to lack the resources to help her do so. Alice's mother, who was still very dependent on her own mother, found it impossible to stand firm in the face of Alice's clinging and tears. Her father was unable to take any position unless directed to do so by his wife. It was decided, therefore, with the parents' agreement that a social worker from the clinic would call at the house each morning and take Alice to school. Along with Alice's principal, her teacher, and the family, the social worker drew up a plan for gradually reintroducing Alice to the school. The first day they would go just as far as the door at a time when no children were in the schoolyard; the next day they would stand in the hall just outside the classroom; and so forth. This process of gradually introducing Alice to increasing exposures to school at a predictable rate that she could tolerate while supported by a kind but determined adult gradually decreased Alice's anxiety about attending school. Twice-weekly psychotherapy sessions were conducted concurrently to prepare the parents to replace the social worker in giving Alice the direction and the support she needed and to help Alice learn to deal with her marked hostility to her parents.

After about two weeks, the parents began to feel that Alice was manipulating them and that anxiety was no longer a major factor in her nonattendance. This, added to their mounting frustration, led them to take the position that Alice would be rewarded if she attended school but sent to her room if she did not. Once Alice was convinced of the parents' ability to hold their position, she returned and remained in school. Unfortunately, once school attendance was no longer an issue, the parents were not motivated to continue to work on the relationship difficulties that had precipitated the school refusal and, against the advice of their therapist, withdrew from treatment.

This example is one in which behavior therapy and psychotherapy were combined in the treatment of the school refusal. The gradual exposure to increasing doses of school was an attempt at desensitization (classical conditioning), while the decision to reward school attendance and isolate Alice in her room for nonattendance in the phase when anger and attention seeking seemed to be the major perpetuating factors was an example of operant conditioning (Hersen 1971; Lazarus, Davison, and Polefka 1965). (For a brief description of the theoretical base and techniques of behavior therapy, see chapter 28.)

As the preceding examples suggest, the management of school refusal usually requires the school, the parents, the child, and the treatment team to work together. Both parents and child require immediate intervention if the disorder is not to become chronic and intractable. Neither simple return to school nor psychotherapy alone can be considered adequate management. In very severe cases that fail to respond to treatment or where suicide, self-injury, or further decompensation are apparent, inpatient treatment may have to be considered. Most children, however, can be returned to school relatively quickly, though frequently this undermines the parental motivation to deal more fully with the underlying psychological and relationship problem.

School refusal in adolescence is both more difficult to treat and has a poorer prognosis. More frequently than with children, it is symptomatic of more serious pathology. It is harder to physically persuade the adolescent to return to school. Often a formerly bright and achieving child becomes, because of repeated absences, thoroughly turned off from academic achievement and doubly difficult to motivate to return.

The picture of school refusal needs to be distinguished from truancy.

GROUP II

In Group II disorders the child avoids anxiety through the excessive use of social withdrawal or psychological defenses. The child is left drained of energy and with a major restriction of the life field. While some degree of restriction accompanies all neuroses, children suffering from Group II disorders automatically avoid any activity, person, or situation associated with even the possibility of anxiety, unpleasantness, or failure. The disorders in this group are represented diagrammatically in figure 12.2. The closest diagnostic category in DSM-III is avoidant disorder of childhood and adolescence (313.21).

Avoidant Disorder of Childhood and Adolescence (313.21)

One example of the avoidant disorder would be that of children who restrict themselves by refusing to try or to participate in major areas of

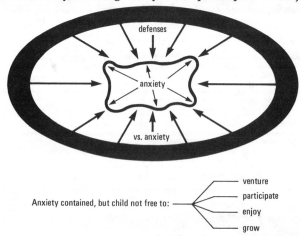

Figure 12.2 The Neurotic Child: Group II—Defenses Restricting.

life because of the anxiety associated with involvement or with the possibility of failure or rejection. Thus withdrawal from activities and restriction of relationships at the cost of impoverishing their life experience and inhibiting further development are the predominant clinical features.

> Gary's parents were concerned about the amount of time he spent watching television alone. He had no problem at home or school but had few interests and no close friends. On examination, Gary, age eleven, showed no evidence of acute distress and in fact expressed an interest in a number of activities and in a few of his classmates. He had never developed these interests or relationships because, he said, it was not worth the effort; he would be a failure and make a fool of himself. In this way he avoided anxiety and any possibility of failure but seriously restricted the scope of his life.

Another example would be constricted children who fear not the anxiety associated with possible failure but a particular activity that has taken on a symbolic significance that, since it is taboo, must then be avoided.

> Stephen, age fourteen, was a fine natural athlete who excelled at skiing and tennis. When playing just for enjoyment, he was almost unbeatable in his own age group. In any major competition, however, he was unable to concentrate or perform anywhere near his level of ability. He recognized the pattern but did not understand it and could do nothing about it. During treatment, the therapist realized that for Stephen, at an unconscious level, winning meant the literal destruction of his opponent. This equation, coupled with Stephen's unrecognized fear of his strong but repressed hostile and aggressive feelings, effectively blocked his ability to compete successfully. When through his therapy Stephen was able to deal appropriately with his aggression, his ability to compete successfully improved.

GROUP III

Group III disorders feature an excessive investment in defenses that, while working, keep the child relatively free of anxiety at tremendous cost. The defenses are used in so exaggerated and inflexible a manner that the child's entire personality and functioning are distorted. The diagrammatic representation of this group of disorders is found in figure 12.3.

Conversion Disorder (Hysterical Neurosis, Conversion Type) (300.11)

In conversion disorder, the conflict is first repressed and then converted (i.e., represented symbolically) via a somatic symptom, usually involving the voluntary muscles or the somatosensory system. Hysterical blindness, paralysis, anesthesias, pain, or vomiting would be examples. A conversion symptom differs from a psychophysiological disorder in that it involves no physiological dysfunction. DSM-III classifies conversion disorders as a subgroup of somatoform disorders, as the symptoms suggest physical disorder in the absence of demonstrable organic findings or known physiological mechanisms (see chapter 16). Although this descriptive definition

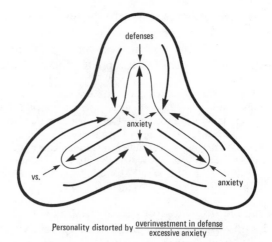

Personality distorted by $\frac{\text{overinvestment in defense}}{\text{excessive anxiety}}$

Figure 12.3 The Neurotic Child: Group III Defenses Distorting.

applies to the conversion disorders, the authors have chosen to discuss them at this point, because they demonstrate the underlying neurotic process common to all the anxiety disorders. A conversion neurosis is more likely to occur in a child with a histrionic personality. (For a definition of histrionic personality, see p. 253.)

> Ten-year-old Nina had one younger brother who, almost a year before, had been left hemiplegic and speechless following a sudden and dramatic illness. Every day after work, Nina's distraught parents would rush to the hospital, leaving Nina in the care of her aged grandmother. Nina too was very upset about her brother's illness, but she also deeply resented it. She felt her parents no longer had time or love for her, but she was called selfish and punished if she complained. She stopped complaining but soon developed pain and a persistent limp in her left knee, which defied investigation. During her third appearance in the emergency room, an intern, noting that the brother was paralyzed on his left side, suspected a conversion reaction. On inquiry, Nina told of a series of repeated dreams. In some of these her brother had died and gone to heaven. In others—and she broke down and sobbed as she told of these—she had killed him. Further investigations suggested that Nina's intense conflict between feelings of love, hate, and guilt had been converted into the leg pain and stiffness that to her symbolized (unconsciously) an identification with the ambivalently loved brother.

Dissociative Disorder (300.12—Amnesia; 300.13—Fugue States; 300.60—Depersonalization)

In a dissociative reaction, there is a temporary marked personality disorganization that results in fugue states (300.13) (i.e., sudden unexpected travel away from home and familiar surroundings, combined with inability to recall the past and the partial or total assumption of a new identity); amnesia (300.12); or depersonalization (300.60) (one or more episodes in which the child experiences so marked a change in self-perception that disorientation and interference with social, academic, or vocational functioning result).

> A twelve-year-old girl, who had always been extremely close to her father and to some extent had taken her mother's place in the unsatisfactory marriage, was greatly upset when the father left home for another woman. In her waking life, the girl quickly regained her composure and continued her academic and social life. At night, however, she had fugue states in which she would wander about, acting-out sexually tinged fantasies that represented unconscious feelings for her father, although she could not recall any of these episodes the next day.

Obsessive-Compulsive Disorder (300.30)

Obsessive-compulsive disorder is characterized by two related groups of symptoms. Obsessions are recurring thoughts, ideas, or fantasies that, often against the child's will, persist in recurring again and again. Associated with them are compulsions, repetitive ritualized acts that the patient is compelled to perform, to participate in, or, conversely, to avoid, often in order to prevent some imagined future situation or event. In actual fact, the activity itself lacks the magical or preventive effect that the child attributes to it. Thus, for example, in spite of a child's fears to the contrary, nothing disastrous occurs if the child is prevented from completing an elaborate and time-consuming bedtime ritual. In other cases it is the degree to which normal behavior must be exaggerated and repeated that makes it compulsive, as in the child who must compulsively wash the hands more than thirty times a day in order to avoid contamination. Often the act is carried out against some internal resistance and is associated with embarrassment or shame, for the child has some recognition that this is senseless behavior even though compelled to perform it to ward off intolerable anxiety. This is particularly true in older children or adolescents, who generally have a more sophisticated and logical sense of casuality. But even if the obsessions and compulsions are recognized as "ego-alien" (foreign) or even crazy by the patient, they must be performed in order to avoid excessive tension.

> An adolescent girl who was struggling to attain a sense of identity separate from her loving but overpowering mother felt compelled to leave the rotating part of the combination on her school locker set at the number sixteen. She felt that sixteen was nice and rounded, the square of a squared number. Fifteen and seventeen were jagged, dangerous numbers. Unless she checked repeatedly that the lock had not been left at a dangerous number, she feared for her mother's safety. She often even phoned her mother to check that she was all right, which annoyed the mother intensely. The girl was unaware of any hostility toward her mother, only feelings of concern. She realized her symptoms were absurd, but if she did not check, she became unbearably anxious.

Breaking the established pattern elicits moderate to severe anxiety and distress. Parents and others important to the child (i.e., peers, teachers), sensing the irrationality and embarrassed by the conspicuousness of the child's symptoms, are often upset by them. As a result they frequently pressure the affected child to control or avoid the ritual. This adds an interpersonal dimension to the child's tension, increasing the level of anxiety or guilt that the child can discharge only via further use of the symptom.

> Sandy, a highly anxious and very angry fifteen-year-old, had a number of compulsive rituals that, the previous year, had made him the laughingstock of his peer group and the butt of one insensitive teacher's jokes. This year he was able, through tremendous conscious effort, to suppress these while in school, although when the tension became unbearable, he would manage to be excused from class and go somewhere where he would privately perform the rituals until he calmed down.
> Each day after school, Sandy would spend hours alone in his room talking aloud about the events of the day while compulsively tugging at his earlobes, although they were sore and red. He was embarrassed by this behavior, but if his upset parents attempted to interrupt it he would become panicky and angry, insisting that he needed to do this in order to settle down to the point where he could do his homework.

According to the DSM-III, the most common obsessions are thoughts of violence, contamination, or doubt (American Psychiatric Association 1980). While even the normal child may develop one or more obsessions or compulsions for brief periods, these usually recede spontaneously within a week or two as long as the parents keep a reasonable perspective and avoid a major battle about them with the child. These "normal symptoms" differ from the obsessive-compulsive disorder, in which the symptomatic behavior is sufficiently severe and lasting to alter and impair the child's normal behavior and social functioning.

Dysthmic Disorder (or Depressive Neurosis) (300.40)

Children are often depressed in reaction to a loss, disappointment, or a physical illness. Depression is neurotic when it becomes a chronic condition maintained largely by internal conflict rather than a transitory response to external circumstances. The depression may be masked, with the clinical picture being dominated by one or more "depressive equivalents," for example, an eating or sleeping disturbance, social withdrawal, antisocial behavior, or academic underachievement. For a more extensive description of depression in children, see chapter 14.

Personality Disorders

In the neurotic disorders just discussed, a specific problem foreign to the child's personality is interfering with the usual mode of functioning. By contrast, in the personality disorders there exists a mental set of thinking, feeling, or relating that is inflexible and maladaptive but that seems to be an intrinsic part of the patient's personality. It is not experienced as a symptom or illness. A personality disorder is an enduring set of characteristics of a person rather than an episodic occurrence like the neurotic disorders. The personality disorders are coded on Axis 2 and may coexist with psychiatric diagnoses such as anxiety disorders, which are recorded on Axis 1 of DSM-III.

Some disorders of childhood and adolescence recorded on Axis 1 have much in common with certain personality disorders recorded on Axis 2. The childhood disorders are not, however, always continuous with the adult personality disorders. The diagnosis of a personality disorder implies not only some degree of subjective distress and impairment in social, academic, or occupational functioning but also that the personality characteristic is a stable (i.e., fixed and permanent) one. As a result, since children's personalities can change considerably in the course of development, a diagnosis of personality disorder is less common in a child. Several personality disorders listed on Axis 2, however, have a corresponding childhood disorder listed on Axis 1, (i.e., it is not yet considered permanent). These are listed in table 12.1.

TABLE 12.1

Disorders in Children and Adolescents Corresponding to Personality Disorders in Adults*

GROUP 1	Paranoid	301.00	Schizoid disorder of childhood	
	Schizoid	301.20	or adolescence	313.22
	Schizotypal	301.22		
GROUP II	Histrionic	301.50		
	Narcissistic	301.81		
	Antisocial	301.70		
	Borderline	301.83	Conduct disorder in child	
			or adolescent	312.00, 312.10, 312.23, 312.21, 312.90
			Identity disorder in child	
			or adolescent	313.82
GROUP III	Avoidant	301.82	Avoidant disorder of childhood	
	Dependent	301.60	and adolescence	313.21
	Compulsive	301.40		
	Passive/Aggressive	301.24		
	Atypical, mixed, or		Oppositional disorder in child	
	other	301.89	or adolescent	313.81

*The diagnostic categories and numbers used in this classification are those used in DSM-III (American Psychiatric Association 1980).

There are three main groups of personality disorders.

GROUP I

Group I disorders are the schizoid disorders of childhood and adolescence, schizoid, paranoid, and schizotypical personality disorders. All disorders in this group are characterized by emotional constriction, rigidity, aloofness, with an inability to participate in free social interaction. Constitutional defects may be significant predisposing factors in these disorders, which show some characteristics seen in schizophrenic disorders though they are not present in sufficient severity or associated with the pathognomic features as to constitute the real break with reality that would allow a diagnosis of psychosis.

Schizoid Disorders of Childhood and Adolescence (313.22)

Distant and seclusive, these children are unable to form close relationships with anyone. They show little apparent interest in making or being with friends and seem indifferent to the feelings or opinions of others, remaining uncomfortable and inept in social situations. Their reality testing remains intact. The disorder, commonly diagnosable at about five years of age, may be self-limited, hence this diagnosis is recorded on Axis I of DSM-III. The trend toward emotional withdrawal may continue, however, developing in adolescence or adult life into one of other personality disorders within Group I or as the precursor of schizophrenia.

Schizoid Personality Disorder (301.20)

The schizoid personality disorder is characterized by marked isolation, indifference to praise or criticism, and an incapacity to experience warmth or empathy for others. Lacking social skills, these individuals often appear cold, aloof, and extremely isolated from intimate relationships.

Paranoid Personality Disorder (301.00)

Those with a paranoid personality are unduly suspicious, excessively jealous, hypersensitive, and overly reactive to any challenge or criticism, which may be been as persecution or attack.

Schizotypal Personality Disorder (301.22)

A person with a schizotypal personality disorder shows marked oddities of thinking (e.g., magical thinking, bizarre fantasy, ideas of reference, superstitiousness), perceptions (e.g., recurrent illusions or depersonalization), speech (e.g., digressive, vague, overly elaborate), and behavior (e.g., social isolation and lack of rapport).

Those demonstrating histrionic, narcissistic, antisocial, identity, and borderline personality disorders are somewhat more socially competent than those in Group I but are dramatic, emotional, self-centered, and unstable in their reactions. These disorders often originate in earlier and more severe developmental defects, especially disturbances in attachment and interpersonal relationships, than do the symptom disorders.

Histrionic Personality Disorders (301.50)

Prone to exaggeration and dramatization, those with a histrionic personality disorder show intense, theatrical behavior that demands constant attention. Emotionally labile and manipulative, their relationships are superficial and demanding. Although at first they often seem socially skilled and sexually provocative, their excitability, irrational outbursts, and manipulative behavior usually end up alienating others and disrupting their interpersonal relationships.

Narcissistic Personality Disorder (301.81)

Those with a narcissistic personality disorder have an exaggerated or even grandiose sense of their own importance. They are continually demanding attention and preoccupied with fantasies of unlimited power and success. Their relationships are manipulative, exploitative, and unempathic. They may respond with cool indifference or catastrophic rage to any criticism from others. They bear a close resemblance to the histrionic but are less likable because of the manifest degree of self-absorption and indifference to others.

Antisocial Personality Disorder

The antisocial personality disorder of Axis II of DSM-III represents the persistence past age eighteen of what, in a child or adolescent, would be diagnosed a conduct disorder under Axis I (see chapter 13). Persons suffering from this disorder typically show a repeated disregard for social norms and are unable to function successfully either in the workplace or in the social environment.

Identity Disorder of Childhood and Adolescence (313.82)

Those with an identity disorder are characterized by the lack of a coherent sense of self. They are frequently troubled by uncertainty about goals, friendship patterns, sexual orientation, moral values, and loyalties. Anxiety and depression are manifest, and social, academic, or vocational functioning are impaired.

Borderline Personality Disorder (301.88)

A person with a borderline personality disorder shows evidence of an identity disorder along with extreme impulsiveness, unpredictability, instability, and intensity of emotion in interpersonal relationships. Underlying these is a profound sense of emptiness and loneliness. Those with a borderline personality show an extreme sensitivity to loss or disruption of key relationships (Shapiro et al. 1975). Self-mutilation and suicidal threats or behavior are common.

GROUP III

Avoidant, dependent, compulsive, oppositional, and passive/aggressive personality disorders seem more closely related to the neurotic (i.e., anxiety) disorders in that they seem to result from the integration into the personality structure of what was once an active intrapsychic struggle between anxiety and defenses against anxiety.

Avoidant Personality Disorder (301.82)

The person with an avoidant personality disorder, the childhood form of which is categorized as avoidant disorder of childhood (313.21) and listed on Axis I, strongly wants affection and friendships but is extremely sensitive to any rejection or humiliation. Such individuals defensively avoid social relationships or challenging situations in order to minimize the risk of rejection or social failure. As a result, withdrawal and restriction of their relationships are the predominant clinical feature.

Dependent Personality Disorder (301.60)

Those with a dependent personality disorder allow others to assume major areas of responsibility, subordinating their own needs to those of others who, in exchange, care for them. Passive and lacking in initiative and self-confidence, they require constant support from others in order to function.

Compulsive Personality Disorder (301.40)

The child or adolescent with a compulsive personality disorder is typically neat, tidy, and respectful, often superficially appearing older than the chronological age. Compulsive orderliness and perfectionism, presumably representing the incorporation into the personality of a successful defense against aggressive and messy tendencies, dominate the personality. Emotionally restricted, often domineering and lacking in spontaneity and creativity, children with a compulsive personality disorder find that the rigidity of their defenses will severely narrow the scope of their potential life experiences unless they manage, as is often the case, to break out during adolescence.

Oppositional Disorder (313.81)

Children with an oppositional personality disorder resist the usual demands for social and academic functioning. Typically stubborn, disobedient, difficult, and negative even when it is clearly in their best interests to cooperate, they either refuse, procrastinate, or become argumentative when asked to do something. They do not, however, show a pattern of repeated violation of the rights of others, or they would be diagnosed as having a conduct disorder. A child showing such behavior that has not yet become a permanent personality characteristic might be diagnosed as having an oppositional disorder under Axis I. The oppositional and provocative attitudes usually persist, often generalizing and becoming, in later life, a passive/aggressive personality disorder.

Passive/Aggressive Personality Disorder (301.84)

The person with a passive/aggressive personality disorder also tends to resist demands for adequate performance in both the social and academic (vocational) areas of functioning. The resistance may seem deliberate as in "intentional inefficiency," dawdling, stubbornness, or it may seem beyond the person's control (e.g., forgetfulness or procrastination). The pattern persists even in situations where it would be to the individual's advantage to be more direct and results in a continuing inefficiency in most areas of performance.

Prognosis

Little is known with certainty about the ultimate clinical course of psychoneuroses in children. The authors agree with Adams (1979) and Barker (1980) that psychoneuroses in children are less clearly defined and also less fixed and chronic than in adults. Both draw attention to the heterogeneity of the group, some of whom recover spontaneously while others appear to carry on at least some of their psychopathology into adult life. Meyer (1980) rightly points out that unlike conduct disorders, which generally become worse during adolescence, the symptoms of psychoneurosis may change but are not routinely intensified during the teenage years. Although Robins reported that children with psychoneuroses have a much better prognosis than those with conduct disorders—neurotic children at thirty-year follow-up were found to be "less of a problem both to society and to themselves" (Robins 1966, p. 73)—Graham, in his short-term follow-up of the Isle of Wight children three to four years after their initial testing, found a markedly increased rate of neurotic problems (Graham and Rutter 1973).

255

Treatment

Treatment is indicated if a neurosis becomes sufficiently fixed to interfere with normal development, as shown by the child not doing well in school, in social or family relationships, or in emotional expression and control. A usual goal of treatment is to enable the child to become sufficiently symptom free to continue a reasonably normal development. The treatment plan will make use of the particular strengths available in the child, the family, and the community. Individual psychotherapy, family therapy, or behavior therapy, all of which are described and illustrated in chapter 28, may contribute to the treatment of the individual child and family.

SUGGESTIONS FOR FURTHER READING

ADAMS, P. L. 1973. *Obsessive children: A sociopsychiatric study.* New York: Brunner/Mazel.
   A detailed study of the obsessive child.
COOLIDGE, J. C., et al. 1960. School phobia in adolescence: A manifestation of severe character disturbance. *Am. J. Orthopsychiat.* 30:599–607.
   An excellent formulation of the dynamics of school phobia, including changes in the dynamic picture as the school refusal becomes chronic.
COOPER, S., AND WANERMAN, L. 1977. *Children in treatment.* New York: Brunner/Mazel.
   A basic psychotherapeutic orientation for mental health trainees of all disciplines, integrating theory with long-term psychotherapeutic methodology of technique.
ELKINS, R.; RAPOPORT, J. L.; AND LIPSKY, A. 1980. Obsessive-compulsive disorder of childhood and adolescence. *J. Amer. Acad. Child Psychiat.* 19:511–524.
   Reviews the evidence supporting a neurobiological hypothesis regarding the obsessive-compulsive disorder, including twin studies, association with Gilles de la Tourette syndrome and brain damage, neuropsychological test data, and psychopharmacological effects.
   Group for the Advancement of Psychiatry. 1973. *From diagnosis to treatment: An approach to treatment planning for the emotionally disturbed child.* New York: GAP Publication 87, vol. 8.
   Easily understood, detailed discussion of the diagnostic process and its relation to treatment planning. Useful clinical examples.
GOODYER, I. 1981. Hysterical conversion reactions in childhood. *J. Child Psychol. & Psychiat.* 22(2):179–188.
   While dealing primarily with what constitutes a sensible assessment of children with conversion reactions, this article warns about the dangers of overinvestigation and comments on clinical outcome.
HERSEN, M. 1971. The behavioral treatment of school phobia: Current techniques. *J. Nerv. & Mental Dis.* 152:99–108.
   Following a review of case histories, this article suggests various behavioral modification techniques that were found effective in managing children with school phobia.
HOLLINGSWORTH, C. E., et al. 1980. Long-term outcome of obsessive-compulsive disorder in childhood. *J. Am. Acad. Child Psychiat.* 19:134–144.
   Reviews seventeen children seen over sixteen-year period with diagnosis of obsessive-compulsive neurosis who had been treated mostly with "intensive"

psychotherapy. Discusses family history, school performance, social adjustment, and relationship of treatment to residual symptoms as well as reviewing the literature on this condition.

LAZARRE, A. 1981. Current concepts in psychiatry: Conversion symptoms. *N. E. J. Med.* 305(13):745–748.
An excellent article highlighting the interrelationships between conversion symptoms and organic disease.

LIPPMAN, H. S. 1962. *Treatment of the child in emotional conflict,* 2nd ed., New York: McGraw-Hill.
This analytically oriented textbook of child psychiatry is notable for its excellent clinical vignettes and discussions of children's responses to psychotherapy.

POZNANSKI, E. O. 1973. Children with excessive fears. *Am. J. Orthopsychiat.* 43:428–438.
Intelligent observation of twenty-eight children with excessive fears, discussing demographic characteristics, the nature and content of the fears, their context, symbolization, and displacement.

RUTTER, M., et al. 1976. Isle of Wight studies, 1964–1974. *Psychol. Med.* 6:313–332.
A summary of the Isle of Wight studies on the prevalence and course of various psychiatric and educational disorders of childhood and adolescence.

WOLFF, S., AND BARLOW, A. 1979. Schizoid personality in childhood: A comparative study of schizoid, autistic and normal children. *J. Child Psychol. & Psychiat.* 20:29–46.
A comparative study of seventeen schizoid, thirteen autistic, and eight normal children. Discusses the similarity of these children to many diagnosed borderline in the United States, the validity of the distinction between the groups studied, and the clinical characteristics of each group.

13 *Clive Chamberlain and Paul D. Steinhauer*

Conduct Disorders and Delinquency

Definition and Introduction

A conduct disorder is a recurrent and persistent pattern of behavior in which the rights of others and major social norms are repeatedly violated. Delinquency, on the other hand, is a legal entity; the delinquent is a person under the age of majority who has been found guilty in court of a breach of the law.

More conduct (i.e., behavior) disorders have been seen in child guidance clinics and child psychiatric settings in Britain and North America than any other group of emotional or behavioral problems (Rosen, Bahn, and Kramer, 1964; Rutter, Tizard, and Whitmore, 1970). In fact, the original impetus for the development of such clinics early in this century was a worldwide concern with chronically misbehaving children and youth that culminated in the establishment of juvenile courts and correctional programs. Now, sixty years after the establishment of these services, we are still left with much controversy regarding causation, classification, and results. Four of the reasons for the persistence of this controversy will be considered.

First, there is no acceptable and generally accepted classification of conduct disorders. The terms conduct disorder and behavior disorder refer to a constellation of behavioral symptoms. In the past this single diagnostic category has grouped together a variety of quite different children who behave the same way for very different reasons and who have not as yet been clearly distinguished from each other. Thus when researchers and clinicians studied and wrote about children with conduct disorders, one could not be sure which subgroup or what mixture of children was being studied or discussed. Recently several classifications that offer greater diagnostic precision have been suggested. While we are not yet at the point where we can agree on the ideal classification of children with conduct disorders, we can at least agree that it should meet the criteria for an acceptable classification listed in chapter 6. It should also be developmental rather than purely descriptive when dealing with children who are still developing and should be widely accepted by the various professions working with this clinical population (Steinhauer 1978).

A second cause of the controversy regarding causation, classification, and results is the variety of agencies and professionals who identify, work with, and study children with conduct disorders. Children with conduct disorders are identified, assessed, labeled, and managed by workers from a variety of services and professional disciplines. Depending on where the conduct disorder was most evident, the socioeconomic group and psychological sophistication of the parents, the training, alertness, and sensitivity of the professionals to whom the child was exposed, or even the services available in the home community, the children might be identified and managed within any one or more of four overlapping service systems: police and correctional authorities; the educational system; child welfare services; or child psychiatric services. Although children with conduct disorders do not make up the whole of the population served by any of these institutions (i.e., not all delinquent, underachieving, neglected or abused, or disturbed children have conduct disorders), they are prominently represented in each, and the overlaps are striking (Robins 1974).

A third factor is the association of conduct disorders with other psychiatric diagnoses. In spite of the common behavioral constellation with which they present, children with conduct disorders are often diagnosed as having a variety of quite different associated psychiatric diagnoses. Thus the child's misbehavior may be just the first or most obvious manifestation of a large range of disturbances, including: hyperkinetic disorder, minimal brain damage or attention deficit disorder; learning disorder; personality disorder; tension discharge disorder; neurotic personality or neurotic behavior disorders; pseudopsychopathic schizophrenia; schizoid disorder; oppositional disorder; borderline syndrome or disorder. Not all children belonging to any of these diagnostic groups have a conduct disorder, although conduct-disordered children are well represented in each. To confuse the picture further, the relationship between the associated psychiatric disorder and the conduct disorder or antisocial behavior is not clear.

We know, for example, that there is a common association between conduct disorders and school failure. We do not yet know, however:
(a) Whether the conduct disorder is a cause of the school failure.
(b) Whether the school failure is a cause of the conduct disorder.

259

(c) Whether school failure and conduct disorder are both symptoms of a third underlying factor.

(d) Whether all of these, in some cases, may be true. (Zinkus 1979)

Fourth, children with conduct disorders are managed differently by the members of the various professional disciplines with whom they come in contact. Since each of these disciplines has its own diagnostic labels, speaks its own language, writes in its own journals, and proceeds in its own often idiosyncratic ways, the potential for confusion is obvious. The inability to agree on and work from a common classification has resulted in the unwitting construction of a professional Tower of Babel (Steinhauer 1978). This has made it almost impossible to interpret satisfactorily or to correlate the vast amount of research that has been done in this area.

Classification

In a discussion of classification, one major caveat is appropriate. The notion of disorder, like that of illness, suggests that the difficulty lies in the individual who is identified and labeled. It has become increasingly apparent that an ecological perspective on behavior dysfunction expands our understanding. Individual behavior can only be understood if we view the child not as an isolated entity but as one node in a network of complex interactions.

> An eleven-year-old boy appeared in juvenile court on his third charge of arson within as many months. Two automobiles had been demolished and a barn burned to the ground. These acts had been carried out alone, and the youngster could not give any reason for his behavior. Quite by chance an adult close to the family was found guilty of sexually molesting another child, at which time it was discovered that a clandestine affair had also involved the young arsonist. Follow-up revealed satisfactory behavior and development following the adult's apprehension.

DSM-III takes a purely descriptive approach to classification and places little emphasis on the historical and developmental dimensions (Rutter and Shaffer 1980). It divides conduct disorders into four main groups, defining each in terms of the common behavior of its members along two major dimensions, aggression and level of social maturity. First it subdivides conduct disorders into undersocialized or socialized groups, depending on whether or not the youngster has been able to establish bonds of affection with and feel empathy toward others. Those in the undersocialized group lack the capacity for meaningful relationships. While they may have superficial relationships, within these they are typically egocentric and manipulative, using others for what they can get and turning on or discarding them without guilt or remorse when it is in their own interest to do so. Thus it is not uncommon for youngsters with an undersocialized conduct disorder to inform on or blame their companions and "friends" whenever they consider it to their advantage. Children with socialized conduct disorders, on the other hand, have a group of friends to whom they are socially attached. They can be just as manipulative, self-serving, and callous whenever anyone outside their particular group is being victimized, but they are unlikely to inform on members of their own group, even when it is to their advantage to do so.

Within these two major grouping, DSM-III divides the population further into aggressive and nonaggressive subgroups. The distinguishing feature of the aggressive subgroup is a repetitive, persistent pattern of aggressive conduct that violates the rights of others, such as physical violence (e.g., rape, muggings, and assaults) and thefts outside the home that involve confrontations with the victim (e.g., purse snatching, extortion, holdups). The nonaggressive subgroup shows an absence of physical violence. Its members generally show more passive behavior such as running away, truancy, stealing, and lying. If they commit thefts outside the home, these typically do not involve confrontations with the victim. The final subcategory, atypical, is essentially residual in nature. The five subdivisions of conduct disorder in DSM-III are summarized in table 13.1.

Additional diagnoses in DSM-III that are commonly associated with conduct disorder and the chapters in this book that discuss them are listed in table 13.2.

When persistent misbehavior is a major characteristic, any of the categories listed in table 13.2 may be appropriate either as added diagnoses or alone, but a judgment has to be made as to the most significant aspect of the behavior pattern. In *attention deficit disorder,* the misbehavior has a random or diffuse character at least early in its development, and seems more disinhibited than purposive. *Schizoid* youngsters may also display a range of antisocial behavior, but their most impressive feature is their so-

TABLE 13.1
Subdivisions of Conduct Disorder in DSM-III

Conduct Disorder	Code
(a) Undersocialized, agressive	312.00
undersocialized, nonaggressive	312.10
(b) Socialized, aggressive	312.23
socialized, nonagressive	312.21
(c) atypical	312.90

TABLE 13.2

Other DSM-III Diagnoses Commonly Associated with Conduct Disorder

Disorder	Code	Chapter
1. Attention Deficit Disorder		Chapter 10
(a) with hyperactivity	314.01	
(b) without hyperactivity	314.00	
2. Schizoid Disorder of Childhood or Adolescence	313.22	Chapter 12
3. Oppositional Disorder	313.81	Chapter 12
4. Specific Developmental Disorders	315.00–.50	Chapter 17
5. Child or Adolescent Antisocial Behaviour	V71.02	
6. Borderline Intellectual Functioning	V62.89	Chapter 18

cial isolation, awkwardness, and aloofness. "Oppositional disorder" describes disobedient, provocative children who confine their behavior to combating authority figures such as parents and teachers but rarely commit offenses. "Childhood or adolescent antisocial behavior" refers primarily to isolated rather than repeated antisocial behavior. Those children with *borderline intellectual functioning* are disproportionately highly represented in delinquent populations and tend to be given harsher sentences, probably because they are less adept at avoiding being caught, less well defended, and because of unrecognized social and legal discrimination (Boone 1975).

Over time, children's behavior and thus diagnoses may shift. Many children with conduct disorders frustrate easy classification. The basic purpose of classification is an applied one, that of enhancing prediction of outcome and choice of management and remedial strategies. Distinctions are useful only if they assist in achieving such goals, either by making group comparisons in research possible or, more immediately, by relating to known differences in treatment response or prognosis. Badly behaved children are not the exclusive province of psychiatry or medicine. Other disciplines and service systems have sought systems of classification for similar practical purposes. One such classification system, developed in conjunction with the California Youth Authority's Community Treatment Project in the late 1950s, is called I-Level (Interpersonal Maturity Level). Warren (1966), T. Palmer (1978), and others studied behavior patterns of large numbers of delinquent youth and developed a typology specifically for the purpose of differentiating between treatment alternatives (Grant 1961).

According to the theory underlying this system, the ways in which individuals perceive the world and themselves change as personality develops and as interactions between them and their environment result in successively new integrations of experience into social-perceptual frames of reference. Warren (1966) describes these frames of reference as "relatively consistent sets of expectations and attitudes, kinds of working philosophies of life." While individuals may simultaneously show some features of more than one level, a level that represents their basic level of interpersonal maturity can usually be selected. Seven levels of interpersonal development are distinguished along a continuum from birth to full maturity (Pauker and Hood 1979). These are:

I_1 This is the level of separation of self from environment.
I_2 Persons and events are viewed primarily as sources of either frustration or short-term pleasure; people are either givers or withholders; frustration tolerance is low, and the capacity for understanding the behavior of others is poor.
I_3 These individuals interact with others mainly in terms of oversimplified, externally determined value systems and assume that others do the same. Those at this level recognize that their own behavior can affect how much they get from others and try to manipulate the environment to provide "giving" rather than "denying" responses. They perceive the world and their part in it largely in terms of power. Although they have learned to assume stereotyped roles, they cannot understand the needs, feelings, or motives of others, and they are unmotivated to achieve in any long-term sense or to plan for the future.
I_4 Those whose understanding and behavior are integrated at this level have internalized a set of standards they use to judge their own and others' behavior. They can appreciate a level of interpersonal interaction in which people have expectations of and can influence each other by means other than manipulation. They have some ability to understand the reasons for behavior and to relate to others on an emotional and long-term basis. Their identifications are with oversimplified models based on black-and-white definitions of good and bad, with little tolerance of shades of gray or ambiguities. They are strongly influenced by those they admire and, because of the rigidity of their standards, prone to feeling self-critical and guilty.
I_5 These individuals have achieved more of a comfortable tolerance of self and others, with an understanding that people are complex and not simply either good or bad. Empathy with different kinds of people becomes possible. Standards for the self and others are less rigid, and there is not one right, easy answer for each problem. Less than 1 percent of the delinquent population falls into this category, and Harris (1978) found only 2 percent of a nondelinquent population had achieved integration at the I_5 level.
I_6 The I_6 person sees self and others in more complex ways, viewing behavior in terms of both general principles and the specific histories of the people involved and distinguishing between a stable self and the role engaged in.
I_7 A hypothetical, ideal level.

In theory all persons can be classified into one or another seven I-Levels. The developers of this system have found that most delinquents tend to fall into levels 2, 3, and 4, within which nine empirically derived subtypes of delinquency have been established, based on the individual's typical ways of conducting relations with others.

I₂ Asocial, Aggressive (Aa)—responds with active demands and open hostility when frustrated.

Asocial, Passive (Ap)—responds with whining, complaining, and withdrawal when frustrated.

I₃ Passive Conformist (Cfm)—responds with immediate compliance to whoever seems to have the power at the moment.

Cultural Conformist (Cfc)—responds with conformity to specific reference groups (delinquent peers).

Manipulatory (Mp)—operates by attempting to undermine the power of authority figures and/or usurp the power role for themselves.

I₄ Neurotic, Acting-out (Na)—responds to underlying guilt with attempts to outrun or avoid conscious anxiety and condemnation of self.

Neurotic, Anxious (Nx)—responds with symptoms of emotional disturbance to conflict produced by feelings of inadequacy and guilt.

Situational Emotional Reaction (Se)—responds to immediate family or personal crisis by acting-out.

Cultural Identifier (Ci)—responds to identification with a deviant value system by living out his or her delinquent beliefs.

This I-Level system is currently used by correctional organizations in various centers in North America, and ongoing research continues to improve its predictive power for treatment and prognostic purposes (Warren et al 1966; Jesness et al. 1972).

Both DSM-III and I-Level make distinctions on the basis of social maturity level (unsocialized—socialized) and aggressiveness. They differ, however, in several important respects. DSM-III is derived from a clinical population (children coming to psychiatric attention) and attempts to avoid theoretical bias and maintain descriptive purity. I-Levels, on the other hand, draw their form from careful examination of a large number of delinquent youth but are shaped by a theoretical preference that takes history and developmental factors into account. Specific subtypes are based on statistical manipulation of observed and inferred characteristics and have been subjected to much scrutiny for validity and reliability. Both systems have their critics and are controversial (Pauker and Hood 1979).

Other systems have been developed over the past twenty years and have currency in various parts of the world or within specific disciplines or service systems. Within the medical sphere, ICD-9 is the chief competitor, being used everywhere except North America and coexisting with DSM-III in Canada. Those correctional services that use classification favor variations of I-Level, as well as other systems based on cognitive development, such as conceptual level (Brill 1977; Harvey, Hunt, and Schroder, 1961) or moral development (Kohlberg 1969), or on less theoretical approaches such as the Quay Factors (Johnson 1977; Quay

1978). (For a summary of these classification systems, see Pauker and Hood 1979.)

All such systems, both medical and correctional, attempt to subdivide a large and diffuse category of problematic behavior into valid and useful subcategories and types, both to permit effective research in a confused field and to enhance the capacity of the clinician and therapist to communicate clearly.

Epidemiology

As with any phenomenon whose definition is fuzzy and shades gradually into normal behavior, reports of prevalence and natural history must be evaluated carefully for error and invalid comparison. Much confusion has resulted from the failure to take into account the fact that there are two separate literatures dealing with conduct disorders, each surveying a rather different population. The self-report literature suggests a high incidence of antisocial behavior, most of it of a mild or occasional nature. This literature contrasts markedly with studies of adjudicated delinquents, whose histories feature more serious antisocial behavior repeated more frequently and over a long period of time. In spite of great difficulty, researchers in many parts of the world have contributed to a progressive clarification of the nature and extent of the group of problems under discussion (Williams and Gold 1972).

Rutter's figures for the Isle of Wight study referred to in the introduction to this chapter stand up well in comparison with studies done in North America (Rutter, Tizard, and Whitmore 1970). In addition to the question of prevalence, the prognostic significance of disturbance of social behavior is one that investigators have addressed.

Robins (1970) reviewed twenty-three studies that followed up antisocial children for a minimum of ten years following first identification. Outcomes were compared with normal, neurotic, and psychotic children. The general finding was that the conduct-disordered group did less well than their normal and neurotic peers but had less maladjusted adult lives than did the children diagnosed as psychotic. Youngsters seen because of antisocial behavior at a child guidance clinic in St. Louis at a mean age of thirteen were followed up by Robins (1966). By age eighteen only 16 percent had permanently "recovered." When interviewed at an average age of forty-three, more than 25 percent had shown sufficient variety and severity of antisocial behavior during their adult years to warrant the diagnosis of sociopath. When social class differences in outcome were sought, none were found.

Supported by other studies, these findings tend to cast doubt on beliefs commonly held over the past few decades. The perception of delinquency as normal masculine aggressive behavior that is merely unacceptable to middle-class authorities or as a product of healthy or normal responses to deviant environments fails to stand up (Robins 1974). Neither is the association with a lower-class population tenable, though it does influence management after detection. Recent reports suggest an increase in female delinquency along with a shift in the nature of the offenses committed, with more girls being convicted of violent offenses and more boys being considered in need of protection by the courts (Warren 1978).

Some studies of delinquent, as opposed to clinical, populations come to similar conclusions, while others seem in some respects contradictory. The President's Commission Report on Juvenile Delinquency, conducted in the United States and published in 1967, surveyed both "official" delinquents (i.e., those found guilty by a court) and the prevalence of delinquent behavior, official and otherwise. Eighty-eight percent of thirteen-to sixteen-year-olds confessed to having committed at least one chargeable offense in the three years preceding the interview. However, the numbers of those who frequently committed serious offenses decreased sharply. Thus while most children may commit the occasional minor offense, the group responsible for serious and persistent misbehavior approximates Rutter's figures.

Reviewing the National Survey of Youth, Williams and Gold (1972) drew attention to the need to be wary of official delinquency as a measure of true rates of antisocial behavior. For example, while social class or racial group do not appear to have much significance as correlates of self-reported delinquent behavior, lower socioeconomic status and ethnicity are overrepresented in most officially delinquent populations.

In summary, in spite of some contradictory findings and methodological difficulties, it is fair to conclude that persistent and serious social misbehavior is a phenomenon with a high prevalence rate and early onset, is highly associated with maleness and serious school difficulty, and persists into adulthood.

Psychopathogenesis

Youths suffering from a serious conduct disorder may be divided into two groups, the first undersocialized and the second socialized. Considering first the undersocialized group, constitutional and organic, cultural, and familial and parental factors can contribute to the failure of socialization.

UNDERSOCIALIZED GROUP

Constitutional and Organic Factors

Especially among those children whose behavior is highly impulsive and aggressive, the incidence of neurological pathology is significant. This has led many investigators to postulate that more subtle cerebral dysfunction may underlie less extreme behavior disturbances. Certainly the under-socialized population, when screened for electrophysiological or psychometric abnormality, shows greater numbers with nonspecific abnormalities than a more random sample (Rutter and Graham, 1966; Rutter, Tizard, and Whitmore, 1970). The well-established strong association between conduct disorder and educational underachievement (Robins 1974), combined with the growing recognition of specific learning disability and attention deficit disorder as real entities has led to more careful clinical assessment of children with behavior disturbance as well as to research to clarify the relationships between these often associated conditions. Thus although constitutional and organic theories have been out of fashion among western criminologists and clinicians, they are overdue for a revival, possibly within an ecological or sociobiological paradigm.

Cultural Factors

Since all human cultures contain a recipe for socialization of the young and a framework for sociability, subcultural delinquency, where behavior antagonistic to general norms seems permitted and encouraged by special groups or communities, is certainly of great concern to the criminologist and sociologist, but it lies outside the area of expertise of the psychiatrist and calls for different interventions. More common in clinical practice is the notion of cultural deprivation, wherein affected individuals may be perceived as not having been adequately introduced to and included in a culture. Working with immigrant children in Israel, Feuerstein, Krasilowsky, and Rand (1974) have developed the notion of failure of cultural mediation. Severely handicapped children, presenting with intellectual, perceptual, and behavioral disturbances, have been treated by methods that involve individually designed programs of instruction and dialogue between child and mediator. This is seen as an institutionalized application of the "built-in" transmission of culture that occurs within intact families and communities and that, due to social and cultural dislocation, these children lacked.

Familial and Parental Factors

Severe undersocialization is usually a cumulative effect of many factors within family life. Poverty and large family size, low intelligence, and parental criminality have been demonstrated to correlate to varying degrees with conduct disorder in children (Hutchings and Mednick, in press; Robins and Lewis 1966). Anything occurring in the life of child and family that interferes with the formation of a primary attachment (see chapter 1) or that undermines the quality and continuity of the child's relationships with major attachment figures will interfere with socialization, especially in biologically vulnerable children. Particularly implicated are family turmoil, especially prolonged and severe marital conflict (Offord et al. 1979); parental depression leading to parental unresponsiveness, irritability, and increased likelihood of neglect or abuse, all of which undermine the quality of the parent-child relationships; multiple moves or especially multiple placements, which interfere with the continuity of a child's primary relationships. Many of these factors often exist together, potentiating each other's effects and blocking the process of socialization. Three results of successful socialization are the ability to contain and control impulses, the internalization of appropriate standards of right and wrong, and the ability to empathize (to perceive and value the needs and feelings of others). Unless these are achieved, socialization and the ability to relate are likely to remain grossly deficient. Some more specific patterns of family interaction are worth illustrating.

A thirteen-year-old boy was charged with attempted murder without apparent motive after stabbing his sleeping mother with a kitchen knife. Both he and his brother had previous records of multiple minor delinquencies, school problems, and assaults against peers. While there was no evidence of gross neglect or abuse, the family resisted investigation by evasiveness, all members "closing ranks" to prevent scrutiny. Persistent effort revealed that the marriage was the result of a premarital pregnancy; its early years were beset by open hostility and physical abuse, while recently the partners had completely withdrawn from each other. Separation was precluded by the discovery that the wife was again pregnant. Her resentment of the second child led to revulsion or nausea when she held or touched him. When he was five, she overcompensated for her feelings of revulsion through overindulgence and favoritism. Thereafter each parent covertly undermined the other and competed for the affection of the children, alternately indulging and rejecting them. However, united by mutual dependency and denial of the emotional reality, the family developed a "fortress mentality" and projected onto neighbors, schools, and police malevolent intentions. While this defused tension within the family, it promoted and sanctioned conflict with outsiders. The parents colluded with the boy's delinquency as it served to discharge their own hostility as well.

In the opening sentence of his great novel, *Anna Karenina,* Leo Tolstoy comments, "All happy families are like one another; each unhappy family is unhappy in its own way." This illustrates why it is difficult to summarize the many possible mechanisms relating parental and family dysfunction to pathological behavior in children. For example, rigid and punitive parental behavior may produce results similar to that which is excessively permissive or uninterested. Families that produce healthy children are open to the world, not closed; parents are parents and seek privacy with each other yet take pleasure in their children, whose need for privacy they also respect. Expectations are usually clear and firm, and conflict, while not feared, is handled fairly. In contrast, overt and covert rejection, whatever its source, undermines the socialization process. Extreme overindulgence, overprotection, and failure to set and enforce reasonable expectations for socially acceptable behavior often represent parental use of reaction formation to defend against recognition of their unconscious rejection of an unwanted or in any way handicapped child. Parents who are inconsistent, either within themselves because of their own psychological conflicts or with each other, so that the child is caught between two warring and polarized parents, undermine their child's socialization. So will the parents who, while consciously disapproving of their child's behavior, unconsciously collude with it, because it discharges their own unrecognized hostile or antisocial needs as they identify vicariously with the child's antisocial behavior (Johnson 1949).

The following vignette illustrates another pattern of undersocialization, less primitive and impulsive than the case previously cited.

> Liberal, well-educated parents consulted a psychiatrist regarding their fourteen-year-old only child. For the previous year, Jamie's attendance at school had been sporadic, he was flagrantly smoking cannabis, and he had disappeared from home for days at a time. Although he was not even civil at home, he expected independence yet continuing material sustenance and support. His parents' threats or denial of privileges elicited volatile tantrums that made them back down to placate him.
>
> Jamie, though bright, charming, and articulate, was badly underachieving at school; furthermore, he had few friends and avoided all forms of competition. He complained that he did not need a high school education and that his parents were old-fashioned and rigid.
>
> Exploration revealed that his mother had always felt guilty and anxious when either separated from Jamie or not meeting his demands. Father, although silently disapproving of this, remained passive because whenever he dealt firmly with the boy, his wife interfered to protect Jamie from his "punitive" approach.
>
> As a result, Jamie had received warmth and nurturance in his early years, but he had never experienced frustration or fear. Thus his infantile omnipotence had never really been challenged; his development was fixed at the tantrum stage, whereby he tyrannized and manipulated his parents. While his verbal fluency and superficial charm were well developed, his academic, athletic, and social skills remained rudimentary. When not in control, he became hostile, then frightened and depressed. Such a youngster could be categorized as falling within the "manipulator" category in the I-Level system, an intermediate position between "unsocialized" and "socialized."

A number of factors—constitutional, cultural, and familial and psychological—contribute to increased aggressiveness in some children with conduct disorders.

Constitutional Factors

Children with strong biological drive, who show the personality traits of high persistence, low adaptability, and low responsiveness, experience more than usual frustration and resultant anger in the socialization process. Correlations between highly aggressive behavior and rare chromosomal abnormalities (such as the XYY syndrome) have further tantalized investigators looking for organic factors, but the association has not been clearly established (Scott and Kahn 1968).

Cultural Factors

At a cultural level, the tendency of socially disadvantaged children toward action rather than verbalization, when combined with the frustration they experience by exclusion from the social and material advantages that their more advantaged peers enjoy, produces in many youngsters a rising resentment of the privileged groups within society, with no verbal safety-valve by which this resentment can be safely discharged.

Familial and Psychological Factors

A major source of aggression is the frustration of not having had basic needs for love and security met. Familial factors that contribute to this are similar to those that simultaneously undermine parent-child relationships and, therefore, socialization. Neglect and abuse, including rationalized forms of abuse such as excessively rigid and severe discipline; chronic and severe family conflict and breakup; placement of the child out of the home and, in particular, a history of multiple placements; consistent failure that results in repeated frustration, rage, and diminished self-esteem for which the youngster strives to compensate by seeking power and status by asserting aggressive superiority over others—all these predispose to the buildup of resentment and rage that plays so prominent a part in the clinical picture of the youngsters in question. Equally important is the tendency toward identification with parental or other role models whose behavior is aggressive, brutal, and assaultive.

SOCIALIZED GROUP

How then do children with socialized conduct disorders differ from those just discussed? The socialized category includes those youngsters whose personality or interpersonal development have reached a stage that permits the inhibition of impulses, at least modest tolerance of strong affects such as fear, anxiety, or anger without immediate discharge, and at least some capacity for taking another person's point of view. Because of these developments, psychic organization is more complex and behavior more flexible and less stereotyped. Conflict between objectives and desires is therefore more likely to be conceptualized and at least partially resolved symbolically within the person rather than immediately being discharged onto outsiders who are perceived merely as frustrators or givers. It is at this stage that the conventional meaning of the word neurotic begins to apply, and the term acting-out can properly be used. Acting-out describes actions that avert the conscious experiencing of unconscious psychological conflict by replacing it with maladaptive and sometimes antisocial behavior which externalizes the internal and still unconscious conflict. Some members of this group at times appear oversocialized, at least in that they seem overcontrolled or overinhibited within a specific sphere of behavior.

The important point is that youngsters in this group may display behavior which superficially resembles that of youth whose socialization is underdeveloped. Failure to distinguish between these two groups is likely to result in youngsters being treated inappropriately. Since we have reason to believe that those with socialized conduct disorders form a significant proportion of persistently misbehaving or delinquent youth, this is a critical consideration.

As with the undersocialized group, socialized youngsters may utilize a variety of mechanisms and have a variety of underlying neurotic conflicts masked by their acting-out behavior. For example, stealing may serve to prevent the experience of manifest depression by symbolically replacing a loss and by venting associated anger. Similarly, some antisocial behavior, particularly that involving aggression or risk, may assist in denial of fear and passivity; this is frequently seen in young males who are defending against anxiety regarding their masculinity. A common variant of these themes takes the form of antagonism toward parents and other authority figures, serving the needs of nascent adults to achieve "escape velocity" as they struggle to undo the ties with those adults on whom they previously depended for support. Where excessive dependent attachment threatens the adolescent drive toward individuation, young persons may unconsciously be driven to extreme and token acts of rebellion against what is seen as an external barrier or antagonist when their real enemy, their own need to remain dependent, lies unrecognized within.

As with all neurotic patterns of behavior, these underlying issues lie outside the awareness of the individual involved, who is either mystified by his or her behavior or rationalizes it, often by means of appeal to some ideological commitment.

A sixteen-year-old boy was eventually sent to training school following repeated car thefts associated with highly dangerous driving. The "last straw" involved a high-speed chase through city streets that endangered his own life and that of others. He had always been a good student and was well liked by peers and adults, who were perplexed by what they called a "split personality." The boy himself could not explain his behavior, offering only half-believed rationalizations that his father would not permit him to obtain a driver's license and drive the family car. His relationship with his father had become strained following his mother's death when the boy was thirteen, and the car thefts had begun the following year.

Although initial clinical interviews were met with resistance, persistence disclosed that the boy had always been close to and somewhat overprotected by his mother, with the father being perceived by both as cold and forbidding. By the age of thirteen, however, the boy began arguing with his mother over her overinvolvement in his choice of clothing, friends, and social activities. She died of a stroke several days after a particularly heated exchange, and there had been no opportunity to make amends before her death. Father and son mourned separately, each taking refuge in activities away from home. The car thefts and reckless driving involved several component unconscious mechanisms, including expression of anger and guilt in symptomatic rather than direct ways, denial of his own mortality, covert attempts to make connections with his father, and denial of dependency. In effect, he was "acting-out" rather than experiencing consciously his grief and his continuing (but dangerous) need to emancipate himself.

Similar neurotic mechanisms often underlie isolated misbehavior that is atypical in terms of family and individual histories. The shy and socially inhibited adolescent who inexplicably becomes involved in sexual activity with a younger child or goes on a rampage of stealing or vandalism will often be surprised by his or her own behavior but may seem powerless to stop it. Such situations often involve excessive suppression of sexual or aggressive themes in fantasy and of their socially acceptable expressions through humor, appropriate sexual sociability and competition, and private masturbation. Lacking the capacity to transmute primitive instinctual drive into socially valued behavior, behavior alternates between overcontrol and inappropriate and unpredictable discharge. The same model used to represent neurotic conflict in chapter 12 can be modified in figure 13.1 to summarize the defensive pattern of the child with a socialized conduct disorder.

Occasionally, similar behavior occurs in the absence of neurotic conflict, fueled by the pressure of extreme environmental circumstances that overwhelm the not yet fully mature individual.

An eleven-year-old girl was referred to a child welfare authority by her school because of persistent fire-setting, which was confined to the school building and environs. Always a polite child with an excellent school record, she had become more reserved and serious over the previous school year and had begun the current year with fire-setting. Her family refused to believe that anything was amiss, asserting that her behavior at home and in the community was exemplary. Subsequent exploration revealed that her mother had been admitted to the hospital eighteen months previously with a diagnosis of paranoid schizophrenia. She had been telling her daughter that her father had sexual designs on her, and no one had told the child that her mother was mentally ill. An explanation of her mother's illness and more support from her father were enough to eliminate the problem behavior and to restore the youngster to her former spontaneous self.

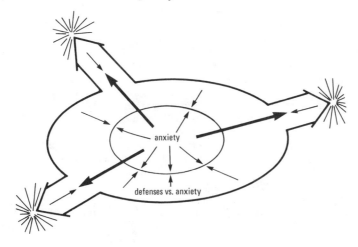

Acting-out behavior $\frac{\text{takes the place of}}{\text{serves to mask}}$ anxiety resulting from inner conflict

Figure 13.1 The Child with a Neurotic Disorder

While the child in this case did not suffer from a neurotic behavior disorder in the usual sense, the abnormal environmental stresses intensified unconscious conflict and provoked symptom formation.

Management and Treatment Considerations

Detailed discussion of management appears in chapters 6, 28, 29, and 30. The following general principles, however, may serve as a guide to assessment and management planning of children with conduct disorders or delinquency.

1. Avoid too narrow a focus in investigation. Data gathering should include information regarding constitutional and organic factors, cognitive and perceptual development, family history and functioning, social and academic achievement, and situational factors. Grandparents, teachers, and others are often valuable auxiliary sources of information and perspective.
2. Decide before initiating treatment the position of the child with respect to degree of socialization. Diagnosis on this dimension is critical for choosing a course of action. Impulse-ridden or manipulative and controlling children need nothing more than an "ego prosthesis"—the function performed by the normal parent for infants and very young children. This involves arbitrary and firm action, not more than necessary but certainly whatever is required, to ensure adequate and consistent control of behavior. With neurotic children, on the other hand, while assistance in controlling extreme and destructive behavior is necessary as part of management, the core of treatment lies in dealing with

273

underlying intrapsychic conflict and situational stresses. Here conventional psychotherapies directed toward restructuring faulty family interaction or resolving unconscious conflict are appropriate.

3. Be aware of the feelings badly behaved children evoke. Manipulative children in particular often leave a trail of ineffective would-be helpers in their wake who were first caught by sympathy and overidentification only to become frustrated and hostile when they, in turn, are manipulated. Neither reaction is constructive, but no therapist working with such children is immune to such entanglement.

4. Unsocialized children and adolescents respond adversely to conflict among the parents, teachers, probation officers, police, and therapists on whom they depend for structure and help. Cooperation among all of these is essential when working with the undersocialized.

5. Be suspicious of panaceas and fads, particularly when these involve separation from the family. Impulsive and manipulative children are often on a slippery slope, and further interruptions in the continuity of care may accelerate a malignant and repetitive pattern. On the other hand, primary-care providers, whether parents or surrogates, need support and, at times, relief. Judicious and tactical removal of a child for a brief time can often buttress family adequacy but avoid the damage of long-term separation.

Delinquency and Its Management

Delinquency, as such, is a legal not a clinical entity. The juvenile delinquent is a child or adolescent who has been charged with a breech of the law and convicted in court. Experts in the social phenomenon of delinquency are sociologists and criminologists, not mental health workers. Yet individual delinquents may suffer from a clinical disorder. Child psychiatrists and other mental health workers have a useful role to play in identifying and contributing to the management of those delinquents whose antisocial behavior is related to a clinical syndrome. Poorly applied, their efforts may even be harmful. In the past some mental health professionals have lost sight of the limits of their expertise and made grandiose and inflated claims that the widespread application of psychiatric or psychoanalytic principles could eliminate delinquency. The clinical professions could not, of course, make good these claims and were generally and understandably discredited when their results fell far short of these aspirations. Shamsie (1981), in his recent review of studies of treatment responses of delinquents, found that the majority suggested that the subjects were highly refractory to conventional remedies. The most promising approaches were the cognitive therapies and those directed to educational and vocational upgrading.

Many of these studies, however, can be criticized on methodological grounds. They suggest primarily the need for further and more tightly designed research on the characteristics and natural histories of the sub-groups of severe conduct disorders in order to select the management of choice for each with greater precision. Failure to do so will only compound the confusion and result in unnecessary failures, increasing pessimism, and even nihilism (Steinhauer 1978). Only with precise and carefully con-trolled studies can we evaluate the result of a specific treatment of specified frequency and duration followed up for an appropriate length of time on a clearly defined and uniform sample of the delinquent population. Only when this has been done will we obtain a valid picture of the effectiveness of the available treatments on each subgroup of delinquents. In the mean-time, the findings now available suggest early assistance to individuals and families affected, greater attention to concrete support (e.g., the provision of jobs and remedial education), and, not least, a long-term involvement of those affected in programs of treatment and support.

SUGGESTIONS FOR FURTHER READING

ALEXANDER, J. F. AND PARSONS, B. V. 1973. Short-term behavioral intervention with delinquent families: Impact on family process and recidivism. J. Abnormal Psychol. 81:219–225.
    Describes a study of different styles of family intervention showing that the short-term behavioral approach obtained superior results.
FEUERSTEIN, R.; KRASILOWSKY, D.; AND RAND, Y. 1974. Innovative educational strategies for the integration of high-risk adolescents in Israel. *Phi Delta Kappan* 55(8): 556–558.
    The integration of psychologically deprived teenagers after World War II involved placement of disturbed adolescents among normal peers and intensive work to correct deficiencies in cognitive functioning.
GLUECK, S. AND GLUECK, E. 1968. *Delinquents and non-delinquents in perspective.* Cambridge, Mass.: Harvard University Press.
    The Gluecks have done the largest, most comprehensive study of delinquent boys and have developed predictive scales. This book also includes a review of their work to date.
JOHNSON, A. M. 1949. Sanctions for superego lacunae of adolescents. ed. K. R. Eissler, *Searchlights on delinquency,* pp. 225–245. New York: International Universities Press.
    Classic paper for the understanding of one group of delinquents relating the delinquency to difficulties in the parents.
NIR, Y., AND CUTLER, R. 1973. The therapeutic utilization of the juvenile court. *Am. J. Psychiat.* 130:1112.
    Describes a collaborative program between a juvenile court and an adolescent psychiatric clinic that has made it possible to deal successfully with otherwise untreatable court-referred adolescents.
OFFORD, D. R.,et al. 1979. Broken homes, parental psychiatric illness and female delinquency. *Am. J. Orthopsychiat.* 49(2):252–264.
    The frequency of broken homes was the strongest distinguishing factor between populations of families with and without delinquent daughters. Parental disability was a weaker factor.
PAYNE, W. D. 1973. Negative labels. *Crime and delinquency* 19:33–40.
    Provocative article on repercussions of labeling gangsters delinquent.
QUAY, H. C. 1978. Classification. In *Psychopathological disorders of childhood,* 2nd ed., ed.H. C. Quay and J. S. Werry, pp. 1–42. New York: John Wiley & Sons.

Good coverage of Quay typology. A discussion of other classification systems (e.g., DSM-III, ICD-9, GAP, I-Level, WHO Multiaxial) and the criteria for evaluating a classification system.

ROBINS, L. N. 1970. The adult development of the antisocial child. *Seminars in psychiatry* 2(4):420–434.

A review of twenty-three longitudinal studies of both clinical and nonclinical populations: patterns of recovery, contribution to adult clinical populations, family backgrounds, theories.

———, AND LEWIS, R. G. 1966. The role of the antisocial family in school completion and delinquency: A three-generation study. *Sociol. Quart.* 7(4):500–514.

A study of the expected rate of problem behavior given deviant behavior in the parents and the extended family.

RUTTER, M., AND SHAFFER, D. 1980. *DSM-III:* A step forward or back in terms of classification of child psychiatric disorders? *J. Am. Acad. Child Psychiat.* 19:371–394.

Issues requiring further discussion and research are derived from an appraisal of DSM-III.

SHAMSIE, S. J. 1981. Antisocial adolescents: Our treatments do not work—Where do we go from here? *Can. J. Psychiat.* 26(5):357–364.

Antisocial behavior should be conceived of as a lack of socialization rather than a sickness. Social learning and behavioral-employment intervention programs are discussed.

WARREN, M. Q., AND THE COMMUNITY TREATMENT STAFF. 1966. *Interpersonal maturity level classification: Juvenile: Diagnosis of low, middle and high maturity delinquents.* Sacramento: California Youth Authority.

A complete description of the I-Level classification scheme, with the treatment plan for each delinquent subtype. A diagnostic interview schedule and diagnostic rating sheet are included.

14
Brian McConville

Depression and Suicide in Children and Adolescents

Suicide and depression in children and adolescents were previously considered uncommon, but these preconceptions have now been corrected. This chapter will outline some more recent concepts and give guidelines to diagnosis and treatment of these two interrelated conditions. Depression will be considered first, since depressive symptoms have turned out to be extremely widespread in children and often form the background against which later suicide or suicide attempts may occur.

Depressive Disorders in Children and Adolescents

HISTORICAL CONTEXT, PREVALENCE, AND DIFFICULTIES IN DIAGNOSIS

Until the late 1960s no major textbook on child psychiatry contained a section on childhood depression. But about this time a number of authors (Group for the Advancement of Psychiatry 1966; Poznanski and Zrull 1970) began to identify and describe depressive disorders in children and adolescents. Childhood depression was soon recognized as often different from full adult depression. Psychomotor retardation was less marked and sleep disturbance less clear. On the other hand, sadness, discontent, and feelings of being unloved were very common. A study of overtly depressed children indicated a high incidence of depression in

277

their parents (Poznanski, Krahenbuhl, and Zrull 1976) and 50 percent of the children remained clinically depressed six years later. There are problems distinguishing children showing only depressive symptoms from those whose depression is part of a major affective illness. A number of studies have demonstrated that up to 50 to 60 percent of children seen in inpatient or outpatient psychiatric clinics have the symptoms of depression, but that only 10 to 25 percent of these warrant the diagnosis of major depressive disorders (Carlson and Cantwell 1979; McConville, Boag, and Purohit 1974; Petti 1981). Others represent minor depressions such as adjustment disorder with depressed mood (DSM-III 309.00), or misery or unhappiness secondary to a wide variety of factors. Other recent studies have attempted to distinguish children with primary depressive illnesses from those whose depression is secondary to such conditions as conduct or attention deficit disorders. In one study about half of the major depressions were secondary to such causes (Carlson and Cantwell 1979). The frequent association of such symptoms as truancy, school phobia, hypochondriasis, or delinquency with depression has led to the concept of masked depression (Glaser 1967; Lesse 1981). Some authors (Carlson and Cantwell 1980) have recently "unmasked" masked depression, suggesting that the term reflects a preoccupation with presenting complaints, while a proper clinical assessment would allow for the diagnosis of major or minor depressions. The concept of masked depression is still useful in that it encourages the examiner to think beyond surface behaviors that are antisocial and manipulative and to consider whether or not these are symptoms of a depressive process. Especially in the child who has not previously shown such behaviors, the possibility of these behaviors reflecting underlying depression resulting from recent cumulative losses and disappointments should be considered.

It is important to distinguish acute from chronic depression. Acute depressive reactions usually follow such major losses as parental death, separation and divorce, or an unexpected move. A key feature is an excessive longing for the lost person and the inability to utilize substitutes. Usually these children appeared to function well before the loss, and generally they improve quickly with the reappearance or provision of a caring person.

In contrast, chronically depressed children usually have been subjected to frequent previous separations from parents or parent figures, often associated with depreciation and rejection, or with the loss of involvement of a central figure (e.g., a best friend or girl friend). Depression is frequently present in one or both parents. This suggests both an inherited predisposition and the likelihood of at least periodic parental emotional withdrawal along with transient frank parental depressions and angry outbursts frequently incomprehensible to the child.

Clearly, childhood depression is an important and common clinical entity. Childhood hypomania, in contrast, is uncommon (Anthony and Scott 1960; Sandler and Joffe 1965; Varsamis and MacDonald 1972).

MEASUREMENT OF DEPRESSION IN CHILDREN

A number of measuring instruments are now available to evaluate childhood depression. These include the Weinberg Scale, the Short Children's Depression Inventory, the Kovacs Scale, the Kiddie-SADS Scale, and the DSM-III, which includes child and adolescent depression with the adult depressive syndromes (American Psychiatric Association 1980; Carlson and Cantwell 1979; Kovacs and Beck 1977; Puig-Antich et al. 1980; Weinberg et al. 1973). The Bellevue Index (Petti 1978) and the Kiddie-SADS may be used to measure therapeutic change, as may the more restrictive DSM-III with some modifications. The overinclusive Kovacs Scale fails to distinguish major from minor depressions. The importance of these instruments is that they provide clinicians with a common language to discuss the depressive syndromes of childhood.

SYMPTOMATOLOGY OF DEPRESSION IN CHILDREN OF VARIOUS AGES

Even with all the available diagnostic instruments, there are still problems in diagnosis. Especially in younger children, the depressive phenomenology varies markedly from time to time. In addition, the depressive process may present in three different ways (Cytryn and McKnew 1979): in fantasy, verbal expression, and mood or behavior.

In fantasy depression may be revealed by play techniques or stories with themes of: mistreatment; being thwarted, blamed, or criticized; loss and abandonment; injury, death, or suicide.

In verbal expression, depressed children talk of: feeling hopeless and helpless; being unattractive, worthless, and unloved; suicidal preoccupations.

In mood or behavior, depressed children exhibit: sadness and crying; sleep and appetite disturbance; loss of former interests, social withdrawal and decreased productivity; such masking behaviors as hyperactivity, aggressiveness, school failure.

Some authors (Cytryn and McKnew 1979) found that depressive fantasy is almost always present in children with a depressive reaction, while verbal expressions of depressive affect occur less commonly and depressed mood and behavior are still less frequent and least stable. Moreover, as the depression improves, mood and behavior improve first, followed by decreased verbalization of depressive themes, while fantasies disappear only after resolution of conflict.

The manifestations of depression in children differ depending on their age and developmental stage (Toolan 1981). Younger (five- to eight-year-old) children verbalize feelings of sadness more directly, whereas older (eight- to twelve-year-old) children are more likely to show increasingly poor self-esteem. The classical theme of extreme guilt common in adult major depression is rare in children before age eleven and

279

twelve, and then seems to follow extreme loss or deprivation. As children enter into adolescence, guilt themes become more common and the depressive syndromes resemble those of adults more. (McConville, Boag, and Purohit 1974).

Young children are thought to have less capacity to verbalize feelings but a greater facility in expressing them nonverbally. Young children's ability to grieve freely and to form attachments to substitute caregivers after parental loss may explain why depression in young children is usually short-lived, except when such substitutes are unavailable (as in some institutions and hospitals). Children from eight to eleven years appear to be in an intermediate position. Their expression of feelings is not as free, and their feelings often seem to be masked and discharged through action. This can lead to the appearance of the so-called masked depressive states previously described, often accompanied by an increase in blaming the self or others.

Clinically it appears that children cannot experience full adult depressive episodes unless they have developed to the point where they are capable of such processes as abstract thinking and a degree of reality testing incompatible with the widespread use of fantasy to deny and escape unpleasant events or feelings. When they reach the point where these criteria are met, the self-criticism of their conscience structure may produce the excessive guilt typical of depression in adolescents.

Some authors (Nagera 1970; Rie 1966; Rochlin 1959; Wolfenstein 1966) have questioned whether children are even capable of maintaining a preoccupation with the lost parent, of experiencing a prevailing sadness and general loss of interests, and of grieving in response to loss. Others (Bowlby 1961, 1963; Furman 1974; Steinhauer 1980) maintain that under ideal conditions, even very young children can experience grief and complete the work of mourning to the point where they can psychologically relinquish the important person they have lost. However, the work of Furman (1974) suggests that this can occur only under the following circumstances:

1. The children's cognitive and emotional development have reached the point where they can retain a memory of the person lost and of their feelings toward that person.
2. They are able to comprehend the meaning, extent, and permanence of the loss.
3. They are psychologically able to tolerate at least periodic continuing sadness.

Further, according to Furman, this is possible in some children as young as three or four provided:

1. The child's need for security is continually met.
2. The key (substitute) adults in the child's life repeatedly encourage the child to face rather than deny the reality of the loss.
3. These same adults can tolerate the child's expression of helplessness, rage, and despair rather than collude with the child in denying its significance.

Children exposed to major losses through parental death, separation, depression, or psychosis for whom the preceding conditions are not satisfied are at high risk of failing to relinquish their psychological attachment to the loved ones they have lost. Often they cannot form new substitute attachments that would provide continuing security and development but show various of the age-appropriate depressive syndromes already described or, frequently, deny and repress their loss and remain vulnerable to depression or conduct or character disorders in later life (Adams et al. 1982; Beck, Sethi, and Tuthill 1963; Wolff 1969), although recent reviews of the literature challenge this relationship in the case of depression (Crook and Eliot 1980; Tenant et al. 1980).

Adams (1982) suggests that where the loss results in persistent disruption of family life, the long-term problems are more lasting and disruptive than when the family life stabilizes; in the latter case the problems were minimal. The more vulnerable the child at the time of the loss—because of constitutional or organic liability, past privation and deprivation, or incompletely resolved separation—the less likely the mourning is to be completed sufficiently to avoid undermining of future security and development. (For a further discussion of incomplete or aborted mourning, see chapter 4.)

ETIOLOGY

Investigation of families of depressed children usually reveals that one or both parents have moderate neurotic or depressive problems but not gross psychopathology (Cytryn and McKnew 1979). The exception is the severely depressed and suicidal child; in that case family pathology may be severe. Sometimes an acute family loss is a precipitant. More often there is a longstanding history of parental discord, depression, emotional withdrawal, unavailability, and constant denigration of the child.

A number of biochemical aspects of childhood depression are currently being investigated. Changes in urinary metabolites occur with age and are more pronounced in those with chronic affective disorders (Cytryn et al. 1974). For example, 3-methoxy-4-hydroxyphenylethylene glycol (MHPG) is excreted less by depressed children (McKnew and Cytryn 1979), while some childhood depressives show cortisol hypersecretion (Puig-Antich et al. 1979). The latter occurs in some children with endogenous depression (major depressive illness) but not in those with secondary depression (Puig-Antich 1980). However, much further clarification of the biochemical aspect of childhood depression is needed. In contrast with those of adult depressives, depressed children's sleep patterns are surprisingly normal. Some studies suggest alterations in REM (rapid eye movement) latencies, but more work is required (Puig-Antich 1980; Petti 1981).

Treatment of Childhood Depression

DRUG TREATMENT

A number of studies carried out on the treatment of depressed children with tricyclic antidepressants (Lucas, Lockett, and Grimm 1965; Weinberg et al. 1973) report a response rate of 75 percent. But the dosages used and the duration of administration have varied. In one study using strict criteria, the 75 percent of children who were severely depressed and did respond had higher plasma levels of the drug than nonresponders (Puig-Antich et al. 1978). A subsequent double-blind study showed no advantage for a group treated by imipramine in doses up to 5 milligrams per kilogram per day over one treated by placebo, but a subgroup with high plasma levels of imipramine and desmethylimipramine (above 152 nanograms/ml) showed 100 percent therapeutic response, compared with 33 percent in the low-plasma-level subgroup (Puig-Antich 1980). Such high drug levels sometimes cause unacceptable side effects such as elevated blood pressure, increased heart rate, and electrocardiographic abnormalities. The usefulness of tricyclic antidepressants, although promising, is not yet fully established. These drugs should only be considered for children and adolescents with quite severe depressive disorders that do not respond to less radical intervention, particularly for those with features closely resembling major affective disorders as defined in DSM-III.

The use of monoamine oxidase inhibitors is also uncertain. British studies (Frommer 1967) suggest their effectiveness in a wide spectrum of childhood depressions, but their use in North America is still limited.

For those children who show intense anxiety as part of their clinical picture, antianxiety agents may prove helpful. Children whose frank schizophrenic psychoses show affective features are best treated with major tranquilizers first, with antidepressants added if needed.

The use of lithium in affective disorders in children is a matter of some controversy (Steinberg 1980; Werry 1977). In adolescents showing clear hypomanic illness, lithium should be prescribed to achieve serum lithium levels in the therapeutic range of 0.5 to 1.5 milliequivalents per liter, as for adults (Cytryn and McKnew 1979). Since children have superior renal clearance function, higher dosages for body weight than for adults are often needed. For the same reason children are reported to tolerate high doses of lithium (up to 1,800 mg. daily) and side effects are rarely encountered. In Europe there has been more interest than in North America in children with frequent mood swings as forerunners of endogenous manic-depressive illness (bipolar affective disorders), and some favorable preventive response to lithium has been reported (Cytryn and McKnew 1979).

Psychotherapy for Childhood Depression

EARLY DETECTION AND INTERVENTION

The most useful approach to the complex and protracted course of childhood depression is to be aware of the clinical entity and to act early. The depression may first be suspected by the family physician or pediatrician, a teacher or parent—especially the nondepressed parent—or a family friend. The observer should consider the possibility of depression when a child is apathetic or withdrawn, seems frequently or constantly sad or frankly depressed, or is described as suddenly lazy, nonproductive, and uninterested. Again, a child who responds to a major loss by becoming delinquent, school phobic, or acting in a troublesome way may be indicating underlying depression.

To this end, the physician or counselor should ask not only about recent loss, separation, divorce, or death but should also investigate changes in living status, long-term depreciation, or scapegoating of the child in the family. In addition, whenever a parent is depressed or alcoholic, the effect of the parental behavior on the children should be explored. Family interviews to determine the effects of the parental mental illness should be routinely conducted in such a situation. Once recognized, the early stages of depression-deprivation syndromes in children may be treated surprisingly easily. Family counseling about the effects of such patterns on the child can prove extremely useful, while if the parent's affective disorder or alcoholism can be treated successfully and there is concurrent therapy to help the child resolve his or her feelings, the child's symptoms may respond dramatically. It seems that the provision of a "good enough" nurturing experience for a child, indicating that help is available, suffices to avert the depressive process.

In some families scapegoating roles and their antecedents may be complex and require full exploration (see chapter 3). In others, where there have been major losses, the family may need encouragement to provide extra support for the depressed child, even during their own individual and group mourning. The essential feature is that clinician and family both agree that the child's depression is real and potentially crippling and that assistance and caring may be essential to the child's future health. At times, a further nondepressed model for identification may be needed. Especially with overwhelmed single parents, a Big Brother or Big Sister can be an invaluable therapeutic asset for the clinician.

PSYCHOTHERAPY FOR LONGER-TERM OR MORE SEVERE DEPRESSIONS

Individual Psychotherapy

Individual psychotherapy is usually necessary in more chronic depressions, often following frequent losses.

Therapy for Predominantly Affectual Depressions. As remarked, while younger children often cry and show sadness more openly, increasing anger and suspiciousness are more common in older and more chronically depressed children. The following case illustrates this.

> Roger, age seven, was admitted for treatment after a series of separations beginning at age four. After his parents separated, Roger had lived with his father. When the father's new partner did not want Roger around, he was placed in foster care and, after a number of brief placements, was referred for long-term residential treatment. The father remained ambivalently in the picture, and Roger insisted he was in the center only temporarily.
>
> Roger had extremely aggressive outbursts toward anyone who frustrated him. At other times he was sad, withdrawn, and cried often. He said he did not trust anybody and could give no clear reason as to why he had been removed from home. In one-to-one therapy, Roger drew a series of unremarkable houses. He used circumlocutions such as "This is a house I drew because I felt like drawing a house," and his diary and conversation consisted of rather flat descriptions of routine daily activities, such as coming downstairs. He denied feeling angry or sad: "I didn't like her hitting me, but I didn't cry since there was nothing to cry about."
>
> After several weeks, some resentment of others "always bossing me around and bugging me to do things I don't want to do" began to emerge. His drawings became increasingly depressive: broken houses with smashed windows falling down on children's playgrounds, making them mad. His pictures of a man named "Time Bomb" who "is going to blow up" symbolized his mounting and excessive anger. After this came another involving scary giants going crazy, as well as one small person afraid of the violent people surrounding him. On the same day Roger remarked: "Nobody cares. I don't care if I kill myself. Everybody picks on me." He therefore showed intense rage and depressive responses, shifting between paranoid and depressive positions and using early denial mechanisms.
>
> As Roger's child care worker reassured him and helped him assert himself more appropriately toward other children and adults, his pictures took on a whimsical tone, with the aggression now partially mastered. He began to express caring for his therapist in his diary: "Sue phoned me from Ottawa; I had a good day." His pictures now became more cheerful; about one he said, "This is a little boy flying his kite. He is happy and the house and kite and sun and smoke and chimney are all happy." He remained ambivalent toward the child care therapist whom he portrayed as having "lots of legs because she is so fat," but finally he described comfort in "being with her" with a drawing showing the sun shining on both of them: "This is Sue and me hacking around. We are both happy because each other is happy and the sun is out."

In summary, Roger was able to let go of his nonreliant and suspicious attitude toward people, to express his intense inner rage and depression, and also to mourn for past losses. Later in therapy he was able to make more realistic plans to be with his father sometime later. He was then ready for discharge from the treatment center to a foster home, having worked through much of his depression and loneliness.

Therapy for Predominantly Negative Self-Esteem Depression. As mentioned, a second chronic depressive response to repeated loss occurs most frequently in middle and late latency children, with thoughts and feelings of being stupid, worthless, and unliked by others. Such distrustful children assume that people will take advantage of and be unfair to them. Most such children have suffered severe and prolonged previous losses, and individual therapy is made difficult by the child's nonacceptance of the therapist. Any relationship is initially resisted, and therapists have to establish their trustworthiness on a person-to-person basis by spelling out in concrete terms in advance what it is worth to the child to risk forming relationships and expressing feelings.

Frank, a ten-year-old with a history of multiple placements, showed excessive anger and depression, with intense feelings of inadequacy and low self-esteem. Cool and distant, he often manipulated his therapist into doing things for him. This was allowed in order to establish in concrete terms the therapist's caring and to prevent paranoid interchanges between child and therapist. Previously Frank had often forced his parents to make up to him for their past failure to meet his needs. In one session he said about them, "I'm going to force them until I see if I can break them; if they break, that's fine by me." In others he angrily verbalized hatred toward himself and the world. Once he said to his therapist, "You think you're so smart. You think you can make me do what you want me to. Well, you aren't going to. One day us kids are going to take over the world and all you grownup bastards are going to get it." These outpourings of rage, bitterness, and hurt, during or after tantrums, alternated with his usual affectionless, cold, manipulating behavior.

At other times Frank had sudden episodes of intense weeping and sadness. He could sometimes talk about feelings of wretchedness and unworthiness, but during these outbursts he was merely overwhelmed by grief. The fixed quality of his depression was shown in one of his pictures, which indicated his obsessive concern with controlling feelings and his hopelessness. The bird, suggested by the Despert fables (1946) as falling out of a tree and requiring nurturance, was described as being dead. The therapist suggested using a watering can to revive the possibly stunned bird, but Frank angrily rejected this suggestion. He not only drew the bird in a graveyard but also put heavy rocks on top of the grave to indicate the death was final. Interestingly, originally he had portrayed the bird as reasonably happy in the nest until forced out by smoke from the chimney, thus again reflecting the basic paranoid belief that catastrophic events happened to him suddenly and without reason. Through his therapy Frank was able to resolve some of his depressive affect, but a residue of persistent low self-esteem continued. Indeed, there is doubt as to how able children are to resolve this type of depression since such residues often remain.

Therapy of Predominantly Guilt Depressions. Guilt depressions in children, although rare, are extremely dramatic.

> Twelve-year-old Charles was playing in a railroad cutting with his younger brother when the brother's foot became caught under a railroad tie just as a train thundered into the cutting. Charles tried unsuccessfully to free his brother and then leaped for safety. The brother was killed instantly.
> Charles was brought to the hospital as an emergency admission with acute suicidal wishes. He had a fixed belief that he should go to heaven to be with his brother and heard voices urging him to do that. He was regarded as an acute suicide risk and placed under close observation and support. He was also started on imipramine, and within ten days the symptoms had lifted dramatically. In psychotherapy he was able to express and work through his guilt and mourning, and was discharged to outpatient follow-up in one month. As often happens, his parents took longer to mourn and continued to blame Charles for several months.

Therapy with Adolescent Depressives

Adolescents frequently experience more severe depressive episodes, often requiring pharmacotherapy. Support and guidance for the teenager is important, and some explanation about the nature and the hopeful prognosis of the illness is required. As with older latency-age children, the therapist should aim to increase self-esteem in teenagers whose chronic depression stems from long-term depreciation or scapegoating. Sometimes this can be done by helping the patient understand his or her inability to communicate with the parent as the result of parental depression or preoccupation. Cognitive therapy designed to alter the patient's thoughts and later perceptions of self is often important as a means of relieving helpless and hopeless ideas. The gradually developing feeling of being accepted and appreciated by a therapist whom the adolescent learns in time to like and respect and who serves as a secondary model for identification, provides the teenager with a basis for beginning to think and feel more positive about him- or herself.

> Harry was a fourteen-year-old boy whose hard-driving father was also depressed with alcoholic tendencies. Harry began to do poorly at school and took drugs. After being reassured through psychological test results that drugs had not harmed his intellectual ability, he continued in therapy, clearly using the therapist as a father figure. About his father he said, "I can't please him. He never talks to me. He is always working." Although he angrily said that he didn't care, his eyes filled with tears. After some hesitation he allowed his father to attend the sessions, and both were able to discuss their own particular concerns and worries. Soon after the father began obtaining help for himself, Harry's chronic depression lifted and his school performance improved markedly.

Family Therapy

Often intervention with parents and child or with the whole family is the treatment of choice. Short-term crises are often easily and best resolved through family therapy, but longer-term problems in attachment, persistent detachment, or depression may require prolonged individual therapy as well as work with the family. Some approaches have been suggested earlier in the section on early intervention.

Summary

Child and adolescent depression is a multifaceted syndrome occurring at many ages and with variable symptoms and outcome. It has been recognized as quite common, and prompt and vigorous intervention, especially during the early stages, is frequently very effective.

Suicidal Behavior in Children and Adolescents

As with depression, suicide was previously considered rare in children and adolescents. However, more recent work shows that suicide is the second cause of death among adolescents and young adults in the United States (Teicher 1979). It is estimated that about 4,000 young people between fifteen and twenty-four kill themselves each year, while 400,000 are estimated to attempt suicide. The rates for teenagers of both sexes are said to have increased greatly (Garfinkel and Golombek 1974; Teicher 1979), and while suicides under age fifteen are infrequent, the fifteen- to nineteen-year group has an incidence of 5.7 per 100,000. Many more girls than boys attempt suicide, but more boys are successful (Bergstrand and Otto 1962; Connell 1972; Pfeffer 1981). While many more attempt suicide than eventually succeed, the majority of those who succeed do so on their first attempt. Those who commit suicide are more isolated, with less opportunity for others to intervene and stop their actions. Suicidal gestures include acts of self-injury without the intent of dying, in an attempt to communicate distress or to punish or manipulate others (Toolan 1975). Some authors have viewed addictions, alcoholism, or the failure to take care of long-term illness such as diabetes as chronic suicide equivalents, while self-mutilation and accident-proneness may be considered as focal suicides. (Garfinkel and Golombek 1974; Pfeffer 1981; Shaffer 1974).

It is difficult to assess how many accidents are basically suicide attempts. Reports by hospitals and physicians often underestimate the true incidence of suicide, perhaps to avoid cultural judgments associated with it or because of excessively conservative estimates or disbelief by the physician or coroner. Nevertheless, accidents remain the leading cause of death in children and adolescents, so that defining the number of unrecognized suicides in this group would be important.

In younger children, the incidence of completed suicide is low, but suicide attempts may be increasing. In the late 1960s, approximately 10 percent of children and adolescents seen in child psychiatry clinics were reported to have made suicide attempts. But in 1979, 33 percent of children randomly selected at an outpatient clinic in New York (Pfeffer et al. 1979) contemplated or had attempted suicide. In part this result may be due to greater skill in case finding, but there may well be an absolute increase.

EPIDEMIOLOGY

Suicide appears to vary with seasons, with more attempts occurring in the spring and early summer; this is perhaps less true in areas showing little seasonal variation, as in California (Shaw and Schelkun 1965). Children are said to commit suicide most frequently between 3 P.M. and midnight, while adult suicides occur more often between midnight and 6 A.M. Most suicides by children take place at home (Garfinkel and Golombek 1974).

The incidence varies between countries, with the overall suicide incidence in Canada being 11.2 suicides per 100,000 per year. Japan, Germany, and Scandinavian countries have rates two to three times higher than Canada, and Moslem and Catholic countries are said to have the lowest suicide rates, although this may be an artifact of underreporting. Stable countries with fixed values may provide some protection against suicide.

The highest reported rates of suicide occur in countries with shifting populations and with families experiencing disruption. Homes broken by divorce, separation, abandonment, alcoholism, or death show significantly increased suicide incidence. With intact families, there is often high marital discord and fewer supportive responses to the child's problems. Schoolwork and peer relationships may worsen before the suicide, and there is more often a history of suicide in the families of those children who do kill themselves (Garfinkel and Golombek 1974). In some studies (Paulson, Stone, and Sposto 1978; Pfeffer 1981), the parents of hospitalized suicidal children have been found to be both depressed and suicidally preoccupied. Forty percent of abused children showed self-destructive behavior (Green 1978), presumably arising from the child's sense of worthlessness, badness, and self-hatred due to parental abuse, harshness, and rejection.

Separations in the child's life appear to be particularly important precursors. These include actual separations or loss as well as threatened loss or emotional detachment by parents. Frequently the father may be absent and the mother, although present, is detached (Schneer, Kay, and Brozovsky 1961).

In adults there is considerable evidence that childhood deprivation is associated with later depressive syndromes (Adam 1982). In one study death of a parent was more common in the histories of those who completed suicide, while in attempted suicides desertion or divorce were more frequent (Dorpat, Jackson, and Ripley 1965). Multiple rather than single separations are important in determining suicide attempts. As an example of cumulative stress the following factors apply for adolescent suicide attempters:

1. Twenty percent have a parent and another 20 percent a relative or close friend who has attempted suicide.
2. Seventy-two percent are living apart from one or both parents.
3. The average number of major environmental changes was 10.4.
4. Sixteen percent have problems with a parent's alcoholism.
5. Families show unusual mobility, and adolescents often are living with persons other than parents.

These findings are significantly different from the experiences of a control group (Teicher 1979).

Often there seems to be a three-stage progression in adolescent suicide attempts (Teicher 1979): (1) a longstanding history of problems as previously listed; (2) recent escalation of stress by adolescent psychological issues, family illness or stress, peer problems, and diminished school performance; (3) a final precipitant such as termination of an important or romantic relationship.

Younger children are often seen with accidental overdosage, while preschool children are not uncommonly involved in a life-threatening event such as drowning, fire, or suffocation. Childhood suicide attempts tend to be more impulsive, a response to being badly treated and an attempt to punish those who have hurt them. In the young child's mind death is not permanent, so that the attempt may be seen as a wish for reunion with the parents (Nagy 1959). The more serious attempts occur in children with major psychiatric disorders. In one study the majority of children threatening to kill themselves were diagnosed childhood schizophrenics, many of whom had compelling hallucinations telling them to do so (Winn and Halla 1966).

Treatment of Suicidal Children and Adolescents

Very frequently the suicidal child or adolescent is brought to the physician or the emergency ward of a general hospital after expressing suicidal threats or making suicidal attempts (Mattsson, Seese, and Hawkins 1969; Teicher 1979). Frank suicidal behavior appears commonly in hospitals. In one study (Mattsson, Seese, and Hawkins 1969), 44 percent of all child psychiatry emergency referrals were made because of suicidal threats or attempts, although in others the percentage of children presenting in emergency departments as psychological crises who were suicidal was considerably less.

A number of clinical subgroups have been described (Mattsson, Seese, and Hawkins 1969):

1. Those suffering from acute loss or grief.
2. Those with marked self-depreciation. (Therapy for these two groups has previously been discussed.)
3. Those with overwhelming external stress due to family chaos, material scarcity, or physical illness. Here the suicide attempt may be seen as a final "cry for help." Rapid postemergency intervention to alleviate sociocultural and familial crises is often effective.
4. Those who are revengeful and angry. The manipulative quality of the act is clear, and there is usually not a high suicidal risk. Support and family counseling are generally effective.
5. Those who are psychotic—either from major affective or schizophrenic illness. These patients may seriously intend to kill themselves, either because of delusions of intense wickedness, or from hallucinations requiring them to act in self-destructive ways. Here the suicide risk is high and prompt hospitalization and pharmacotherapy with supportive psychotherapy to the child and family is mandatory.
6. Those who see suicide as flirting with death or as a thrilling and preoccupying game. Such children and adolescents often show extreme denial of expected fears and may be difficult to treat, especially following repeated attempts. The therapist must be able to spell out the degree of risk clearly and calmly, to be available, and to indicate both the extent and limitations of his or her support. A related subgroup consists of adolescents who mutilate themselves, especially by wrist cutting. Often there is little pain experienced during this action and a subsequent feeling of tension relief, which makes the action more likely to be repeated. Again, provision of adequate medical care and "good enough" support during these episodes is important. Usually the disorder is limited over time as considerations of discomfort and cosmetic appearance begin to establish themselves.

In all cases, there must be a detailed assessment of the overall suicide risk. This may be explored in the following areas (Garfinkel and Golombek 1974).

1. Means selected: If pills, how many and did the patient know of their effects? If other means, their potential lethality?
2. Was there premeditated, careful planning?
3. The circumstances of the attempt—likely to be discovered, announcing it in time, or when no one was around?
4. Recent precipitants?
5. Expression of continuing suicidal intent on examination?
6. Degree of depression? Particular inquiries should always be made about preceding and continuing depressive symptoms and their intensity and degree of discomfort.

7. Previous attempts?
8. Family history?
9. Availability of supportive and safe arrangements?

In cases where the assessment leaves particular questions in the psychiatrist's mind about a child or adolescent's danger to him- or herself, hospitalization is necessary. Frequently removal from the stressful situation will clarify the clinical condition while also decreasing the level of emotional distress.

In one study (Mattsson, Seese, and Hawkins 1969), a large number of families had failed to effect follow-up recommendations. Repeated and vigorous contacts with the child and family are therefore needed.

Prevention of Child and Adolescent Suicide

Given the centrality of depression in determining the onset of most suicides, there is a need for increased public and professional awareness of the scope of childhood and adolescent depression. Awareness by school teachers of the premonitory and frank symptoms leading to suicide attempts is very useful. A close working relationship between physicians, public health nurses, and teachers can often be of assistance. So far community-based services such as suicide prevention centers have not been shown to reduce overall suicide incidence, but further research in this regard is needed.

A number of measures have been suggested to offset the risks involved with drugs (Garfinkel and Golombek 1974). Barbiturates should be used only when no alternatives are available and then prescribed in smaller quantities (Barraclough 1974). Other safer hypnotics are available, including the benzodiazepines. For younger children the various safeguards by pharmacists to avoid accidental ingestion of pills from bottles are useful, and drugs and other harmful substances should be kept out of reach. Alcohol abuse is also common in both children and adolescents, and educational programs and restrained adult modeling of sensible drinking could be of considerable advantage.

Summary

Suicide, once thought rare, is the second most common cause of death among adolescents and young adults. Since many suicides are impulsive acts rather than symptoms of profound depression, early and adequate clinical assessment and prompt intervention are clearly indicated not only for youngsters who have experienced loss or who manifest low self-esteem, but also for those whose families are in crisis.

SUGGESTIONS FOR FURTHER READING

ANTHONY, E. J., AND SCOTT, P. 1960. Manic-depressive psychosis in childhood. *Child Psychol. & Psychiat.* 1:53–72.
A classic early paper on the subject.

CARLSON, G. A., AND CANTWELL, D. P. 1979. A survey of depressive symptoms in a childhood and adolescent psychiatric population. *J. Am. Acad. Child Psychiat.* 18:587–599.
Makes the distinction between depressive symptoms and full depressive illnesses.

CYTRYN, L., AND McKNEW, D. A. 1979. Affective disorders. In *Basic handbook of child psychiatry*, vol. 2, ed. J. D. Noshpitz, pp. 321–340. New York: Basic Books.
An overview of affective disorders, from a wide perspective.

GARFINKEL, B. D., AND GOLOMBEK, H. 1974. Suicide and depression in children and adolescents. *Can. Med. Assn. J.* 110:1278–1281.
A brief and excellent summary from a Canadian perspective.

KASHANI, J., et al. 1981. Current perspectives on childhood depression: An overview. *Am. J. Psychiat.* 138:143–153.
A thorough recent review.

MATTSSON, A.; SEESE, L. R.; AND HAWKINS, J. W. 1969. Suicidal behavior as a child psychiatry emergency: Clinical characteristics and follow-up results. *Arch. Gen. Psychiat.* 20:100–109.
A well-known study from the viewpoint of hospital emergency services.

PFEFFER, C. R. 1981. Suicidal behavior of children: A review with implications for research and practice. *Am. J. Psychiat.* 138:154–159.
A wide-ranging recent review, stressing various etiologies and treatments.

POZNANSKI, E. O., AND ZRULL, J. R. 1970. Childhood depression: Clinical characteristics of overtly depressed children. *Arch. Gen. Psychiat.* 23:8–15.
An excellent description of childhood depressive symptoms.

PUIG-ANTICH, J. 1980. Affective disorders in childhood—A review and perspective. *Psychiat. Clin. N. Am.* 3:403–424.
Another excellent review article, more from the perspective of major affective disorders in childhood.

SHAW, C. R., AND SCHELKUN, R. E. 1965. Suicidal behavior in children. *Psychiatry* 28:157–168.
An early and widely quoted paper.

TEICHER, J. D. 1979. Suicide and suicide attempts. In *Basic handbook of child psychiatry*, ed. J. D. Noshpitz, vol. 2, pp. 685–697. New York: Basic Books.
A broad and balanced overview of the subject.

TOOLAN, J. M. 1975. Suicide in children and adolescents. *Am. J. Psychother.* 29:339–344.
A general overview from an author who has been a pioneer in this field.

15 *Michael Thompson and Milada Havelkova*

Psychoses in Childhood and Adolescence

Psychosis is a mental disorder that impairs a person's mental capacity, ability to perceive reality correctly, communication skills, affective responses, and capacity for relating to others so badly that the person cannot respond age-appropriately to the demands of everyday life.

The term *childhood psychosis* includes a heterogeneous group of disorders meeting these criteria. The nomenclature has varied: Kanner (1944) described infantile autism; Bender classified what she termed childhood schizophrenia into pseudodefective, pseudoneurotic, and pseudopsychopathic types; Mahler wrote of the autistic and symbiotic psychoses; Rand (1963) of the atypical child; Kolvin referred to early- and late-onset childhood psychosis. Despite the considerable efforts made by these and other workers to identify specific disorders with a defined etiology, specific diagnostic criteria, predictable course, and, ideally, a specific treatment, no real unanimity of opinion has emerged. There does, however, appear to be reasonable agreement on the following points.

First, an organic and, for some, a genetic vulnerability is probably a necessary but possibly not always a sufficient condition for the emergence of psychosis. Second, all these disorders involve a pervasive disruption in multiple areas of functioning (motor, cognitive, perceptual, language, affective, self-concept, and interpersonal) and in the interrelationship and integration of these areas (Fish and Ritvo 1979). Third, unlike the retarded child, psychotic children show great variation in the degree of developmental retardation, with severe deficits in some areas contrasting with normal or even advanced functioning in others. Fourth, the child's capabilities may fluctuate markedly from one testing period to another. Fifth, for many of these children, the specific disorder diagnosed will depend on the age at which the child is seen. The diagnosis may change over time, so that the autistic infant or toddler may show a symbiotic psychosis later as a preschooler and may develop a pseudoneurotic psychosis in the grade-school years.

Prevalence

The incidence of infantile autism is about 4.5 per 10,000. Approximately half of these children show symptoms of organic brain damage (Lotter 1966; Treffert 1970; Wing, O'Conner, and Lotter 1967).

The ratio of males to females for autism varies from 2.5 to 1 (Lotter, 1966) to 6 to 1 (Bender and Grugett 1956); for psychosis with onset after two years the ratio is about 2.6 to 1. There appears, however, to be a higher male to female ratio, about 5 to 1, for cases of later onset (age eight to nine) childhood schizophrenia (Fish and Ritvo 1979).

Reported social class distribution has varied considerably, largely because of the diagnostic criteria used and other sampling biases. Except for Kanner (1944), most studies have found the highest prevalence in the middle class (Kolvin et al. 1971; Ritvo 1971).

Havelkova (1968) reports that, whereas twenty-five years ago practically no lower- and only a few lower-middle-class psychotic children were seen, over the years the case distribution has altered and is now spread across all classes. Probably in lower-class families, the autistic children were diagnosed retarded or behavior disordered, and, as a result, they were not referred. She finds a similar phenomenon currently occurring with non–English-speaking immigrant families.

Signs and Symptoms in the Childhood Psychoses

BIOLOGICAL SIGNS AND SYMPTOMS

Disorders of Development

Psychotic children demonstrate a rather chaotic variability in their level of functioning from one developmental line (e.g., motor development, language acquisition, etc.) to another, and within any one line, from one observation to another. A few higher functions may be attained, although similar but more primitive functions cannot be mastered.

> Kevin, age four, could not walk up the stairs alternating his feet or feed himself with a spoon, yet he could keep two objects running in a twirling motion at the same time. Mary, age five, could not throw or catch a ball but was able to draw intricate patterns that required good fine-motor coordination.

Homeostatic Vegetative Functions

Psychotic children may exhibit lability and poor regulation of such functions as temperature regulation, flushing or pallor, sweating, appetite and temperature maintence (flushing or pallor)(Bender 1947; Bender and Helme 1953). Bender described excessive fever with minor infections, or normal temperatures with severe illness. She also recorded abnormal responses to pain, illness, and noise, as well as abnormal vascular responses, none of which occurred in any of a group of matched controls. At least one such abnormality was seen in each of the psychotic children in her sample.

> Tommy, age three, had a white translucent skin. When anxious or excited, his right ear would turn bright red. Ronny, age four, used to develop an extreme dilatation of his pupils, which upset him more than what had frightened him originally. He would go to the mirror, look at himself, and scream that his eyes were turning black.

Growth

Fish (1959, 1975, 1977) has demonstrated that some schizophrenic children, more commonly those with early onset and retardation (Fish and Ritvo 1979), show definite growth failure in serial measurements of growth. These periods of retarded growth appear to correspond to periods of abnormal visual, motor, and postural development.

Physical and Neurological Abnormalities

Various authors have reported an increased incidence of physical (Walker 1977) and particularly neurological abnormalities along with a higher prevalence of abnormal electroencephalograms and seizures (Chess 1971; Treffert 1970; Wernar and Ruttenberg 1976). Virtually all studies have noted soft neurological signs such as transient esotropia (squint), unsteadiness of the outstretched hand, hyperreflexia, abnormal plantar responses, awkwardness, poor balance, mixed laterality (e.g., a right-handed child with a left eye dominance), minor degrees of incoordination, and other signs noted in the following sections.

Gross Motor Development

Some psychotic children have doughy or flaccid muscle tone and joints that appear hyperextensible. Gross motor development may be uneven.

Gross awkwardness is sometimes seen along with a heavy-footed, wide-based gait and poor coordination on finger-nose and finger-to-finger tests, as well as poor balancing on attempts to walk along a narrow rail (Engelhardt 1974). Some walk in erratic spurts and on their toes, while others are both graceful and well coordinated. Fish and Ritvo (1979) have emphasized that some such children show not a specific neurological deficit but disorders of timing and integration. For example, head control may lag months behind control of arms and legs. Higher functions may remain intact, while more primitive ones such as motor ability are severely retarded (Birch and Walker 1966), the reverse of the picture seen with diffuse chronic brain damage. At some point during their illness, most psychotic children demonstrate bizarre and stereotyped gross motor movements and ritualistic mannerisms such as hand clapping, repetitive rhythmic head banging, twiddling of the fingers, twirling (Bender and Helme 1953; Rachman and Berger 1963), rocking, hand and arm flapping, toe-walking, darting movements, and other rather bizarre postures. Although some of these may occasionally and briefly be noted in normal infants and toddlers, in psychotic children, particularly those with early-onset psychosis and lower IQs, they are exaggerated and persistent. With maturation, these bizarre movements and postures recur mainly in response to personally perceived environmental stress.

Responsiveness and Activity Level. As infants, many psychotic children are abnormally quiet, even with vigorous manipulation (Fish and Ritvo 1979; Eisenberg and Kanner 1956; Rimland 1964). They may be totally unresponsive to cuddling and maternal vocalization. They may fail to reach out for mother when being picked up (Mahler 1961) Some of these abnormally quiet infants, however, show normal or increased responsiveness to visual, auditory, and tactile stimuli. On the other hand, quite the opposite extreme, that of gross irritability, has been recorded by the authors. Activity levels may also be at either extreme, and some of these children alternate between hyperactivity and hypoactivity.

Attention, Adaptability, and Perception. Although their visual and auditory acuity are normal, psychotic children show poor integration of auditory, visual, and proprioceptive perceptions. They may be inattentive to both visual and auditory stimuli on one occasion yet respond at another. Toys may be examined briefly and aimlessly without any real interest and then discarded. Psychotic children need to preserve sameness and may be very upset by even minor alterations in the environment. Some toddlers, seemingly completely oblivious to verbal stimulation, are diagnosed as deaf until this is ruled out by extensive testing. Others may respond, but only to different tones or melodies or to sharp commands or overly kindly encouragement. Condon (1975) has demonstrated that for some children, sounds appear to register only after a delay, so that the nonverbal communication, including the speaker's lip movements, are then out of phase with the registration of the sound.

Visual inputs also appear to be distorted. Experiments have indicated that some psychotic children are underattentive to visual stimuli. They have difficulty learning visual discrimination of shapes or direction and cannot seem to use visual cues to accomplish visual motor tasks (Hermelin and O'Connor 1970). During formal testing they appear to use trial and error or manipulation to solve problems. They also have difficulty recognizing simple visual patterns: for example, they have trouble placing squares in size order (Hermelin and O'Connor 1970). Visual inputs also appear distorted, and their drawings of human figures may be highly detailed in some areas of the body, whereas others remain primitive and at the level of a much younger child. With some psychotic children, bizarre inclusions are found in their drawings or a preoccupation with certain body parts can be demonstrated.

> Ann, age six, was an intelligent child who spent two years in treatment. Following discharge, she was enrolled in a normal school where she did very well academically although her behavior was often quite unusual. During a period of several months durint which she was preoccupied with elimination, whenever she was asked to draw a person, she would include the whole digestive system with feces coming out. The people she drew were dressed, but their organs appeared through their clothing, like an x-ray.

Finally, some psychotic children show grossly bizarre distortions of perceptual functioning. Toys may be sniffed or mouthed (Alderton 1977). Objects such as wheels of carts, tricycles, or even plates may be spun endlessly very close to the child's face. Some such activities may later become necessary rituals before the child can attempt another activity (e.g., closing the door three times before entering). Objects may be manipulated without regard for their physical properties or usual functions, and the child may become totally preoccupied day after day with a single activity (Creak 1964; Kolvin et al. 1971; Rutter 1972).

> Johnny, age three and one-half, was preoccupied with doorknobs, which he would handle and turn endlessly. He spent much time playing with a toy tractor but, instead of "driving it" and making tractor noises like a normal toddler, he would repeatedly sniff it, mouth it like an infant, and twirl the wheels endlessly. (Alderton 1977)

Psychotic children's perception of their body often appears distorted. They may repeatedly try to fit themselves in a tiny toy chair or may not understand even after repeated trials that there is no danger of their being flushed down the drain.

> Jane, age four, always became panicky when her mittens and hat were removed. It was only after she learned to speak that she could explain that she used to be afraid that her head and hands would come off with the hat and mittens.

Visual Motor Functioning. Some psychotic infants show severe delays in fixating on objects held in front of them, in reaching and manipulating objects, and in integrating the functioning of both hands at the midline.

Cognition

A number of difficulties are found in the linkage of perception and cognition. Hermelin and O'Connor (1970) concluded that autistic children have difficulties discerning patterns within a series of stimuli. Others have noted that psychotic children may behave as if structured visual inputs or auditory information, such as the meaningful aspects of language, are just random and meaningless. They do not seem to interpret stimuli meaningfully: These authors hypothesize that this integrative defect may be responsible for the ignoring of verbal signals and the stereotyped and inappropriate responses to complex visual patterns and other sensory input (Hermelin and O'Connor 1970).

Individual children show great variability in performance on general intelligence tests. In these, islets of near-normal, normal, or high intelligence differentiate psychosis from mental retardation (Wechsler and Jaros 1965). Intratest variability is demonstrated by tests of verbal skills (such as information, comprehension, similarities, and vocabulary), which may be either significantly higher or lower than tests of performance (such as block designs or object assembly). In psychoses that develop during the preschool years, however, performance scores are more likely than verbal scores to approach the normal. Intratest variability is also shown by the children's tendency to succeed on difficult items while failing some of the easier ones. Many psychotic children are retarded, yet some test at the normal or superior level in a number of subtests. In one review of children diagnosed as suffering from infantile psychosis who probably meet the criteria for early infantile autism Fish and Ritvo (1979) state that from 62 to 78 percent had IQs of under 70, with 42 to 51 percent of these being under 50. Only one-third to one-half as many children in the same review who were diagnosed as having childhood schizophrenia had IQs under 70 and only one-tenth as many had IQs under 50, leaving a much higher proportion of this group with IQs over 70.

Rutter, Greenfeld, and Lockyer (1967) have shown considerable stability of IQ on five-to fifteen-year follow-ups, although tables of serial IQs do demonstrate variability over the years. Others such as Bender (1970), Goldfarb (Goldfarb, and Pollack 1969), and Havelkova (1968) have found that a few children, particularly those having early treatment as preschoolers, showed quite remarkable IQ changes of up to 40 to 50 points, which they managed to maintain, although the role of the treatment in the preservation of the intelligence could not be proven.

Perhaps the most characteristic feature of cognitive functioning in the childhood psychoses is the rather chaotic variability in maturation, with occasional islands of higher functioning being attained even though many lower cognitive functions cannot be accomplished.

> At age four Jim, while unable to play with toys in an age-appropriate manner, mastered jigsaw puzzles that would challenge the average eight-year-old. While still lacking communicative speech, he could identify correctly all makes of cars passing by.

Hermelin and O'Connor (1970) note that the rote memory and recall of autistic children exceeds that of a group of matched mentally retarded children but that it appears to depend purely on the acoustic and phonetic rather than on the semantic aspects of speech. They also note that coding and categorization of information are deficient in psychotic children and that nonsense is almost as easily remembered as things that make sense. The autistic children could not associate words semantically, and even when they seemed to have learned a specific task they had great difficulty generalizing that recognition, understanding, or accomplishment to other similar situations.

Recognition of one object did not stop the autistic child from retesting each other similar object in the same manner. Similarly, more complex tasks had to be completely relearned in each new context.

> Johnny, age four and one-half, played with pegs, which often remind children of candy. While a normal child may taste one or two before realizing that these are not candy, Johnny repeatedly tasted a whole box of them in turn without coming to the same conclusion.

Because their judgment is also impaired, some psychotic children seemingly unwittingly place themselves repeatedly in dangerous situations. Their thought processes appear concrete, and the ability to abstract is deficient. Even a child who has language and some areas of above-normal intelligence will have great difficulty extracting meaning from several inputs, synthesizing that information, and producing a response that is both different from, yet meaningfully derived from, the inputs.

Observation of those psychotic children who have language gives some understanding of defects in their form of thinking. Many of them demonstrate a loosening of associations that causes ideas to shift from one frame of reference to another without any logical connection between them. This, plus their distortions of grammar, incomplete sentences, and idiosyncratic metaphors culminate in incoherent speech. Thoughts that seem logical and realistic to the child may be quite bizarre.

> Ricky, age fourteen, who was fascinated with airplanes, suddenly announced that he would get a job at the airport. His father remarked that the airport was seventeen miles away and wondered how he would get to work. Ricky replied that he would just get into a plane, fly it home, and land in the

middle of his street. Further questioning established that he could see nothing illogical or unrealistic about this proposal.

All of the preceding text suggests that to some of these children the world may seem like an endless succession of randomly juxtaposed events, devoid of meaning or predictability in a confusing or incomprehensible experience that cannot be shared by other children or adults (Fish and Ritvo 1979).

Thought content may include excessive preoccupations. These will vary from child to child but may include either preoccupation with the details of maps, bus schedules, or with a class of objects, such as the manner in which doors close, or with fantastic or bizarre fantasies that seem undifferentiated from reality.

> Samuel, age five, who "knew" he was really a horse, insisted on eating grass or hay at every opportunity. One day when asked to draw a picture of himself, he drew a head from which protruded two large legs with hoofs rather than feet. When asked what they were, he replied that they were hoofs. When asked what the picture was, he said, "It's me, a horse."

Although well-formed paranoid delusions may emerge, they are usually not seen except in a fragmented fashion before age ten (Fish and Ritvo 1979). These rarely meet the criteria for schizophrenic delusions (i.e., thought insertions, thought broadcasting, and thought control) before adolescence. Although all children at times have fantasies of being able to fly or of having supernatural powers, such thoughts hold an unusual fascination for psychotic children. Occasionally bizarre delusions completely beyond the norm—for example, belief in peculiar lacerations of their body, or having a machine or other objects inside the body, are reported. These seem to take on the quality of reality for these children.

Language.

In some infants who later become psychotic, babbling is retarded from the start and the child is mute (20 to 40 percent of autistics) (Fish and Ritvo 1979). In a second group, both babbling and the first words may develop normally or with minimal delay, only to become arrested or to regress in the latter half of the second year or the beginning of the third. However, even with the autistic group, Kolvin has reported that 88 percent acquire three-word sentences after three years (Kolvin et al. 1971a). Most of these children are also deficient in nonverbal communication. For the most part, they do not use gestures or pantomime. Although this failure to imitate is in itself a serious learning difficulty, with intensive teaching even those children with serious speech retardation can often learn signing in order to communicate, and from this language frequently evolves. In a third group, language develops slowly but shows peculiarities: echolalia (Ekstein 1964); a reversal of pronouns so that the child says "you" when he or she should say "I"; singsong or melodic intonation or a monotonous voice; abnormal cadence and rhythm; irregular volume or pitch; extreme literalness; prolongation of sounds, syllables, or words; and stacatto sentences (Fish and Ritvo 1979). These children also use idiosyncratic terms, that is, utterances that have a specific meaning only to them but may be understood if the original context of the child's association is known. Fish and Ritvo (1979) use the example of a little boy to whom a saucepan became a "peter eater." It remained so even three years after it had been dropped on his foot while his mother was reciting to him the nursery rhyme about Peter, Peter Pumpkin Eater.

As speech develops, it may first be limited to naming objects, later to using simple adjectives or using the present tense to refer to the past. Children may copy precisely the question asked of them, using the same intonation as the speaker. There may be distortions of syntax and fragmentation of speech. With more developed speech, difficulties with the following may be observed: words that have more than one meaning; the use of similar sentences in different contexts; the creation of sentences to fit new situations (Shapiro et al. 1972; Shapiro, Roberts, and Fish 1970); the formation of long sentences; the use of complex syntax; and the comprehension of subtle and abstract meaning (Fish and Ritvo 1979). At each stage of speech development, it is not primarily the retardation of language that is so characteristic of these disorders. It is, rather, the coexistence of the peculiarities of speech already cited with varying degrees of retardation in different speech functions (Goldfarb, Braunstein, and Lorge 1956; Pronovost, Wakestein, and Wakestein 1966; Shaprio and Fish 1969; Wolff and Chess 1965). Indeed, these latter discrepancies make it particularly difficult for many parents to initially accept the seriousness of the condition.

> Several mothers of autistic children reported their early hopes that everything would be just fine once the child learned to speak. Yet after their child did develop speech, they wished that the child had never done so. Only then did they understand how strange were the thoughts and how bizarre and disorganized the child's thinking.

In contrast to all the preceding information, it should be noted that a small but definite group of psychotic children may show precocious language and may be preoccupied with word play (Bender 1947).

PSYCHOLOGICAL SIGNS AND SYMPTOMS

Emotions

Anxiety, at times of panic proportions in response to minimal stimuli, and the defenses against it have long been regarded as one of the hallmarks of the psychoses of childhood. It significantly differentiates psychotics from controls (Bender 1953). Psychotic anxiety is acute, excessive, and illogical (Creak 1961), with an unmodulated quality that distinguishes it from that of less disturbed children. It may be precipitated by minimal environmental change or by separation from a caring figure.

> Ruth, age four, had seemed normal until her third year when she began to panic whenever her mother left her sight. Even the mother's going into the next room was at times enough to precipitate panic. After the mother returned or whenever a stranger came into the room, Ruth would cling frantically to her mother. Unlike the shyness of the normal child who may briefly cuddle or cling when a stranger appears on the scene, Ruth clung endlessly rather than letting go and getting on with her play once the stranger had demonstrated that he or she did not constitute a threat. Ruth would also panic if her hair or toenails were cut, even by her mother, as if she were losing a vital part of her body on each occasion.

On the other hand, some children appear aloof, displaying shallow affect and a blank expression. Other psychotic children exhibit gross lability of affect, with abrupt shifts from flat, unresponsive, and shallow to explosively angry, silly, or panicky feelings without any obvious precipitant. In still other, usually older children, the affect may seem incongrous.

> Michael seemed unaware of what the group was doing. Suddenly one of the boys threw a balloon into the air. Michael virtually exploded into spasms of silly giggling. Flapping his hands in the air, he began to whirl himself round and round.

In those psychotic children who progress psychosocially, some control over this state of pananxiety may be achieved. Initially panic underlies the autistic withdrawal and inability to relate. Later these children handle their anxiety either by frantic clinging to the mothering figure at any threat of separation or, in still more developmentally mature cases, through numerous phobias and compulsions.

> Douglas, age three and one-half had shown all the symptoms of infantile autism. In his early development he had failed to form an attachment. In treatment, however, he formed a very close relationship with his therapist. Instead of ignoring her as he had on admission, he began to cling to her and had tremendous difficulty separating from her at the end of the day. Gradually his clinging subsided but was replaced by more specific anxieties. These became specific phobias that changed after a period of months.

SOCIAL SIGNS AND SYMPTOMS

Social Responses

Through infancy and childhood autistic withdrawal of interest from all social contact is a hallmark of early-onset psychosis. As infants, psychotic children fail to play the usual childhood games of peek-a-boo or waving bye-bye. They do not imitate. This, in toddler and early childhood years, makes teaching and training exceedingly difficult. In other children development arrests or regresses at about thirty months of age. These children appear preoccupied and oblivious to the presence of other children.

In both groups the child's behavior seems motivated by inner fantasies that have little if any relation to what is going on around. During play, other children or the examiner may be moved about as if they were pieces of furniture.

> John, age five and one-half, was playing with a small wooden track and train. When the examiner put her arm across the track as the train approached, Douglas quite matter-of-factly and without obvious communication lifted the examiner's arm and propped it up so that the train could pass under it.

Even the better functioning children establish cooperative interactions with their peers only with difficulty. Friendships of any real depth are a rarity.

Organization of Symptoms for Clinical Use

Since the causes of childhood psychosis are still unknown, treatment has to be symptomatic. It is often difficult to decide which symptoms should be treated and what goals can realistically be set. Most psychotic children can attend to only one activity at a time, and too many demands result in withdrawal, negativism, and sometimes in an increase of psychotic symptoms. With a patient and persistent approach, many children can be helped considerably, but there are no real "cures." Some symptoms have to be tolerated or the child has to be helped to replace troublesome and unacceptable behavior by more acceptable behavior in order to decrease social isolation.

To assist in understanding the symptoms, to facilitate the setting of appropriate and realistic goals, and to devise treatment strategies, the most common symptoms have been divided here into three fairly distinct groups.

PRIMARY SIGNS AND SYMPTOMS

The primary signs and symptoms listed in table 15.1 are considered to result from a serious developmental and functional disorganization of the central nervous system. This disorganization is thought to be the primary source of the extremely high, pervasive anxiety, the severe delays in language acquisition and social functioning, and the marked cognitive deficits present in these children. The primary symptoms dominate the early picture (up to three years). They continue as the child grows older but often

TABLE 15.1

Primary Signs and Symptons of Childhood Psychoses

These dominate the picture in the early years (up to age 3). They continue as the child grows older but become partly masked by secondary or tertiary symptoms.

Major Areas of Disturbance	Signs and Symptoms
Biological	
Disorders of development	Grossly disorganized, distorted, uneven development (physical, speech, emotional, intellectual and social).
Disorders of physical functions	Abnormality of tonus; poor patterning such as reverse sleep rhythm, uneven body temperature, colic; abnormalities of gross motor functions such as tics, choreoathetotic movements, rhythmic headbanging, handflapping, jumping, twirling, and other bizarre movements. Coordination and balance may or may not be affected
Disorders of memory	Memory may be poor or abnormally good for selected subjects; photographic memory may be present.
Disorders of attention	Attention span may be short or abnormally long. The latter may be due to preoccupations or preservation.
Disorders of activity level	Hyper- or Hypoactivity may be present; they may follow each other or alternate.
Biophysical	
Disorders of adaptability	Resistance to change and poor adaptation with, at times, catastrophic reactions to alterations in the environment.
Disorders of perception	Disturbances of body image perception; hallucinations (rare); distortions of both visual and auditory input.
Disorders of intellect	Uneven intellectual functioning from mental retardation to islets of superior intellect.
Disorders of Learning	Failure to learn from experience or specific learning defect. Yet some children may demonstrate specific talents far above their age level (music, math, memory tasks).

TABLE 15.1 *(continued)*

Major Areas of Disturbance	Signs and Symptoms
Biophychological	
Disorders of thinking and breaks of contact with reality	Speech delay, spurts, and regression; autistic use of speech (ability to use speech for communication may be lacking; developmental stages of speech distorted, prolonged, and greatly overlapping). Use of different voices, singsong, or lack of normal intonation.
Psychological	
Disorders of emotions	Extreme and sustained generalized anxiety and pleasure; inappropriate emotions, lack of normal fear, emotional flatness.
Social	
Disorders of relationship	Primary autism, self-centeredness, no apparent need for physical or emotional contact, "enjoys isolation."

are partly obscured by the secondary and sometimes tertiary symptoms. The primary symptoms are not greatly affected by environmental treatment. They may, in some children, be partly controlled by medication through a decrease in anxiety and better organized thinking.

SECONDARY SYMPTOMS

Secondary symptoms are considered defensive in nature. The child, troubled by the everpresent pervasive anxiety, develops defenses to contain this anxiety or, at least, to attain some degree of personal predictability in spite of it. Since these defensive behaviors may be the most obvious features of the child's illness, they have become the basis for many of the labels given to these syndromes (e.g., autism, symbiotic psychosis, pseudoneurotic psychosis, etc.).

The choice of the defenses seems partly due to the child's imitation of parental defenses but probably is mainly influenced by the child's developmental level. Autism, the most primitive form of withdrawal, is used by the youngest, the most affected, and the most seriously disorganized children. Symbiosis requires at least a recognition by the child that he or she functions better when supported by an adult. The child then clings to the adult and becomes first panicky and then autistic when separated. While not all children develop symbiosis, those who do are more able to relate later and to benefit from parenting, therapy, and teaching. Later, in

TABLE 15.2

Secondary Symptoms of Childhood Psychoses.
These are considered to be defensive manoeuvres to control anxiety. The form they take depends on the
child's age, intellect, degree of illness, and the parents' defenses. Some appear to be learned.

Type of Defense	Secondary Symptoms	Age When Usually Present
Secondary autism	In contrast to primary autism in which child has never related, here the child withdraws actively to avoid anxiety-producing situations.	Develops after age two to three. May last for lifetime in different forms and degrees.
Symbiosis	Child uses another person to enable him or her to function in contrast with reality. Becomes openly psychotic (autistic) when separated.	Develops after age two to three and lasts for months to years.
Pseudoneurosis	Phobic-compulsive-obsesssive syndrome. Rigid adherence to schedules; somatization of anxiety.	Usually after age four, typically age six into the teens. May continue to adulthood as pseudoneurotic schizophrenia.
Controlling behaviour	Decreased ability of the child to adapt causes anxiety in response to change. Child tries to keep environment constant by domination.	After two or three years of age. May last for life. Both degree and form may vary with time.
Pseudo-psychopathy	Lack of emotional attachment, self-centeredness, complete lack of consideration for others, paranoid ideation, ruthless pursuit of personal goals.	Teenage and older.

the preschool years, children often begin to focus their diffuse anxiety into a variety of fears (e.g., dogs, doctors, loud noises, and so on) similar to those of normal children. In the psychotic child, however, the fear is extremely intense and takes the form of a phobia. Then as long as the "dangerous object" is removed or avoided, the child can relax when it is out of sight. (See chapter 12.) As the defense develops further, the child frequently becomes preoccupied with the phobic object, repeatedly approaching it for reassurance until, instead of fearing it, the child returns to it whenever anxious for any reason.

Sally, age four, was terrified whenever the furnace turned on. Her therapist took her to see the furnace and showed her how to switch it on and off, explaining that the furnace is needed to keep people warm. Reassured, Sally would return to play in the playroom. The sequence repeated itself many times, until Sally began to go to the furnace on her own, not only when it was turned on but also when she became anxious about an airplane noise or a stranger coming into the room. She would approach the furnace, seem reassured, and return happily to the playroom until something else made her anxious.

These fears, obsessions, and compulsions, called pseudoneurotic defenses, are most commonly a part of the psychotic pathology of the school-age child.

Psychotic adolescents typically defend via pseudopsychopathic behavior. The teenager, wanting but not knowing how to have friends or how to relate to people, imitates the behavior of others. In the psychotic child this imitation, however, fails to serve the intended purpose because of the patient's inability to empathize with others, lack of judgment, extreme self-centeredness, and lack of guilt. Some of these youngsters—usually adolescents with a milder form of psychotic illness that may previously have gone unrecognized—commit serious antisocial acts. The pseudopsychopathic psychotic uses grandiose ideas and persecutory trends to defend against an anxiety that has arisen from feelings of inadequacy, impotence, and unknown dangers. These feelings seem to result from these children's difficulty understanding normal cause-and-effect relationships.

Pseudopsychopathy differs from true psychopathy in that in pseudopsychopathy there is an underlying psychosis. Longer observation and a good history are needed to distinguish these two conditions. However, they may be harder to distinguish between than neurosis and pseudoneurosis, possibly because pseudopsychopathic patients are older and better developed psychologically when this overlay of reactions to the environment occurs.

The part played by secondary symptoms in the course of treatment differs from that of primary symptoms. Some degree of defense is helpful, as without it the child would not be able to function at all. The essence of therapy in each case, then, is to ensure that at each given age and stage of treatment the therapist understands whether the defenses should be supported, left alone, or decreased. When they increase to the point of interfering with the child's functioning, something should be done to decrease the child's anxiety or to change the type of defense the child has been using.

> Terry, age four, was progressing quite well in treatment. In one and one-half years he had developed a relationship with his mother and his therapist that they could use to teach him routines and structures. When his therapist started to take him to the nursery, his anxiety increased and he reverted to relying on his old prop, a large truck that he would hold tightly and cling to while at the nursery. His therapist replaced the large truck first by a smaller one, which he could hold in one hand, and later by one that he could just keep in his pocket.

Sometimes both environmental support and medication may be needed during a period of stressful adaptation. Supportive psychotherapy may be used in selected cases.

TABLE 15.3

Tertiary Symptoms of Childhood Psychoses

These are considered reactive to, and designed to control, the environment or to retaliate against key persons who frustrate the child.

Type of Behaviour	"Purpose"	Age
Vomiting, paralysis, malingering illness	To avoid school or to attract attention particularly when jealous	School age
Panics and fears, increase of bizarre behavior, masturbation, screaming	To be removed from crowds or other anxiety-provoking situations, or for attention getting	After five
Temper tantrums	To defend against pressure put on child	Later preschool, ages four to five
Repetitive questioning, nonsensical speech or changes of subject	To avoid either answering questions or revealing feelings	School age
Antisocial acts: stealing, breaking in, physical attacks on others	Often the child's way of attempting to copy or identify with other teenagers	Later adolescence

TERTIARY SYMPTOMS

Tertiary symptoms, which resemble the conduct disorders of normal children, often make the diagnosis of psychosis very difficult, as they may appear to be evidence against the diagnosis of psychosis. In order to develop tertiary symptoms, the child must be sufficiently organized and have enough contact with the environment to be able to want to relate, even if in a distorted way. While the symptomatic behavior in itself makes sense and seems from its context to serve a purpose, (i.e., is not psychotic), it is grafted onto the underlying psychosis and is often self-punishing or self-destructive.

Although tertiary symptoms may occur in early–school-age children, they are more typical in better-functioning adolescent psychotics. They form a major part of the clinical picture of pseudopsychopathic schizophrenia. The treatment program for these children may require a residential setting or a carefully supervised home-care program.

Subgroups of Childhood Psychoses

DSM-III provides a reasonably detailed list of diagnostic criteria, some flexibility, the possibility of multiple diagnoses, and some indication of the child's level of functioning. (See chapter 6.)

DIAGNOSTIC CRITERIA FOR INFANTILE AUTISM (299.0x)

Infantile autism may be diagnosed in the following cases. Onset of the illness is before two and one-half years of age. The child exhibits extreme failure to respond to others (i.e., autism). The child's language development is grossly defective. If there is speech, it is unusual and characterized by: echolalia, immediate or delayed; and/or reversal of first- and second-person pronouns (e.g., says "I" for "you" and "you" for "I"); and metaphorical language. In addition, the child shows a bizarre response to the environment exhibiting extreme resistance to change and a preoccupation with and attachment to animate or inanimate objects. A last consideration in diagnosing infantile autism is the absence of evidence for a schizophrenic thought disorder as seen in adults; there are, no loosening of associations, incoherence, delusions, or hallucinations.

CHILDHOOD–ONSET PERVASIVE DEVELOPMENTAL DISORDER (299.9x)

Children with a pervasive developmental disorder exhibit pervasive and persistent disturbance in relationships to others, including inappropriate emotional responses, extreme and excessive clinging, lack of social interest and activity, incapacity for empathy, along with at least three of the following behaviors: (1) sudden outbursts of panic, including all-pervasive anxiety, extreme overreactions to normal life events, inability to be comforted; (2) inappropriate affectual response (emotional constriction alternates with unexpected and unexplained outbursts of rage, extreme variability of mood, absence of normal fear reactions); (3) profound and persistent resistance to environmental change (e.g., upset if solitary play is interrupted), inability to tolerate any change in normal routines (e.g., eating in the dining room instead of in the kitchen as usual); (4) bizarre motor movements such as posturing, hand flapping, toe-walking; (5) speech abnormalities, flat, singsong intonation; (6) over- or underreaction to sensory stimulation; (7) self-mutilating behavior, including extreme headbanging, biting, or scratching of the self.

In addition, the age of onset of the full-blown syndrome is between two and one-half and twelve years of age. Finally, there is no evidence of a schizophrenic thought disorder as seen in adults (i.e., no loosening of associations, incoherence, delusions or hallucinations.

ATYPICAL PERVASIVE DEVELOPMENTAL DISORDER (299.8x)

The diagnosis of atypical pervasive developmental disorder is reserved for children with widespread distortions in many aspects of psychological functioning essential to the development of social and language skills which, nevertheless, fail to meet the criteria for diagnosis either of infantile autism or childhood-onset pervasive developmental disorder.

If the child has delusions, hallucinations, loosening of association, and incoherence, it may be necessary to use the diagnostic criteria for schizophrenic disorders for adults. (See chapter 19.)

Assessment of the Child

A playroom or office setting should allow some spontaneous behavior by the child along with some chance to observe the child's responses to normal directions and limits, thus revealing both strengths and weaknesses. The strengths provide the keystone around which treatment is built. The examiner should observe the child in a systematic attempt to determine the developmental level in each of the following areas: physical, motor, and perceptual functioning; intellectual capacities; language; and emotional and social adjustment. The child's speech and language should be observed and the possibility of a hearing defect explored. Along with the parents' history, the medical history, and the examiner's observation, descriptions of the child's behavior should be obtained from others who have known the child longer, such as school or nursery school teachers who can compare the child with their normal pupils. Additional consultations should be sought depending on the particular symptoms presented by the specific child. The following professionals may therefore contribute.

1. The teacher or day-care worker, who can provide information about the child's ability, learning patterns, and day-to-day functioning over an extended period. This allows a comparison of the child's motor, intellectual, emotional, and social functioning with that of other normal children.
2. The child psychologist, who can assess developmental, motor, and conceptual functioning, and can delineate and measure various defects.
3. The speech pathologist, who can evaluate, diagnose, and quantify disorders of speech or language.
4. The otolaryngologist, who can exclude peripheral defects in auditory perception and arrange for audiometry if hearing loss is suspected.

5. The opthalmologist, who can exclude peripheral defects in visual perception.
6. The neurologist, who through clinical examinations and other procedures such as electroencephalography may help clarify a confusing clinical picture.
7. The pediatrician, who, if not already consulted, may add clarity by excluding other conditions in the differential diagnosis.
8. The occupational therapist, who can assess the child's motor and perceptual functioning by comparing them to the norm for any given age.
9. The public health nurse, who, through home visits and as a result of contacts with the school and health agencies whom the family has known in the past can help assess the level of family functioning both within the home and within society.

Problems in Making the Clinical Diagnosis

FLUCTUATING PICTURE

There are a number of problems in making the clinical diagnosis. Not all psychotic children have impaired reality contact all the time. The psychotic child may alternate between relatively normal or neurotic adjustment and periods where reality contact is definitely and seriously impaired. This fluctuating picture makes the diagnosis more complicated.

FAMILY PROBLEMS

In addition, less obviously psychotic children who could benefit from treatment are often misdiagnosed as suffering from a conduct disorder in response to family rejection, scapegoating, overindulgence, and so forth. The physician or psychologist must remember that these family problems may or may not have been present earlier in the child's life. Indeed, they may be to a large extent the result rather than the cause of some of the secondary and tertiary symptoms. Unfortunately it sometimes takes months or even years of unsuccessful treatment before an underlying psychosis is discovered.

Differential Diagnosis

See table 15.4 for guidelines for differential diagnosis between childhood psychosis and the organic syndromes.

311

TABLE 15.4

Guidelines for Differential Diagnosis Between Childhood Psychosis and Organic Syndromes

Symptoms and Signs	Psychotic	Organic
Biological		
Physical and developmental signs	Mild	Clearly present
BioPsychological		
Usual presenting symptoms are:	Secondary symptoms*	Primary† (younger child) or tertiary symptoms‡(older child)
Thought disorders	Present	mild, if present
Psychological		
Reality contact, including eye contact	Poor or none	Good or only mildly impaired
Diffuse and abnormal anxiety	Extreme	High
Affect inappropriate	May be present	Absent
Emotional flatness	Present	Absent or minimal
Social		
Bizarre behavior	Marked	None or minimal
Social relationshios	Grossly distorted or absent; negative motivation	Less impaired: positive motivation

* Secondary defenses.
† Primarily from central nervous system.
‡ Reactive to environment.

DEAFNESS

Deafness should be suspected in all children who fail to speak and answer to their name. Nerve deafness in particular can mimic early infantile autism and can also be a cause of autism. Deafness can also be an additional handicap to the autistic child. Because of the importance of the early introduction of a hearing aid to a deaf child's general management, the possibility of deafness is not to be taken lightly. It is often very difficult to test these children's hearing. Frequently clinical indications of hearing problems must be relied upon: singing or dancing to music suggests at least some hearing, but routinely listening to the radio or television at a volume so loud that others are uncomfortable suggests substantial hearing loss, as do enjoyment in making a lot of noise and responding, but only when in eye contact and not to directions given from behind. Sometimes in confusing cases electroencephalogram audiography or a trial with a hearing aid may be helpful. Finally, all professionals should be aware that deaf infants make early babbling sounds that are often considered a language by the parents but which disappear by the age of one and one-half. Their presence does not exclude deafness. Their absence suggests developmental delay, abnormality of the central nervous system, or autism.

MENTAL RETARDATION

Many children with autistic symptoms are also retarded. As they get older these children are likely to end up with the signs of retardation predominating. Psychological test results may be difficult to interpret. Too frequently, a child's inability to perform tasks is misinterpreted as unwillingness or an "emotional problem" instead of being recognized as evidence of mental deficiency. Variability, as previously described, remains the key to the accurate diagnosis of psychosis. The nonpsychotic retarded child does not show the test variability or the fluctuations in functioning that the psychotic does. In addition, retarded children usually respond socially; their conversation is uniformly simple and limited to concrete subjects related to their immediate environment; their affect is not incongruous; their thoughts seem simple rather than disorganized. Bizarre behavior is absent or minimal. Parents of retarded children tend to report their child's highest level of functioning, in an attempt to avoid having to face what they fear is evidence of mental defect. If the highest level of functioning the parents report is far below that which would be expected for the age, mental defect is very probable. To make the necessary school placement decisions for a child who is not testable, the psychiatrist must rely on combined reports from parents and other professionals (e.g., psychologists, occupational therapists) place the child in what seems to be an appropriate class, and try again to test him or her later. Retarded, autistic children are even less responsive to treatment than children who are merely retarded.

THE BRAIN DYSFUNCTION SYNDROME (314.01)

The brain dysfunction syndrome includes organic brain syndrome, minimal brain dysfunction, and attention-deficit disorder. It can be very difficult to distinguish brain dysfunction associated with specific learning disabilities or a maturational lag with aphasia from a mild psychosis. Psychotics have an organic core, while the child with brain dysfunction sometimes has a psychotic overlay. Borderline psychotic children, when in contact with reality, often show to a variable extent the signs and symptoms of brain dysfunction. However, since the treatment of both conditions is similar—that is, intensive, concrete, and directed toward relief of specific symptoms—in the beginning it is not necessary to distinguish between the two in order to start treatment. The final diagnosis can be made over an extended period of observation and symptomatic treatment.

All types and degrees of brain dysfunction resemble childhood psychosis and may show as primary symptoms poor organization, uneven maturation, and a high level of anxiety. Brain-dysfunctioning children who are extremely anxious may also develop secondary symptoms such as withdrawal resembling mild autism or, more often, pseudoneurotic defenses of a phobic-compulsive-obsessional or somatic nature. The main distinguishing features are the psychotic children's lack of relationships and bizarre behavior.

DEVELOPMENTAL APHASIA

In developmental aphasia, which appears to represent a lag in neurological maturation, speech may not begin until the child is between four and six years old. None of the other symptoms of childhood psychosis are present, however, and the child communicates well nonverbally.

CENTRAL COMMUNICATION DISORDERS

Central communication disorders include expressive aphasia (315.31). In these disorders the child is able to communicate nonverbally and may understand complex commands.

REACTIVE BEHAVIOR DISORDERS

Reactive behavior disorders are responses to environmental stress. "Folie-à-deux" with another family member belongs in this category. The main feature distinguishing these disorders from psychosis is the absence of primary signs and symptoms of childhood psychosis. To rule out their presence, prolonged observation, additional reports from teachers, psychologists, occupational therapists, and other specific consultations may be needed. Removal of a child to a treatment or other setting may lead relatively quickly to the decrease or disappearance of symptoms. Complete disappearance of a symptom in preschoolers is of diagnostic significance. In children past age six to seven, however, some of the abnormal response is usually fixed, so that residual symptoms may remain even when the child is away from the family.

Elective mutism must also be distinguished from childhood psychosis but here the other signs and symptoms of the latter are lacking and the child's symptoms are clearly a tool for the manipulation of the environment.

REACTIVE ATTACHMENT DISORDERS OF INFANCY, OR ANACLITIC DEPRESSION (313.89)

Reactive attachment disorders of infancy represent yet another group of environmentally caused conditions. The history of extreme deprivation combined with signs of failure to thrive, depression, and absence of bizarre behavior differentiate these children from the autistics.

ORGANIC CONDITIONS

Autistic psychotic behavior may be imitated or caused by other organic conditions, many of them resulting from prenatal or perinatal damage. These include the following categories of disorders.

1. Genetic: Schilder's acute disseminating sclerosis, Hurler's disease, tuberous sclerosis, trisomy 21, phenylketonuria, neurolipoidisis (Knobloch and Pasamanick 1975).
2. Infectious: congential rubella, toxoplasmosis, neurosyphilis, meningitis, encephalitis (Benda 1952; Chess 1971; Desmond et al. 1970).
3. Toxic: toxemia, thyrotoxicosis, conditions due to drugs taken during pregnancy.
4. Traumatic: injuries with or without obvious organic sequelae (Janou 1971; Montagu 1962; Owen 1976).
5. Degenerative and multiple etiologies: neonatal ataxia, epilepsy, retrolental fibroplasia, hydrocephalus, and cerebral palsy (Schain and Yannet 1960).

The three most common conditions imitating infantile autism or other childhood psychosis are congenital rubella syndrome, phenylketonuria, and tuberous sclerosis. With the possible exception of tuberous sclerosis these conditions usually present no problem in diagnosis since practically all children suffering from them have been diagnosed for their primary condition by a neurologist. This is understandable, since tuberous sclerosis usually starts in the preschool years and develops slowly.

A progressive neurological degeneration should be suspected from indications of steady rather than a fluctuating deterioration with increasing motor and intellectual impairment. Headache, anorexia, vomiting, fatigue, and loss of previous interests are particularly important indications for prompt referral to a pediatrician or neurologist. Seizures, twitching, the development of squint or even mild paralysis and loss of balance also call for immediate consultation.

In all cases, it is good practice for the psychiatrist to keep in touch with the family physician. Psychotic children are even more difficult to examine than normal children. They do not communicate well about pain or distress, and if they do, they may just give signs of general distress without localization. The family physician, with firsthand knowledge of the child's physical development, is usually best able to evaluate any changes in physical condition, thus assisting in making the diagnosis.

Etiology

The etiology of childhood and adolescent psychoses is by no means clear. Even in isolated clinical subgroups, no conclusion can be drawn in spite of considerable research. The hypotheses have run the gamut from early environmental factors, organic predisposition with environmental stress, to genetics. To date, it is not even clear whether there is a connection between the psychoses of childhood and adult schizophrenia.

GENETIC AND ORGANIC ROOTS OF PSYCHOSIS

Basic organic defects may be caused either by a genetic abnormality; a prenatal or perinatal event such as infection, trauma, or poisoning; or a combination of the two. As to the possible genetic component, Fish has noted that three subgroups of children with childhood psychosis have an increased number of schizophrenic relatives (Fish and Ritvo 1979): (1) those with onset after age five who show a formal thought disorder, (2) those with onset before age five who have developed a thought disorder, and (3) those children who fit the criteria of early infantile autism or pervasive developmental disorder and show no evidence of organic brain syndrome but are later diagnosed schizophrenic. Nonspecific intrauterine and perinatal factors (including nutritional, circulatory, traumatic, infectious, and other insults) have been reported in one-third to one-half of those with infantile autism and one-sixth to one-quarter of those with later onset psychoses (Knobloch and Grant 1961; Kolvin, Ounsted, and Roth 1971c; Taft and Goldfarb 1964). Minor signs of brain dysfunctioning also have been described in up to one-quarter of the children with infantile autism (Anthony 1958; Creak 1963; Dahl 1976). Gross organic pathology is rare. It is not possible at this time to say where the dividing line between organic brain syndromes and the childhood psychoses should be placed. Even differentiating clearly between these so-called syndromes is a thorny task. Alderton (1977) notes that there is an essential continuity between the various syndromes subsumed under the rubric of childhood psychosis and that each represents a variety of possible etiological clusters acting together to produce a clinical picture. Fish and Ritvo (1979) and Havelkova all have made similar comments (Ornitz 1969, 1976).

Different genetic studies have had diametrically opposite results. Bender's children, for example, showed a high incidence of schizophrenia in the parents (Bender and Faretra 1972; Bender and Grugett 1956). Kanner's sample, on the other hand, indicated an absence of psychosis in the parents (Kanner and Eisenberg 1955). Bender and Grugett (1956), Fish (1975, 1977), and Rosenthal (1970; Brown 1963) have stated that childhood schizophrenia (i.e., pervasive developmental disorder, not autism) is genetically continuous with adult schizophrenia. Studies on adult schizophrenics (Gottesman and Shields 1972; Slater and Cowle 1971) point to genetic factors as a necessary but not sufficient condition for the development of schizophrenia. Concordance in monozygotic twins (Kanner 1953; Stabenau and Pollin 1967) is from 35 to 58 percent, and children from schizophrenic parents reared in adoptive homes have a similar risk to children reared with their schizophrenic relatives (Heston and Denny 1968). Children from nonschizophrenic parents reared by schizophrenics have no increased incidence of schizophrenia (Wender et al. 1974). The rates for schizophrenia in parents of childhood psychotics are the same or higher than those for adult schizophrenics—4.2 to 4.4 percent (Rosenthal 1970; Slater and Cowie 1971), and, in a later and comprehensive review, Alderton (1977) found that from 10 to 40 percent of the parents of psychotic children were schizophrenic. If later-onset schizophrenic disorders were included, an 80.2 percent concordance rate is found for monozygotic twins (Kallman and Roth 1956), while dizygotic twins show rates of 17 percent for childhood schizophrenia and 22.9 percent for all schizophrenic disorders.

The results for psychosis before age two are less clear (Hanson and Gottesman 1976). Kanner (1953); Rutter (1972); Rutter and Lockyer (1967); Rutter, Greenfeld, and Lockyer (1967), and Kolvin et al. (1971) have all stated that early-onset psychosis is not continuous with adult schizophrenia. On the other hand, 44 percent of Kanner and Eisenberg's (1955) autistics with speech around four years of age were considered psychotic in adolescence; Brown (1963, 1969) and Reiser and Brown (1964) found that 11 percent were psychotic in adolescence, with a further 30 percent severely disturbed. In viewing these statistics, the problem arises of comparing studies where the precise criteria used for diagnosing infantile autism originally and schizophrenia on follow-up are not always clear. Also, it is almost impossible to obtain a sense of that important aspect of psychosis—its quality and its severity.

The results of studies of the parents of infantile psychotics have also been contradictory. The proportion of parents who are themselves psychotic is clearly higher than expected but figures vary from 5.7 percent (Fish 1977) to 21 percent (Meyers and Goldfarb, 1962). However, Kanner (1953), Fish (1968, 1976), Rutter (1967, 1970) Coleman and Provénce (1957), and Lotter (1967*b*), in looking at parents hospitalized for schizophrenia, did not have similar results.

These differences become somewhat comprehensible when viewed in the light of the aforementioned biases (Goldfarb 1961; Lotter 1967*b*). Rutter and Kolvin's group are generally lower functioning and include a higher percentage of children with brain disorders. In addition, there is a higher prevalence of adult schizophrenia in the lower socioeconomic classes (Kohn 1968). Bender's and Fish's (Bender and Faretra 1972; Fish 1976; Fish et al. 1968) samples include a higher proportion of lower social class patients than do those of Kanner, Rutter, Creak, and Kolvin. It appears that eliminating the confusion introduced by the inclusion of organic brain syndromes and socioeconomic bias might allow a clearer picture to emerge. The authors speculate that such future studies will show a definite genetic loading for at least subgroups of psychotic children.

BIOCHEMICAL STUDIES

Studies of the biochemical roots of psychosis are also limited and inconclusive. They suffer from the lack of established norms for some of the measures and from differences in the biochemical assay techniques employed. Nevertheless, a number of studies suggest differences between psychotic and normal children. Serotonin levels may be higher in a subgroup of patients with florid psychosis and in those with lower IQs (Brown 1960). There also appears to be a lower rate of serotonin uptake by platelets in autistics than in nonautistic psychotic children and other patient groups and these lower levels are similar to those found in younger children (Ritvo et al. 1970*b*; Siva-Sankar 1970).

Studies with catecholamines have revealed increased homovanilic acid (HVA) and 5-hydroxyindoleacetic acid (5-HIAA) in cerebrospinal fluid and a greater urinary excretion of 3, 4-dimethoxyphenylethylamine (DMPEA) (Widelitz and Feldman 1969). These studies require replication.

HEMATOLOGIC STUDIES

Hematologic studies have revealed the following: atypical leucocyte patterns (Fowle 1968): low levels of magnesium and potassium (Saladino and Siva-Sankar 1969); differences in red blood cell cholinesterase activities (Lucas, Krause, and Domino 1971); increased variability of free fatty acids and plasma glucose levels (Demyer, Ward, and Lintzenich 1968; Demyer et al. 1971); and, in one group of autistics, increased blood levels of lead (Cohen, Johnson, and Caparulo 1976).

NEUROANATOMIC STUDIES

Enlarged lateral ventricles with widened left temporal horns have been observed (Hauser, DeLong, and Rosman 1975).

Psychoses in Childhood and Adolescence

PSYCHOLOGICAL STUDIES

These studies have looked at a large number of different areas: Ornitz investigated perceptual inconsistencies (Ornitz and Ritvo 1968); Bergman, unusual sensitivities (Bergman and Escalona 1949); Goldfarb (1956), receptor preferences; Schloper (1965), receptor processes and the preference for proximal over distal receptors. Electroencephalographic (EEG) studies have been largely noncontributory (Bradley 1941; Hermelin 1968; Hertzig and Birch 1968; Ritvo et al. 1970*a*), but eye movements during sleep appear more like those of normal infants than of age-matched controls (Ornitz et al. 1971; Tanguay 1976). Studies of auditory-evoked responses during sleep have also been largely equivocal (Ornitz et al. 1968; Ornitz et al. 1974), as have studies of galvanic skin responses (Bernal and Miller 1970; Miller and Bernal 1971) and of contingent negative variation responses, or CNV (Small, Demyer, and Milstein 1971; Small 1971). Autistics do not show, however, a differential response to familiar versus unfamiliar faces in a series of slides (Lelord et al. 1973). Another report has shown larger, slow, negative or positive potentials in response to stimulus coupling. Tests of vestibular function have revealed a significant reduction of the duration of postrotatory nystagmus in a lighted but not in a dark room (Ritvo et al. 1971; Ornitz et al. 1974).

Hauser and colleagues (1975), in a sample of seventeen children diagnosed as autistic, found abnormalities in half of the EEGs and fifteen of the pneumoencephalograms. In the latter, the temporal lobe was implicated. Condon (1975) found delays in auditory apperception. He postulated that the autistic child may see the lips of the speaker form a word but does not "hear" the word until after a short delay and/or more than once in a reverberating manner.

A number of authors have hypothesized that the biological clock mechanism governing normal maturation and development is grossly disturbed in psychotic children. In healthy children each developmental line (postural, motor, visual motor, verbal, physical growth, etc.) develops in an orderly manner and each area is predictably linked with development in all others. In psychotic children there appears to be a delinking, so that spurts of development in one area are completely dissociated from the rates of development in all others. Sequences within any developmental line may be out of step, and reversals may occur (Fish and Ritvo 1979).

Many factors contribute to the confusion in defining the etiologies of these disorders: poorly delineated syndromes, each of which is relatively rare, so that each author can observe only a limited number of cases; fluctuating picture; changes with maturation. Comparisons with adult schizophrenia adds to the problem, as that condition probably also has multiple

319

etiologies and many forms and degrees. Follow-up studies of psychotic children into adulthood should provide some help in this regard.

Clinical observations and past follow-up studies suggest that infantile autism and childhood-onset pervasive developmental disorder are groups of conditions with an organic core, probably due to a number of different etiological factors. There appears to be a group with genetic etiology, which is related to adult schizophrenia. This group has a positive history of relatives, including parents and siblings who suffer from conditions falling within the schizophrenic spectrum. While it is necessary for classification and research to clearly distinguish between infantile autism and childhood-onset pervasive developmental disorder, there is not much difference between the groups with regard to family history of schizophrenia. Other cases seem related to attention deficit disorder, brain dysfunction, or mental retardation, which may be either a primary or a secondary result of the psychosis.

Prognosis

Prognosis is poor for most of these children. Rutter's (Rutter, Greenfeld, and Lockyer 1967) sample of severely impaired children did poorly on follow-up; 71 percent showed an IQ of less than 70 (with approximately 63 percent less than 35), and 35 percent had organic brain syndromes. Fifty-nine percent were in institutions and only 8 percent were in regular schools or employed. Havelkova's (1968) sample showed a bimodal distribution and, although 76 percent were in institutions on follow-up, 24 percent were in regular school or employed and some, though markedly disabled, were doing well academically and had begun to maintain some meaningful social relationships.

Havelkova found that the most common outcome of infantile autism was a mixture of different degrees of intellectual defect ranging from profound retardation to specific learning disorders combined with different degrees of autism. Some of these patients were quite bizarre, not fitting into any adult diagnostic category. Others were like hebephrenic schizophrenics. Some, but not all, of those with normal intellect had a psychotic breakdown in adolescence or young adulthood.

Because the samples are different, comparisons and conclusions concerning the prognosis of these disorders are very difficult. There does, however, appear to be a general agreement that a better prognosis is found in children with an IQ greater than 60 (Rutter and Lockyer 1967) and some language before five (Eisenberg 1956; Havelkova 1968). Both Bender (1942) and Havelkova have shown that in those children who adjusted well to the community, the IQ rose during their childhood as much as 40 points. At the other end of the spectrum, 87 percent of those of Bender's group whose IQs remained less than 70 were chronically institutionalized. In addition, those children who developed a pseudoneurotic form of psychosis did better (Havelkova 1968). Finally, a poor outcome is probable if, even by the age of three to four, there is an inappropriate use of toys and a complete lack of speech (Brown 1960).

Some symptoms are more likely to respond than others. With time and treatment, attention, goal directedness, abstract thinking, language, bizarre activities, resistance to change, and relating to others all tend to improve, and hyperactivity tends to decrease. On the other hand, hypoactivity, thought disorders, unusual intonations of speech, inappropriate affect, and brittleness of adaptation all tend to remain or increase. With age the discrepancies between various areas of functioning tend to become less marked. Most of the secondary and tertiary symptoms tend to remain. Where they do subside, relapses are common, particularly during stressful periods.

In conclusion, even those psychotic children who experience the best outcomes are left with some social and emotional problems. They often long for friends at about age eight or nine but are usually unable to go about making and keeping them. This may be helped by group therapy. However, since their progress is much slower than that of other children, they sometimes require as long as three years in treatment before any progress can be seen. Some psychotic children improve in their early teens. Those with learning problems may need remedial education, either temporarily or on a long-term basis. For some, intellectual development and academic progress begin to deteriorate after two to three years' schooling, until they finally require placement in schools for the retarded. Those with emotional problems are sometimes helped by individual therapy, but since their progress is slow, they are not often selected for psychotherapy. Even those who improve greatly with psychotherapy may break down in late adolescence or young adulthood. This breakdown may take the form of schizophrenia or of an atypical depression. In the mildly retarded patient with childhood psychosis, the breakdown may at first appear just as normal adolescent self-assertion, only to evolve later into completely uncontrolled behavior requiring residential care. Lack of social judgment, need for sexual relationships, and grandiose or persecutory ideas can lead to bizarre and dangerous situations. The dangers have increased with the philosophy of keeping everyone in the community rather than in hospital, a trend that sometimes goes against the best interests of the patient.

A number have overcome their illness enough to function independently in the community. Some of those followed by Havelkova have graduated from college or university, while others are self-supporting. A few are married. On the whole, however, even those who do relatively well tend to remain introverted loners dependent on their families for company, advice, or financial support. While far from ideal, in view of the seriousness of their original condition, this represents a successful adjustment.

Treatment

The first consideration in treatment is the family and, in particular, the parents. The parents must be assisted through the stages of mourning for the child who might have been until they are eventually able to accept their child's disorder and assume a client role. Concurrently, they should be helped to find support systems in the community, both for their child and for the family as a whole. Often introduction to a local group of parents dealing with the same or similar problems can be helpful. In addition, parents are encouraged to become involved in treatment for any existing problems in the family system or for personal intrapsychic problems (a patient role). Finally, the parents should be taught to become proficient in applying specialized techniques to help their child at each stage of the treatment process (a colleague role).

In treatment, therefore, parents must deal with the denial, protest, and bargaining phases of mourning and come to terms with the fact that: something is wrong; it is serious; it is not something else; it is not anyone else's fault that it has not been diagnosed, stopped, or cured; another center, a new miracle cure won't change the probable outcome. They must withstand the despair that will follow working through the earlier phases and come to genuinely feel that: the family still exists; they are not helpless; they are not completely abandoned; some assistance is available; they can redesign their thoughts, expectations, and hopes; they and their child can continue to function, although this illness will be a controlling factor for the remainder of the child's life, regardless of how well he or she adjusts to these limitations or compensates for the disabilities. This is a process that any parent of a retarded or otherwise handicapped child has to go through. However, the denial in the parents of a psychotic child is often more intense because of the child's normal appearance and occasional islets of higher functioning.

The therapeutic staff should recognize that one to two years is a normal amount of time for mourning and that even twice as long is not very abnormal for these parents. In addition, the mourning process is exacerbated as their child reaches the age where such milestones as choice of school, puberty, choice of career, separation from family, and marriage are usually considered.

The factors that appear to govern the negotiation of this mourning process include: first, the family's characteristic patterns for handling stress, its coping style, and problem-solving ability (see chapter 3); second, the personal meaning of the child's psychosis to the parents' self-esteem; third, the support they can glean from significant others; fourth, the collective vulnerabilities of the family system; fifth, the sum of other stresses impinging on their family; and sixth, the quality and extent of the child's disability.

Having carried out a full assessment of both child and family and having begun a program to assist the parents, the educator/therapist's attention can then be focused on the treatment of the child. Treatment of these children is essentially symptomatic. It demands, therefore, that the professional first make a clear, succinct list of objectives; second, decide on priorities and the sequence in which these objectives should be worked upon; and third, devise a treatment strategy for attaining each of the objectives. The simplest approach is to set graded objectives for each biopsychosocial area of functioning, as outlined earlier in the section on symptoms. An objective in this context consists of what the child must achieve in order to demonstrate the necessary predefined level of functioning. Having thus decided what the child must be able to do and the order in which these skills will be taught, a specific treatment program may be devised. In so doing there are several basic principles to keep in mind.

1. The child's strengths are used to facilitate gains in weaker areas.
2. For each specific area of malfunctioning, the stated treatment objectives are worked on in sequence.
3. In designing individual, child-specific therapeutic programs, learning principles are at all times coupled with a dynamic understanding of the psychosocial development and the biological strengths and weaknesses of that particular child.
4. The parents are involved in teaching the child at every stage of the process.
5. Where behavior modification methods are used, they should always be coupled with a determined attempt to encourage a relationship between the principal therapist and the child.
6. It is the relationship between the teacher/therapist and the child that motivates development in the child; it activates and maintains the drive toward growth.
7. Treatment activities should be part of or blend into the natural play of the child and should be appropriate to the child's developmental level.
8. For the most part, the teaching of each new skill will proceed according to the following pattern: attention; imitation; use of gestures and/or signs; reciprocation with adults; reciprocation with children; self-initiated action with adults; and self-initiated action with other children.

Common features of most treatment programs are structure, consistency, security, limit setting, reduction of anxiety-provoking situations, reinforcement of necessary contingencies toward goal-directed behavior, and the formation of an emotionally meaningful bond between the therapist and the child.

No single therapeutic modality is sufficient. The application of play therapy, behavior modification, education, physiotherapy, and medication must all be considered within a total treatment atmosphere that is appropriate to both the cognitive and the emotional developmental level of the child. With the autistic child, the first major thrust of therapy is toward forming a single emotionally meaningful personal relationship with the therapist. When this is accomplished, involvement with others, peer relationships, and social expectations are slowly embarked upon. Anxiety is kept at a minimum. Slow and gradual changes are introduced into the environment as the child appears ready to handle them, in order to help the child adjust to change. Meanwhile behavior modification and medication may be introduced to undermine stereotyped rituals and make the child more amenable to relating appropriately with the therapist. Early in treatment a symbiotic relationship with the therapist is encouraged, and only later are separation and independent functioning made the focus of therapeutic efforts. Treatment is always carried out at a pace that the child can tolerate, in order to minimize disruptive anxiety and the need for pathological defenses (Mahler 1961). The child is helped to test reality within the security of the therapeutic relationship, and anxiety is further minimized by providing structure, predictability, safe limits, clear reality-oriented communication, and supportive relationships with others. When anxiety is marked, phenothiazines may facilitate overall treatment planning.

As the child grows, a relatively satisfactory adjustment may be maintained except at times of external stress. Stress may result from family disequilibrium, rapid changes in the child's life, such as a move to a new school or neighborhood, and feared or actual relationship loss. The emphasis is on reducing stress to a tolerable level and encouraging social relationships and involvement. If decompensation is marked, brief hospital admission may be necessary with a return to the family at the earliest opportunity. Concurrent work with parents in family therapy may help clarify family communication and facilitate members deriving adaptive ways of dealing with and resolving disturbing affect. Medication may again be helpful to reduce the disorganizing effects of anxiety or to control severely impulsive behavior. Because of the relative instability of the neurotic defenses, psychotherapy when indicated is generally of a supportive nature. In adolescence the emphasis may have to be on reducing paranoid interpretation of the environment by establishing feelings of trust and security within the therapeutic relationship. Once trust can be secured, either by residential treatment or intensive individual psychotherapeutic work several times a week, it may then become possible to help the youngster discover what it is that he or she does that evokes hostility and rejection from the environment and find more adaptive ways of dealing with stress. These children are often very hard to reach because of their suspiciousness and their ability to disguise symptoms. Individual psychotherapy with them requires great skill and persistence on the part of the therapist and frequently needs to be prolonged because of the fragility and instability of the child's defenses. Psychotherapy seems useful for the higher functioning children, particularly when combined in a total treatment program for the child (Barrett et al. 1971, Havelkova 1968; Ward 1970). It is, however, generally agreed that psychotherapy alone is not the treatment of choice. Studies of its effectiveness are equivocal, with some authors such as Rutter (1965; Rutter, Greenfeld and Lockyer 1967), Eisenberg and Kanner (1956), Goldfarb (1956), and Fish (1975) finding that improvements are not related to the length or type of psychotherapy.

At all stages of therapy, behavior modification has proven useful and has been incorporated into educational approaches for dealing with psychotic children. The therapist/educator rewards socially adaptive behavior and ignores and/or punishes maladaptive functioning. In teaching language, for example, a definite hierarchical sequence is followed. The child's behavior is shaped through positive reinforcement of behaviors in the following sequence: pay attention; imitate gross, then fine motor movements; imitate oral movements; use meaningful gestures; vocalize; match therapist's vocalizations; make difficult vocal discriminations; and so on. This slow, stepwise procedure is carried out until, it is hoped, the child is able to initiate conversation and improve the use of language for his or her own gratification.

The same principles may be applied to increasing socially acceptable behaviors such as dressing, table manners, social greetings, personal hygiene, and for learning progressively more difficult cognitive concepts.

Aversive therapy, that is, the release from an undesirable stimulus, is sometimes used. For example, forcibly and repeatedly turning the child's head toward the therapist in order to maintain attention may cause a child to maintain attention in order to bring an end to the unwanted procedure. On the other hand, most aversive procedures where, for example, the child is forced to react to the therapist to avoid a shock, have not proved successful. Behaviors learned this way remain specific to the exact situation and the therapist and are not generalized to other situations or areas of functioning. In addition, as Tinbergen and Tinbergen (1976) have pointed out, therapists should be attempting to reduce anxiety-provoking situations, while aversive methods have exactly the opposite effect. One exception would be the use of shock to eliminate specific self-mutilatory behaviors that have proven resistant to other procedures or are of an emergency nature. Here, too, however, overdiscrimination may leave the child still self-destructive in other settings.

Reinforcement of unacceptable behaviors has worked in some cases. For example, the child who flaps his hands may be given food that can only be eaten when he is not flapping. Having the child spend time out with the removal of all attention, reinforcement, and stimulation, while useful in the modification of behavior in children with conduct disorders, may reinforce withdrawal and self-stimulation in these children.

The autistic child's deficiency in generalizing and the phenomena of overselectivity in discriminations make learning difficult. An example of the latter is the child who, having learned to pick up the red truck on command, may, when challenged with a number of objects, pick up a red ball, because she appears to have discriminated the colors and not the objects. Generalization of what is learned in treatment to other contexts is greatly assisted by involving the parents as coeducators. It is also helped by carrying out treatment in the home as well as in the therapeutic setting. This has the desirable secondary effect of being cost effective and increasing the parents' confidence in their own ability to help the child (Lovaas et al. 1973; O'Dell 1974).

Psychoactive medications are used as a temporary adjunct in the total treatment of the psychotic child. Phenothiazines such as chlorpromazine and thioridazine* have been found somewhat useful, though unwanted effects such as excessive sedation, worsening of the psychosis, catatonic-like states, insomnia, motor excitation, and irritability may be observed. Trifluoperazine, a less sedating phenothiazine, has produced in preschoolers increased alertness, social responsiveness, motor initiation, and language production (Fish et al. 1968) and, along with thiothixine, has been found useful in reducing withdrawal and stereotyped behavior (Wolpert, Hagamen, and Merlis 1967). Both the phenothiazine fluphenazine and the butyrophenone haloperidol improve self-awareness and constructive play while reducing compulsions and self-mutilation (Englehardt et al. 1973; Faretra, Dooher, and Dowling 1970). Newer classes of neuroleptics such as molindone and loxapine are not proving any more effective in early trials (Campbell et al. 1971; Pool et al. 1976).

Lithium carbonate is effective in reducing hyperactivity, aggressiveness, and stereotyped behavior (Gram and Rafaelson 1972). It does not appear very effective in preschoolers (Campbell et al. 1972*b*). The effectiveness of megavitamins has not been demonstrated (Greenbaum 1970). Amphetamines may worsen behavior (Campbell et al. 1972*a;* Campbell 1976*b*). However, the authors have found methylphenidate useful in some hyperactive children with short attention spans. Because of its low toxicity and quick action compared to phenothiazines, a trial is worthwhile. Fish has suggested that diphenhydramine, which is effective in some children, be tried first with preschoolers because of its relative safety (Fish 1960; Fish and Shapiro 1964). Campbell (1976*a*) has noted that the good of psychopharmacological treatment may be different for adults than for children. In the former, decreased reactivity, particularly in the acute phase, may be desirable (Himwich 1960). In children, particularly the listless, apathetic, withdrawn preschooler, this may be detrimental. For this reason drugs such as haloperidol and thiothixine may be preferred for use with preschoolers. On the other hand, sedating effects may allow some of these children to focus their attention on a task, making them more amenable to learning and to joining constructively in social situations. This in turn

---

*See Campbell et al. 1972*b;* Campbell 1976*a;* Fish 1960; Fish et al. 1965; and Korein et al. 1971.

may lead to other gains. The neuroleptics do, however, have potential undesirable side effects: skin rashes, agranulocytosis, liver damage, and extrapyramidal effects, though infrequent, are possible (Dimascio 1970; Dimascio, Shader, and Giller 1970; Dimascio, Soltys, and Shader 1970; Shader and Dimascio 1970).

In addition, phenothiazines lower the seizure threshold (Lowery and Wright 1957) and affect the neurotransmitters that control the secretion of hypothalamic neurohormones. The latter effect may influence growth, and abnormalities such as menstrual irregularities, amennorhea, galactorrhea, aspermia, and weight gain all have been noted, as have effects on the IQ (Campbell 1976a; McAndrew, Case, and Treffert 1972). In addition, tardive dyskinesia-like symptoms including involuntary movements of the upper extremeties with akathesia have been recorded after the abrupt withdrawal of phenothiazines (Polizos et al. 1973; Schiele et al. 1973).

In the treatment of childhood psychoses, there is certainly a place for medication, but it should be used with care, reviewed frequently, and limited to a relatively short-term intervention.

In summary, it can be seen that all the approaches to treatment overlap. Each treatment has different strengths: physiotherapy for areas of fine and gross motor coordination; medication for attention and for decreasing some bizarre behaviors; behavior modification for increasing socially appropriate behaviors; learning language for purposes of communication and reducing undesirable behaviors; and psychotherapy for helping the child learn to form emotionally meaningful relationships with others and for reducing anxiety.

As to the therapeutic setting, stimulation by other preferably normal children is an important part of treatment. Grouping psychotic children together without including any normal, less disturbed, or mildly retarded children is far from satisfactory. All psychotic children socialize poorly, and most are poorly motivated to interact with other children. Even a good therapist finds it hard to provide the stimulation and modeling that normal children provide, though a supportive adult is needed in any group.

In communities lacking specialized psychiatric facilities, mental health workers would attempt to interest and involve special teachers who have worked or are working with mildly retarded children in special education classrooms or in nursery schools. Sometimes an additional staff person can be hired for the nursery to help the psychotic child function within that group. Some parents ask whether, for the child's sake, they should move to a city where treatment is available. Such decisions represent a major upheaval for the family, and parents should be given as realistic a prognosis as possible, since some children are extremely unlikely to benefit from any treatment while others may derive only minimum benefit. The effects of such a move on the rest of the family may be disastrous.

Inpatient treatment for the young psychotic child is usually not indicated. Separation from the family may interfere with progress. Exceptions would include admissions during family crises or, on occasion, short-term admission for assessment. Some children insist on sameness so stubbornly that outpatient treatment grinds to a halt. A brief admission makes it possible to see whether the child can respond favorably to a new environment or different treatment methods. Sometimes initiation and regulation of medication, impossible or unsuccessful on an outpatient basis, can be achieved through a short-term admission.

In conclusion, such a multimodal yet holistic approach to diagnosis and treatment is beyond the scope of any single professional. A team approach with inputs from many additional consultants is required. At the same time, however, a single principal therapist should be designated who, given the team's input concerning highly specialized therapeutic techniques, will maintain a psychotherapeutic relationship with the child for as long as it takes the child to form an emotionally meaningful relationship with him or her. When this is accomplished, the treatment regimen may be broadened to include group processes, with their greater emphasis on individuation and the forming of relationships with peers.

Summary

The childhood psychoses are caused by an as yet unknown organic pathology that has some genetic basis in at least a subgroup of the early-onset cases and in the majority of those whose onset is later in childhood. Boys appear more vulnerable than girls. These psychoses represent forms of pandevelopmental retardation characterized by fluctuations in development along individual lines with great variations in the degree of maturation along different lines of development. From a practical standpoint, it is essential that the professional document these levels of functioning in an orderly manner and record the changes in each developmental line (e.g., motor, cognition, language, social functioning, etc.) over a considerable period of time before making predictions about the prognosis for an individual child. The precise clinical picture varies from case to case and appears to depend on the developmental level of the child at the onset of the psychosis, the major areas of dysfunction, and the types of ego defenses utilized to maintain psychological homeostasis (Mahler 1951; Schain and Yannet 1960). No symptoms are pathognomonic.

If the problems are clearly specified for each line of development, then specific symptom-oriented treatment programs can be applied concurrently and altered independently as progress is achieved. With good leadership and full collaboration between the parents and the treatment team, approaches of this kind can be both holistic and multimodal and may be reasonably effective. Nevertheless, the ultimate prognosis for a psychotic child must always remain guarded.

SUGGESTIONS FOR FURTHER READING

BENDER, L. 1970. The life course of schizophrenic children. *Biol. Psychiat.* 2:165–172.
A thirty-three-year follow-up study of 100 individuals showing one-third able to make a social adjustment. Favorable and unfavorable influences are discussed.

CAMPBELL, M. 1976. Pharmacotherapy. In *Autism: A reappraisal of concepts and treatment,* ed. M. Rutter and E. Schopler, pp. 337–355. New York: Plenum Press.
A thorough, well-referenced review of the psychopharmacological treatment of psychotic children.

CREAK, M. 1961. The schizophrenic syndrome in childhood: Progress report (April 1961) of a working party. *Br. Med. J.* 2:889–890.
A brief communication in which nine diagnostic criteria for childhood psychosis are offered.

FISH, B. 1977. Neurobiologic antecedents of schizophrenia in children. *Arch. Gen. Psychiat.* 34:1297–1313.
Findings show that pandevelopmental retardation is significantly related to the severity of later psychiatric and cognitive disorders and provides a "marker" in infancy for the inherited neurointegrative defect in schizophrenia.

——— AND RITVO, E. R. 1979. Psychoses in childhood. In *Basic handbook of child psychiatry,* vol. II, ed. J. D. Noshpitz, pp. 249–304. New York: Basic Books.
A general review of psychoses in childhood. Focuses primarily on children with psychosis in which there is no definite evidence of a specific organic brain syndrome.

HANSON, D. R., AND GOTTESMAN, I. I. 1976. The genetics, if any, of infantile autism and childhood schizophrenia. *J. Aut. & Child Schiz.* 6(3):209–234.
A critical examination of the data for and against genetic factors in early infantile autism and childhood schizophrenia.

HAVELKOVA, M. 1968. Follow-up study of 71 children diagnosed as psychotic in preschool age. *Am. J. Orthopsychiat.* 38:846–857.
Ultimate intellectual deficit in psychotic children is only partially prevented by treatment. In less severe cases, the clinical form of the psychosis changes on a maturational basis irrespective of therapeutic procedures.

KANNER, L., 1944 "Early Infantile Autism," *J. Pediatrics* 25: 211–217
The original description of early infantile autism as a clinical syndrome.

KNOBLOCH, H. AND PASAMANICK, B., 1975. "Some Etiologic and Prognostic Factors in Early Infantile Autism and Psychosis," *Pediatrics* 55: 182–191.
Describes a group of autistic children examine in infancy and the early preschool period and considers the relationship of 'autism' and 'infantile psychosis' to parental complications and associated disorders. Feelings are compared with those of two studies of older children.

KOLVIN, I., et al. 1971. Studies in the childhood psychoses, I–VI. *British J. Psychiat.* 118:381–419.
Six studies by a prominent British researcher dealing with (1) diagnostic criteria and classification; (2) phenomenology; (3) family and social background; (4) parental personality and attitude; (5) cerebral dysfunction; and (6) cognitive factors in childhood psychosis.

MILLER, R. 1975. Childhood schizophrenia: A review of selected literature. In *Annual Progress in Child Psychiatry and Child Development,* ed. S. Chess and A. Thomas, pp. 357–401. New York: Brunner/Mazel.
Though somewhat dated, this remains an excellent clear review of the literature on childhood psychosis up to the time of publication. The review is organized around

concepts central to an understanding of childhood psychosis, focusing on a number of key questions that remain unresolved today.

ORNITZ, E. M., AND RITVO, E. R. 1976. The syndrome of autism: A critical review. *Am. J. Psychiat.* 133(6):609–621.

The clinical factors and behavioral characteristics of autism and its medical management and treatment are reviewed.

RUTTER, M.; GREENFIELD, D.; AND LOCKYER, L., 1967. A five to fifteen year follow-up study of infantile psychosis: II: Social and behavioural outcome. *Br. J. Psychiat.* 113:1183–1199.

Reports a five- to fifteen-year follow-up study of sixty-three children with infantile psychosis and sixty-three control children attending the same clinic and closely matched for age, sex, and IQ.

RUTTER, M., et al. 1976. Isle of Wight studies, 1964–1974. *Psychol. Med.* 6(2):313–332.

Summarizes a few of the main findings from the educational and psychiatric studies of schoolchildren on the Isle of Wight. It includes a complete list of books and articles on the subject as well as summaries of major studies then in progress.

16

Rose Geist

Conditions with Physical Presentations and Their Psychosomatic Relationships

Introduction

Emotional states produce physical changes. Anxiety is reflected in heightened blood pressure, pulse rate, sweating, and frequency of urination. Physical illness is often accompanied and complicated by concurrent or consequent emotional problems.

These interrelationships have fascinated practitioners for the last fifty years. Various theories have been propounded—for example, attempts to relate specific personality profiles to specific physical disorders, the general concept of stress and its activation of the autonomic nervous system. Recently attention has been given to the effects of stress on the immune system, particularly the concept of cumulative stress effects. Interestingly, these stress events relate to the onset of even such clearly organic conditions as cancer. Rees in his 1976 address emphasized the interrelationship among stress, distress, and disease.

While this chapter could legitimately cover most of the psychiatric and many of the physical illnesses, it will confine itself to that area where there is general agreement as to concurrent and coequal physical and psychological factors—the psychosomatic and psychophysiologic disorders.

331

Classification

There are three groups of disorders with which children present with what seems at first glance to be a physical complaint. These can be classified as physical disorders, physical symptoms, and physical behaviors.

PHYSICAL DISORDERS

The child with a physical disorder presents with a condition that satisfies these criteria:

(1). There is demonstrated organic pathology or a known pathophysiological process.
(2). There is a clear temporal relationship between psychological stress and the physical condition.

PHYSICAL SYMPTOMS

The child with a somatoform disorder presents with physical symptoms, but:

(1). There is no demonstrable organic pathology or known pathophysiological process.
(2). There is evidence of psychological conflict and stress.

PHYSICAL BEHAVIORS

The child with physical behaviors has no demonstrable organic pathology or known pathophysiological process. The child's behavior, however, has in the past been seen as an expression of psychological conflicts or stress.

Physical behaviors can be further classified into three subgroups:

1. Physical behaviors associated with postulated psychological profiles (e.g., eating disorders: anorexia nervosa and/or bulimia).
2. Physical behaviors in which psychological conflicts and associated psychopathology were once believed to play a primary role. More recently, however, these are increasingly seen as resulting primarily from developmental lags or neurological influences, with psychological factors playing a secondary role in aggravating and perpetuating them, (e.g., enuresis, stuttering, sleepwalking, night terrors).
3. Movement disorders in which psychological factors have been suggested as the cause of the physical behavior (e.g., tic disorders, Gilles de la Tourette's disease). Current thinking holds that these are primarily neurological conditions, although secondary psychological factors may play an important role in perpetuating them and interfering with development and self-esteem.

Those in the latter two groups are discussed in chapter 9, since they are frequently considered as disorders occurring in the course of development.

Physical Disorders

DEFINITION OF PSYCHOLOGICAL FACTORS AFFECTING PHYSICAL
CONDITION (316.0)

> When a population of individuals is exposed to the same environmental pathogens, only some individuals manifest disease. (Ader 1980)

Conditions fall into category 316.0 when we can demonstrate (1) organic pathology or a known pathophysiological process [classified under Axis III], and (2) a temporal relationship between psychologically meaningful stimuli and a physical condition.

Diseases traditionally considered psychosomatic fall into this category. Over the last fifty years, research in psychosomatic medicine has turned away from looking for psychological issues specific to certain psychosomatic diseases. Despite the recent tendency to acknowledge the potential importance of psychological factors in all physical disorders, a number of medical conditions remain that have traditionally been seen as resulting from the interaction of psychological and physiological factors more closely than others. These include bronchial asthma, neurodermatitis, rheumatoid arthritis, inflammatory bowel disease, peptic ulcer, essential hypertension, and hyperthyroidism (Alexander 1962). A great deal of literature, mainly by psychoanalysts, has attempted to correlate specific conflicts with particular diseases. This literature has been widely criticized since conclusions, often broadly generalized, were based on few case studies that lacked control groups and as replication of findings was extremely difficult. Methodological approaches varied, ranging from chart reviews to long and short psychotherapeutic interviews and psychological testing with nonstandardized use of terms such as depression, personality, and stress. Physiological variables were highly speculative, with very little evidence or scientific validation. In spite of these limitations, this early psychosomatic literature made a major contribution in that it focused attention directly on a consideration of psychological variables in physical diseases. Although specificity theories have largely been abandoned, most physicians are very much aware that some physical conditions appear to demonstrate a closer association between psychological factors and physical disease than others. But the concept of a linear cause-and-effect relationship from psychological conflicts to physical disease (e.g., conflict A leads to disease B) has proven unsatisfactory. A systems model—one that considers psychological, social, and physical factors as interacting with each other as part of a system—has proven useful. Depending on the patient, the contribution of each of these components will vary.

PREDISPOSING FACTORS—PSYCHOLOGICAL

Loss

One of the important theoretical models used today has been most clearly described by Engel (1968), who believes that many diseases begin as a response to the real or threatened, assumed or imagined loss of a significant person. This loss creates a sense of extreme insecurity and results in what Engel calls the "Giving up/Given up" state, one of helplessness and hopelessness. He believes that loss resulting in the "Giving up/Given up" complex is associated with disease onset in 70 to 80 percent of all patients, not just those with the classical psychosomatic diseases. Real or threatened, loss has been described as a predisposing event to many diseases including cancer (Bahnson 1969; Leshan 1966), tuberculosis (Day 1951), congestive heart failure (Perlman 1971), juvenile diabetes (Leaverton, et al. 1980; Stein and Charles 1971), and diabetes mellitus (Hinkle 1952). There is so far, however, no proven model of how the physiological changes accompany the psychological state.

Dependency is frequently described in many patients with classical psychosomatic diseases. Not everyone reacts to loss in the same way. Prior life experience as well as personality types will determine the nature of the individual's reaction. Not everyone is immobilized, becoming helpless and hopeless in response to loss. Nevertheless in those cases where these reactions do prevail, Engel suggests that physical disease is likely to occur. Engel's theory seems a reasonable way of understanding a dependent person's reaction to threatened or imagined loss of an important nurturant figure. Moreover in children and adolescents, for whom dependency and the struggles against dependency are such major universal developmental themes, loss—symbolic or real—is especially significant psychologically.

Finally, in considering the role of dependency, the regressive potential of any disease must be taken into account. Disease promotes dependency. It is often difficult to decide whether the dependency conflict is primarily a precursor to or a consequence of the disease process; in fact, it is usually both.

Alexithymia

In 1963, Marty and DeMusan (1963) described a group of patients suffering from psychosomatic diseases for whom verbalizing or imagining feelings was very difficult. They labeled this problem *pensee operatoire*. The term implies a style of cognition in which there is little affect or imagination. These patients thus find it easier to describe physical pain than painful feelings. Sifneos (1973, p. 255) adopted the term *alexithymia* to mean "a relative constriction in emotional functioning, poverty of fantasy life and inability to find the appropriate word to describe their emotions." Translated literally from the Greek, this word means "no words for feelings" (*a*—no; *lexis*—word; *thymos*—emotion).

Alexithymia was considered the result of defects in early personality formation that are neurophysiological, neuroanatomical, and developmentally based and are not explained in terms of psychoanalytic theory. Its proponents believe that the inability to express emotion verbally combined with a diminution of fantasy life predispose to the somatization of emotions. This concept is still controversial and not universally accepted. Alexithymia is difficult to measure, and measuring instruments have varied with researchers. The Beth Israel Hospital psychosomatic questionnaire has been used by some researchers to assess alexithymia, while others have used psychological tests and interviews. Nakagawa and associates. (1979) studied alexithymic features in digestive diseases. A comparative study using interviews and psychological testing was conducted on patients with chronic pancreatitis, peptic ulcer, ulcerative colitis, and irritable colon syndrome. It was found that patients with chronic pancreatitis and ulcerative colitis presented prominent alexithymic features. Taylor, Doody, and Newman (1981) studied alexithymic characteristics in patients with inflammatory bowel disease and psychoneurotic patients, using clinical observations, self-assessment questionnaires, and quantified projective tests. They found that their psychoneurotic patients were more able to verbally express emotions than were their patients with inflammatory bowel disease.

The concept of alexithymia has significance not only for the understanding of patients but for patient management as well. Sifneos (1973, p. 261) suggested that alexithymia patients are poor candidates for psychotherapy. "Their inability to express their emotions verbally and their diminution of fantasy life would jeopardize a form of treatment which would emphasize verbal expression and require the capacity for emotional interaction."

The Psychosomatogenic Family

The family therapy literature, especially the work of Minuchin (1978), broadens the focus beyond the identified patient. Minuchin suggests a consideration of family structure and recurrent transactions as relevant psychosomatic variables. He describes in psychosomatic families the common occurrence of the process of enmeshment, overprotectiveness, rigidity, and lack of conflict resolution that combine to cause a physiologically vulnerable child to decompensate. He feels that psychosomatic medicine has been handicapped by the use of models that focused too narrowly on

335

the individual and did not take sufficiently into account the transactions of ongoing patient-family life. Minuchin claims excellent results, especially with diabetics and some asthmatics, with the use of family therapy to address the possible psychosomatic family unit. He does not attempt to "cure" the disease with family therapy but rather to influence perpetuating familial factors and to alter positively ongoing management.

PREDISPOSING FACTORS—PHYSIOLOGICAL

A person may be physiologically predisposed to a particular disease process. Predispositions include the consideration of genetic, psychoendocrine, autonomic, physiological, biochemical, immune, and latent virus factors.

In considering inherited physiological factors, the difficulty lies in determining what is genetically inherited and what is environmentally determined in any familial disorder. Many chronic diseases run in families. Monozygotic and dyzygotic twin studies have attempted to sort out purely genetic from environmental influences.

Psychosomatic research has concentrated heavily on the autonomic nervous system and on consideration of the neuroendocrine processes. Ader and Friedman (1965) suggest that the immune system may be a potential mediator of psychosomatic phenomena. Immune mechanisms, active in many of the chronic diseases, are especially evident in the classical psychosomatic diseases, including bronchial asthma, inflammatory bowel disease, and rheumatoid arthritis. Although it is not a universally accepted premise that the nervous and the immune systems are directly related, there is some evidence to support this view. Sklar and Anisman (1980) have shown that the capacity to cope with environmental circumstances can influence tumor growth and mortality in rats. Immunological reactivity has been observed among bereaved subjects (Bartrop et al. 1977). Pierpaoli (1981) and Murphy and Brown (1980) have data that describe the parallel development of neuroendocrine and immune functions.

PERPETUATING FACTORS—PSYCHOLOGICAL

As was stated in the introduction, most diseases, especially serious chronic illnesses, have psychosomatic relationships, in that both psychological and physiological factors will be operative at various points throughout their course. The psychological responses and contributions to chronic physical disease will be discussed in chapter 21. The precise nature of this contribution in an individual case will be determined by multiple factors including the child's age, premorbid personality, family system, and the nature of the disease itself. It should be noted, however, that not all chronically ill children develop emotional disturbances.

Pless and Roghmann (1971) found that while chronically ill children demonstrated more emotional and behavioral disturbance than did healthy children, only 30 percent of the chronically ill children that he studied developed secondary emotional maladjustments. He felt that the assessment of family functioning and family structure was crucial in identifying those children who were at risk. Hamilton (1979), studying children with inflammatory bowel disease, found that the adaptive potential of both the children and the family was readily apparent. Those families who maintained a supportive relationship with the child without promoting extreme dependency coped best. The same families continually sought information and kept the communication lines open between themselves, their physician, and their child.

Often patients and families, anxious about the disease, tend to deny, resist, or misinterpret information. This can be avoided if the doctor repeatedly reviews the family's understanding of the disease, taking special note of how the information is understood.

We may conclude that the development of a chronic disease may increase the vulnerability to psychosocial difficulties. It does not, however, automatically result in psychosocial maladjustment, as is often assumed. Some suggestions for preventive measures have been mentioned. More research in this area is indicated.

PERPETUATING FACTORS—PHYSIOLOGICAL

Sometimes drugs that are medically indicated have both direct and indirect psychological effects. The *steroids,* drugs commonly used in the management of many chronic illnesses, have many troublesome side effects. For the child or adolescent, they can cause hirsutism, acne, and a moon face that can be particularly hard on the child's self-image and self-esteem. This can perpetuate increasing isolation and social withdrawal from peers. Moreover, acute psychotic reactions that have been described as dose-related occur in patients receiving greater than 40 milligrams of prednisone per day. Falk (1981) states that at 40 milligrams or less per day, the incidence of psychosis is less than 1 percent. The psychiatric reactions are usually manic in type, although depression and a full-blown organic psychotic picture have also been described. Psychoses can occur in patients with no prior history of psychiatric illness, although some investigators believe there may be increased sensitivity to mood-altering effects in patients with affective disorder. This has not been clearly supported in the literature. Early symptoms include frontal paresthesias (feeling of heaviness, fullness, or fuzziness), moderate insomnia, and restlessness. Although the onset of psychosis may begin the first week of treatment, more commonly it occurs in the second and third weeks. These patients can be managed by close clinical observation for early signs of psychosis, followed by the use of phenothiazines, if necessary. Most physicians are aware of the potential difficulties of the management of psychotic patients on steroids. They may be much less aware of what, in the long run, can prove to be the even more deleterious effects on self-esteem that result when hirsutism, moon facies, and acne that occur as side effects of treatment are poorly managed or ignored.

PHYSICAL DISEASE

Although many chronic diseases may be understood in terms of their psychosomatic relationships, this chapter will use inflammatory bowel disease, bronchial asthma, and obesity as examples.

Inflammatory Bowel Disease

The term inflammatory bowel disease describes two conditions of unknown etiology—ulcerative colitis and Crohn's disease. In both of these, especially in ulcerative colitis, psychosomatic relationships have been studied for years. These diseases have strong familial associations. They may begin at any age, including infancy and middle age, but their incidence rises in adolescence. Both are characterized by bloody diarrhea, pain, fever, and variable degrees of delayed growth. Although similar, they do represent pathological and clinical patterns distinguishable from each other. Extraintestinal problems are multiple and may involve the eyes, mouth, liver, spine, and large joints. Diagnosis is often delayed for weeks and sometimes months from the onset of symptoms. The diagnosis is made on the basis of the symptoms and signs of significant intestinal illness, a definite intestinal lesion shown on barium contrast examination, and the findings on sigmoidoscopy and biopsy. Other possible causes of inflammatory bowel reaction must be excluded. Medical management consists of attention paid to the nutritional status of the patient. No specific diet is recommended, but it is important to maintain the nutritional status despite patients' difficulties with the disease itself. Sulfasalazine (2–4 gm daily) and corticosteroids orally (sometimes in doses more than 40 mg per day) or parenterally have been used. More recently, antimetabolites such as azothioprine have been tried. When surgery is required, it is a radical procedure, and the care of the ileostomy or colostomy may present an additional physical and psychological burden.

The pathogenesis of inflammatory bowel disease remains a mystery. Investigators have considered microbiological, viral, toxic, and immune mechanisms. Psychological studies addressing potential etiology have been done mainly on ulcerative colitis patients, but the findings have been generally extended to apply to those with Crohn's disease as well.

Psychological studies of children with inflammatory bowel disease have demonstrated serious difficulties in their relationships to their mothers (Arajarvi, Pentti, and Aukee 1961, 1962; Sperling 1949, 1960). The children have been described as unusually passive and compliant, with an intense desire to be taken care of by the mother (dependent). Since psychological studies are often done after disease onset, it is difficult to determine whether the features described result primarily from the disease or from premorbid characteristics that "predispose" to the illness. These children have also been described as having difficulty expressing their feelings verbally. Conflicts over aggression have been particularly noted. Although many of these children have been described as having obsessive personality types, many other personality styles have also been described (Weiner 1977).

> Fred was a fifteen-year-old adopted boy with ulcerative colitis. He had been hospitalized many times since the age of eight and maintained episodically on high doses of steroids. Recently he had been moody and withdrawn and his condition particularly difficult to manage.
>
> Fred was adopted at seven weeks by parents with severe marital difficulties. He was a very isolated child, distant from his younger adopted sister and fearful of his father, but he had a close special relationship with his mother. Even before his colitis he was sickly and weaker than other children. He remained aloof, spending hours in his room reading science fiction and fantasizing ideal worlds. His best friend, he said, was his mother, who tried to protect him "from his disease, the world, and his father."
>
> During assessment, Fred appeared very withdrawn and depressed. He had the severe acne typical of a steroid user and displayed feelings of hopelessness about his disease. It was clear that these feelings extended to the rest of his life. He was extremely angry with both parents, but all such feelings were highly controlled. He was more interested in and able to focus on his physical symptoms than on feelings about other aspects of his life.

In approaching this case, the focus is not on understanding which psychosocial factors specifically caused the symptoms but rather on appreciating the situation of the child in whom the disease occurs in the context of his family. An adopted boy entering adolescence, he may have been predisposed organically to develop the disease. The adolescent issues of separation, identity formation, and the development of peer relationships confronted a child who had long felt isolated and inferior. These feelings may have been accentuated by his physical appearance, which was affected by the disease and its treatment. The patient dealt with his conflicts by developing a dependent and protected relationship with his mother. His parents had marital difficulties, and the mother encouraged a dependent stance in her son even before he developed colitis. Normal adolescent conflicts with parents were colored by his feelings of being adopted as well as by his feelings of exaggerated dependency. He withdrew increasingly from involvement with peers into his world of science fiction, in which characters were super strong. He thus developed feelings of hopelessness and helplessness when faced with the adolescent conflicts around giving up dependency en route to autonomy. He focused these feelings on the disease, remaining unaware of their psychological origins. He then presented to his medical doctor as much sicker than he should have been for psychological reasons that needed to be recognized and addressed.

Carol was a thirteen-year-old living with both parents and a younger brother. She had been diagnosed as having ulcerative colitis eight months previously. Her mother was very concerned at the change in her daughter from being an extremely eager and independent child to one who was lethargic, withdrawn from family and friends, uncharacteristically dependent, and demanding of special attention. Usually a top student, Carol had been unable to attend school for the last four months because of her symptoms.

Carol's mother had been abandoned by her own mother in infancy and raised by her grandmother. She experienced difficulties in marriage and had sought psychiatric help. During treatment she became aware of conflicted feelings over her own dependency wishes and their expression in her relationship to her husband. She had been pleased by her own daughter's independence and was all the more upset by Carol's present behavior.

Carol was an ill-looking girl who related in a mature manner. She denied any depression or concern about her disease, clearly enjoying the status it brought her. She did not miss her school or her friends and said that she liked the new-found closeness with her mother.

Carol's mother took great pride in seeing her daughter as an independent child. She had great difficulty tolerating, let alone responding to, her daughter's dependent needs and tended to minimize them. Carol's frustration in response to her unmet dependency needs was expressed via her physical illness. Her mother's own conflicts over dependency were reactivated and causing problems in the management of her daughter's disease. Carol was encouraged to return to school as soon as possible. The family was referred for family therapy, with the hope of pinpointing and resolving some of the major interpersonal conflicts.

Bronchial Asthma

Bronchial asthma is a term that applies to a heterogeneous disease characterized by reversible airway obstruction. Clinically it presents as wheezing or dry cough. Extremely common in childhood, it has a strong familial component. The exact cause of asthma is unknown, although in childhood it is usually associated with IgE (Reaginic–Antibody)—mediated immune response. The term extrinsic asthma is applied to those patients in whom an allergic component has been identified. In childhood, asthma has been associated with a higher than usual incidence of childhood infections and is thought to be more common in children of families where one or both parents smoke. The child develops hypersensitive airways. An acute attack can be precipitated by emotional factors as well as exposure to allergens, sudden stretching of the bronchial tree, and so forth. The diagnosis is made on history with supporting evidence provided by a positive family history and pulmonary function tests, which may be abnormal even in a symptom-free period.

Medical treatment involves the use of inhaled Beta 2 specific-sympathomimetic bronchial dilators (e.g., salbutamol [Ventolin]) but disodium chromoglycate (i.e., Intal) can be a useful adjunct, especially when there is a large exercise-induced component. Steroids are used only when necessary; in general, they are to be avoided when possible because of the well-documented deleterious side effects on children.

Asthma is a disease in which psychological factors play a prominent role. Many studies have addressed the psychological characteristics of asthmatic patients, describing their conflict over dependency (Weiner 1977). This conflict is expressed as a wish to be protected and enveloped by the mother. Knapp (1960) has observed that asthmatic children have difficulty in expressing their emotions verbally. No unique personality type has been described, but a fear of separation from mother or of the loss of maternal approval is often described as precipitating an asthmatic attack in children. Many authors have noted that a variety of aroused emotions, both pleasant and unpleasant, correlate with the onset of the asthmatic attack (Rees 1956; Weiner 1977).

> Jonathan was a ten-year-old boy, adopted at age four weeks, who had suffered from severe eczema and asthma from infancy. His mother had adopted her children after fifteen years of marriage and was extremely unsure and anxious in her mothering. Jonathan presented as an isolated and angry child, in constant conflict with his mother. Her attempts to discipline him often led to serious asthma attacks. Jonathan had developed an attachment to the hospital and would deliberately not take his medication in order to precipitate a hospital admission, after which his symptoms would clear within twenty-four-hours.

This patient had an extremely conflicted relationship with his mother. Her doubts and insecurity about her mothering ability were aggravated by her son's asthma attacks when she tried to discipline him. Her conflicts were clearly reflected in her hostile and distant relationship with her son. She avoided contact with him except for disciplinary purposes. He, in turn, began to use his asthma as a weapon against her.

Obesity

Obesity is a physical condition characterized by excessive fatty subcutaneous tissue. The judgment is usually made visually, however; people are obese if they look obese. Clinically a patient is considered obese when the weight/age or weight/height ratio exceeds two standard deviations from the mean.

In North America, the prevalence of obesity has been given as 5 to 13 percent of preschool children, 10 percent of school-age children, 9.5 percent of adolescent males and 12.9 percent of adolescent females (LeBel and Zucherman 1981). Medical conditions occasionally causing obesity include endocrinological disorders (Cushing's syndrome, hypothyroidism), rare syndromes (Willi Prader syndrome), and brain lesions, among others. Most obesity has a multifactional etiology, with environmental, psychological, social, and genetic factors contributing.

One of the most important predisposing factors in childhood obesity is the presence of one or two obese parents. If one parent is obese, the risk of an obese child is estimated at 40 to 50 percent (LeBel and Zucherman 1981). The risk increases if both parents are obese. Both genetic and environmental factors have been hypothesized to explain this correlation.

Psychological factors may contribute to the etiology of obesity or may result as a consequence of it. Although there is no distinct conflict or personality associated with obesity, some people use food to alleviate psychological tensions including depression, anger, loneliness, or anxiety. There have been psychological explanations of why food reduces tension for these individuals (Bruch 1973). More recently it has also been suggested that some of the relief is related to an increase in the central levels of serotonin secondary to a high carbohydrate load that may then lead to a change in mood (Wurtman and Fernstrom 1976).

Regardless of the diverse potential causes of obesity, once established, three factors almost universally apply.

1. Obese people suffer major personal and social consequences secondary to their obesity and invariably wish to lose weight. They are also at risk medically of hypertension, diabetes mellitus, and metabolic abnormalities.
2. Obesity is extremely difficult to treat, medically and psychotherapeutically. The best approach is a preventive one.
3. Obesity is particularly painful for children and adolescents. Peer relationships and body image are invariably affected by the obesity. Moreover, obese children often mature sexually earlier than the norm, and the struggles with body change and body image become particularly intense and complicated.

MANAGEMENT

1. The obese child requires a complete medical and psychological evaluation.
2. The family should be evaluated with special attention paid to the role of food in alleviating psychological tension in all family members. It is important to examine the mother-child relationship and to understand the mother's use of food in her relation to her child.
3. The physical activity of the child should be increased.
4. The goal for children should be the maintenance of weight rather than weight loss.
5. Many overweight adults are involved successfully in group weight reduction programs that use behavior modification principles. Group programs of this type are not generally available for children. However, this approach, quite successful for adults, should be considered for children.

Ten-year-old Sally lived with two obese parents and an eleven-year-old normal-weight sister. Both parents had become increasingly obese as adults. Presently in the midst of separation, they had had marital difficulties since Sally was a baby.

Sally had always been overweight. Extremely passive and compliant, she would become angry or assertive only when her parents tried to control her food intake. Unlike her independent and aggressive sister, Sally did not express any feelings of pain or anger about the deteriorating marriage. In the last six months she had gained an excessive amount of weight while continuing to deny the impending separation.

Both parents were concerned about Sally's obesity. An extended family assessment revealed the parents' use of food to mitigate depression and anger. As Sally became more verbal and more aware of her rage, she realized that she too used food to reduce anxiety, but she did not lose weight nor did either of the parents. It was suggested that once the parents separated, Sally might be more able to control her eating but that the impact of having obese role models for so many years might make the treatment of her obesity more difficult (Guggenheim and Uzogara 1981).

Physical Symptoms

CLASSIFICATION OF SOMATOFORM DISORDERS IN DSM–III

Somatoform disorders include somatization disorders (300.81), conversion disorder (300.11), psychogenic pain disorder (307.80), hypochondriasis (300.70), and atypical somatoform disorder (300.71).

DEFINITION

In somatoform disorders a physical symptom is the somatic experience and expression of a difficult psychosocial event. The patient's difficulty lies both in experience and communication; that is, the patient presents with a physical symptom, unaware that the symptom is related to psychosocial phenomena. However, there may be evident psychological distress in the form of anxiety or depression, or a temporal association between a perceived difficult psychosocial event and the physical symptom. In addition, there is primary or secondary gain (i.e., advantage) from the symptoms. The physical symptoms suggest a physical disorder, but there are no organic findings or known pathophysiological mechanisms to explain the symptoms.

In childhood the physical experience and expression of emotion is particularly intense. Parents, in their daily interaction with their children, connect for them the physiological and the psychological experiences of emotion. They verbalize that the child is angry when she has temper tantrums, or that he is sad when he cries. Ultimately children learn to identify and to verbalize to themselves and to others the psychological experience of their emotion. This is a major developmental task. Unless it is successfully achieved, the child may be left to experience only the somatic component of emotional responses, remaining unaware of the psychological components. This phenomenon, termed alexithymia when studied retrospectively in children who have developed psychosomatic disorders, raises

343

the question of whether the child with a somatoform disorder is vulnerable to the later development of a psychosomatic disease. At any rate, the child or adolescent with a somatoform disorder appears unaware of psychosocial tensions and experiences and expresses feelings primarily via physical symptoms.

Somatoform disorders must be distinguished from malingering, which, despite common belief, is rarely seen in pure culture in children. Malingering children are aware of using a physical symptom to avoid an unpleasant situation. They are often evasive in describing their symptoms as they do not wish to be "found out."

ASSESSMENT

Communication

It is important to ascertain how a child communicates feelings. Children who have difficulty recognizing and communicating feelings verbally may resort to somatic expressions of emotion. The way feelings are typically expressed in the family is also important. Is the child identifying with or modeling himself on others in the family who somatize their anxieties? Is verbal communication spontaneous and easy, or are important and affectively loaded areas avoided or communicated nonverbally?

The Family

The child must be understood in the context of the family system. (See chapter 3.) Is the child responding to family problems or tensions by physical symptoms? Is there an "unspeakable" family problem?

Psychosocial Stressors

Any recent stresses affecting either the child or the family should be identified. Are difficulties at school causing tension that the child is experiencing as a somatic complaint? Any family stress may also be expressed by the child via somatic symptoms.

The Child

In performing a complete assessment of the child, the focus should be not just on potential conflicts and actual stressful events but also on the symbolic meaning and stress associated with these experiences.

Some children may have genetic predispositions to anxiety and its physical expression. Based on studies of animals, physiological studies, and clinical work, Slater and Shields (1969) have suggested that some patients are genetically predisposed to anxiety. Such children may show more intense physiological responses and therefore be more aware of the somatic experience of their anxiety. The genetic predisposition would be activated in a response to psychosocial stresses.

CLINICAL SYNDROMES

Somatization Disorder (300.81)

Lipowski (1968, p. 413) defined somatization as a "tendency to experience, conceptualize and/or communicate psychological states or content as bodily sensations, functional changes or somatic metaphors." Somatization disorders usually involve multiple organ systems and may include symptoms that are pseudoneurological (paralysis, blindness), gastrointestinal (abdominal pain), psychosexual, cardiopulmontary, or involving the female reproductive system (severe dysmenorrhea), or pain. Somatization disorders are usually first diagnosed in adolescent females and rarely in males. The diagnosis may not be made, however, until symptoms have been present for several years.

> Marie was a sixteen-year-old living with her mother, stepfather, and eight siblings. She was under medical investigation of a two-year history of anorexia and diffuse abdominal pain, as well as headaches, insomnia, leg and lower back pain. Marie presented as a withdrawn girl with psychomotor retardation. She appeared clinically depressed but denied feelings of depression or any difficulties at home or school, focusing entirely on her somatic complaints. There was no history of a preoccupation with food, but she had been a very dependent child. Menarche coincided with the onset of symptoms, and she became even more clinging and afraid to be left alone, staying home continually. Extensive hospital investigation showed no evidence of organic pathology.

The patient was diagnosed as having a somatization disorder. She presented as a dependent adolescent whose symptoms began at puberty. Adolescent conflicts involving autonomy and separation were reflected in her increasing clinging to her mother and avoidance of school. She appeared clinically depressed but was subjectively unaware of her depression. She focused on her physical symptoms as a defense against dealing with psychological conflicts.

Conversion Disorder (300.11)

A conversion disorder occurs when there is a loss or alteration in physical functioning suggesting a physical condition. The psychological factors involved in conversion disorder are discussed further in chapter 12. It may be difficult to distinguish conversion symptoms from an organic illness (Lazarre 1981). It is not unusual for a patient whose initial diagnosis is conversion disorder to have that changed to an organic illness as the condition is better understood. Also, a significant number of patients have organic illness in combination with conversion disorders. Studies that have addressed misdiagnosed conversion reactions are discussed by Lazarre (1981). Positive psychological criteria that support a diagnosis of conversion reaction include:

1. The concomitant presence of a somatization disorder.
2. The presence of associated psychopathology, including depression, schizophrenia, or personality disorder.
3. The presence of a psychological conflict, symbolically expressed in the patient's symptoms.
4. The temporal relation of a psychological stress to the conversion disorders.
5. Primary or secondary gain as a result of the symptom.
6. The absence of organic pathology.

Conversion disorders usually begin in adolescence. The need for caution in the use of this diagnosis is illustrated by the following case.

> Sean was a ten-year-old boy who, for two weeks, had been vomiting every morning at breakfast. He was a sickly child with numerous somatic complaints that were often diagnosed as psychogenic in origin. His parents were in the process of separating, and just before the onset of the vomiting, Sean had accidentally found his father having sex with another woman. His mother arranged a psychiatric assessment, convinced his symptoms were psychogenic.
>
> Sean appeared extremely depressed and tearful. He was relatively nonverbal and uncooperative. His play was characterized by depressive content and themes of loss of parental figures.

This child presented as a depressed boy with a past history of somatization. There was a clear psychosocial stress in the separation of his parents. Although the vomiting superficially suggested a conversion disorder, further investigation revealed the presence of a brain tumor. This case emphasizes the importance of a complete medical assessment in combination with a psychological assessment before a diagnosis of conversion disorder is made.

Psychogenic Pain Disorder (307.80)

DSM-III describes psychogenic pain disorder as pain occurring as a predominant complaint in the absence of adequate physical findings or known pathophysiological mechanisms but in the presence of psychological factors that appear etiologically involved.

Abdominal pain is extremely common in childhood. Yet organic disease is found in less than 10 percent of all children investigated for recurrent abdominal pain (Apley 1976). Psychogenic abdominal pain can begin at any age but is more common in preadolescence and early adolescence. The pain is usually vague and variable in location. Apley (1976, p. 185) suggests the rule of thumb that "the further the pain is from the center, the more likely it is to be organic." There is often, but not always, an absence of associated symptoms such as vomiting or nausea. Many children who present with psychogenic abdominal pain have families with a high incidence of family pathology, in which one or both parents also suffer from recurring pain, usually abdominal. Apley found that the earlier the symptoms were treated, the better the prognosis.

> Risa was an eleven-year-old admitted to the hospital for the investigation of diffuse abdominal pain of five years' duration. The pain had increased in the last six months. After extensive investigation, no organic pathology was found.
>
> During her psychiatric assessment Risa appeared as an irritable, egocentric girl. She was an emotionally labile child who argued continually with all members of her family. Attacks of pain would generally end these arguments, with either parent or the older sister attending to her pain. Both mother and sister reported that they had abdominal pain when upset.

In addition to her diffuse abdominal pain and other complaints of long duration, Risa was an emotionally labile, egocentric girl who had difficulty handling aggression. Extremely insecure, she needed continued reassurance from others. Her abdominal pain, which usually occurred in the company of others, enabled her to interrupt conflict situations and to gain support from and control the environment.

Hypochondriasis (300.71)

Hypochondriasis occurs when an individual is preoccupied with physical sensations and in continual fear of having a serious disease or diseases. Sometimes a physical disease may be present, but the patient's reaction exaggerates its extent, limitations, and disability. The fear of serious disease despite medical assurance may lead to impairment in social or occupational functioning. Hypochondriasis usually begins in adolescence, although it may occur in the third or fourth decade. The patient often attempts to use the symptoms to control others. Such patients may resist attempts at psychiatric intervention, often responding to the suggestion by changing doctors.

> Nancy was a sixteen-year-old girl referred for psychiatric assessment by her family doctor. For years she had complained of numerous physical problems. A simple cold was enough to take her to bed for weeks, and dysmenorrhea accompanying her period would keep her home for a week each month. Nancy expressed her resentment of the referral by being extremely uncooperative. She refused to give a personal or social history, insisting she only had physical problems. Information obtained from her family doctor described Nancy as extremely hostile in her interpersonal relationships. A poor student at school, she had few friends. There was gross family pathology and the patient had a very difficult relationship with her alcoholic mother.

This patient presents with a picture of typical hypochondriasis. Psychological problems were extremely difficult to address, as she was highly focused on her physical experiences. She resisted further psychological intervention and eventually changed her family doctor.

Atypical Somatoform Disorder (300.70)

The diagnosis of atypical somatoform disorder is reserved for atypical symptoms for which no organic cause or pathophysiological mechanism is found.

Mrs. L, nineteen and recently married, was referred for psychiatric consultation by her plastic surgeon. She complained of a birthmark on her chin that she had begun to feel was disfiguring her face. Objectively, it was almost unnoticeable. She realized that her feelings were unrealistic but found herself avoiding social engagements because of it. Mrs. L had married to escape a difficult and belittling relationship with her parents. She described a troubled sexual relationship with her husband, which she attributed to low self-esteem secondary to the scar. She had wanted plastic surgery but had accepted her surgeon's referral to a psychiatrist.

This patient's low self-esteem was clearly developmentally determined. Her inability to face her conflicts directly was reflected in her unconscious use of the scar on her face to avoid dealing with her feelings about herself and her relationship with her husband.

MANAGEMENT

Patients with somatoform disorders are often extremely unpleasant and hostile in their relationships with their physicians. Demanding and difficult, they can put great pressure on their doctor to "do something," becoming angry and attacking if they sense that their doctor does not believe how intensely they are suffering. There can be a challenging quality to their "You don't believe me" that all too often provokes harassed doctors to respond in one of two equally unfortunate ways. Some become angry or rejecting, at times rationalizing this with some statement such as "There's not a thing wrong with you! Your problem is just tension (or nerves). You need to see a psychiatrist!" This usually succeeds only in making the patient feel misunderstood and belittled and in undermining the relationship with the physician. The other equally unproductive response to the hypochondriac's demands and accusations is to overinvestigate, overprescribe, overdiagnose, and overconsult in an attempt to appease the patient, even though the doctor is convinced that hypochondriasis is the problem. By taking this tack, the physician reinforces the patient's conviction that there is indeed a mysterious organic problem that has so far eluded identification. In such cases, an iatrogenic component often begins to play an increasingly prominent role in perpetuating the hypochondriasis. This is particularly likely since such patients invariably pick up subverbally the doctor's ambivalence to them and feel patronized rather than cared for.

A more useful approach is for the physician to acknowledge to the patient that he or she recognizes that the patient's symptoms are real and distressing but that at times real physical symptoms can be precipitated by emotional tension and distress. The physician should point out that stress affects different people in different ways: some feel nervous and upset, others have trouble sleeping or lose interest in food; some respond by drinking excessively; while still others develop physical symptoms in response to pressure. Often an example of other patients who, while under extreme psychosocial pressure, developed physical symptoms may help patients accept in general terms the concept of physical symptoms resulting from stress, even when defensiveness still makes them deny that their symptoms are in any way stress-related. Such general examples can, at times, help patients feel sufficiently understood and believed to free them to join the doctor in a search for possible sources of tension and for alternative ways of dealing with it.

SUGGESTIONS FOR FURTHER READING

ADER, R. 1980. Psychoimmunology. *Psychosom. Med.* 42(3):307–321.
   Discusses the need to consider the immune system in its relationship to the central nervous system. Makes an excellent case for the possible mediation by the CNS of the immune system.

FALK, W. E. 1981. Steroid psychosis: Diagnosis and treatment. In Psychiatric medicine up-date: *Massachusetts General Hospital Reviews for Physicians,* ed. T. C. Manschreck, pp. 147–154. New York: Elsevier.
   Presents a clear and practical approach to the consideration of potential psychological effects of steroids, a difficult problem that may often confront physicians dealing with chronic physical disease.

HUNTER, R.C.A. 1979. Psychoanalysis, somatization and psychosomatic disease. *Can. J. Psychiat.* 242:383–390.
   Discusses the concept of somatization and reviews and discusses the psychoanalytic theories of the somatization process.

LESSER, I. M. 1981. A review of the alexithymia concept. *Psychosom. Med.* 43:531–545.
   Comprehensively reviews the concept of alexithymia in terms of its historical background, clinical presentation, measurement, etiology, and treatment considerations.

LAZARRE, A. 1981. Current concepts in psychiatry: Conversion symptoms. *N. E. J. Med.* 305 (13):745–748.
   An excellent article that highlights the interrelationships of conversion symptoms and organic disease.

SIFNEOS, P. 1973. The prevalence of alexithymia: Characteristics in psychosomatic patients. *Psychotherap. & Psychosom.* 22:255–262.
   Provides a clear description of alexithymia and includes a sample of the psychosomatic questionnaire often used to assess alexithymic characteristics.

WEINER, J. 1977. *Psychobiology and human disease.* New York: Elsevier.
   Outstanding, comprehensive review of all the psychological and physiological literature on the subject of peptic ulcer, essential hypertension, bronchial asthma, Graves disease, rheumatoid arthritis, and ulcerative colitis. The review is thorough and critical and also suggests areas of potential psychosomatic research.

17 *Arlette Lefebvre and William Hawke*

Learning Disorders in Children and Adolescents

The term learning disorder refers to a child's failure to meet society's expectations of academic achievement. This chapter will present current knowledge and speculation about the prevalence, diagnostic features, etiology, and remediation of learning disorders.

Prior to the 1960s, school underachievers were usually considered either slow learners or simply lazy. But over the past twenty years, despite repeated multidisciplinary investigations, considerable confusion and contention remain regarding learning disorders in general and specific learning disabilities in particular. Few authors agree on the definition of learning disorders, and there is even less agreement about their etiology and treatment. Learning disorders currently account for one-third of all referrals to mental health and pediatric developmental clinics.

Definition of Terms

Children are referred for investigation of a learning problem because a teacher, a parent, or, occasionally, a physician thinks they are "underachieving" in school. This can be concluded by comparing the child's work with that of classmates (e.g., by using report cards) or with the average level expected for the grade (e.g., by using achievement tests). But children identified in this way may or may not be truly underachieving. It is only when each child's achievement is compared with a reliable estimate of his or her potential that true underachievement can be established.

The suspected underachiever, then, is referred for answers to the following questions: (1) Is the child really capable of a higher level of achievement? (2) Is the child in the right class for one of similar general potential? (3) If the answer to both of these questions is yes, why then is the child underachieving, and what can be done to help?

In this chapter, the following definitions will be used.

- *Learning Disorder* (or learning problem). Children have a learning disorder if their academic performance and/or classroom behavior cause concern to the parents, the teacher, or the child.
- *Underachievement.* Students are underachieving if their academic performance falls short of their potential.
- *Learning Disability.* If underachievement persists and the child's performance falls two grades below the average expected level for his or her age and grade in one or more subjects, that child is described as learning disabled.
- *Specific Learning Disability.* If a child's learning disability is confined to circumscribed areas of academic functioning (e.g., reading, math, printing), the child is said to have a specific learning disability (SLD).

Prevalence of Learning Disorders and Disabilities

PROBLEMS IN ESTIMATING TRUE PREVALENCE

There is a tremendous variation, ranging from 1 to 40 percent, in quoted prevalence figures (Gottlieb, Zinkus, and Bradford 1979). There are a number of reasons for this.

First, there is a lack of standard universally accepted definitions. Some studies define learning disability broadly as any discrepancy between potential and performance, such as problems in oral or written expression (Schere et al. 1980). Others define it much more narrowly. Whereas the broad definition includes all except underachievement due to mental subnormality, the latter one restricts the field by focusing just on one particular type of specific learning disability.

Others (Blakely 1969; *Journal of Abnormal Child Psychology* 1980) argue that "learning disabled" has become a meaningless term conveniently used by school administrators to segregate a variety of poor learners into "special" classes. Those who believe this consider prevalence statistics highly artificial figures that describe a heterogeneous group of children with many different problems who just happen to be in special classes within a particular year. As knowledge and diagnostic skills improve, theoretically, at least, it becomes increasingly possible to place children with a variety of learning problems and specific learning disabilities into remedial programs or classes tailored to their individual needs.

A second reason for the tremendous variation in prevalence figures is the different methods used to reach a diagnosis. A wide range of procedures and tests can help determine the proportion of schoolchildren with learning disabilities. One study (Adelman 1978) found that half the learning disabled identified in one prevalence estimate were diagnosed only by clinical observation and that one-third were so labeled in spite of contradictory evidence.

A third reason for the variation is the fact that different populations have been studied (Meier 1976). Some investigators examine a cross-section of children identified as having academic problems enrolled in all public schools during a specified time. In such studies, average socioeconomic status of the district studied has been shown to be a critical factor (Rutter 1975). Others record the number of children referred to special education services, the frequency of learning disorders or specific learning disability in children referred to psychological or psychiatric services, or the frequency of learning disabilities in a known delinquent population.

Other environmental and ecological factors play a part in the variation found in prevalence rates (Meier 1976). The diagnosis of learning disabilities requires that a variety of specialists be available to identify and treat specific learning problems. In school districts in which remedial educational resources are made available, referrals to "special" classes increase, and so the prevalence rate for that board rises dramatically.

PREVALENCE FIGURES

American studies (Barrows et al. 1977; Gottlieb, Zinkus, and Bradford 1979; Myklebust and Boshes 1969; Suran and Rizzo 1979) report that 20 to 25 percent of all school-age children show academic underachievement at some time. There are an estimated 8 million learning disabled children in the United States today (Kinsbourne and Caplan 1979). Ten to 15 percent of children have learning disabilities severe enough to make them fall two grades behind in at least one subject (Hallahan and Kauffman 1976; Kinsbourne and Caplan 1979; Suran and Rizzo 1979). However, only 1 to 3 percent of the school population are enrolled in special education classes (Hallahan and Kauffman 1976).

Canadian studies are fewer in number than American ones and are based on smaller numbers of subjects. *Statistics Canada* quotes an unpublished figure of 5 to 7 percent of all school-age children with learning disabilities, with 1 to 3 percent requiring special education.

Regarding the male/female ratio, boys with mild learning disorders outnumber girls four to one, and the ratio approaches eight to one in severe disorders. The male prevalence is even more pronounced—ten to one (Gottlieb, Zinkus, and Bradford 1979; Graham and Sheinker 1980)—in specific reading and spelling disabilities, while girls outnumber boys in mathematical disabilities. As the cultural bias that places a greater value on achievement for boys than for girls diminishes (Rutter 1974), it becomes hard to assess the validity of these sex-ratio figures.

Diagnoses Commonly Associated with Learning Disorder

Learning disorders are more common in two groups of children:

1.) Those with a diagnosis of *hyperactivity or attention deficit disorder*. Fifty-three percent of hyperactive children are reported underachievers. Different authors suggest that from 4 percent to 42.6 percent of children with an ADD meet the criteria of specific learning disability (Kinsbourne and Caplan 1979; Millichap 1977).
2.) *Juvenile delinquents*. At least one-third of all delinquents of average intelligence satisfy the strictest criteria of learning disability (Kinsbourne and Caplan 1979). This figure rises to 70 to 90 percent if one includes delinquents of below-average intelligence who show any type of learning disorder, including unexplained school dropout.

Classification of Learning Disorders

Unlike a visible symptom, learning is an internal psychological process that cannot be observed directly but can only be inferred after it has taken place. Although the nature of the process is not fully understood, the circumstances necessary for learning to occur can be described. There must be: (1) the opportunity to acquire knowledge; (2) the ability, capacity, and emotional maturity to understand what is being taught; and (3) the wish to acquire a new skill or information.

A number of factors can interfere with one or more of these prerequisites.

GENERAL INTELLECTUAL DEFICITS

The child of borderline or below-average intelligence usually does poorly in all academic subjects and is frequently described by teachers as socially and emotionally immature.

Although moderate or severe mental retardation is usually identified prior to or during kindergarten at the latest, the borderline or mildly retarded child may reach first or second grade and fail before retardation is suspected and tested for. This is especially true since most of the work in these grades is achieved via rote memory. The child who is well behaved, eager to please, and trying hard to keep up with the work can utilize rote memory to compensate for mild intellectual defects until the work becomes more difficult at and after the third-grade level. Such children may, in fact, overachieve, that is, perform up to 10 or 15 percent beyond their expected performance level by compensating for a lower intellectual ability through application, organization, and motivation.

Other mildly retarded children soon realize that the tasks of a regular classroom are beyond them and become so frustrated, restless, and unmotivated that they cannot achieve even at their expected performance level. Some even stop trying to read or write, although they are capable of learning such basic skills in a special class tailored to their needs. Some of these children remain in regular classrooms throughout primary school, especially if they also have a minor physical handicap on which their low performance can be blamed. Sooner or later, especially at the secondary school level, their ability to cope with such stress becomes too much for them, and a vocational school placement is necessary. (See chapter 18.)

PHYSICAL IMPAIRMENTS

Developmental Immaturity or Delay

The child may be among the youngest and least mature in the class, especially if born just before the deadline for acceptance in a particular grade. For example, in Ontario the child who turns six in December of a given year enters first grade and is expected to compete against many six-and-one-half or almost seven-year-olds born in January, February, or March of the same year.

Other children, though of average age for their class, are developmentally immature and temporarily underachieve because they have not yet caught up with their peers in motor coordination, language skills, or social competence.

Physical Handicaps

Sensory deficits may cause a number of problems. A mild or moderate hearing loss may affect speech development and reading skills and may contribute to an aggressive behavior problem before being diagnosed and treated. Similarly, visual impairment can affect a child's spatial orientation, motor coordination, and ability to discriminate between letters and words.

Chronic illness or major handicap can be at the root of many learning problems. The frequently hospitalized child, especially if repeated outpatient tests, physiotherapy, or treatments are required, may miss a great deal of school as well as lacking the stamina and self-esteem required for active concentration on learning. (See chapters 21 and 22.)

The child with a less noticeable *nutritional deficit* or *sleep disorder* may be weak, drowsy, and confused for part or most of the school day. In particular, sleep apnea, a newly recognized condition that sometimes presents with nightly snoring and daytime hypersomnolence as its only symptoms, can impair intellectual functioning and short-term memory in both adults and children and can indirectly cause learning problems, depression, and even psychosis (Martin and Lefebvre 1981).

Disease of the central nervous system, with or without an associated intellectual impairment—for instance, a previously undetected mild cerebral palsy—may undermine a child's coordination, writing, and elocution skills, while remaining unnoticed except by a neurologist. (See chapter 11.)

The child with an *attention deficit disorder* will have learning problems. (See chapter 10.) The distractible, impulsive, and/or hyperactive child may underachieve because of an inability to sit still or concentrate long enough to learn or to finish the work. Such children may also have specific learning disabilities.

EMOTIONAL FACTORS THAT INTERFERE WITH LEARNING

Emotional problems can either cause or contribute to and perpetuate learning problems. This section will deal only with the primary emotional factors involved in learning problems (Rutter 1974, 1975). The secondary factors will be covered after the clinical picture of the learning disabled child has been discussed, since they result from the learning disabilities.

Temperament

The restless, "difficult to handle" child often has difficulty concentrating, especially when expected to regulate his or her own behavior and work pace (e.g., in an open-concept classroom). A self-motivated, creative, persistent child may excel in the same situation. Conversely, the shy, sensitive, "slow to warm up" child may do poorly in an overly structured, highly competitive environment in which praise and encouragement have to be earned with confident, aggressive achievement excellence.

Anxiety

A little anxiety stimulates learning and achievement, but too much for any reason can be paralyzing. In addition to general sources of anxiety (e.g., a recent move, a marital separation), some children show specific anxiety due to fear of failure. Examples include the child afraid to disappoint the parents with a poor report card; the child whom the teacher, school, or classroom competition have made anticipate failure and rejection; the child reluctant to speak up and answer questions because to do so draws attention to a physical defect or handicap.

355

Whether generalized or specific, excessive anxiety monopolizes the child's energy and attention, decreases concentration, and interferes with short-term memory and organizational skills.

Depression

Academic underachievement is a common symptom of depression in children and adolescence. It is described in more detail in chapter 14.

Avoidance of Learning

From hostility, defiance, and a wish to assert their independence, adolescents may rebel against adult values by skipping school or adopting an "I don't care" attitude about school achievement. This primary refusal to learn may be difficult to differentiate from hostility secondary to repeated failures and an underlying learning disability. In many adolescents who are rebelling against school, a thorough investigation reveals undiagnosed learning disabilities.

Psychotic Disorganization

Relatively few psychotic children are initially referred for assessment because of a sudden drop in academic achievement. Unfortunately, some drift and eventually drop out of the school system before being recognized as seriously disturbed. (See chapter 15.)

Lack of Motivation

Lack of motivation is the most intangible and hardest to define of all the emotional factors contributing to learning disorders, perhaps because it is so hard to prove and so intertwined with the child's family and social context. Interest and wish to succeed are important variables in school learning (Rutter 1974). They are increased by identification with the teacher or the wish to please an encouraging parent. But some children lack or, more commonly, lose interest in schoolwork despite the best of family and classroom conditions. We know little about why this sudden drop in motivation occurs, or how to prevent or deal with it, as there has been little systematic investigation in this area. It is not clear whether there is a critical period during which motivation to learn must be acquired, or whether motivation needs periodic "booster shots" of school success, community and family support, or varied stimulation.

SOCIAL FACTORS ASSOCIATED WITH UNDERACHIEVEMENT

Not all first-grade children of similar intelligence have an equal opportunity to learn what they are being taught in the classroom. Learning starts in the home well before school entry. Children's behavior patterns (e.g., the ability to sit still and concentrate on a task, attitudes toward authorities such as parents and teachers, social skills, self-esteem and familiarity with learning tools and materials [books, art supplies, vocabulary, etc.]) are crucial determinants of future learning (Abrams 1976).

Teachers' evaluations of children's social competence in first grade are an even more important predictor of academic success in later years than intellectual ability as measured by IQ scores.

Social Deprivation—Too Little Stimulation

A significant number of disadvantaged (i.e., lower socioeconomic class) children do not learn at the same rate as upper- and middle-class children (Rutter 1974, 1975). This was once attributed to a generally lower intellectual potential due to genetically inherited subnormality. However, recent studies indicate that such children may have normal intelligence levels through the preschool years but show a gradual drop in the early school years particularly in the verbal areas but also, at times, associated with weaknesses in auditory memory and visual motor skills (Tarnopol 1977). This may be accounted for by:

1. Lack of intellectual stimulation during preschool years (e.g., fewer books and nursery school experiences, multiple day-care experiences of variable quality).
2. Lack of parental time, energy, and interest in motivating children to learn, because of preoccupation with multiple family problems.
3. Large family size (Rutter 1975), resulting in less time available for individual child-adult contacts.
4. High mobility of families and teachers.
5. Lack of behavioral controls within the family (e.g., lack of consistent discipline to promote self-discipline, frustration tolerance, persistence at a task, pride in learning achievements).
6. Action-oriented problem-solving attitudes (punching instead of talking problems out) that do not fit teacher expectations and therefore lead to reprimands, resentment, and decreased motivation.
7. Programs directed toward the stimulation of the child alone are less beneficial than dual programs that involve both the child, and the family such as Project Headstart.

Cultural Differences

The child raised with a different language who comes from a differing cultural background until kindergarten or first grade is at an obvious disadvantage in competing with English-speaking peers. Those who speak with an accent, wear different clothes or eat different lunches, have a socially isolated mother or father who cannot communicate well with the teacher or other parents may feel different, unworthy, and misunderstood in the school milieu. Similar feelings are typical of the child who feels victimized, with or without parental support, because of belonging to a racial or religious minority.

The adolescent who has grown up in a small town and is suddenly transplanted into a big, cosmopolitan high school may suffer from a more subtle culture shock. However, as it occurs at a particularly vulnerable time of life, it can seriously undermine self-confidence.

357

Overstimulation or Excessive Expectations

The average child of bright, upwardly mobile parents and siblings may be placed in an enriched, highly academic program. Expected to read and write in at least two languages as well as cope with swimming, skating, ballet, music lessons, Brownies, and so forth, such children may not be able to compete with very bright classmates or siblings, or may do so only at the cost of a tremendous expenditure of energy and effort. These children are not underachievers; they are normal children who simply cannot meet the inflated expectations of their families. Such unrealistic pressures usually produce an increasing dislike of school, resentment of parental or school pressures, and loss of self-esteem.

Specific Learning Disabilities

Specific learning disabilities are usually defined as circumscribed areas of academic deficit in spite of at least average intelligence and in the absence of physical disorder, primary emotional or social factors, or cultural differences sufficient to explain the failure to learn. They can, however, occur in children at all levels of ability; an obvious example is the child with a mental age of four years whose language skills are barely at the one-year level because of a specific disability of language development. The DSM-III includes these disabilities under developmental disorders, implying a physical etiology and eventual recovery. However, the authors feel that they deserve separate consideration because their etiology and prognosis remain controversial. A minority of these children appear to have a lag in the development of those skills needed for learning. After several years in school, they begin to learn at a normal or near-normal rate. In the majority, however, evidence of the specific learning disability persists throughout life.

DEVELOPMENTAL READING DISORDER (315.00)

The developmental reading disorder, still frequently referred to as dyslexia, is the most common learning disability. It is defined by DSM-III as:

> Performance on standardized, individually administered test of reading skill is significantly below the expected level, given the individual's schooling, chronological age and mental age (as determined by individually administered I.Q. test). In addition, in school, the child's performance on tasks requiring reading skills is significantly below his or her intellectual capacity. (American Psychiatric Association 1980, p. 94.)

DEVELOPMENTAL ARITHMETIC DISORDER (315.10)

The developmental arithmetic disorder has the same definition as the developmental reading disorder, substituting the word arithmetic for reading.

MIXED SPECIFIC DEVELOPMENTAL DISORDER (315.50)

The mixed specific developmental disorder category should be used when there is more than one specific developmental disorder (reading, arithmetic, language articulation), but none is predominant.

ATYPICAL SPECIFIC DEVELOPMENTAL DISORDER (315.90)

Atypical specific developmental disorder is a residual category used for other specific learning disabilities not covered by the previous three categories. An example would be the child with dyspraxia, that is, poor fine motor control.

Description of Clinical Syndromes

GENERAL COMMENTS

There is no typical clinical picture of a learning disorder. The learning problem may be the presenting complaint or may be associated with any number of behavioral or emotional symptoms for which clinical intervention is sought. Children with learning problems may be referred initially because of aggressive behavior; distractibility or lack of motivation in the classroom; anxiety, moodiness, or school phobia; nightmares, enuresis, tics, or migraine, to name just a few of the most common symptoms. The underachievement may last a month, a year, or a lifetime. If it persists and becomes a learning disability, it may be severely incapacitating or may be missed completely, depending on its severity and on the expectations of the child's parents and teachers.

Primary underachievement, present from the time of the first report card, commonly results from general or specific intellectual deficits or chronic social deprivation. Secondary underachievement, which follows a sustained period of average or above-average performance, is generally, though not always, reactive to life stresses or emotional factors. Exceptions to this rule exist, such as specific disabilities that may only become apparent when the subject matter becomes more complicated in second or third grade or basic emotional conflicts that interfere with learning from the start.

COMMON FEATURES OF CHILDREN WITH SIGNIFICANT, PERSISTENT
LEARNING DISABILITY OF ANY TYPE

By the time a learning disability is diagnosed, the child has usually suffered a crucial blow to self-esteem and social competence, even if a grade has not yet been repeated. Gottlieb, Zinkus, and Bradford (1979) describe the typical defensive behaviors used by such children during a clinical assessment to cover up or postpone an expected failure on tests.

1. Anticipating failure, they frequently avoid answering by "I can't" or "I don't know." Such replies are more typical of fear of failure than of deliberate defiance.
2. If they do attempt a task, they become frustrated and angry easily with their shortcomings, real or imagined. This can be mistaken for defiance or destructiveness but is usually the behavior of children with high expectations who are upset by what to them is one more bit of evidence of their own inadequacy.
3. The child may try to avoid the test by asking to go to the washroom, complaining of fatigue or headaches caused by the length of the interview.
4. Alternately, some children hide behind a facade of not caring about school performance or parental disappointment. They insist that they just don't like school and that nothing or no one can hurt their feelings. This type of denial is often the hardest to overcome. The rare child who truly does not care about adults' opinions is usually either too depressed and hopeless to show enthusiasm about any subject (see chapter 14) or, alternatively, refuses to believe any adult could be genuinely concerned and therefore protects and distances himself with a wall of silence or lies (e.g., some antisocial adolescents). Psychotic children are usually erratic or evasive, not only on the topic of school performance or during tests but in their general conversation, thought content, and mood swings (see chapter 15).

The majority of learning disabled children are very aware of their problems. If undiagnosed and untreated, on school days, at least, they live in a constant state of anxiety, frustration, and fear. Perhaps the major reason that early diagnosis and effective intervention are so crucial is to avoid these feelings.

Clinical Features of Specific Learning Disabilities

TYPES OF LEARNING DISABILITIES

Specific learning disabilities are circumscribed learning and behavioral deviations severe enough to require special teaching procedures (Epstein 1980). While their origin has not been established, clinical experience suggests that in many or most cases the basic problem appears to be a deficit in either long-term or short-term memory, auditory or visual. The inability to remember the sound or shape of the letters appears as a problem in perception, and hence for some time these children were considered perceptually handicapped. The three most commonly described kinds of specific learning disabilities are reading and spelling difficulties, difficulties in mathematics, and fine motor disabilities.

Reading and Spelling Difficulties

The typical history (Rutter 1974) of a child with reading and spelling difficulties is that of a boy who first shows a delay in learning to speak (either as a late talker or later due to poorly articulated speech) and then has great difficulty learning to read, along with severe, persistent spelling difficulties. Often some other family member has similar difficulties, and the child may have a history of poorly defined ambidexterity early during development. A number of these children show associated difficulties in the following areas of function.

1. Expressive language.
   a. Persistent language problems, for example, faulty pronunciation (Chess and Hassibi 1978; Critchley 1968) of vowels, such as "big" for "bag" and of consonants, such as "sad" for "sat."
   b. Primitive syntax, for example, confusion of Mr., Mrs., he, she; of present and past tenses (Critchley 1968).
2. Receptive language.
   a. Inability to discriminate between the auditory properties of letters or words (Chess and Hassibi 1978), such as "bat" and "but" that leads to confusion of words with minor differences, like "quiet" and "quite."
   b. Reversal of letters or entire words, such as reading "big" for "dig," or "saw" for "was."
2. Verbal coding and sequencing. The child has trouble remembering categories of concepts or words (e.g., months or seasons) and particular difficulty keeping straight the order of items in a given category (e.g., the days of the week, numbers, months of the year).
3. Right and left confusion. How this relates to learning disorders has always been a point of contention. If children with mixed dominance are examined, a significant number with academic problems may not be found. If, on the other hand, a specific type of disability is examined in the child with problems due to an inadequate long-term visual sequential memory for letters, almost invariably a history of ambilaterality and poor fine motor control is found in the child or in the family background (Rutter 1975).

There are two clinically different types of reading and spelling disabilities. One, involving audiovocal (spoken) language, usually develops during the preschool years. The other, more evident in visuomotor (written) language, is acquired later, during the fourth, fifth, and sixth years.
Audiovocal Deficits The child with an audiovocal deficit usually has a history of delayed speech development, poor articulation, and deficient vocabulary. Difficulties in understanding and retaining verbal instructions are less

obvious and may be mistaken for disobedience or distractibility. These children usually do poorly in verbal subtests of the Wechsler Intelligence Scale for Children (WISC). They have great difficulty learning to read phonetically, since they cannot remember a sequence of letter sounds long enough to blend them into a word.

The result is a more profound deficit than a visuomotor one. Remediation is generally less effective in overcoming audiovocal deficits. As a result, because of the inability to utilize phonics, the inability to read persists through the child's educational career, and special programs may be required throughout high school. Added to the obvious reading and spelling problems, these children usually have great difficulty organizing their thoughts sequentially, so that projects, essays, and written assignments present major problems. Even if they are allowed to type essays or to be examined orally, these children have difficulty presenting an organized approach.

Visuomotor Deficits. Children with visuomotor deficits usually develop speech normally but have a strong individual or family history of ambixterity or left-handedness, and in most cases one parent, usually the father, has had life-long problems in spelling. In kindergarten or first grade, the children can usually match letters but have trouble naming them and learning the sound associated with each. They cannot recognize even simple words either by sight or, initially, through phonics. With application, however, most do eventually learn to read phonetically. In later years many can read, often with great skill, although slowly and phonetically, so that their persistent reading disability is often overlooked.

Spelling remains a problem; except for very familiar words, children with visuomotor deficits spell phonetically and thus have great difficulty spelling words that are structurally nonphonic. This seems a fairly specific deficit in sequential long-term visual memory for shapes. Since many of these children have excellent long-term visual memory for past events, many parents have trouble believing that a disability in long-term memory exists. These children have a better prognosis than those with an audiovocal deficit and generally do well with treatment. Well-motivated and intelligent visuomotor-handicapped children often progress to high school, while the occasional one, with understanding and support, may even complete college.

Although their verbal scores on the WISC, which tests immediate visual memory and, to a much lesser extent, long-term visual memory, are usually average, in general their performance scores are lower, although occasionally exceptions occur.

A simple and practical way to assess long-term visual sequential memory is to have a child prepare for a spelling test and then, four or five days later and without warning, repeat the same test. Children with problems will show a markedly decreased ability to remember the shape of words and to spell them correctly.

Difficulties in Mathematics

Difficulties in mathematics are more common in girls. They occur less frequently than reading and spelling difficulties, which are more common in boys. Whether or not cultural expectations contribute to this sex-related prevalence remains unproven, although an adequate family history of mathematical difficulties in other female relatives is frequently obtained. Recently it has been suggested, though not proven, that sex-related differences in right- versus left-brain hemisphere development (*Journal of Abnormal Child Psychology* 1980) contribute to girls having more weaknesses in spatial orientation.

Some mathematical deficits can be partially compensated for in early grades and become apparent only at the secondary school level when the child faces the more involved challenges of geometry and calculus. On the WISC these children typically have fairly good verbal scores but do poorly in the performance area. They often have demonstrable deficits in spatial localization, right/left discrimination, short-term auditory memory, and digit retention.

Problems in Printing and Writing

Often termed dyspraxia, poor fine-motor control leading to problems in printing and writing is presumed due to poor organization of activity at the level of the cerebral cortex, though a cortical lesion can rarely be demonstrated. Most children with this disability are ambidextrous, often with a family history of left-handedness or ambilaterality. Rather than having clearly defined dominance with good fine-motor skills, these children have only relative dominance of one hand, which therefore lacks the fine-motor control of a truly dominant hand.

In the classroom these children, even when highly motivated, are slow and sloppy in their written work, appearing at their worst on written examinations. Teachers often interpret the messiness or failure to complete assignments as evidence of lack of care or effort. Drawings, maps, and graphs are usually sloppy, poorly centered on the page, and difficult to recognize.

Cognitive Impairments Associated with Specific Learning Disabilities

MEMORY IMPAIRMENTS

There are three types of *memory impairments:* (1) decreased visual memory: short term or long term; (2) decreased auditory memory: short term or long term; and (3) both.

Children with specific learning disabilities may be less able to rehearse newly acquired knowledge (Bauer 1979) and associate it with previous experience (Swanson 1979). This may interfere with either short- or long-term memory.

ATTENTIONAL DEFICITS

Attentional deficits include distractibility (Myklebust and Boshes 1969) or difficulty in differentiating (Koppitz 1977) and paying attention to the relevant aspects of a situation (Adelman 1978), although some hyperactive children who appear to have a short attention span have a surprising ability to retain most of what has been discussed.

There are two factors in attention. One is quantitative, that is, how hard a person concentrates on a stimulus (e.g., the way one listens to background music as compared to a concert). The other is qualitative, that is, the ability to focus selectively on certain aspects of a stimulus (e.g., the melody or words of a song). Children with specific learning disabilities may have trouble in both these areas.

MOTOR IMPERSISTENCE AND WEAK INTERSENSORY INTEGRATION

Due to motor impersistence and weak intersensory integration, it is hard for some children to repeat with the hand and pencil a pattern registered with the eye. Others have trouble coordinating what they see with what they hear, for example, sounding out a word they see on the chalkboard (Rutter 1974).

MOTOR IMPULSIVITY

Children with motor impulsivity are unable to take their time in order to print (or whatever task they set out to do) carefully, and thus their work is careless and sloppy (Epstein 1980).

DECREASED CREATIVE THINKING

Some children exhibit decreased creative thinking—they are less able to generate new ideas and change their approach to problems (Graham and Sheinker 1980).

IMPAIRED ABSTRACT REASONING

Due to their inability to comprehend abstract concepts, some children have trouble following class discussions. They get lost and frustrated unless they constantly have a concrete example (e.g., a picture; a specific concept) to relate to (Richman and Lindgren 1980).

DIFFICULTY INTERPRETING SOCIAL CUES

Children who have difficulty interpreting social cues, both verbal and nonverbal, ramble on inappropriately, oblivious to the boredom and annoyance they evoke in others and unable to utilize the responses of others to modify their own behavior. The resulting insensitivity, which may directly contribute to the frequency of emotional and social problems in these children, is often a secondary emotional reaction rather than part of the basic disability, except in those children whose disability is caused by organic brain damage (Bryan 1978; Bryan and Bryan 1977; Ozer 1980). The loss of self-esteem that complicates their learning problems (Chapman and Boersma 1979; Epstein 1980; Foley 1979) further undermines their self-confidence, especially in social situations.

Secondary Emotional and Social Problems Associated with Specific Learning Disabilities

PROBLEMS

Repeated failure and frustration lead to anger, hopelessness, and sadness in the child. These feelings, in turn, may contribute to school refusal, truancy, and destructiveness in the classroom, or avoidance and battling at home when it is time to do homework.

Parents' and teachers' initial failure to recognize the child's limitations and their criticism or pressure to "try harder" often cause resentment and mistrust of adults, along with defiant behavior (talking back, clowning, disrupting the classroom, making fun of the teacher). Peers' lack of respect for children with learning disabilities further undermines their self-esteem, contributing to a sense of alienation and often causing fights that invite further labels (e.g., "aggressive" and "belligerent"). Eventually some such children identify with antisocial peers in order to get some support and restore their prestige in the schoolyard.

PROBLEMS

The parents' negative, rejecting attitude is often blamed for having caused their child's learning problems. In fact, this negativism and rejection are often the response to unrecognized learning disabilities. When the parents' universal wish for a well-adjusted, successful child is threatened by poor report cards or teachers' complaints, parents usually proceed through certain stages in coming to grips with the reality of the child's handicap.

1. Initial denial of the problem. "He's just so stubborn," or "She'll grow out of it."
2. Anger at the school or teacher who first identified the child's learning problem. Some parents defend by blaming the school system (e.g., the teacher's personality or methods, the child's classmates) to which they can attribute the problem. The danger at this stage is that parents may merely change schools rather than look into the problem carefully, thus postponing diagnosis and remediation.
3. Anger at the child for not trying harder. It is easy to confuse the child's unhappiness or resentment about school assignments with intentional laziness or forgetfulness. Such misinterpretation only increases the child's resentment toward parents and teachers.
4. When the severity of the underachievement can no longer be denied, and especially when a handicap is detected during psychological testing, common family reactions include anger at the professional who confronts them with the potential permanence of the child's limitations, (e.g., "How can she be so sure in half an hour?"), followed by anger at those (family doctor, pediatrician, first teachers, etc.) who did not diagnose the problem earlier. This anger is symptomatic of guilt the parents feel for having passed on a learning disability or for not having recognized and dealt with the problem and the child's limitations differently. While a second professional opinion can be beneficial at this stage, the danger is that parents, still rejecting the diagnosis, may shop around endlessly for other opinions, indefinitely postponing treatment. Alternately, they may look for instant remedies or "cures," such as a pill or dietary solution that will rapidly eliminate the problem and allow the child to learn in a regular classroom. Whether or not such measures may temporarily improve the child's attention span and decrease impulsivity, they alone cannot overcome cognitive deficits or restore damaged self-esteem and social isolation. When at last they realize that the hoped-for panacea does not exist, the parents may return to whoever made the diagnosis to seek direction on how to help the child with both academic and social problems.

Associations of Specific Learning Disability with Hyperactivity and Juvenile Delinquency

SPECIFIC LEARNING DISABILITIES AND HYPERACTIVITY

Kinsbourne estimates that over 50 percent of hyperactive children are underachievers and that up to 42.6 percent also have specific learning disabilities (*Journal of Abnormal Child Psychology* 1980). However, many hyperactive children are not learning disabled, and some with learning disabilities are not hyperactive, so that the relationship between the two conditions is not clear. The restless, hyperactive child who disrupts the classroom attracts more attention than the quiet underachiever and is therefore more likely to be tested and diagnosed than the latter.

LEARNING DISABILITIES AND DELINQUENCY

Repeated studies on the personality profile and school histories of delinquents have shown a strong association between learning disability and delinquency (Ross 1976). The finding that a vast majority (90 percent) of delinquents have a history of academic failure and/or school dropout (Compton 1974*a, b;* Poremba 1974, 1975) has been used as evidence of "learning disability." When the current learning status of incarcerated youth is studied, the figures drop to between 50 percent (Henderson 1968; Jacobson 1974) and 70 percent (Berman 1974 *a, b, c*). A further breakdown (Kinsbourne and Caplan 1979; Stenger 1975) reveals that one-third are poor achievers because of low-average or below-average overall IQ, and an additional one-third have specific learning disabilities as suggested by a discrepancy of 15 points between verbal and performance IQ and specific underachievement in reading or mathematics. Reading failure associated with weak symbolic sequencing and defective sensory motor integration are particularly common (Hurwitz et al. 1972) and, in one study (Hogenson 1974), correlated highly with aggression in delinquent boys. Adolescents referred because of delinquency or conduct disorders frequently reveal unsuspected and untreated learning disabilities, often in marked contrast with their more successful siblings whose greater effectiveness and acceptability to the parents is a common source of resentment.

Several authors (Jacobson 1974 *a,b*; Matthews, n.d.; Poremba 1974, 1975) have used these figures to suggest a causal relationship between specific learning disability and juvenile delinquency. Poremba describes a vicious cycle of early school failure leading to frustration, acting-out, and truancy that intensify the child's sense of failure, lower the self-image, and promote a sense of alienation, predisposing to an early dropout by overwhelming the youngster with a sense of defeat and hopelessness. This, however, is an oversimplification; the fact that delinquency and learning disabilities are associated does not prove that either causes the other. (See chapter 13.) Learning disabilities or even general underachievement are not the only predictors of delinquency (Elliott 1974). Not all children with learning disabilities become delinquents (e.g., Winston Churchill), and not all delinquents are learning disabled (Mauser 1974 *a, b*).

These studies linking learning disability and delinquency are significant in that they point out the vital importance of early identification of learning disabilities and conduct disorder in order to interrupt the learning disability/juvenile delinquency cycle (Berman 1974*c*). Schools and communities should be alerted to the potential significance of a sudden drop in achievement and the onset of truancy by the sixth grade. Every effort should be made to prevent truancy or dropout through active intervention of a guidance counselor (Matthews, n.d.), social worker, or, if necessary, the courts. Probation officers should be alerted to the special problems faced by delinquents with learning disabilities so that they can appreciate the desirability of motivating the individual delinquent toward regular school attendance and remedial education wherever possible (Love and Bachara 1975; Mulligan 1969, 1972, 1974).

Diagnostic Assessment of the Child with a Learning Disorder

A multidisciplinary assessment is often essential to a full understanding of learning disabilities (Koppitz 1977; Muir 1975). The team may include: teacher; family physician; pediatrician; neurologist; psychologist; speech therapist; occupational therapist; psychiatrist; special education consultant; as well as the parents, siblings, and child.

A guide to taking a psychiatric history has been outlined in chapter 7. In taking the history of a child with a learning disorder, particular attention should be paid to the developmental history of the child; the child's attitude to school, schoolwork, and the teacher; the attitude of the parents to the child and his or her work and to the school. Two particular areas to be explored are those of the child's handedness (i.e., right, left, or ambilateral) and the presence of similar disabilities (i.e., learning, speech, or handedness) in other family members. In a one-to-one office examination, the child is usually less active and distractible than in the classroom, where there are many more visual and auditory stimuli to compete with the examiner for attention. As a result, in an office examination children often cooperate and perform better and with much less evidence of attentional deficit than is typical of their classroom behavior. An adequate physical examination, including a careful assessment of vision and hearing, a neurological examination and electroencephalogram, and, occasionally, a study to rule out sleep apnea, begin the examination. They are followed by a psychological assessment of the child and family. (See chapter 7.)

A number of simple office tests help assess a child's developmental level and provide a rough screening for possible learning impairments. Table 17.1 lists those tests.

The Fit Between Child and School

Learning difficulties may reflect the child's reaction to an unsatisfactory school placement or teacher or to a poor fit between child and school.

The best way to assess this is to visit the school, meet the teacher, and observe the child in the classroom. At the very least, the professional should attempt to communicate with the teacher or principal by phone to get the clearest possible picture of the child's areas of success and underachievement, the typical classroom behavior, attitude toward peers and teachers, and particular behavioral difficulties. School reports stating that the child shows "aggressive behavior" or "poor attention span" are insufficient; the professional needs to know who starts the fights and how, or what has been tried to increase the attention span and with what results. The teacher's attitude toward the child and the relationship be-

TABLE 17.1

Diagnostic Tests

Test	Information Provided	Norms
1. Draw a person or draw yourself	Handedness, pencil grasp, fine-motor performance, eye-hand coordination. Body image and self-concept: size, expressed mood, activity portrayed, missing body parts. Manner of execution may suggest presence or lack of self-confidence, self-esteem, obsessional defences, organization, and use of space.	*Pencil grasp*: Until age three, pencil may be grasped with the whole fist. By age five, pencil should be held between thumb and fingers (adult tripod grip).
2. Print your name	Confirms the above. Indicates letter reversals and any directional problems.	*Printing name*: Should be possible by the end of kindergarten. *Letter reversals*: Some reversals are normal in child first learning to print. Should end by grade 3. *Mirror-image writing*: May persist to age seven and one-half.
3. Describe a picture	Provides sample of vocabulary, sentence formation, articulation, and general knowledge.	
4. Remember your name and phone number	Tests long-term auditory memory.	The child should know this information by age five.
5. Remember a short list	Tests short-term auditory memory. (The child is given something to memorize and recall after fifteen minutes— e.g., "the name Sally, the color blue, the number 4, etc.")	

TABLE 17.1 *(continued)*

Test	Information Provided	Norms
6. Copy a shape	Tests visual perceptions and hand-eye coordination.	A child should be able to copy: a standard circle by two and one-half years; a cross by three years; a square by four and one-half years; an angle by five to six years; a diamond by seven years.
7. Demonstrate left and right		A child should be able to demonstrate left and right: on self by 6 years; on others by 9 years.
8. Pick up pencil, kick a ball, peek through a hole	Tests laterality. If one hand and the other foot or eye are preferred, the mixed laterality is indicated.	
9. Hop, walk on tiptoes, stand on one foot	May reveal minor degrees of gross motor incoordination.	The child should be able to walk on tiptoes or heels by age five. Eightly percent can balance on one foot for ten seconds by age five, on one foot for twenty seconds by age six. Eighty percent can balance on either foot for thirty seconds by age eight.
10. Imitate rapid hand movements	Tests fine motor coordination. The child is asked to imitate such movements as tapping with each hand in turn, a rapid screwdriver motion, touching finger to nose. Not only the hand that is performing should be observed but also the other limbs for evidence of accessory overflow or parallel movements. When present, these suggest neurological immaturity.	

tween teacher and parents should be assessed; these are important topics almost never recorded in official school reports. It helps to know how early the school expressed its concerns to the parents and with what result. How often have the teacher and parents met, and how have they been able to cooperate in helping the child? Conferences with school personnel are as useful to mental health professionals as they are to those from the school, since the discussion often gives the clinician a more realistic awareness of child and parents than may have been obtained in an office setting.

Psychological Tests

After the history is taken and the child is examined, a psychologist usually administers psychological tests, which are particularly useful in delineating the nature and extent of the learning difficulties.

THE WIDE RANGE ACHIEVEMENT TEST

School achievement is usually surveyed by "achievement tests" such as the Wide Range Achievement Test (WRAT) of Jastek and Jastek, which measures how much a child has learned in various subjects. The WRAT is standardized to compare a given child's score to the average for that child's grade level, so that the child can be described as "below," "above," or "at grade level." The mean is 100 and the standard deviation is 15. Like all tests, achievement tests are subject to various distortions, the most common of which is better performance in a one-to-one testing than in a busy classroom (Ross 1976).

THE WECHSLER INTELLIGENCE SCALE FOR CHILDREN

A child's intellectual potential is usually assessed by measuring that child's performance on a standard test of intelligence, such as the Wechsler Intelligence Scale for Children (WISC). This assumes that the child's test score bears some relationship to his or her actual potential. Although IQ tests are no more than a measure of performance on tasks where prior learning affects how well one does (Ross 1976)—not necessarily the same as native intelligence—IQ scores remain the best predictors of school success (Gold and Berk 1979). Other tests, such as the Wechsler Preschool and Primary Scale of Intelligence, the McCarthy, and the revised Binet are more suitable for children of kindergarten or preschool age.

The WISC is composed of ten sections or subtests plus two supplemental tests. Five of these (the verbal scale) call for verbal responses, while the other five (the performance scale) involve the child doing things manually. The verbal and performance scales are scored separately, then combined to obtain a full-scale IQ score. If the overall score is average but one or more subtests are significantly below average, the results show a "scatter" and a specific learning disability is suspected. However, certain subtests, such as "digit span" (i.e., the number of digits recalled in a sequence) are particularly hard for the anxious or distractible child, who may not perform reliably in any test situation. Only one subtest, "coding," specifically looks at ability to learn new material, and this scale bears less relationship to overall IQ scores than any other subtest (Ross 1976). The Information Subtest is the scale most influenced by cultural factors.

In children with learning disabilities, repeated test scores using the WISC often show a definite but gradual drop, particularly in the verbal areas. Such areas as information, vocabulary, and/or arithmetic are obviously affected in an individual unable to progress at the normal rate, since that person's scores are compared to those of children whose learning has progressed at the expected rate.

THE ILLINOIS TEST OF PSYCHOLINGUISTIC ABILITIES

The Illinois Test of Psycholinguistic Abilities (ITPA) is usually administered by a speech therapist to confirm and complement the assessment of specific cognitive functioning whenever a specific learning disability is strongly suggested by the history, the examination of the child, or by the WRAT and WISC. It often correlates well with the results of intelligence testing.

The ITPA assesses both the spoken (audiovocal) and written (visuomotor) language. It provides quotients comparing functioning in each area to norms for children of the same age. Subtests provide additional information about specific linguistic skills essential to learning, such as the reception of spoken or written language and expressive ability in both the audiovocal and visuomotor areas.

Diagnostic Feedback and Recommendations

After the assessment is complete and a diagnosis has been made (e.g., specific reading disability or underachievement due to hyperactivity), one designated team member must:

1. Explain this diagnosis to the child, family, and teachers.
2. Be specific about what the child can or cannot be expected to do.
3. Find out what remediation techniques are known to the school, suggest the possibility of a special placement if necessary, and arrange to find out how the teaching strategies are working.
4. Supervise medication if necessary.
5. Explore strategies to increase the child's self-esteem, social skills, and motivation to learn.
6. Last, and at least as important, maintain a supportive relationship with the child and parents. The diagnosis should be a first step in treatment rather than a sadly self-fulfilling prophecy.

Etiological Theories About Specific Learning Disabilities

There are numerous unproven opinions and theories about the origin of specific learning disabilities, which fall into three broad categories or schools of thought: psychophysiological theories, psychological information-processing theories, and theories of dyspedagogia (Epstein 1980).

PSYCHOPHYSIOLOGICAL THEORIES

Psychophysiological theories about specific learning disabilities have the longest history, going back to Orton, who in the 1930s spoke of developmental word blindness to describe dyslexia. These theories argue that:

1. There is a frequent association between learning disabilities and pre- or perinatal complications such as toxemia, blood incompatabilities, induced labor, and pre- or postmaturity (Smith and Wilborn 1977).
2. There is often a family history of learning disabilities (Rutter 1974), suggesting a genetic pattern of inheritance.
3. Specific learning disabilities present the same clinical picture as developmental delays, except that they tend to persist throughout the child's and often the adult's life, whereas developmental delays are transient by definition (Rutter 1974).
4. Retrospective studies describe children with specific learning disabilities as having been temperamentally different as infants (Scholom and Schiff 1980), that is: either below or above average in activity level; biologically irregular in their patterns of sleep and wakefulness; less positive or more negative in mood; and less approaching in their attitudes than "average" babies.

Of all these arguments, the first two are the most convincing, though it could be argued that perinatal complications predispose children to a whole gamut of neurological and psychiatric disorders and that not all children with audiovocal learning disorders have parents who were similarly affected. On the other hand, retrospective studies are hard to evaluate since they depend on the recollections of parents whose recall may be biased since they already know their child is "different" (has a learning disability). The similarity between developmental delays and learning disabilities is noteworthy but occurs only occasionally and does not prove a causal link.

There is no doubt that learning takes place in the brain and that a number of children with damaged brains also have trouble learning. But current knowledge does not clarify whether or not specific learning disabilities are due to irreversible minimal brain damage or to temporary dysfunction or delay. The current psychophysiological hypotheses postulate a structurally based dysfunction of the central nervous system, a metabolic abnormality, or a biological hypersensitivity to certain substances.

PSYCHOLOGICAL INFORMATION-PROCESSING THEORIES

Psychological information-processing theories hold that specific learning disabilities are caused by specific intellectual or cognitive weaknesses, without speculating as to their origin. Deficits have been postulated in visual perception and memory, auditory perception and memory, sensory integration, communication, general or particular deficits in psycho-linguistic ability, selective attention, and motor development. However, to state that a child who has difficulty copying a pattern on a marble board or repeating a rhythmic series of taps has a "perceptual-motor" problem, that a child who cannot find pictures hidden in a diffuse background has "poor figure-ground discrimination," or that the child who reads words backward or mirror-writes has a "visual perception difficulty" or "faulty sensory integration" tells us little more than what has already been observed in the classroom (Ross 1976), except that the child has failed at the same tasks in the psychologist's office. However, even if these theories do not explain the etiology, they can help the teacher select an appropriate remedial method.

DYSPEDAGOGIA

Those who believe in dyspedagogia argue that there are no learning disabilities, only teaching disabilities (Ross 1976). A child's failure to learn is seen as just as much the fault of the education system as a problem within the child, either because of inappropriate techniques used by the teacher (e.g., trying to teach a child with a visuomotor deficit by the sight system instead of by phonics) or an unsatisfactory relationship between child and teacher. Many children do well with one teacher but poorly with another, for many reasons including the "fit" between teacher and pupil. Examples include: a gentle teacher who, failing to structure the classroom, has difficulty teaching a child with an attention deficit disorder; a rigid, perfectionistic teacher who demands fine-motor skills of a child who cannot supply them; a power struggle between a determined child and an equally determined teacher; a timid, passive child who needs a warm and supportive teacher but functions less adequately with one who is shrill and demanding.

Dyspedagogia is based not on scientific evidence but rather on the lack of knowledge about what can be done about learning disabilities. Dyspedagogists argue that the type of specific cognitive or metabolic abnormality decided on as a diagnosis does not matter if the label only adds to the child's and parent's sense of irreversibility and hopelessness.

On the other hand, assuming that any child could have a learning problem if placed in the wrong class and that any learning-disabled child can improve in the right environment carries with it the promise of eventual improvement. To the extent that it is realistic, such optimism may be an essential ingredient of treatment.

Treatment

PRIMARY PREVENTION

It is impossible to prevent learning disabilities as long as their etiology remains obscure. However, many of the general prevention principles outlined in chapter 27 have particular application in the field of learning disorders, namely:

1. Reduction of perinatal complications by good prenatal counselling and obstetric care.
2. Provision of high-quality day care and nursery school programs for all children, especially for those of disadvantaged and minority social groups at increased risk of starting school with the disadvantages of intellectual understimulation and emotional immaturity. (See chapter 5.)
3. Education of future parents, especially those who themselves have a history of learning problems, about how to prepare preschoolers for formal education by developing social and self-help skills, attention span, motivation, and pride in accomplishment.
4. The continuing education of teachers, guidance counselors, social workers, and physicians on ways to promote learning by increasing motivation, self-esteem, and social competence. These three areas are particularly important, since children's early ratings of social competence, self-esteem, and classroom behavior are important predictors of future academic performance in particular (Feldhusen 1971) and invulnerability to stress in general.

SECONDARY PREVENTION

Early Identification Programs

The goal of early identification programs is to specify which preschoolers or kindergarten children are vulnerable to learning disorders, in the hope that early intervention can help them catch up with their peers before a cycle of failures leading to discouragement and aversion to school becomes established. These programs are based on the findings that 70 to 90 percent of learning disabilities can be predicted by screening students in kindergarten and first grade (Mercer et al. 1979). Some screening projects such as recent ones in Ontario (Schickler 1981) and Pennsylvania (Reider and Portnoy 1977) attempt to identify children at risk at the even earlier age of three to five (i.e., nursery school or junior kindergarten). However, these programs have the following shortcomings.

1. They focus narrowly on the early identification of specific learning disabilities, while failing to identify other equally vulnerable children such as those who are culturally deprived, overactive or underactive, aggressive, or socially immature.
2. Screening at such an early age invariably yields a higher number of "false positives," that is, children who are simply developmentally immature in one or more psychological functions (e.g., spatial orientation, motor coordination) but socially well adjusted and actively learning. The danger of falsely labeling these children as learning disabled, thereby increasing their parents' anxiety and decreasing their teachers' expectations, is that such labels may become self-fulfilling prophecies.
3. It is a luxury to spend so much professional time exclusively on diagnostic screening programs when there remains a serious shortage of resources and long waiting lists for children already diagnosed as learning disabled. Some argue that the money might be better spent providing more small diagnostic first-grade classes that could thoroughly evaluate children's learning capacities and attitudes as well as provide the first steps of individualized teaching programs.

Educational Remediation

The key to effective remediation is early intervention (Adamson and Adamson 1979). For years, children with learning difficulties were placed in "special classes" with programs that were essentially the same, regardless of the nature and extent of their disabilities (Ozer 1980). These early classes, containing a mixture of slow learners, behavioral problems, and children with specific learning disabilities, proved of doubtful value (Rutter 1974).

Special Education. Some general principles are applicable to the management of all learning disorders (Rutter 1975). The basic goal is that of changing the usual emphasis on failure to an emphasis on success (Stanton 1981). To do this the teacher must appreciate the nature and extent of the child's capacities, weaknesses, or limitations, in order to know what can reasonably be expected. The teacher must gain the child's trust and interest and restore confidence in his or her ability to succeed. How this is done depends largely on the personality and sensitivity of the teacher and on the structure of the academic program designed to ensure early success. For example, the curriculum can be broken down into a series of small steps, both to facilitate learning and to demonstrate to the child that learning is occurring, or progress in concentration as well as in accomplishments could be systematically rewarded (Ross, 1976) in an attempt to lengthen the attention span. There must be good communication between student and teacher on all academic and social aspects of the program in order to integrate affective and cognitive education (Berman 1974: a, b, c). The sensitive, perceptive teacher can help some children learn to make friends without clowning, and teach alternatives to punching when a child is hurt by teasing or criticism. Close cooperation between parents and teacher is essential, both to support the child's involvement in the remedial classroom by offering encouragement and praise for any school progress and to reinforce progress by promoting good work habits and encouraging responsibility and self-discipline at home (Scranton et al. 1978).

If a child is on medication, teachers should meet regularly with the key physician (family practitioner, pediatrician, or psychiatrist) following the child. Teachers are perhaps the most reliable source of information on the child's school behavior and may be best able to judge the effect of medication on concentration and learning. Finally, the special education teachers' experiences with behavior modification principles can help "restructure parental attitudes," that contribute to anxieties about learning and to behavior problems (Kinsbourne and Caplan 1979; Scranton et al. 1978).

Specific Teaching Programs for Children with Specific Learning Disabilities. The ideal academic program is a completely individualized one-to-one program (one teacher, one child) (Rutter 1975). The format varies according to the type and severity of the child's handicap and the school facilities available. Some such children require a full day in a special class. Others may remain with their peer group in the mainstream for some subjects (e.g., gym, music, art) but require "withdrawal help" or "special instruction" in reading or math. Still others can remain entirely in a regular classroom and receive intensive tutoring after school. Because academic segregation can intensify feelings of social isolation and further undermine self-esteem, a happy medium between total segregation and total integration is sought. If a full-day special class is required, the placement should be reevaluated yearly to be sure the child reenters the mainstream when ready to do so.

The Method

Despite a lack of solid evidence about the relative merits of different teaching approaches (*Journal of Abnormal Child Psychology* 1980; Ross 1976; Rutter 1975), it seems unlikely that there is one single "right" approach. Some programs emphasize training activities to strengthen areas of weakness, providing, for example, intensive tutoring in reading until the student catches up to grade level (Ross 1976; Rutter 1974), while others stress the need to avoid areas of weakness and take advantage of the child's strengths (Epstein 1980), by allowing the child to type or tape record essays instead of writing them out, for example. Still others advocate first strengthening the child's preferred sensory pathway, for example, by stressing auditory learning in the child whose disability is primarily a visual one, and then attempting to strengthen the visual pathway by simultaneously presenting a visual stimulus paired with an auditory or tactile one that the child can more easily deal with (e.g., flash cards for reading, Montessori colored blocks for math) (Ross 1976). In all of these approaches, certain "targeting procedures" are used to focus all the child's attention on a stimulus word or number concept and to reward the child for selectively attending to certain aspects of this stimulus. The type of disability as well as the child's age and general ability level must be considered in selecting the appropriate remediation program. The child with an audiovisual deficit can often be encouraged to read through the use of pictures and color-coding, although if the sound becomes associated with the color rather than the shape of the letter, there may be difficulties reading type that is not color-coded. The child with a visuomotor deficit requires a phonetic approach to reading and will have to learn to summarize material and use a typewriter in high school to avoid becoming overwhelmed by details. The impulsive, distractible child may be helped by training in self-command (Bachara and Zaba 1978). For instance, such children can be taught to give themselves verbal instructions such as "Stop, look, and think" before doing anything. Children with poor fine-motor control that causes difficulties in printing or writing may be instructed in the use of a typewriter at an early age, while children with specific mathematical difficulties can often obviate them by the early use of a calculator.

It is not helpful to the impulsive child to be told to "take your time" or "be careful," since such children may never have learned to do this step by step. They may require concrete instructions on how to look for similarities and differences between stimuli, how to eliminate alternative answers until the correct one remains, how to check the result obtained.

For many years remedial education programs were confined to primary schools. Now, however, there is a wider range of secondary schools tailored to the needs of a broad variety of adolescents. These include college preparatory, general, accelerated or enriched programs for adolescents preparing for college; secondary schools where the child is withdrawn from the regular class for periods of individual remediation, for children of normal or near-normal ability; vocational schools for slow learners that provide basic and remedial programs within the intellectual capacity of the slow learner plus an intensive program in industrial arts to introduce the student to a trade that can provide a living in adult life.

Behavior Modification

The basic principle of behavior modification is that by rewarding children immediately by praise or with a token (e.g., star or checkmark) that they can collect and exchange for concrete rewards, the rewarded behavior is encouraged and motivation is increased. Unlike most children who can work independently with only occasional encouragement, many learning-disabled children cannot continue to work without immediate "reinforcers," especially if academic work has provided little gratification in the past.

The basic rules of any behavior modification program are:

1. What kinds of behavior are required in order to earn a token must be explicitly defined (e.g., the number of minutes spent quietly in one's seat, the number of problems correctly solved, etc.).
2. These requirements should be minimal at first to ensure early success and can be gradually increased as children's proficiency increases.

3. Reinforcers (tokens, points, or stars) must be dispensed regularly, consistently, and systematically—for example, at the end of each school day or half day.
4. The ultimate reward, obtainable in exchange for a certain number of tokens can be decided on:
   a. unilaterally by the teacher (e.g., pens, awards)
   b. jointly by the teacher and class (special activity)
   c. together with the family, in the case of an individualized token system for a particular child
5. The program must be continued until the child begins to obtain some intrinsic reward from the satisfaction of doing homework, obtaining good marks, being proud of report cards, being admired by peers, and so forth.

Psychiatric Therapies

See chapter 22 for a discussion of learning problems caused by primary physical handicaps or emotional disturbances.

The learning-disabled child with significant secondary emotional and social problems may need both individual psychotherapy to restore a sense of faith in self and others and to repair damaged self-esteem (Epstein 1980; Rutter 1974; Chapman 1979) and group psychotherapy to provide insight into socially inappropriate responses as well as training in skills required to get along with others and in communication strategies by modeling, coaching, and rehearsal techniques (Duplessis and Lochner 1981; LaGreca and Mesibov 1981).

In addition, the child's parents need access to ongoing supportive counseling offered by someone they trust, someone who can understand their frustration and help them recognize and manage their feelings toward the child's problem, while providing practical suggestions to increase their own sense of competence as well as the child's self-esteem. Gottlieb, Zinkus, and Bradford (1979) emphasize the importance of lowering unrealistic parental expectations and of stressing the learning-disabled child's need for structure and discipline at home as well as in school. At times, family tensions and parents' individual psychopathology or marital problems may require marital or family therapy.

While teachers and school psychologists might be trained in the skills of counseling parents (De Quiros and Schrager 1979), they are often too closely identified with the school system to be accepted by the family as truly objective advisors. Furthermore, due to school changes throughout the school years, the family physician, pediatrician, social worker, or psychiatrist is in a better position to offer the family continuity of care.

Biological Therapies

Medication. It is important to identify that group of attention-disabled children and adolescents most likely to benefit from methylphenidate (Clampit 1981). (Details of dosage and monitoring are given in chapter 29.) While this medication is widely used for all kinds of distractible children with learning disabilities, there is considerable controversy regarding its effect on learning. Some studies suggest that behavior alone is improved (see chapter 10), while others report an increased ability to learn secondary to improved concentration and attention (Kinsbourne and Caplan 1979). It is particularly important to clarify for parents that while the drug can help the child sit still and concentrate, thus making him or her more manageable in the classroom and easier to teach, it cannot correct any specific learning disability and there is no good evidence that medication ultimately improves long-term academic and occupational achievements. (See chapter 10.)

Motor Training. Programs of motor training, initially proposed in the hope that improved motor skills would be accompanied by an increased capacity to learn, are controversial. Current thinking holds that such programs improve motor skills and may enhance self-confidence, which may then be reflected in improved motivation and, secondarily, better work in school (Hawke and Lesser 1977). This is also true of therapies that promote better ocular control or improved listening skills. However, there is currently little evidence that improving either basic motor or ocular skills will directly increase learning capacity.

Recent Theories. At the present time, a number of additional therapies based largely on biochemical concepts are sometimes recommended for children with learning disabilities. One such program recommends a low-glucose diet on the grounds that some children, given normal amounts of dietary glucose, respond with a rebound hypoglycemia, which produces fatigue and interferes with learning (Hawke and Lesser 1977). Another approach, considering hyperactivity a manifestation of an allergic reaction to certain dyes and other food additives, relies on a rigorously controlled diet (Feingold 1975). Still another, the so-called megavitamin therapy, holds that a number of these children have unrecognized vitamin deficiencies despite what most physicians consider adequate diets (Sieben 1977). Proponents of this therapy therefore regularly administer multiple vitamins in extremely high doses (Kershner 1978).

Unfortunately, most of these approaches have not had carefully controlled studies, so that their value is at best unproven. The interference with learning caused by certain food additives, such as red dye, is currently under investigation in several centers, including Toronto. The role played by sleep apnea in other learning difficulties is also under investigation.

Prognosis

Most, if not all, children with a learning disability can be helped. The learning disability itself may not be corrected, as the improvement may be less in the educational than in the social and emotional areas of the child's life. With increased experience, it seems clear that many children are left with serious persistent educational deficits that, as yet, we have no way of correcting. In many cases, therefore, limited academic progress must be accepted while significant improvement in other areas of function (i.e., tertiary prevention) is sought.

For a given child the prognosis depends on a number of factors, the most important of which are:

1. The child's overall intellectual ability. The more intelligent the child, the greater the capacity to compensate for a deficit.
2. The type of deficit. The prognosis is better for those with a visuomotor language deficit than for those whose deficit is in the audiovocal language system.
3. The severity of the deficit as determined by the diagnostic assessment as well as by the academic progress.
4. The emotional stability and motivation of the child and the family and the support given to the child. These factors are particularly important to older children.
5. The early detection of the disability and the prompt provision of an adequate remedial program before secondary psychological reactions occur and become fixed.

Remedial education has not yet yielded the dramatic successes that were at first hoped for, perhaps partly because it was indiscriminately applied without individual tailoring of programs or perhaps because in the past it dealt only with one aspect of the child's problem, namely the academic underachievement (Shelton 1977) without paying sufficient attention to the secondary emotional and social problems that can only be helped in a climate of close cooperation between teacher, family, and physician. Perhaps the whole question of what causes learning disorders should be revised to ask "What makes children learn?" that is, what are the social and emotional prerequisites of the motivation to learn in the intellectually normal first-grade child, and how can the school, family, and community maintain this high level of motivation throughout the child's adolescence and adulthood?

SUGGESTIONS FOR FURTHER READING

CHESS, S., AND HASSIBI, M. 1978. *Principle and practice of child psychiatry.* New York: Plenum Press.
   A particularly good review of the cognitive problems associated with dyslexia.
EPSTEIN, M. H., et al. 1980. Understanding children with learning disabilities. *Child Welfare* 59(1): 2–14.
   An excellent article on the basics of early identification of learning disorders for pediatricians, family physicians, and educators.

GOTTLIEB, M. I.; ZINKUS, P. W.; AND BRADFORD, L. J. 1979. *Current issues in developmental pediatrics: The learning disabled child.* New York: Grune & Stratton.

An excellent, up-to-date review of the interaction of physical, cognitive, and emotional aspects in development. Addresses the controversial link between learning disability and juvenile delinquency.

ROSS, A. O. 1976. *Psychological aspects of learning disabilities and reading disorders.* New York: McGraw-Hill.

A comprehensive text that explains to parents and educators the complicated terminology in the field of learning disorders and provides practical, positive guidelines to management.

RUTTER, M. 1974. Emotional disorder and educational underachievement. *Arch. Dis. Child.* 49: 249–256.

The best review of research up to 1974 in this field. Problems of definition, epidemiology, and measurement with standard psychological tests are discussed.

Psychiatric Aspects of Mental Retardation

Society's Attitude Toward the Mentally Retarded

From earliest times the retarded have been subject to prejudice, discrimination, and harsh penalties. The laws of Sparta and ancient Rome provided for the extermination of severely retarded children and infants. In medieval Europe the retarded were used as objects of ridicule, such as court jesters, or were viewed as "possessed" and subjected to exorcism and torture. Despite isolated pockets of humanism such as the town of Gheel in Belgium and the Monastery of St. Nicholas of Pyre, until near the end of the eighteenth century the retarded shared with the mentally ill the stigma of being regarded as social outcasts. Since World War II, some cases of active euthanasia have raised major bioethical controversies. There has been only tepid medical interest in the retarded, despite Hippocrates' early description of some specific forms of severe mental retardation involving cranial malformation (Menolascino 1970).

By publishing in 1801 his report on educating the mind of Victor, the "Wild Boy of Aveyron," Jean-Marc Gaspard Itard sparked the beginnings of scientific and professional concern with mental retardation. Simultaneously, however, in 1798 Thomas Malthus predicted the domination of the world population by the poor and reintroduced a philosophy of "survival of the fittest" that discouraged medical and social assistance to the poor or their children. In 1865 Gregor Mendel founded the science of genetics, which led to our present understanding of the causes of some types of mental handicap. In 1871 Francis Galton founded a subscience that he termed eugenics, to study "how more suitable races or strains of blood" would stand a better chance.

The development of both negative and positive climates toward the mentally retarded continued into the twentieth century. Breakthroughs in understanding some causes of mental retardation have resulted in successful primary prevention (Fotheringham and Morrison 1976). The development and application of learning theory has ameliorated retarded people's lives and improved their living conditions. A tragic interlude of only twenty years (1900–1920), however, produced a radical shift of psychiatric interest away from mental retardation. The eugenics scare (i.e., the fear that the retarded who were criminal and sexual menaces would overpopulate the world) ushered in large, isolated custodial institutions. Unfortunately, psychiatrists and other professionals led the way into the institutional wilderness. The mirage of "mental age" and the bias of middle-class professionals against lower socioeconomic groups led to a climate in which a mildly retarded lad from a lower-class family would be described as bearing "cultural-familial mental retardation," while similar functioning in a middle-class child would be diagnosed as "minimal cerebral dysfunction." Only recently, through the public efforts of the retarded and their families, has it been demonstrated that the response of the mild and moderately retarded to their environment resembles less that of the more severely retarded than that of normal children. Many physicians, among them psychiatrists, have recommended institutional care because they were unaware of the major expansion of community resources for the retarded since World War II.

Following World War II, possibly in reaction to Nazi Germany's attempted extermination of the mentally retarded, a rise in humanism spurred the beginnings of a parents' voluntary movement and encouraged the development of alternative community resources for the retarded, particularly in Scandinavia and Western Europe. The "normalization principle" enunciated by Bengt Nirje and N.E. Bank-Mickelson in the 1960s (Nirje 1976) underlies the thrust to community care. It states, "the patterns and conditions of everyday life [for the mentally retarded person] should be as close as possible to those which are the normal patterns of the mainstream of society. These should be made available to any individual within an institutional setting." A 1970 landmark case in the United States, stimulated by Dr. Stonewall Stickney, a progressive psychiatric commissioner of mental health, resulted in the United States District Court of Alabama ordering, in *Ricky Wyatt versus Stickney,* that institutions must be linked with community services, that there be individual habilitation plans, that the least restrictive alternatives should be used in treatment, and that there should be qualified staff in sufficient numbers (Prigmore and Davis 1973).

It is clear from prevalence studies that most mentally retarded persons have always lived in the community. Institutions are gradually and painfully taking their place as only one component within comprehensive care and rehabilitation systems.

TABLE 18.1

Components of Special Need

Life Stage	Physical and Mental Health	Shelter, Nurture, Protection	Intellectual Development	Social Development	Recreation	Work, Economic Security
Infant	Specialized medical follow-up Special diets, drugs, or surgery Home nursing	Residential nursery Child welfare services	Sensory stimulation Home training Environmental enrichment			
Toddler	Correction of physical defects Physical therapy	Foster care Trained baby sitter	Nursery school		Playground programs	
Child	Psychiatric care Dental care	Day care Homemaker service Short-stay home	Religious education Classes for slow learners Special classes—educable Work-school programs		Scouting Swimming Day camps Residential camps	"Disabled child's" benefits
Youth	Psychology Halfway house	Boarding school	Occupational training Speech training	Youth groups Social groups		
Young Adult	Facilities for retarded in conflict Long-term residential care		Vocational counseling—Personal adjustment training	Guardianship of person Marriage counseling	Bowling	Health insurance Selective job placement Sheltered employment Total disability assistance Sheltered workshops Guardianship of property Life annuity or trust
Adult		Group Homes Boarding Homes	Evening school	Social supervision	Evening recreation	
Older Adult	Medical attention to chronic conditions					Old-age assistance

Following the Scandinavian model (Goldberg 1975, 1980a, b), services for the retarded are gradually moving from specialized to generic agencies. Despite public education programs, fear and prejudice are still evoked when someone is labeled retarded or a community living facility is associated with mental retardation. These attitudes are the leftovers of past mythology and fears, combined with a failure to recognize current knowledge. Concerns still exist that the mentally retarded as a group constitute a potential sexual and criminal menace, despite evidence that a relatively small minority are involved in such crimes.

There are three prevailing and persistent societal attitudes about the retarded (Morgenstern 1973). While often latent, these attitudes are easily made manifest by a sensational incident.

Particularly after a sex crime, society's reaction is to view all the retarded with suspicion and to reaffirm that all their characteristics are inherited. This view decreases compassion and enlightment, and the retarded are even considered *subhuman*. The *child innocent*, paternalistic view regards the retarded as eternal children to be pitied and cherished. If the retarded person's sexuality comes to the attention of those who hold this view, its expression must be negated and his or her innocence made to prevail.

Some consider the retarded to be *developing persons*. This optimistic view holds that the retarded have good potential for inclusion within the mainstream of society. This has led to the normalization principle and the movement for civil rights for the retarded. This attitude favors access by the retarded to programs in sex education, birth control, maternal and infant care, and individual counseling on sexual problems. It encourages parents and administrators to allow the retarded the same degree of freedom and sexual expression as the rest of society.

Definitions

Mental retardation is defined in DMS-III as requiring: (1) significantly subaverage general intellectual functioning—an IQ of 70 or below on an individually administered IQ test (since available intelligence tests do not yield a numerical value for infants, a clinical judgment of significant subaverage intellectual functioning is required); (2) concurrent deficits or impairment in adaptive behavior, the person's age being taken into consideration; (3) onset before age eighteen.

The upper age limit of eighteen has been set to differentiate mental retardation from the decreased intellectual functioning that accompanies the later onset of presenile dementias. This definition is similar to that provided by the 1973 American Association on Mental Deficiency. The World

Health Organization (WHO), however, recommends the use of the term mental subnormality, which in turn is divided into two distinct categories: mental retardation and mental deficiency. "Mental retardation" is reserved for subnormal functioning caused by environmental factors in the absence of central nervous system pathology. "Mental deficiency" describes subnormal functioning resulting from pathology of the nervous system. The WHO definition, however, continues to reinforce the therapeutically nihilistic concepts of absolute and relative feeblemindedness (Kanner 1948) or curable and incurable mental retardation (Doll 1941).

The British Mental Health Act of 1959 uses a parallel differentiation that defines two separate levels of mental retardation: severe subnormality (SSN) and subnormality. These terms do not reflect the continuous distribution curve of intellectual functioning. The term oligophrenia is commonly used in the Soviet Union, Scandinavia, and other European countries, usually for retardation associated with brain damage. Terms such as amentia, feeblemindedness, moron, imbecile, and idiot, historically used to denote the degree of intellectual handicap, are regarded as pejoratives in North America.

Classification According to Severity of Symptoms

There are four degrees of intellectual impairment: mild, moderate, severe, and profound. IQ levels that distinguish the four subtypes are given in table 18.2.

Mental retardation should not be diagnosed unless the IQ is at least two standard deviations below the mean, that is, below 70. The term borderline mental retardation, once used for those with IQs in the range of 70 to 90, has been discredited by the recognition that many of those in this category are culturally disadvantaged rather than retarded.

Intelligence tests and quotients have been under substantial attack in recent years and are even banned in some states (Tarjan and Keeran 1974). Most tests in current usage have been standardized in the United States,

TABLE 18.2
Distinguished by IQ Level
Subtypes of Mental Retardation

	IQ Levels	DSM-III/Diagnosis
Mild Mental Retardation	50–70	317.0 (x)
Moderate Mental Retardation	35–49	318.0 (x)
Severe Mental Retardation	20–34	318.1 (x)
Profound Mental Retardation	Below 20	318.2 (x)

primarily on middle-class individuals with a good command of English. Culture-free and culture-specific tests have been designed only recently. Individual testing, performed and interpreted with sophistication by a skilled, professional psychologist with knowledge of the child from a variety of sources, considers the test score as but one index of intellectual functioning. The tests measure general intelligence, which consists of a number of factors, fairly well. IQ tests remain reliable and have good predictive value if used for their original purpose—the determination of the likelihood that an individual child will or will not succeed in a classroom.

In general, intelligence test scores indicate variable rates of growth in the first three or four years but become more stable thereafter. Verbal scores stabilize earlier in girls. Such personality characteristics as drive, perseverance, and attention span may enhance or retard the development of mental abilities. Mental growth, especially in boys, seems to be facilitated in a supportive, "warm" emotional climate that provides positive reinforcement for specific cognitive efforts and successes.

Within mentally retarded populations, the IQ can also predict significant events such as morbidity, mortality, the presence or absence of secondary handicaps, and the chance for admission or release from institutional settings (Tarjan et al. 1973). Although the label of mental retardation may evoke rejection by a child's peers and may undermine that child's self-concept and self-esteem, level of aspiration, teacher's expectations, and the chance for a healthy adult adjustment in marriage or employment (Macmillan, Jones, and Aloia 1974), these dangers can be minimized by recognizing each child's individuality and helping all achieve their own personal limit of social competence and adaptive behavior. (See table 18.3.)

"Impairment of adaptive behavior" implies unsuccessful or incomplete coping. "Coping" can be assessed by examining the retarded person's degree of independent functioning and assumption of personal and social responsibilities. Scales exist that measure different facets of coping or adaptive behavior, such as: self-help skills; communication skills; socialization or interpersonal skills; locomotion; self-direction (i.e., initiative, attending); occupational skills; economic activity; neuromotor development (i.e., motor control, mannerisms); personal responsibility (i.e., trustworthiness, care of own property); social responsibility (i.e., care of others' property); emotional adjustment (i.e., prevalent mood, control, reaction to criticisms); health.

During infancy and early childhood, the emphasis is on self-help skills. During childhood and early adolescence, academic and social skills are emphasized; during late adolescence and adult life, vocational capability and social responsibility are measures of coping. While it is misleading to use precise categorization of adaptive behavior as a predictive device, a realistic assessment of coping skills and deficits provides a more balanced view of achievements and shortcomings than IQ alone in preparing a goal-directed treatment plan.

TABLE 18.3

Developmental Characteristics, Potential for Education and Training, and Social and Vocational Adequacy

Level of Retardation	Preschool Age 0–5 Maturation and Development	School Age 6–21 Training and Education	Adult 21 and Over Social and Vocational Adequacy
Profound	Gross retardation; minimal capacity for functioning in sensorimotor areas, needs nursing care.	Obvious delays in all, areas of development; shows basic emotional responses; may respond to skillful training in use of legs, hands, and jaws; needs close supervision.	May walk; needs nursing care; primitive speech; usually benefits from regular physical activity; incapable of self-maintenance.
Severe	Marked delay in motor development; little or no communication skill; may respond to training in elementary self-help (e.g. self feeding).	Usually walks barring specific disability; has some understanding of speech and some response; can profit from systematic habit training.	Can conform to daily routines and repetitive activities; needs continuing direction and supervision in protective environment.
Moderate	Noticeable delays in motor development, especially in speech; responds to training in various self-help activities.	Can learn simple communication, elementary health and safety habits, and simple manual skills; does not progress in functional reading or functional arithmetic.	Can perform simple task; under sheltered conditions; participates in simple recreation; travels alone in familiar places; usually incapable of self-maintenance.
Mild	Often not noticed as retarded by casual observer but is slower to walk, feed self, and talk than most children.	Can acquire practical skills and useful reading and arithmetic to a third or sixth grade level with special education; can be guided to social conformity.	Can usually achieve social and vocational skills adequate to self maintenance; may need occasional guidance and support when under social or economic stress.

SOURCE: The President's Panel on Mental Retardation, *Mental Retardation, A National Plan for a National Problem: Chart Book* U. S. Department of Health, Education and Welfare (Washington, D. C.: U. S. Government Printing Office, 1963) p. 15.
NOTE: Classification developed by the American Association on Mental Deficiency

Epidemiology

Approximately 3 percent of the population score below 70 on standard IQ tests. Most of the mildly retarded are not diagnosed during preschool years since parents, unless unusually alert, do not detect maladaptive behavior before school begins. Mildly retarded children are likely to develop at the same rate as other children. Most of the mildly retarded live in marginal social circumstances and disappear into the general population upon reaching adulthood. It is principally the moderately, severely, and profoundly retarded who are spotted in the preschool years. The recorded prevalence of mental retardation is therefore much closer to 1 percent.

Dugdale's study (1877) of a notorious family called the Jukes (see Robinson and Robinson 1976) and Goddard's study (1912) of the Kallikak family attributed to inheritance the low intelligence in these families. In England Sir Cyril Burt (1958) argued for a polygenetic inheritance of intelligence, although his studies have been severely criticized as predicated on contrived results. The modern-day study by Reed and Reed (1965) also concluded that 1 to 2 percent of the population is composed of fertile retarded individuals who produce a third of the retarded population of the next generation.

There is an unevenness in the distribution of IQ in the population, particularly at the lower end of the normal statistical curve. This arises because specific pathological processes, such as major genetic abnormalities or brain injury, begin to influence IQs below 50, and also because of the large number of cultural and multifactorial familial factors that affect the normal bell-shaped curve above IQ 50 (Dingman and Tarjan 1960). The Isle of Wight study (Rutter et al. 1970) revealed a rate for mild retardation of 21 per 1,000 and for severe retardation of 3.9 per 1,000. Other studies (Hansen, Belmont, and Stein 1980) confirm the prevalence of mild mental retardation as ten times greater than that for severe mental retardation.

The largest segment of the retarded (the mild or educable group composing 75 percent of the total retarded population) can acquire basic skills and symbolic communication. They encounter major difficulties only when called upon to think abstractly or to pass complex judgments. The smaller moderate group, making up approximately 20 percent of the retarded, is able to distinguish between safety and danger but fails in daily tasks requiring symbolic communication such as reading, writing, and arithmetic. A much smaller proportion, approximately 5 percent of the diagnosed retarded, is so severely impaired that they require constant care for survival.

As causes of severe mental retardation are identified, some conditions become accessible to prevention and treatment, such as vaccination programs against rubella in the mother and amniocentesis for detection and consequent termination of abnormal pregnancies. In the developing countries, estimates suggest that a 15 percent reduction in severe mental retardation is an immediate possibility. The sociocultural context in which mild mental retardation occurs makes it less amenable to specific preventive strategies of the sort outlined for severe retardation. Various North American attempts such as Project Head Start (Bronfenbrenner 1974) and the Wisconsin Project with disadvantaged children (Heber, Garber, and Falender 1975) have been aimed at the mildly mentally retarded with modest success.

In highly socialized countries such as Sweden, where major efforts at physical, functional, and social integration have been made, the prevalence rate for the entire retarded population, including those only mildly retarded, is only 0.44 percent. The mildly retarded make up only 23 percent of this group, reflecting the high degree of social integration (Grunewald 1979).

Etiological Factors

CHROMOSOME ABNORMALITIES

Many cases, particularly of moderate and severe mental retardation, result from chromosome abnormalities. The disorder may be in a single autosomal chromosome or in the female sex chromosome. In some cases there may be an extra chromosome (i.e., trisomy), a deletion of chromosome material, or the displacement of material from one chromosome onto another (i.e., translocation). In cases with chromosome abnormalities, the retardation is often combined with other obvious physical abnormalities to form a well-defined clinical syndrome. The most common of these is Down's syndrome, but many other well-recognized but less frequent syndromes exist. These syndromes are summarized below.

The single most common chromosomal cause of moderate to severe mental retardation is *Down's syndrome,* formerly called mongolism. At least 10 percent of moderately to severely retarded children exhibit Down's syndrome, which is known to be associated with an extra number 21 chromosome, so that the condition is often called trisomy 21. The average incidence of Down's syndrome is 1 per 800 live births. The condition occurs equally in all classes of society. Too much has been made of the epicanthic folds at the corners of the eyes, which gave rise to the term mongoloid. Because "mongoloid" carries negative connotations, "Down's syndrome" or "trisomy 21" is the preferred terminology. In 80 percent of cases, the parental source of the extra chromosome is the mother. This is particularly true of older mothers, whose ova are more vulnerable to the harmful effects of endogenous and exogenous agents, including x-rays. The risk for a mother over age thirty-five having a child with trisomy 21 is about 1 in 100, but when the mother shows a translocation chromosome 21 the risk is about one in three. Forty percent of Down's children show associated cardiac abnormalities, particularly septal defects, and about 20 to 30 percent do not survive the first few years. After these critical early years, the mortality is like that of others with the same IQ. Although a placid, cheerful personality has been described, this stereotype is by no means universal. Those with Down's syndrome are subject to early aging associated with Alzheimer's disease.

Trisomies of the large chromosomes are unusual, though frequently found in spontaneous miscarriages. Two other commonly encountered trisomies of autosomal chromosomes, trisomy 18 and trisomy 13, are both associated with multiple malformations and severe mental retardation. In addition, deletions of chromosome material may be associated with severe syndromes. In the "crie-du-chat" syndrome, named after the characteristic high-pitched, catlike cry in infancy, there is a partial deletion of the short arm of chromosome 5.

In the past, the higher prevalence of mental retardation in males (2 to 1) has been attributed to social and behavioral variables. Recent surveys suggest that X-linked mental retardation may account for 20 percent of the moderate retardation range. A subgroup of X-linked retardation associated with the so-called Marker-X or Fragile X chromosome may account for a quarter of all X-linked retardation. This would make it the most frequent genetic cause of retardation resulting from chromosome abnormality. Affected males commonly show an enlarged head, enlarged testes, and protruding chin. Female carriers of the abnormal X chromosome are said to have a high incidence of mild mental retardation.

Other abnormalities of the sex chromosomes are more compatible with survival, often with relatively unaffected mental development. Examples are Klinefelter's, XYY, and Turner's syndromes.

Klinefelter's syndrome (XXY) occurs in chromatin-positive males with one or more additional X (i.e., female sex) chromosomes. Testicular atrophy becomes evident at puberty and is associated with signs of feminization, such as breast enlargement (gynecomastia). Mental retardation, usually mild, occurs in about 50 percent of such patients. The greater the number of X chromosomes, the higher the risk of significant mental retardation. Replacement therapy using testosterone may prevent the secondary social immaturity and psychopathology that frequently occur in postadolescent years.

Turner's syndrome (XO, gonadal dysgenesis) describes females with only one X chromosome and no other sex chromosomes. The main physical features include small stature, web neck, broad chest, coarctation of the aorta, and deformed elbow. Only a minority of patients are retarded, and then only mildly. They have a special perceptual-motor difficulty in space-form visual reception and construction.

Single Dominant Gene Abnormalities

Single dominant gene abnormalities are characterized by variability in a number of features and are often associated with only mild mental retardation. Skull, limb, skin, and visceral abnormalities are frequently involved.

Tuberous sclerosis, or epiloia, is characterized by severe mental retardation, seizures, and a peculiar butterfly rash across the cheeks.

Neurofibromatosis, or von Recklinghausen's disease, is the condition made famous in the nineteenth century by John Merrick, the Elephant Man. The main features are café-au-lait spots over the trunk and extremities, with multiple tumors of the skin and nervous tissue that may become large, grotesque skin polyps. Only about 10 percent of these patients are retarded.

Sturge-Weber disease, or cerebral trigeminal angiomatosis, in its classical form includes a facial nevus along the distribution of the fifth cranial nerve, enlarged eyes, hemiparesis, convulsions, and mental retardation associated with intracranial neurangiomata, which may become calcified.

Various other cranial abnormalities have been described that combine variations in the shape of the skull with other congenital abnormalities. These are usually named after the clinician who first described them: Crouzon, Apert, Greig. These conditions, along with various forms of hydrocephalus, may be of sporadic and presumed genetic origin.

Single Recessive Genes

Single recessive genes affect 1 in 4 children born to parents who are heterozygous carriers of the defective gene and who themselves produce only half the normal level of the relevant enzyme. The first single gene metabolic enzyme defect, alkaptonuria, was described by Garrod in 1908. Although the incidence of most of these inborn errors of metabolism is less than 1 in 10,000 live births, the total of all known hereditary metabolic defects probably accounts for about 4 to 5 percent of the moderate to severely retarded group. It is estimated that with further biochemical research, this figure would approach 10 percent.

The classic condition of *phenylketonuria (PKU),* first discovered by Folling in 1934, is responsible for interesting organically oriented physicians in mental retardation. The information gained from the study of PKU serves as a model of investigation for other hereditary biochemical disorders, more of which are now detectable through amniocentesis. Prompt early intervention is now possible in some of these conditions. PKU is associated with eczema, severe retardation, and convulsions. It occurs in young children with blond hair and blue eyes, because of an associated relative deficiency of melanin. Screening tests depend on the reaction of urine to ferric chloride solution or bacterial inhibition using the Guthrie test and must be done soon after birth. Paper chromatography has made the detection of this and other metabolic disorders much easier. The basic defect of PKU is the inability to convert phenylalanine to tyrosine because of a deficiency of the liver enzyme phenylalanine hydroxylase. This results in toxic levels of phenylalanine and disturbances of tryptophan and tyrosine metabolism. With the careful monitoring of phenylalanine in the diet, mental retardation can be prevented if treatment is begun before three months of age.

Other *amino acid disorders* have also been described with varying success using dietary controls. These include maple syrup disease (Menkes' disease), hyperammonemia, histidinemia, citrullinuria, homocystinuria, and Hartnup's disease. This latter condition is of special interest to psychiatrists since it is associated with defective tryptophan transport, marked amino aciduria along with a photosensitive rash, episodic cerebellar ataxia, mental deficiency, and psychosis.

Disorders of *carbohydrate metabolism* have also been discovered that follow the model of PKU. A particularly striking example is *galactosemia,* first detected in 1956 and associated with severe mental retardation, cataracts, and convulsions. A milk-free diet, at least until school age, will prevent mental retardation in these children, although recent evidence suggests a continuing subtle learning disability.

There are several types of genetic defects in thyroid hormone synthesis. Screening tests have been initiated in Quebec, Ontario, and other provinces to detect *congenital hypothyroidism.* Cretinism, the term given this type of mental retardation, is associated with dwarfism, a large tongue, and mental retardation. The condition may also be due to congenital absence of the thyroid gland. Treatment with thyroid extract instituted early in life may avert most of the symptoms.

Mucopolysaccharide storage diseases are a group of conditions formerly known as gargoylism. At least six subtypes have been described. Two major types are referred to as Hurler's syndrome and Hunter's syndrome. The large head and coarse features in all types are associated with the accumulation of mucopolysaccharide and related substances in the skull. The condition, which may present originally as hyperactivity in a normal-appearing child, is progressive, causing death before adolescence. Active research is currently underway to find replacement enzymes.

Wilson's disease, or progressive hepatolenticular degeneration, is associated with a diminished blood level of copper-containing ceruloplasm. The associated excess copper in the liver and brain results in emotional and mental deterioration and the classic greenish-brown ring in the iris (Kayser-Fleischer ring). The juvenile form begins during the school years, and psychiatric symptoms may precede the mental deterioration. The condition responds to heavy metal chelating agents.

INTRAUTERINE ENVIRONMENT

Only a few recognized but significant infections cross the placental barrier and cause variable degrees of multisystem damage to the fetus and neonate (Boone 1975). *Syphilis* can be detected early enough in pregnancy so that it can be treated appropriately. *Maternal rubella* causes a high incidence of multiple abnormalities including microcephaly, hearing loss, cataracts with visual loss, heart defects, and retardation. This syndrome seriously affected some 15,000 children in the United States during the last rubella epidemic in the 1970s. Mass administration of rubella vaccine to all school children to produce herd immunity or, more recently, to all children by one year of age is designed to immunize them before they reach childbearing age. However, recent evidence suggests that a single inoculation of rubella vaccine does not necessarily produce life-long immunity. In many children immunity begins to wane so markedly that reinfection (often asymptomatic) is necessary to rebuild antibody levels. Unfortunately, this reinfection can be associated with viremia and may infect the fetus in utero.

Although the typical rubella baby, the so-called blueberry muffin infant, is covered with round bluish bruises associated with thrombocytopenia, it has been recently recognized that rubella infants may also be quite normal in size, appearance, and function, though suffering continued infectious activity that can cause a sudden progressive neurological deterioration as late as two or three years of age.

A similar syndrome, with a very obvious and severe multisystem and microcephalic neurological defect, has been described in association with *cytomegalovirus infection* in mother and father. It may also present as simple microcephaly in a child with a variable degree of intellectual failure. The incidence of cytomegalovirus infection in newborn infants may be as high as 1 percent of all children. One-tenth of this group demonstrates severe neurological sequelae. Immunity does not appear to prevent subsequent teratogenesis associated with a dormant virus.

All *chemicals and drugs* cross the placenta. It is important for physicians to review the most recent literature about fetal drug effects before prescribing for the pregnant mother. Hypoglycemic and antithyroid agents, sulfonamides, aspirin, vitamin K, diazepam, and phenobarbital and narcotics have well-known effects on the fetus. More recently described is the association of multiple defects with phenytoin use in the epileptic mother. Even more serious is the newly recognized association of congenital abnormalities in alcoholic and even social-drinking mothers, resulting in the so-called fetal alcohol syndrome.

Smoking during pregnancy causes a distinct lowering of the birth weight by an average of 180 grams (6 ounces), apparently through the same mechanism of increased catabolism as in the smoking mother. The father who smokes also places his offspring at risk. Associated with this lowered birth weight is a small but significant increase in perinatal mortality and in the incidence of congenital abnormalities.

Studies in developing countries and in poverty areas in North America have clearly demonstrated that the newborn infant can suffer from the effects of *maternal malnutrition,* especially in the third trimester when the central nervous system is undergoing one of its periods of rapid development. The very restricted weight gain fashionably imposed to prevent toxemia not so long ago in North America also reduced significantly the birth weight of offspring. Such restrictions may have led to an increase of "small for date infants" at risk for hypoglycemia, hypocalcemia, and secondary damage to the central nervous system. Today's mother is not only allowed but encouraged to gain twenty to thirty pounds during her pregnancy.

Other complications of pregnancy, such as toxemia, maternal diabetes, and placental abnormalities, may sometimes result in mental retardation.

PERINATAL FACTORS

Low birth weight (less than 2,500 grams) "small for date" but born close to term infants, while not prone to the anoxia of the respiratory distress syndrome, must be actively monitored for low blood sugar and low calcium. The infant who is "premature for date and weight" is more prone to anoxia and the respiratory distress syndrome, along with other complications.

Neonatology has vastly improved both the rate and quality of survival for neonates larger than 1,000 grams. In 1965, 30 percent of this group developed cerebral palsy, whereas with intensive neonatal care this has virtually disappeared. The improved result stems primarily from the prevention of anoxia and secondary acidosis, from maintenance of normal temperatures, early feeding and nutritional support, along with freedom from infection. Follow-up studies, however, indicate that 50 percent of these children will have problems associated with learning disabilities or mental retardation (Boone 1975). This problem group comes, however, from significantly poorer social environments.

Kernicterus, associated with pigmentation by bilirubin of various components of the brain, can result from Rh incompatibility, severe infection, prematurity, and toxic effects of various medications during the neonatal period.

POSTNATAL FACTORS

Infections of the brain (i.e., either bacterial or viral meningo-encephalitis) have diminished as a result of the advances in antibiotic therapy. The effects of the resulting brain damage can vary from learning disorders to severe mental retardation. Seemingly "ordinary diseases of childhood" such as chicken pox and mumps can prove fatal or cause severe brain damage.

Head injuries in children seldom produce serious brain damage and consequent mental retardation. Automobile accidents and child abuse are among the most frequent causes of brain trauma when it does occur.

Cerebral palsy is a condition defined by the presence of pyramidal tract and extrapyramidal motor disorders. Spastic quadriplegics are most likely to have associated mental retardation; those with the athetoid type of cerebral palsy are least likely. Because of associated speech and hearing disorders, however, athetoid-type children may have their intelligence underestimated, with consequent frustration and high suicide rate. The same organic factors that are associated with mental retardation can also result in cerebral palsy.(See chapter 22.)

The association of *childhood psychosis* and mental retardation has been known for several years, although the causes of childhood psychosis are still undetermined (see chapter 15). It is not uncommon to see children who, sequentially or in any combination, have acquired a series of diagnoses that included early infantile autism, atypical child, childhood schizophrenia, mental retardation, brain damage, or minimal brain dysfunction.

Current research into causation follows two main lines of investigation, one biochemical and the other neurophysiological. DeMyer and associates (1972), for example, noted the presence of body imitation failure (traced to neurophysiological deficiencies) combined with severe central language disorders in the psychotic group. This results in more abnormal visual-motor or language processing than is present in most mentally retarded children. Recent treatment approaches emphasize total communication and/or behavior modification techniques.

PSYCHOSOCIAL DISADVANTAGE

Psychosocial disadvantage, the most frequent cause of mental retardation, is associated with environmental influences. There may be no associated organic disease or pathology. This group gives rise to the major controversy regarding nature versus nurture. Genetic components and variations in IQ became deeply embroiled in the racial turmoil in the United States, particularly through Jensen's 1969 publication.

The *continuum of reproductive casualty* is a term introduced in 1953 by Pasamanick and Knobloch (1966) to describe the sequelae of harmful events in pregnancy and parturition that result in damage to the fetus or newborn infant, primarily localized in the central nervous system. They showed that children affected by these events may demonstrate features ranging from fetal or neonatal death, through cerebral palsy, epilepsy, mental deficiency, to all types of behavioral and learning disabilities, with the latter originating from lesser degrees of damage that are still sufficient to disorganize behavioral development and lower thresholds to stress. Pasamanick and Knobloch stated that the majority of the mentally retarded and of those

397

suffering these other relatively less severe mental disabilities come from the economically and psychosocially disadvantaged segment of the population. In their careful epidemiological studies, the authors made a compelling case for environmental and life experiences (poor nutrition, health, perinatal care, etc.) as opposed to genetic disorder as the major cause of reproductive casualty. Critics of the concept of "reproductive casualty" indicate that it is difficult to differentiate whether a "poor passenger" (i.e., genetic) or a "poor passage" (i.e., environment) initiates the sequence (Pasamanick and Knobloch 1966).

Currently polygenetic and environmental factors are considered interrelated in a way yet to be determined. Because of the controversy the term cultural-familial mental retardation has fallen into disuse. In the absence of other causative factors, specific environmental deprivation, such as maternal or sensory deprivation if present, is to be noted as a psychosocial stressor.

Sociocultural retardation is usually not diagnosed until school entrance. The label is usually shed upon reaching adulthood (Tarjan and Keeran 1974). The retardation is mild, with IQs somewhere between 50 and 70. The economically, educationally, and socially disadvantaged segment of society is heavily overrepresented in this IQ range. The families of such children generally do not notice any major difference between their affected child's performance and that of other family members. The diagnosis is externally imposed on school entry; this has led to such controversial issues as the appropriate and inappropriate use of intelligence tests, the positive or negative impact of labeling, the usefulness or futility of special classes, the appropriateness of defining these children as "retarded." Such children are frequently unwanted, unplanned, and raised in broken homes with absent fathers and emotionally or physically unavailable mothers. "Sensory deprivation" is considered the most important causative factor and includes a deprivation of tactile and kinesthetic stimuli, a suppression of exploratory behavior, inconsistency between the child's responses and physical and social reward, and poor stimulation of language development. Shifting these children from the disadvantaged family to an adequately stimulating environment has been shown to result in at least average intellectual performance and social adaptation, thus demonstrating the reversibility of these factors.

Diagnostic Evaluation and Formulation

Assessment of a mentally retarded child to evaluate accurately the etiology and those social factors contributing to the current status requires the skills of a multidisciplinary team. This includes a pediatrician, child psychiatrist, neurologist, other medical specialists, clinical psychologist, social worker, public health nurse, speech and hearing clinician, nutritionist, teacher, physiotherapist, child care worker, and laboratory technician. The leader of this team has the task of integrating a wide variety of information, possibly utilizing a conceptual model similar to that of Garrard and Richmond (1965), as shown in table 18.4.

A thorough assessment should point toward an individual treatment plan for which the family assumes responsibility. A detailed medical and psychiatric history is followed by a physical and neurological examination and an assessment of the child's mental status. Laboratory procedures include routine blood count, urinalysis, paper chromatography, electroencephalogram, skull and wrist x-rays for bone age, buccal smears, and chromosome analysis. Brain scan and tests for cytomegalic inclusion virus and toxoplasmosis may also be indicated.

Although the "fairness" of psychological tests has been questioned, they are standardized and less subject to the vagaries of clinical intuition than the usual mental status examination. The physician should become familiar with one of several screening instruments, such as the Denver Developmental Screening Test, Gesell, or Illingworth, which are useful for

TABLE 18.4

Etiological Mechanisms

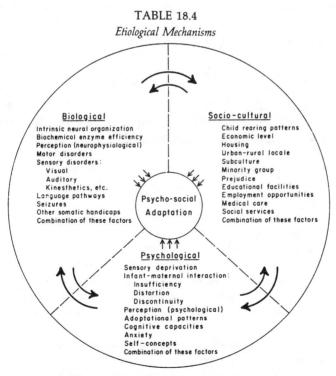

SOURCE: S. D. Garrard and J. B. Richmond, "Mental Retardation with Biological Manifestation," in *Medical Aspects of Mental Retardation,* ed. C. H. Carter (Springfield, Ill.: Charles C Thomas, 1965), p. 34.

preschool children. The Goodenough Draw-a-Person Test and the Bender Gestalt can measure visual-motor development as well as detecting brain damage, particularly in mildly retarded children. More complex testing by an experienced psychologist may include the Stanford-Binet, the Wechsler Intelligence Scale for Children, the Peabody Picture Vocabulary Test (which overcomes language barriers), and the Illinois Test of Psycholinguistic Abilities (which tests specific auditory, verbal, and motor responses). The simplest test for adaptive functioning is the Vineland Social Maturity Scale, from which is derived a Social Quotient. The IQ scores derived are merely summary indices of the child's performance. The child's motivation, personality pattern, and nonintellectual ability, the life situation and available opportunities within the family, community, and society may do more than IQ alone to determine immediate and eventual level of function.

The Family of the Mentally Retarded

As described in chapter 3, the development and growth of any family are never smooth. For the family of a retarded child, the complications and hazards may be greater and the rewards of parenting less obvious than the inevitable crises of family living (Robinson and Robinson 1976). All of the complications—the child's specific handicap; the slow and limited development; the special arrangements needed for physical care, training, and companionship; the disappointments and the lost dreams; the additional financial problems; the continued tensions and immature self-control; the problems in communication; the parents' guilt and self-doubt; and the prospect of life-long emotional and economic dependency—may lead to periodic overwhelming of the usual coping mechanisms at crisis points in the retarded person's life (Willer, Intagliata, and Atkinson 1979).

These crisis points commonly occur: at the first suspicion of retardation; at the final diagnosis; at school entrance; in response to rejection by peers; in sibling relationships; with acute illness or general family crises; soon after puberty; related to complicating problems of vocational adjustment and decisions regarding marriage and institutionalization. Additional crises may complicate separation following institutionalization or, in recent years, discharge from an institution and return home (Solomons 1979).

These crises have also been conceptualized as: *novelty shock,* as the parents' expectations are suddenly shattered, forcing them to begin the process of mourning for the child who might have been; *value conflict,* due to culturally mediated attitudes toward defect or deviance; and *reality stress,* resulting from the situational demands of raising or caring for a retarded person. (Wolfensberger and Menolascino 1970).

It has been assumed that families of the mentally handicapped invariably react by a combination of denial of the handicap; irrational guilt; chronic sorrow, anger, and attempts to fix blame on others; shopping for invalid diagnoses and cures; rejection of the child with unnecessary institutionalization; or family dissolution.

Recent studies, however, indicate that family emotional disintegration and social isolation may be exaggerated by professionals (Matheny and Vernick 1969; Reynolds 1979). This may reflect a changing social climate. It is becoming more evident that the impact of the various crises resulting from having a retarded child is closely related to the level of family integration before the retarded child's birth. It has been demonstrated that families' capacities for solving existing problems and dealing with crises do not necessarily improve significantly after institutionalization of the retarded child (Fotheringham, Skelton, and Hoddinott 1972). If anything, institutionalization may precipitate a new crisis.

Overprotection is, however, more common among parents of children with any chronic disability. This may stem from the lack of parental reward obtained in teaching a child self-help skills so that the parents find it less frustrating to do things themselves, from prolonged dependency that encourages more mutually gratifying indulgence, or as a reaction formation to underlying feelings of rejection and hostility (Grebler 1952).

The more dependent the retarded child and the greater the major burden that falls on the siblings, particularly the normal sisters, the greater is the siblings' resentment (Farber 1959). Parents who themselves have adapted well to the presence of a retarded child convey this acceptance to their normal children (Grossman 1972). If anything, the siblings in such families are more tolerant, more compassionate, and more focused, both occupationally and personally, than other young adults (Lewis et al. 1976). However, when siblings are expected to assume unusual responsibilities in response to irrational, overprotective, or rejecting attitudes of the parents, then unhappiness and tension result (Lewis et al. 1976). (See chapter 21.)

Karen, a girl with Down's syndrome, was the daughter of a deeply religious professional family in northern Ontario. When the diagnosis was confirmed, the parents stated that if God willed that their daughter should remain a child all her life, they and their children would accept this. They undertook to provide her with all the love and affection they could in order to help her develop her full potential.

On reassessment twelve years later, it was obvious that both parents and siblings had been able to accept Karen and provide a warm, understanding, and supportive environment. Karen appeared a happy girl, who related well to the family and in the community, presenting no problems either in the home or in the special day school that she attended.

The Role of the Professional in Families

The first person with whom families discuss their problems with a retarded child is usually their family doctor or pediatrician. Thus it is the primary physician who will usually be expected to make the diagnosis and to help them deal with the emotional disturbances, behavioral difficulties, and added responsibilities that may arise secondary to the retardation. As the child grows older, a counselor associated with the community facility in which the retarded child is placed often assumes the major role in helping the family deal with current difficulties and plan for the future. At this stage the role of the primary physician depends on the degree of the doctor's interest and the family's trust. It can vary from that of a coordinator and advisor consulted at points of crisis or proposed change of management to someone who is consulted only around problems of physical health.

The mother of a retarded child gives the following advice to professionals:

> Tell us the nature of our problem as soon as possible; see both parents; don't use jargon; let us make decisions; help us to understand it is our problem; know your resources; never put us on the defensive; remember that parents of retarded children are just people; remember that we are parents and you are professionals; remember the importance of your attitude toward us." (Patterson 1956, p. 14.)

Parents react favorably to: an appreciation of their love and caring for the retarded child; careful planning and an uninterrupted and unhurried discussion of the findings; allowing parent contact with a child before the diagnosis is told; sharing extensive information at an appropriate time with them but without making absolute predictions; making specific practical recommendations. The more severe the defect, the more likely parents are to follow the physician's recommendations (Rubin and Rubin 1980).

Some physicians who know little about even the more common specific disorders may minimize the child's potential or pressure the family against raising the baby. They may stress the special burdens posed by the retarded child and deemphasize the normal need for mother-infant bonding. In order for professionals to counsel parents of retarded children or adults regarding institutional care, they should be aware of modern concepts of the role of institutional care in the management of the retarded.

Before recommending a potential institutional placement, professionals should be aware whether the proposed placement offers custodial care that protects and isolates the retarded individual or, through rigidity of programming and block treatment of inmates in groups, contributes to depersonalization of the resident population by failing to respect the personal identity of each and by creating social distance between the caregivers and the patients (Tizard 1970). Menolascino (1970) eloquently described the life in such an institutional backwater:

> Residents are awakened en masse very early in the morning so that night attendants can . . . get them toileted before hustling them down to a barren dining room in which they are seated on benches before lengthy tables. They are placed in close proximity to the sloppy mess in their steel or unbreakable plastic plates, and are only given large spoons because we surely "know" that they cannot be trusted with forks and knives. . . . Once in the day room, they are again seated on benches or chairs and allowed the grand pleasure of viewing TV, or simply one another, until mid-morning. . . . In the "play yard" they wander around aimlessly; stereotyped behavior is commonplace, and the attendants busy themselves maintaining a watch for the "hole-diggers," the "excessive masturbators" (there is a degree of distinction!), and anyone subject to overt seizures. This same routine—appropriate for the separation and temporary maintenance of cattle at a livestock yard—is repeated in the afternoons. (p. 722.)

Facilities that are homelike rather than like a large sterile barracks and ones in which patients are grouped to meet the individual's needs represent a viable alternative to the family as part of a continuum of services. With changing community attitudes and increasing availability of modern diagnostic treatment and training facilities in larger communities, the need for centralized long-term institutional placements has been reduced. These are currently reserved for severely and profoundly retarded patients who are multiply handicapped or for those with severe emotional and behavioral difficulties.

In the absence of a spectrum of community programs (see table 18.1), regional or nearby alternative living arrangements may be needed in order for the retarded children of families in smaller or rural centers to be close to training or vocational programs. A hierarchy of least restrictive alternative living situations should include living with family, living with relatives outside the nuclear family, foster care, supervised apartments, group homes, residential treatment facilities, community-based nursing homes, and small regional mental retardation centers (Menolascino and Eaton 1980).

Several sessions may be required to help parents overcome feelings of irrational guilt, for example regarding the influence of heredity. Genetic counseling may, in some situations, be indicated. The likely impact on normal siblings may need to be anticipated. Parents who find the child embarrassing or feel stigmatized by the child's disability may benefit from discussing their feelings with their physician or counselor. Exposure to other parents with similar children may be extremely helpful, though parent groups should not be introduced prematurely, as they may be rejected by families still preoccupied with working through their personal anguish.

Each particular crisis should be accurately identified as it occurs. As with all crises, the quicker and more available the professional's response, the more successful the intervention may be. Realistic difficulties should be determined accurately. Physicians who are personally unable to give practical day-to-day support should involve other professionals who can assist with specific advice, treatment, or training related to associated physical or neurological defects, financial burdens, and remedial training for developmental defects in motor, communication, or sexual development. If there are gaps in needed community services such as relief, baby-sitting services, group homes, or transportation, parents should be encouraged to join with others to organize and lobby to fill these gaps (Strider and Menolascino 1979). Such community advocacy may do much to help the family overcome feelings of helplessness and depression, as well as broadening the spectrum of community services.

The importance of providing therapeutic support for families of retarded children is highlighted by reports indicating an increased incidence of child abuse in children with developmental disabilities (Solomons 1979). The additional stresses introduced by the handicap dramatically increase the potential for abuse and therefore make it incumbent on the clinician to ask three simple questions: "Is this child difficult to handle?" "Does the child drive you up the wall?" "What do you do when this happens?"

The physician must be aware of personal feelings about the mentally retarded before entering into a counseling situation. The clinician who is pessimistic or caught up in societal attitudes of rejection described earlier may overreact by providing an immediate prescription without listening to the family's problem, by defining the condition as a nonmedical problem and making a quick referral, or by making a premature or inappropriate recommendation for institutional care.

There will, however, always be a minority of parents whose distress at having produced a retarded and/or multiply handicapped child will make it impossible for them to accept the demands and frustrations of caring for that child. To force or shame them into doing so will be damaging to them, to their normal children, and, in the long run, to the retarded child forced to grow up in a family where he or she is unwanted, unloved, and potentially neglected and abused. The personal feelings of the professional counseling the family must not interfere with that counselor's sensitivity to the needs of both child and family. Such a counselor will help the family appreciate the needs of the child as well as their own needs but will respect the family's right to make the final decision.

The effectiveness of a clinician in dealing with families of the retarded depends on: a positive attitude; a thorough knowledge of the medical syndromes; the ability to describe diagnostic and prognostic information in a clear manner, appreciating and taking into account the family's shock and other reactions even when these are not immediately and overtly expressed; and an understanding of the dynamics of the specific family at hand (Group for the Advancement of Psychiatry 1963; Morgenstern 1973).

Emotional and Behavioral Disturbances in the Mentally Retarded

Common myths about the typical personality of the retarded person range from the stereotype of the happy, innocent child to that of an uninhibited, sexually aggressive menace. Studies, mainly on retarded individuals in institutions, have described their personalities as passive and withdrawn; anxious and impulsive; rigid; suggestible; lacking in persistence; immature; low in frustration tolerance, self-concept, and level of aspiration; self-pitying, hopeless, and possessive; having strong and contagious feelings of insecurity; hungry for attention and affection (Beier 1964; Heber 1964).

Despite attempts to describe a primary constitutional psychopathology of the mentally retarded, it is clear that while the brain dysfunction may be of organic origin, it is the interpersonal relationships that determine whether the delayed development leads to adaptive or maladaptive behavior. The mentally retarded child is more vulnerable to the development of maladaptive behavior than the normally endowed child at all periods of life (Philips 1967; Robinson and Robinson 1976).

In *infancy,* major problems generally involve the parents' reactions to the diagnosis and their difficulties coping with the feelings that follow from the child's failure to develop normally. The child's slow responsiveness and, in some cases, unusual appearance may interfere with mother-infant bonding. The mother's withdrawal, in turn, may lead to the sequelae of maternal deprivation, with resultant autoerotic play, infantile depression, and even greater defects in intellectual and language development. Continuing family pathology, including maternal depression, inconsistent care, rejection and hostility, and inhibition and fear may produce in the infant signs of emotional tension and/or developmental disorder including vomiting and spitting up, frequent episodes of infection and diarrhea, head banging, blanket and finger sucking, rocking, and sleep disturbances.

Delayed acquisition of skills such as walking, toilet training, and speech will interfere with the normal development of independence, separation-individuation, and a sense of mastery. It is crucial that parents have realistic expectations in order to avoid the extremes of hopelessness or unrealistic optimism and to prevent overprotection or overstimulation. At this point a satisfactory parent-child relationship may do much to keep the retarded child from developing a lifelong sense of low self-esteem and failure.

Parents who make excessive demands and rigidly seek to enforce them may do well with a retarded child who is basically passive, but a more aggressive child is likely to rebel. Resistance to discipline, refusal to conform, and rebellion are frequent responses to parental rejection expressed through excessive expectations or continued nonacceptance.

Infancy is the most crucial stage for counselors to work through with parents. Yet most studies indicate that this is the stage least successfully dealt with (Robinson and Robinson 1976). As a result, the mentally retarded tend to be more anxious than nonretarded children. Many have come to accept failure as a way of life and show excessive sensitivity to environmental cues, a high degree of defensiveness, or denial of their incapacity.

In most *preschool* and some *older children,* family complaints center on hyperkinetic and undisciplined behavior often associated with a short attention span, lack of concentration, and distractibility. Such children require almost constant supervision, and their short attention span causes much difficulty and frustration for those trying to teach them to control their behavior and respond to discipline. Some parents are left feeling hopeless and overwhelmed by the child's hyperactivity, which fortunately often seems to settle gradually as the child enters adolescence (see chapter 10).

The moderately or severely retarded school-age child may have to remain at home under continuous parental supervision. This may further intensify parental frustration and increase the child's sense of isolation and unworthiness. Some are fortunate to be enrolled in a special nursery with other retarded youngsters. In a regular school, the retarded child may be shunned and teased by peers and forbidden to play with other children.

As retarded children of higher ability grow older, they sense the gap between themselves and normal children. This often results in their feeling different and developing a poor self-image. In the community, retarded children make friends with children of their own intellectual age who are chronologically younger, but within a year or two, they have been surpassed in their development, leaving them to find new friends within an even younger age group. This pattern, repeated over the years, frequently ends in their giving up even trying to make friends in the community and restricting their friendships to family or special school, where they are associated with the same children over a period of years. This may be a source of great concern to parents sensitive to the loneliness and isolation of their children.

In spite of their increased need for group identification, socialization, vocational choice, and separation from parents, retarded *adolescents,* may become even more dependent on their parents and fearful of their sexual and aggressive impulses. Alternatively they may handle their frustrations through increased aggressivity, sexual indulgence, or delinquent behavior. If their sexual impulses are met by parental fear, dread, disgust, or panic, the adolescents are more likely to indulge in irresponsible behavior.

Mildly retarded youngsters who learn slowly and are poor in language and communication skills fall behind in school. This results in absenteeism, immature and impulsive behavior, lack of motivation, and a variety of other emotional disturbances that stem from their sense of rejection and their confrontation with their academic limitations. These may be compounded by the likelihood of their living in psychosocially disadvantaged families, in which case the emotional energy of coping with harsh family and economic realities may lead to apathy, distrust, and suspicion.

Because they have learned to distrust their own resources, retarded children and adults look to adults and normal peers when they encounter challenges. Adults who are retarded value conformity and are more likely to be helpful and cooperative than to be independent and competitive (Severy and Davis 1971). The older retarded person, well aware of his or her intellectual handicap, may continue to deny, become defensive, or even to develop fantasies to cover up deficiencies in an attempt to hide behind a "cloak of invisibility" (Edgerton 1967).

There is a misconception that emotional disorder in the retarded is different from that seen in children of average intelligence. It is true that there is a higher incidence of behavioral disturbance among the mentally retarded than in the general population (Beier 1964). But the same gamut of psychopathology occurring in children of average intelligence is also seen in mentally retarded children, including transient, psychoneurotic, character, personality, psychophysiological, and psychotic disorders (Philips 1967). With increasing age and higher intelligence, there is increased clarity of definition of the behavioral disturbance. Conversion, anxiety, and obsessive-compulsive disorders are the most frequent psychoneuroses in the retarded (Beier 1964). Depression is diagnosed less frequently than in those of normal intelligence, although it may present in masked form. Schizophrenia is the most frequent major psychosis, with the affective psychoses occurring much less frequently than in the normal population. Episodes of psychotic excitement seem more common in the retarded population (Beier 1964). There also seems to be an increased incidence of attention deficit disorder, with hyperactivity occurring in 5 to 10 percent of mentally retarded schoolboys, a rate significantly higher than in the normal, non–brain-damaged population.

The presence or absence of behavioral disturbance complicating mental retardation is important, since this is the most frequent cause of institutionalization. This higher incidence of behavioral disturbance in the retarded may be associated with the disturbed interpersonal relationships described earlier, or there may be an expectation of psychopathology by the caregivers. Mentally retarded children may behave in ways that in a normal child of the same mental age would not be considered pathological. For example, repetitive motor activity, which occurs frequently in younger children, may be considered "hyperactive" in an older retarded child (Kugel, Trembath, and Sagar 1968).

The same factors that produce criminal or antisocial behavior in the general population may also produce delinquency and criminality in the retarded. Particularly in the more severely, institutionalized retarded, there is, however, an increased capacity for aggressive and violent behavior. Lack of verbal communication skills aggravated by developmental and interpersonal problems may lead to a decreased frustration tolerance. Criminal populations exhibit a higher incidence of mental retardation, varying from 3 to 24 percent in some jurisdictions (Eyman and Padd 1980). The retarded are less efficient criminals; they may be poorly represented by counsel, are more likely to plead guilty, and are less likely to be examined for competence to stand trial. They are also more likely to confess to crimes, whether or not they committed them. The retarded also serve about twice as much time in prison as do nonretarded inmates (Brown and Courtless 1971), a reflection of their continuing second-class status.

When it comes to sexual behavior, society demands of the retarded a standard of conduct not observed in society as a whole. A common reason in the past for institutionalization of retarded boys between eleven and twenty years of age was homosexuality. Promiscuity commonly led to the institutionization of mildly retarded girls. By themselves, neither of these activities in someone of normal intelligence would provide sufficient reason for segregating the individual from family and society. One must assume that the fear of producing further retarded children by parents who cannot provide for them lies behind this concern.

Most studies of sexual activity in the retarded deal with those in institutions and therefore can provide only indirect conclusions about the mentally retarded population as a whole. In institutions, retarded children are involved in more homosexual and less heterosexual play than are prepubertal children of normal intelligence. This is probably associated with delayed psychosexual development and less opportunity for heterosexual play. There is also a higher incidence of homosexual play and fantasies in older age groups. In institutions, the retarded are less responsive to psychological and visual erotic stimuli. The moderate and severely retarded participate in less heterosexual, homosexual, and autoerotic activity but have more nocturnal emissions than the mildly retarded. Rape by the mentally retarded is rare (Kugel, Trembath, and Sagar 1968).

Successful marriages of retarded adults parallel those of adults of normal intelligence in regard to number of children, adequacy of income, marital relationship, and, particularly, the mental health of the mother. Usually a mildly retarded woman marries a somewhat brighter man. In one large-scale study, the average number of children in such marriages was only slightly higher than that in the normal population (Scally 1973). With additional external child care assistance, the average intelligence of the children was higher than that of both parents—that is, approaching normal—an example of the psychometric principle of reversion to the mean. None of the children had committed offenses, and most were growing up in a loving, caring environment (Scally 1973). There are no studies indicating a higher incidence of child abuse or neglect by retarded parents.

Retarded individuals should not be sterilized merely because they are retarded. The myths and individual case examples of genetic transmission, excessive fertility, or inability to parent cannot be generalized to the whole group. While there may be special indications for such sterilizations, they should occur only after there has been a multidisciplinary determination that less restrictive alternatives are not viable. Legal protection of the rights of the retarded is currently required in most provinces in Canada, although compulsory sterilization laws remain in several American states. Much of the concern around this issue would be diminished with adequate sex education for both the retarded and their families (Goldberg 1979).

Severely retarded children and adults, particularly within institutions, may demonstrate repetitive, stereotyped behavior. These are more common in blind nonambulatory retardates and may range from forms of self-stimulation to self-mutilation or self-injurious behaviors including head banging, eye gouging, biting, and rectal digging. They may become severe enough to lead to fatalities. Although self-mutilation occurs in normal children before age three, the normal child finds other types of attention-seeking behavior, while the severely handicapped child does not develop an expanded repertoire of rhythmic behaviors. In specific organic syndromes, such as the Lesch-Nyhan syndrome, this symptom may be prominent. Stereotyped behaviors may later develop into rituals or compulsive phenomena, such as turning light switches on and off, taking clothes off and on, or periodic noisiness. This type of behavior needs to be differentiated from early infantile autism or Gilles de la Tourette syndrome (see chapters 9 and 15).

Although it was stated earlier that affective psychosis or manic-depressive illness is rare in the retarded, these diagnoses may be difficult because of lack of verbalization of depressive mood. The diagnosis of depression may need to be considered in moderately or severely retarded individuals with cyclical mood changes every one to two months, or if apathy, irritability, eating, or sleep disorders are present (Reid 1980). The possibility of a superimposed dementia in older retarded patients, particularly those with Down's syndrome, should be considered.

Psychotherapeutic Management of the Mentally Retarded

Obstacles to psychodynamic involvement by professionals include the problems that the mentally retarded have with abstraction and communication skills needed for insight and dependency, and the evidence of the clear success of behaviorally oriented therapists. Professional bias ignores the importance of feelings of the retarded person. "Curing" retardation is not the goal; rather the aim is to ameliorate a complicating mental disturbance to permit the retarded person to live a more normal life (Szymanski 1980).

Psychotherapy with a retarded patient cannot be an isolated procedure. It must be accompanied by casework with the family or behavioral management within a residential center or school. Every experience, activity, and personal relationship should be regarded as having therapeutic potential. The patient is accepted as a worthy individual, permitted expression of feelings, taught emotional control through the provision of role models or specific, concrete standards for control. Self-confidence is enhanced by demonstrating success, which can be encouraged by training the retarded person to seek help when encountering obstacles or challenges.

Very young retarded children who are uncomfortable in a playroom may feel less anxious when given a concrete evidence of affection such as candy or physical contact. Structured play, such as with a doll family, may serve as a neutral "icebreaker" with the older, moderately retarded child. Play not only helps decrease anxiety but may also serve to teach communicative, motor, and social skills (Leland and Smith 1965).

The retarded patient particularly requires personal warmth from the therapist, along with a helpful attitude and frequent reassurance. Occasional misbehavior within the interview should be limited. Clear, simple, and concrete language and goals should be utilized to avoid criticism or confrontation. Phrases that can be used to motivate patients to utilize therapy include ones like "becoming happier," "troubles in learning." The therapist will need to be more directive with children of limited intelligence. This will include setting structure and limits and keeping the focus on relevant issues. While allowing an opportunity for the expression of feelings, the therapist should also lead the patient in the desired direction, periodically checking the patient's comprehension, since retarded patients sometimes try to conceal their lack of understanding. Fantasy material should be avoided. The patient's frustration tolerance can be improved by exposing him or her to gradually increasing degrees of frustration, while simultaneously engaging patients in tasks in which they are proficient. Long periods of silence are likely to be interpreted as rejecting and critical by retarded patients (Szymanski 1980).

Goal-directed or group psychotherapy for retarded adolescents can be helpful. The therapist must be active, serving as a bridge to reality, a teacher, a model for restraining impulses. This can help adolescents express their feelings about authority, grievances, running away, sexual concerns, dreams, future plans, cooperation, sharing, friends, peer interests, peer standards, peer personal traits. All of these may require specific advice by the therapist. Such techniques help patients learn to verbalize feelings rather than to act them out, while reversing self-depreciation and failure cycles (Slivkin and Bernstein 1968).

Behavior modification, based primarily on the operant conditioning model of Skinner as well as the classic conditioning theories of Pavlov and

Hull (Gardner 1970; Eyman and Padd 1980), attempts to alter human behavior by dealing systematically with the relationship between changes in the environment and in the subject's responses (see chapter 28). This technique has had a major impact in demonstrating that many of the behavioral limitations of the retarded come more from an inappropriate or limited learning environment than from a helpless/hopeless manifestation of the individual's retardation. Through the systematic application of such behavior modification techniques as positive shaping and time-out procedures for inappropriate behavior, even some of the severely and profoundly retarded can develop language, motor, perceptual, cognitive, affective, and social skills that can make possible a more worthwhile personal and social existence.

Types of behavior modification in which environmental activities and communication input are enriched and desirable behavior is positively reinforced are less controversial than: overcorrection (those procedures in which patients are required to repair destruction or to practice desirable behavior repetitively); confinement time-out (in which violent patients are isolated in a special room); and strongly aversive stimuli (such as shock-sticks used to decrease severe self-destructive responses). These punishment procedures, although controversial, have nonetheless demonstrated effectiveness in highly controlled circumstances, particularly for the control of severe and repeated self-mutilation that fails to respond to other forms of intervention. Token economy programs have been used with the mentally retarded. Each person receives a token (i.e., a reward) as an immediate reinforcement. Tokens can be exchanged later for snacks, toys, or privileges. Such programs have also been successful in improving classroom and vocational performance. Parents and siblings have also been utilized as behavior modifiers (Tarjan and Keeran 1974). Opponents of behavior modification criticize it on the grounds that it is restricting, controlling, manipulative, and punitive. On ethical grounds, such programs should be monitored to ensure that the least restrictive alternative is used.

The major and minor tranquilizers, sedatives, stimulants, antidepressants, and anti-Parkinsonian agents must be considered with special caution in treating the mentally retarded. Parents should be told that medication will not affect intelligence directly and that it can only control certain target symptoms, such as seizures, hyperactivity, or psychotic behavior. Drugs should not be the sole form of treatment, but rather one part of a comprehensive program that utilizes the assets, liabilities, and feelings of the children, parents, or caregivers. Drugs should never be used as a substitute for adequate programming. There are too many reports of excessive drug use, both in terms of numbers medicated and in duration and amount of dosage (Colodny and Kirlander 1970; Cytryn and Lourie 1967; Freeman 1970) on institutionalized children. Anticonvulsant medications may also be abused in the mentally retarded. Most require only one anticonvulsant drug. The conjoint use of anticonvulsants and psychotropic medication is usually ineffective and unnecessary (Tu 1981).

Retarded patients should have their medication explained to them in simple language. They should be told that the pill cannot make them learn better or please the family more or have better control of themselves, although the medication will make it easier for the child to accomplish these tasks. Unrealistic expectations should be avoided, and the children should be encouraged to take pride in what they have accomplished for themselves. "Just as we all sometimes overlook a retarded child's or adult's sorrow over his shortcomings, his shame and failures, his humiliation at his bad conduct, his discouragement at being himself, we may disregard his wish to be better, and the joy he feels when he can make some progress" (Colodny and Kurlander, 1970, p. 385).

SUGGESTIONS FOR FURTHER READING

CHESS, S., AND HASSIBI, M. 1970. Behavior deviations in mentally retarded children. *J. Amer. Acad. Child Psychiat.* 9:282–297.
An old but easy-to-read descriptive review of the clinical problems that mentally retarded children present with.
COLODNY, D., AND KURLANDER, L. F. 1970. Psychopharmacology as a treatment adjunct for the mentally retarded: Problems and issues. In *Psychiatric approaches to mental retardation,* ed. F. J. Menolascino, pp. 368–386. New York: Basic Books.
A practical guide to management.
CYTRYN, L., AND LOURIE, R. S. 1967. Mental retardation. In *Comprehensive textbook of psychiatry,* ed. A. M. Freedman and H. I. Kaplan, pp. 817–856. Baltimore: Williams & Wilkins.
A general overview. Includes history and social aspects of mental retardation. Discusses various causes and syndromes (with illustrations), the effects of mental retardation, its diagnosis and treatment.
FOTHERINGHAM, J. B.; SKELTON, M.; AND HODDINOTT, B. A. 1972. The effects on the family of the presence of a mentally retarded child. *Can. Psychiat. Assn. J.* 17:283–298.
An old but good description of the impact of mental retardation on the family. Describes the emotional phases that parents go through in their adjustment to having a mentally retarded child.
FREEMAN, R. D. 1970. Psychopharmacology and the retarded child. In *Psychiatric approaches to mental retardation,* ed. F. J. Menolascino, pp. 294–368. New York: Basic Books.
A good review of the use of psychopharmacotherapy for retarded children.
HANSEN, H.; BELMONT, L.; AND STEIN, Z. 1980. Epidemiology. In *Mental retardation and developmental disabilities: An annual review,* ed. J. Wortis, pp. 21–54. New York: Brunner/Mazel.
An up-to-date review concentrating on issues relevant to public health policy in developed countries. Contains interpretative reviews of studies of incidence and prevalence in mental retardation, a critical account of selected causes for which new evidence has accrued, and a general estimate of attributable risk to mental retardation of these causes at present. Intended to furnish a quantitative basis for those involved in planning for care and for prevention in mental retardation.
PASAMANICK, B., AND KNOBLOCH, H. 1966. Retrospective studies on the epidemiology of reproductive casualty: Old and new. *Merrill-Palmer Quart.* 12(1):7–26.

Discusses the epidemiology of reproductive casualties and its preventive implications.

ROBINSON, N. M. AND ROBINSON. H. B. 1976. The Mentally Retarded Child; A Psychological Approach. New York: McGraw-Hill Book Company (2nd edition).

One of the most comprehensive textbook in the field, dealing with etiology, syndromes, psychological development, psychotherapy, practical problems of retarded individuals and their families.

19

Saul Levine, Marshall Korenblum, and Harvey Golombek

Disorders Commonly Appearing First During Adolescence

Disorders of Identity (313.82)

Over the past several decades an increasing number of late adolescents and young adults have been experiencing and articulating considerable subjective distress focused mainly on problems surrounding their identity. Instead of arriving at a clear sense of their own identity and a workable educational and vocational plan for the future—what Erikson would term identity resolution—they remain unable to reconcile opposing interests and personality features into a coherent and acceptable sense of self. Instead these issues continue to be debated constantly—what Erikson terms identity diffusion—and the individual stagnates while peers begin moving ahead personally, scholastically, vocationally, and socially (Erikson 1968). Meanwhile those young people whose identity remains diffused have increasing difficulty making life decisions. Rather than regarding the future with enthusiasm and optimism, they experience apprehension and confusion over where they fit in academically, socially, and sexually. They exhaustively and painfully rehash values, tentative goals, career aspirations, and life-style decisions without achieving any resolution.

Accompanying this is a growing sense of alienation—feelings of not belonging, of lacking control over their immediate life or their destiny, and a sense of being isolated and alone. This leads to a creeping demoralization, pessimism, and a sense of futility and emptiness. Associated with these is low self-esteem. The individual feels too lacking in self-respect and confidence to be worthy of anything better (Levine 1982).

Identity diffusion must be differentiated from more serious conditions such as borderline states or affective or schizophreniform disorders. Some of the feelings just described may occur in these conditions, but their severity is much greater and the accompanying psychopathology stands in marked contrast to that of disorders of identity (American Psychiatric Association 1980*b*).

Some anxiety and depression do occur as part of an identity disorder, but they seldom become the predominant clinical feature. Occasionally the young person, in an attempt to find or define the self, acts impulsively—leaves home, quits school, abuses drugs or alcohol for a prolonged period. This rarely resolves the problems and often makes the situation worse.

Young people whose identity remains diffused are particularly susceptible to the seduction of intense communal belief systems such as cults, pop therapies, or political movements. These allow the individuals at least temporary relief from the alienation, demoralization, and low self-esteem that have been so distressing. They provide a powerful belief system, a meaning and coherence to life, a raison d'être, surrounding the young person with an intense, supportive, and receptive group sharing common ideals, goals, and values. In addition to providing a source of belief and belonging, they raise the young person's sense of self markedly and dramatically. This makes it very difficult to persuade someone to withdraw from a movement that provides such relief and a sense of purpose to a previously drifting soul (Levine 1979).

Identity diffusion, as just defined, represents one extreme of the normal adolescent process of questioning and modifying values, goals, and family relationships described in detail in chapter 2. This self-searching, frequently associated with brief periods of being "down" or confused, only becomes a disorder if the suffering is marked and prolonged (longer than six months), if confusion and indecision persist, if scholastic performance deteriorates, or if impulsive behavior begins to dominate the personality (Offer 1969; Rutter, Graham, and Chadwick 1976).

Just as individuals with identity diffusion are vulnerable to the lures of cults with charismatic leaders, they are also very accessible to support, constructive leadership, and therapeutic intervention. During this stage a mentor or older role model can have major influence on a young man or woman's current life and future development. Various forms of psychotherapy can be extremely helpful to the young person with an identity disorder, and in a relatively short time.

In psychotherapy the young people learn to see themselves in new perspectives, to confront their limitations, and to begin to appreciate their strengths. The therapy redirects and expedites the process of identity resolution that went awry. Yet psychotherapy with these adolescents is often but not always successful. Some are too disturbed to be helped readily; others have already committed themselves to choices that prevent a smooth return to family, friends, or school, but these are the exception. Most can be helped to resume happy, productive lives.

Borderline Personality Disorders (301.83)

The borderline syndrome is a personality disorder whose essential feature is "stable instability" in a variety of areas—interpersonal behavior, mood, and self-image. Patients with this disorder are like chameleons, appearing differently to different examiners at different times. But they are neither as sick as they look at their worst nor as healthy as they look at their best. What is distinctive is their ability to regress and reconstitute with astonishing ease (a quality not seen in other functional psychiatric conditions), the fact that their overall symptom pattern forms a stable core at the heart of the patient's long-term functioning, and the very multiplicity of their symptoms, which cut across the spectrum from neurotic to psychotic.

In North America this disorder is being diagnosed with increasing frequency in adolescents. Because so many borderline teenagers present with "existential crises" or severe identity diffusion, it is possible that the syndrome reflects the rising uncertainties and shifting values of modern society.

EPIDEMIOLOGY

The prevalence of this disorder is unknown, largely because standardized diagnostic criteria have become available only recently. It makes its clearest appearance in adolescence, occurring more frequently in females of all social classes.

CLINICAL PICTURE

Impulsive, angry, and confused—these are the key descriptive features of the borderline syndrome. The borderline population is heterogeneous; antisocial behavior, anorexia nervosa, school refusal, and some minimal brain damage may all be superimposed on an underlying borderline personality disorder. In fact, the term itself reflects early investigators' opinion that the syndrome lay on the "borderline" between psychosis and neurosis.

DSM-III has clarified the situation by providing the following operational diagnostic criteria: self-damaging impulsivity in at least two areas (spending, sex, drug abuse, over- or undereating, gambling); extreme mood changes; a pattern of unstable and inadequately controlled anger; identity disturbance (uncertainty regarding career goals, choice of friends, and gender identity); chronic feelings of emptiness/boredom; intolerance of being alone; physically self-damaging acts.

> S. was fifteen when she made her first suicide attempt. Bright, attractive but prone to uncontrollable outbursts of anger, she slashed her wrists after being jilted by a boyfriend. She made six further attempts over the next two years, each precipitated by a separation from or perceived rejection by someone close to her. At one point she thought she was a lesbian and frequently asked, "Who am I?" She was unpredictable, especially regarding her mood and choice of friends. She experimented with drugs (amphetamines) for six months.
>
> In therapy, she alternated between romantic love for and tremendous rage at her psychiatrist. Once she cowered in the corner of the office, apparently hearing voices, and accused the therapist of being a rapist who intended to kill her. As the end of the hour approached, however, she quickly "pulled herself together," stood up, and said, "Thanks, Doctor, see you next week." After four years of psychotherapy, she still had an unstable self-image but was living on her own, attending a university, and doing well. She had a steady boyfriend and had made no suicide attempts in two years, viewing that part of her life as "tempestuous and silly." Throughout her illness she had maintained good marks at school and worked successfully as a part-time waitress.

This case graphically illustrates how, despite a picture of severe disturbance, the borderline patient can continue to function at a high level in certain areas. This split between their public (school, work) and private (mood regulation, interpersonal relationships) selves is characteristic. It distinguishes them from psychotics who usually, if schizophrenic, function at uniformly low levels and from neurotics who function more consistently at high, albeit constricted, levels. Typical, in response to major stress, are transient periods of extreme decompensation and apparently psychotic behavior with loss of reality-testing followed by equally rapid reintegration, which Gunderson and Singer (1975) have referred to as micropsychotic episodes.

Anxiety attacks and multiple "neurotic" symptoms (obsessions, phobias) may also be present. These patients often confuse their own thoughts and feelings with those of others around them and use the defense of splitting, viewing events or others as well as themselves as either "all good" or "all bad." For them there is no gray area in between.

There are no specific physical or laboratory findings. The diagnosis is made on the basis of history, mental status examination, and reports of behavior from others. A series of interviews, with the family being seen as part of the assessment, is usually required.

The most common ancillary diagnostic tool is psychological testing. On structured tests, such as the Wechsler Adult Intelligence Scale

(WAIS)/Wechsler Intelligence Scale for Children (WISC), responses are generally normal. On unstructured ones, like the Rorschach, the results are often bizarre, sometimes resembling those of schizophrenics.

PATHOGENESIS

Multiple etiologic factors appear to contribute to the development of the borderline syndrome in an as-yet-unclear interaction between nature and nurture.

Early genetic studies emphasized the proximity of the disease to schizophrenia (Siever and Gunderson 1979; Wender 1977). More recently, however, studies using biological markers, follow-up studies, and new data on family pedigrees have suggested that the entity is closer to affective disorders (Stone 1979). This is supported by the positive response some borderlines show to antidepressant medication or lithium (Klein 1977). The fact that up to one-quarter of patients have histories of minimal brain dysfunction (now called "attention deficit disorder") also suggests that organic components are important (Andrulonis et al. 1981). Ten to 15 percent have had head trauma, encephalitis, or epilepsy, and some show signs of an "episodic dyscontrol syndrome"—outbursts of explosive rage with abnormal electroencephalograms (Andrulonis et al. 1981).

The families are pathological. They communicate more via actions than words. Unable to perceive borderline children as they are, the parents project their own conflicts onto them, relating to them in a distorted fashion that often reflects their own upbringing. This suggests a boundary disturbance (i.e., an inability to achieve and maintain a clear and stable distinction between self and nonself on the part of the parent) that interferes with that parent's ability to continue to see children as separate from him- or herself. As a result, the parent is unable to help or even allow the child to individuate, and the parental boundary defect is mirrored by a reciprocal defect in the child (Rinsley 1981). (See also chapter 3.) The mother may be unable to tolerate autonomy, and histories often show that the mother encouraged dependence when the child was in the separation-individuation stage (age one and one-half to two years). Fathers often neglect these children, creating a vacuum and depriving the child of an appropriate role model. Masterson (1972) has suggested that the core conflict is one between autonomy and dependency. Having had repeated experiences where moves toward autonomy were met with shaming and rejection, the young person is forced to choose between repudiating the normal drive toward independence in order to remain accepted and secure or continuing toward autonomy at the unbearable cost of badly needed acceptance and support. This dilemma, he suggests, is responsible for the basic core of emptiness and depression that resurfaces in adolescence, the accompanying rage, and the vulnerability to decompensation especially in response to separation. Many of the other symptoms he sees as the individual's pattern of defending against the core conflict and the feelings arising from it (Masterson 1980).

The relationship between borderline pathology in childhood and adolescence is unclear. Most patients have a curiously quiet latency. Upon reaching puberty, increased expectations of and demands for independence probably expose the latent vulnerability already described. Cognitive maturation (attaining "formal operations") is delayed or blocked, so the teenager's thinking remains egocentric and excessively concrete (Korenblum 1979). The marked awareness of personal inadequacies so typical of even normal adolescents may be a necessary precondition for the precipitation of the syndrome.

DIFFERENTIAL DIAGNOSIS

Because of the continuing lack of diagnostic clarity, it is important to carefully distinguish the borderline disorder from other psychiatric disorders. When the diagnosis is in doubt, possible alternatives to be ruled out include schizophrenia, primary affective disorder, other personality disorders, neurosis, and organic brain syndrome. A borderline disorder may develop in a child with a preexisting attention deficit disorder. DSM-III allows for multiple simultaneous diagnoses through its multiaxial approach.

Evaluating the degree of personality integration, the capacity for reality-testing, and the level of defenses used helps distinguish these conditions from borderline disorders. In each case, the borderline patient, while showing characteristic fluctuations, will occupy an intermediate position along these parameters.

MANAGEMENT

In keeping with the clinical and etiologic heterogeneity of the syndrome, treatment approaches vary considerably. In life-threatening situations such as suicide attempts, crisis intervention with brief hospitalization must be considered.

In the longer term, psychotherapy is the keystone of outpatient treatment. An initial phase of testing that requires limit-setting to control acting-out is usually followed by the working through of abandonment fears and, ultimately, by the patient's achieving the ability to live and function independently. Frequently individual therapy is combined with parental counseling or conjoint family therapy. Pharmacotherapy, behavior modification, and environmental manipulation can all be useful adjuncts at times, if they are indicated for the management of specific symptoms. Extended hospitalization and/or residential treatment is usually reserved for the more severe cases. Clearly, treatment programs must be individualized and based on a thorough assessment of the unique factors present in each patient's situation and background.

PROGNOSIS

Unfortunately, there are few systematic follow-up studies of border-line adolescents. According to one source (Masterson 1980), roughly 60 percent of patients show symptom reduction and improved achievement of independence, peer relations, and increased ability to cope emotionally and behaviorally following long-term hospital/milieu therapy followed up by psychoanalytically oriented individual psychotherapy. Positive prognostic factors include absence of early life stress, good premorbid social functioning, the ability to evaluate symptoms realistically, and motivation for outpatient therapy. Studies of borderline adults show that job performance can be quite good, though interpersonal relationships and mood regulation continue to present serious problems at times.

Since their maladaptive functioning can be so severe at times, border-line adolescents are better managed by psychiatrists familiar with their complexity than by primary physicians or nonmedical therapists. Otherwise these patients tend to trap well-meaning but inexperienced professionals into feeling so intensely responsible for them that the professionals feel totally accountable yet, at the same time, incapable of controlling their patients' demanding or outrageous behavior. Then when the professionals seek to extricate themselves from the no-win situation, either by a burst of personal anger or an attempt at withdrawal, the patients feel abandoned and precipitate another crisis that intensifies the caregiver's sense of responsibility, guilt, and entrapment.

CONCLUSION

The borderline syndrome is currently a fashionable diagnosis in North America. The uniqueness of the syndrome and its usefulness as a diagnosis are being vigorously debated, as is the justification of the resources required to treat these patients when clear verification of the value of psychotherapy for this condition is not yet proven.

Nevertheless, the term encompasses a frequently seen constellation of personality factors and manifest behaviors. Its clinical manifestations may vary, but its core features—extreme instability and changability of functioning in the context of intense anger, poor impulse control, and severe identity disturbances—are actually stable and form part of the patient's long-term life pattern. Hopefully, researchers and clinicians will rise to the challenge and proceed to clarify the various unresolved theoretical questions and management issues that have made the borderline syndrome the subject of such ongoing dispute.

Anorexia Nervosa (307.10)

Anorexia nervosa is a unique syndrome, not only because its onset is specific to adolescence but because of the anorexic's stated aim of self-preservation through voluntary weight loss, sometimes to the point of death. Case reports date as far back as 1689, but it was not until the 1870s that Sir William Gull gave the syndrome its name which, unfortunately, is somewhat of a misnomer since anorexia is neither a necessary nor a constant feature of the disease (Gull 1974).

The syndrome's defining characteristics are the relentless pursuit of thinness and an intense fear of becoming obese. Other diagnostic criteria include: a disturbance of body image (claiming to feel fat even when emaciated); loss of at least 25 percent of original body weight; refusal to maintain weight over minimal norms for age and height; absence of physical illness to account for the weight loss; onset under twenty-five years of age; and amenorrhea (American Psychiatric Association 1980*a*).

EPIDEMIOLOGY

Anorexia nervosa is primarily a disease of middle- and upper-class adolescent females. Only 5 to 10 percent of patients are male. The age of onset is usually between twelve and eighteen years. The incidence may be as high as 1 per 200 high school girls, and in the last decade the condition has become even more widespread (Crisp et al. 1976). In certain subgroups such as ballet students, the rate has been reported as at least ten times as high as in the general population (Garner and Garfinkel 1978).

CLINICAL PICTURE

Anorexia nervosa is probably not a homogeneous entity. Two groups have now been identified—restricters, who lose weight solely by dieting, and bulimics (307.51), who binge-eat and then vomit or use laxatives to become thin (Garfinkel, Moldofsky, and Garner 1980). This latter group is more extroverted, sexually active, and impulsive than the restricters. The bulimics are also more likely to have a family and personal history of obesity, and a poorer prognosis. Bulimia can occur in the absence of anorexia, in which case the weight can remain normal or nearly so.

Most anorexics, however, share certain symptom clusters: (Bruch 1973).

1. Food related: preoccupation with food and bizarre eating behaviors (food fads, hiding food, and enthusiastically cooking for others).
2. Perceptual disturbances: overestimation of body size, denial of thinness, lack of awareness or denial of hunger, and early satiety.
3. Behavioral: hyperactivity.
4. Cognitive: poor concentration, magical thinking, all-or-nothing logic, egocentrism, and a sense of ineffectiveness and powerlessness associated with an intense preoccupation with gaining control over themselves.
5. Biological: amenorrhea (which may precede weight loss in up to one-third of the cases), constipation, and insomnia.
6. Affective: irritability, anxiety, lability, depression, or inability to identify feeling states (which may resemble *la belle indifference*).
7. Social: withdrawal or highly ambivalent relationships with others.

Physical findings are largely related to the degree of starvation. Slow heart rate, low blood pressure, and a carotene-pigmented skin may all be present. Laboratory tests often reveal a decreased number of white blood cells and a decreased sedimentation rate. The blood urea nitrogen level depends on the state of hydration. Low serum potassium levels occur in bulimics who use purgatives. Low fasting blood sugar, normal or decreased thyroxine and triiodothyronine levels, elevated growth hormone levels, activation of the hypothalamic-adrenal axis, and suppression of the hypothalamic-ovarian axis are associated findings (Halmi 1981). All of these abnormalities are reversible upon the restoration of weight, except for the secretion of the hormones that regulate menstruation (i.e., follicle-stimulating and luteinizing hormones), which may lag behind.

PATHOGENESIS

The specific etiology of anorexia nervosa is unknown. Its probable pathogenesis is hypothesized in terms of multiple predisposing and precipitating factors.

Genetic studies suggest a hereditary predisposition, and family histories are often positive for eating disorders, (Garfinkel 1981), but the relative contributions of nature and nurture remain undetermined because studies on siblings raised in different environments have not been done (Halmi and Brodland 1973). There is also tentative evidence of hypothalamic dysfunction (Garfinkel et al. 1975), but no lesion has ever been found, and the effects of nonspecific factors have not been teased out.

Sociocultural factors, such as the ubiquitous emphasis on thinness as an ideal for females, are important (Garner and Garfinkel 1978). Anorexia may represent an attempt to take over internal control of the self in the context of a family or society that cannot tolerate or support this (Bruch 1973; Selvini 1974). Some argue that psychological conflicts centering around the struggle to internalize control, and the regressive and self-destructive use of that control, once achieved, represent the nuclear problem of which the aversion to food is but a symptom (Bruch 1973;

Selvini 1974). Many authors feel that disturbed family relationships represent an important, if not an essential, predisposing factor (Minuchin et al. 1978). Even those who disagree concede that once the condition is well established, characteristic patterns of pathological family interaction develop. These can prove devastating to family members, who are openly consumed with anxiety, resentment, depression, and guilt, and to the anorexic, whose control of the family in defense of the symptom may leave her as depleted of emotional support as she is of food.

Minuchin has described the families of anorexics as rigid, enmeshed, and frequently overprotective (Minuchin et al. 1975). The enmeshment, usually between mother and anorexic although both parents may be involved, is frequently associated with an emotional disengagement between husband and wife. The mother may also have somehow interfered with the anorexic's developing the ability to recognize hunger and satiety by responding inappropriately to the patient when she was very young (Bruch 1977).

During middle childhood, these often overly compliant, "perfect" children fail to show the exploratory behaviors, the growing sense of autonomy and self, and the social skills appropriate to their age (Goodsitt 1977). This in turn reinforces the enmeshment. Since these families often experience considerable latent rage but have great difficulty tolerating the direct and open expression of anger, their children develop strong psychological defenses favoring the repression and introjection of rage (Minuchin et al. 1978). This latent defect is activated in adolescence, presumably by hormonally induced body changes and socially reinforced pressure toward sexuality and independence. In the face of this threat the youngster, who is prepared for neither, regresses emotionally and cognitively. The latent defect in the autonomy/control area is activated and, for some reason, the taking in and spitting out of food becomes the battleground on which the struggle for control is primarily fought. Other secondary benefits may be afforded by the condition, however. Depending on the needs of the individual patient, anorexia may provide immense power and control over the family; a way of punishing ambivalently loved parents; a method of dealing with internalized rage and depression; a way to safely avoid many of the unwanted opportunities for independence commonly associated with adolescence for which this particular adolescent feels unprepared, such as expanding social and sexual activities; high parental expectations; the search for an independent identity. The final precipitant is often an environmental event that further stresses the patient's psychological vulnerability—for example, the loss of a boyfriend or girl friend; a first sexual encounter; a separation from the family; some teasing about weight, physical development, or bodily proportions.

These psychological and familial factors, while commonly present, constitute only a part of the total picture. The cognitive defects (i.e., distorted body image and distorted ideation in the area of control) and the

423

physiological sequelae of starvation (Walsh 1980), including hypothalamic malfunctioning, decrease in intestinal hormones and stomach size that cause true anorexia and postprandial bloating, irritability, and insomnia, do much to perpetuate the condition once established, even in the patient who is trying to eat. Similarly the amenorrhoea, smaller breasts, and weight loss allow the patient to avoid essential areas of psychological conflict and provide an illusion of increased self-control.

DIFFERENTIAL DIAGNOSIS

Physical conditions that can mimic the syndrome include hypothalamic tumors, anterior pituitary insufficiency, Addison's disease, hypo/-hyperthyroidism, and occult cancer.

Psychiatrically, anorexia must be differentiated primarily from schizophrenia and depression. Paranoid delusions in the former can cause a voluntary restriction of food intake. A psychotic agitated depression can produce many of the same signs and symptoms as anorexia, but the prominence of the disturbed mood helps to distinguish the two. Anorexia occuring in the course of these illnesses is often called secondary anorexia nervosa, and DSM-III, in these cases, suggests that two diagnoses be given.

MANAGEMENT

The initial approach involves ruling out other biological and psychological causes of weight loss. This requires a proper functional inquiry, physical examination, and appropriate lab tests on the one hand, and a complete psychiatric history including mental status examination and family interview on the other.

Once the diagnosis of primary anorexia nervosa has been established, the short-term management is first concerned with whether or not hospitalization is needed (Russel 1977). This is indicated if the patient's medical or psychological condition is life threatening and/or if outpatient treatment has failed or cannot be implemented.

Anorexic patients can be extremely difficult, provocative, and disruptive on a pediatric or medical ward not experienced in caring for them. They often evoke extreme anxiety and rage in the staff by their refusal to cooperate and by the manipulations they use to avoid weight gain. Unless ward staff remain acutely aware of their subjective reactions to the patient, there is real danger of their retaliating punitively by rejecting them, by forcing feedings when these are not medically indicated, or by other forms of unrecognized attack. The key to successful hospital management consists of avoiding getting caught up in power struggles around food or eating on the patient's terms. The patient should be weighed regularly and given the responsibility for gaining weight at a prescribed but gradual rate. If tube feeding is medically required, it is undertaken automatically and in a matter-of-fact manner. Attempts are made to establish relationships with the patient, and, when she is sufficiently beyond the effects of starvation to tolerate this, psychotherapy can be initiated in an attempt to help her begin examining the emotional, cognitive, familial, and social difficulties that underlie preoccupation with eating.

There are two main approaches to management of anorexia nervosa. Some authors recommend behavior modification and dietary counseling (Halmi and Larson 1977), while others consider the short-term gain more than offset by the patient's reaction to having control taken out of her hands (Bruch 1973, 1977). Some settings attempt to avoid this by dividing the responsibility for care between two physicians. The family doctor or pediatrician is responsible for physical care, while a psychiatrist or other mental health professional deals with the psychological component of the treatment. This may help the therapist avoid getting caught up in struggles around eating on the patient's terms, but it is not without its drawbacks. Issues of cognitive and emotional significance can be stirred up by weigh-ins. The experienced therapist who can use these productively while still avoiding a struggle on the patient's terms may find taking total charge of the case advantageous. For example, once the patient recognizes that she has lost control of her weight, she may find it helpful to have the therapist take control of it for her. In view of the excessively concrete and at times magical thinking that these patients show, it often helps to set limits within a range (e.g., "If your weight drops to between eighty-five and ninety pounds, we may have to consider . . ." rather than "If your weight goes below the eighty-five-pound mark, then we will automatically . . ."). This further takes the weight issue out of the patient's hands, placing it in the hands of the therapist. As the patient begins to do better, greater freedom of choice and activity is handed over in a steplike manner, so that self-control is increasingly handed by the therapist to the patient as she shows her readiness for it. If control is split between psychotherapist and pediatrician or primary physician, whoever takes responsibility for the weigh-ins should recognize and utilize their psychological impact, and good and regular communication between physician and psychotherapist is essential. For outpatients, it may be important to have the family throw away its scales and have the patient weighed only in the doctor's office.

Long-term management is aimed at maintaining appropriate weight and ameliorating those factors that contributed to the development and perpetuation of the illness. In less severe cases, a consistent relationship with a family physician may prove sufficient. Education, support, reality-testing, and allowing ventilation of fears of growing up are the hallmarks of such a relationship. Those who do not respond to such an approach may need referral to a psychiatrist. Treatment is then individualized, often combining individual psychotherapy, family therapy, and environmental manipulation in order to address the multifactorial pathogenesis. Younger adolescents show more problems in their family relationships, while in older patients the internalized (psychological) aspects of the problem predominate.

OUTCOME

The prognosis is mixed. Three quarters of patients are able to regain their normal weight. A similar number, however, retain a disturbed body image and morbid attitude toward eating for years afterward. At least 25 percent may remain amenorrheic for some time despite weight restoration (Hsu 1980). Their work histories are generally good but their interpersonal relationships are poor and psychiatric morbidity, in the form of depression, obsessionality, and social anxiety, commonly persists. Although the initial normalization of weight is usually successful, this does not necessarily ensure freedom from relapse. Older age at onset, long duration of illness, and the presence of bulimia are poor prognostic indicators (Crisp 1981). The mortality rate is 5 to 10 percent, with death usually due to electrolyte disturbance or suicide (Hsu 1980).

CONCLUSION

Anorexia nervosa is a complicated and sometimes tragic illness. Pleasant, high-achieving, "no-problem" children become oppositional, defiant, self-starving adolescents. They fast in an attempt to gain a greater sense of control but end up losing control over themselves or, in response to their distorted body image and persistent somatic delusions, use that control to destroy themselves. Their bodies push them in one direction—maturity—while their minds pull them in another—back to the comfort of childhood.

If the incidence of this syndrome is to decrease, research efforts ought to shift from secondary to primary prevention. This may require a greater understanding of normal adolescence and a joining of forces with our colleagues in the sociological fields toward a greater understanding of the developmental stresses of coping with modern society.

Substance Abuse

Throughout the history of man, drug use has permeated all societies and all age groups and is a firm and accepted part of our culture. Ours is a drug-oriented society. People of all ages utilize a variety of prescription and nonprescription chemicals to alter symptoms, feelings, moods, or mind-states. "Drug or substance abuse" refers to taking drugs in a way that is organically or psychologically destructive, either because of the nature of the drug or the quantity consumed. The term abuse, unfortunately, has been used pejoratively at times to criticize any drug use that is threatening, for real or imagined reasons, to the dominant society and its mores. Drug abuse is not restricted to contemporary youth. The distinguishing feature between the generations in our society is that each has its "own" favorites. Alcohol, nicotine, tranquilizers, sedatives, stimulants, and pain relievers—traditional drugs—are as susceptible to abuse as the drugs more commonly favored by the younger generation.

The drug scene is not static. It changes markedly and unpredictably, often within weeks and months. Even in times of relative quiescence and stability, a sizable proportion of high school and college students experiment occasionally with "illicit," chemical, mind-altering substances. If alcohol and nicotine are included, the percentage of young people who utilize drugs at least occasionally exceeds 90 percent. This is not to say that anyone who ever uses drugs has a problem. Before a psychiatric or medical label is affixed, one should know a number of facts about the user and the particular drug.

The User Mental health professionals should learn about the user as a person, not merely as a drug-swallowing machine. How successfully is the user handling major life areas? How does he get along with his family? If she is no longer living at home, was leaving the family painful and chaotic, or natural? Are there friends, and what is the quality and stability of the friendships? How comfortable and successful are his relationships with girls, or hers with boys? How does each user respond to authority? Is she responsible and productive in work and school performance? What can be learned about his moods, his energy level, his interests, his feelings and how he handles them? What are the user's ideas, values, and aspirations? Does the user have a goal and direction in life, or is life one of aimless drifting or erratic changes of direction? What role do drugs play in her life and in the lives of friends? Why do they use drugs, and what do they feel drugs do for them?

The Substance. In assessing the extent of a "drug problem," the substance —the exact drug or drugs being utilized—should be known. This may involve chemical analysis, since street samples are notoriously prone to adulteration. Aside from the specific substance, it should be determined how long the individual has used the particular drug, in what dosage, by which method (ingestion—"popping"; intravenously—"cranking, shooting, hitting"; nasally—"snorting"; etc.) and with what frequency. What other drugs have been used, and how old was the user at the onset of drug use? In addition, an attempt should be made to determine the social context of the drug taking—alone or with friends, at home or outside, and so forth. Where does the user get the supply—from friends, underworld, peer-group dealers? How was he or she involved initially?

Most young people who use drugs do so only occasionally and not because of serious psychopathology, utilizing minor substances (e.g., marijuana) with no ill effects. Further, often when drugs are abused, the abuse is symptomatic of other, more significant problems. Indeed, in most cases where drug abuse and serious emotional problems coexist, the emotional difficulties preceded the drug use. Using any substance to excess can denote psychological problems. The specific chemical chosen is but one of the variables to be considered.

REASONS FOR DRUG USE

There are almost as many reasons for drug use as there are drugs. These reasons can be divided roughly into social and personal categories.

Social Factors Contributing to Drug Use

Pressure of Living in Contemporary Society. Few people are immune to the effects of rapid change on tradition, lifestyle, stability, and predictability. All industrialized societies are showing the effects of rampant technological growth, often associated with a blind push toward materialistic acquisition or expansion, without sufficient concern for the quality of life. The population explosion is a source of concern, especially in view of the earth's limited resources and deteriorating ecological environment. The intact, cohesive, extended family is much less common than in the past, and we may be witnessing the demise of the nuclear family (see chapter 5). At the very least, the stresses on it are enormous. There is a growing feeling of alienation in crowded, dehumanizing environments, which increases when the pace of life exceeds thresholds tolerable for physical or emotional health. People of all ages, not only youth, are reacting to these multiple pressures by searching for relief of some kind. Drugs offer, temporarily at least, the illusion of such relief.

Cultural Ethic. Chemicals have been used for mind alteration for centuries, but never has there been such public and media preoccupation with drug use. Never have so many substances, both legal and illicit, been available. The ongoing redefinition of the work ethic and the increasing trends toward narcissism and hedonism as more acceptable alternatives make experimentation with drugs difficult to prohibit.

There is also a well-defined counterculture made up in part by those who have rejected the pressures, uncertainties, conventions, and hypocrisies of the outer world by turning inward and emphasizing the subjective experience, which is elaborated on at times to a point that approaches the mystical. This has generated its own art, literature, and music, much of it philosophically committed to the principle of pharmacological mind alteration and "consciousness expansion." Within this subculture, certain groups value "tripping," putting pressure on those who wish acceptance to join in these activities.

428

Personal Factors Relating to Drug Use

An individual motivational state cannot be categorized merely on the basis of drug use or abuse. Those who use drugs do so for their own reasons, some of which will be listed. While any of these reasons may stem from psychological problems, the last four are more usually associated with emotional disturbance. Reasons for drug use include:

1. *Intellectual curiosity.* Some adolescents use drugs to experiment and try out new experiences in order "to see what it's like."
2. *Recreation.* Many youth "light up a joint" just as many adults take a drink at a cocktail party, as their way of enhancing the social experience.
3. *Ignorance.* This includes situations in which drugs are "slipped" to an individual or ones in which the individual is unaware of the implications of particular drug use.
4. *Philosophy.* Some individuals use drugs for consciousness expansion or in the search for truth, in keeping with their or others' theoretical rationale.
5. *Ritual.* Here drugs are used to provide a mystical experience, which at times may have religious implications.
6. *Self-awareness.* Some adolescents attempt to achieve an understanding or resolution of recognized personal problems by trying to increase their self-awareness or to free themselves emotionally through drug use.
7. *Rebellion.* For some adolescents, parental or societal prohibitions make the taking of illicit or illegal drugs even more attractive. In such cases, the drug use is an acting-out of feelings of resentment against authority.
8. *Escape.* Some use drugs to find relief from intolerable real or imagined stresses or situations. The drug is used in an unrealistic attempt to discover a personal utopia or to avoid personal problems.
9. *Compulsiveness.* With some drugs (alcohol, heroin, etc.) true addiction can occur. The compulsive reliance on even nonaddictive drugs to meet neurotic needs may reach the point of psychological dependence (habituation).
10. *Self-destructiveness.* The repeated use of drugs in spite of knowledge of their potential danger may represent either a conscious or an unrecognized suicide attempt or equivalent.

THE DRUGS

The following is a brief review of the various substances under discussion. Technical terms used are defined later on pages 432–433. For more information, refer to those works listed in the suggestions for further reading.

Alcohol (303.00)

Alcohol abuse is by far the greatest drug problem in our society, both in its frequency and in the short- and long-term deleterious physical, emotional, social, and economic effects of alcoholism (Vista Hill Foundation 1982). Social encouragement through advertising makes alcohol attractive to those most susceptible to irresponsible use. Alcohol is addictive and dangerous, leading to physical dependence, tolerance, and withdrawal symptoms in response to abstinence. Alcohol is more widely used and abused than any of the drugs about which our society is much more concerned.

Marijuana and Hashish (305.20)

Marijuana and hashish are the second most popular intoxicants among high school and college students, although their use seems to have leveled off. They do not cause physical dependence, and no significant tolerance is developed. Increasing reports have suggested deleterious organic effects after prolonged usage (Cohen 1981). Marijuana is not particularly associated with crime or violence, but the "amotivational syndrome" in chronic users has caused concern (Dupont, Goldstein, and O'Donnell 1979). As serious as the possible direct effects of the drug are the legal consequences, which involve a criminal record in many jurisdictions.

Heroin (and Other Opiates) (305.50)

While less commonly used by this age group, the proportion of users of heroin and other opiates who become dependent is high. Although increasingly common among middle-class youth, heroin still appeals primarily to relatively socioeconomically deprived young males. While they frequently use minor crimes to support their habit, most addicts have a history of antisocial behavior preceding their opiate use but are associated with violent crime less frequently than alcohol or amphetamine users. The best forms of therapy thus far include (1) replacement medication (Methadone); (2) time spent in a treatment milieu; or (3) medical dispensation of opiates. Methadone treatment is not without danger. Methadone is more highly addictive than heroin and should be reserved for true addicts under strict controls (Lowinson and Ruiz, 1981). Milieu therapy involves intense confrontation in the context of a belief system bordering on the religious (Cohen 1981). The medical dispensation of opiates is a British form of treatment not permitted in North America.

Barbiturates (Long- or Short-Acting) (305.40)

Barbiturates (downers) are addictive substances, dangerous and ubiquitous. Their increasing use is due partly to the frequency with which they are prescribed by physicians as sedatives. Barbiturates are frequently used in suicide attempts and completions. There is cross-dependence and potentiation with many other drugs, especially alcohol. An extremely strong psychic dependency develops in addition to a true (physiological) addiction. Though they are primarily central nervous system depressants, barbiturates are often associated with violence, since initially they lessen behavioral inhibitions.

Methaqualone

Introduced as a sedative in the late 1960s and widely known by the trade name Quaaludes, this drug gained notoriety in the 1970s among college students for its hypnotic and supposed aphrodisiac qualities, especially when ingested with other central nervous system depressants. Users describe a loss of physical and mental self and a euphoria associated with ataxia and paresthesia of the arms, fingers, lips, and tongue. Other effects include an increased pain threshhold and a sense of indestructibility that can lead to physical accidents (Ager 1972). Reported similarities between methaqualone and opiates make it an attractive substitute for heroin.

Methaqualone was originally prescribed as a sedative because it was nonbarbiturate and thought to be nonaddictive, but this is not true of the current methaqualone, which is both psychologically and physically addictive. A tolerance to the drug develops, so that the quantity required to get high increases and approaches the lethal dose (Pascarelli 1973). Overdose victims and those attempting abrupt withdrawal face serious complications (*Journal of the American Medical Association* 1973; Pascarelli 1973; Swartzberg, Lieb, and Schwartz 1973).

Amphetamines (327.30)

Amphetamine abuse varies from time to time and place to place. Many governments strictly control amphetamine use and have successfully curtailed middle-class abuse by stopping doctors from prescribing it for the "wrong" reasons (obesity, depression, fatigue). Strong psychological dependence often develops, although there is no evidence of physical dependence. Chronic use, especially intravenously, is particularly debilitating and associated with cachexia, intercurrent infections, exhaustion, depression, paranoid tendencies, and violence that may reach psychotic proportions.

LSD and Other Hallucinogens (327.56)

Use of the hallucinogens such as LSD, MDA, STP, mescaline, peyote, psilocybin, DMT, and so forth, largely by middle-class senior high school and university students, seems to have peaked. Hallucinogens have been employed mainly for self-exploration or experiencing a psychedelic "high." Occasional use is more common than habitual use even among "heads" (habitual users). There is little evidence of true dependence, and those who do become habitual users show evidence of obvious disturbance before taking hallucinogens. Hallucinogens can produce drug-induced panic, which can precipitate a psychosis or suicide attempt or, rarely, toxic reactions. There is a great deal of unresolved controversy—and ignorance—regarding the long-term effects (psychological, physical, and genetic) of their prolonged use.

Solvents (327.90)

A "high" or disorientating effect is achieved by inhaling ("sniffing") glue, gasoline, and nail-polish remover, often by placing a plastic bag containing the inhalant over the nose to obtain a higher concentration. Their use is largely restricted to lower-class youngsters between the ages of eleven and fourteen. Repeated inhalation can cause brain and liver damage, toxic delirium, and an acute brain syndrome. The frequency of abuse waxes and wanes periodically. Strict controls and the addition of odoriferous chemicals to solvents are important preventive procedures.

Tobacco (327.71)

Nicotine is found in all cigarette tobacco. Psychic dependency rapidly develops, and physical dependence (addiction) occurs in many smokers. The most pernicious physical effects (lung cancer, arteriosclerotic changes, etc.) are caused by the inhalation of smoke, with or without nicotine. In spite of extensive advertising about the dangers inherent in smoking, the incidence of smoking in adolescents is steadily increasing, and the drug has effects on the next generation through its effect on birth weight (see pages 19 and 395–396).

"Legal" Tranquilizers, Sedatives, Stimulants

These drugs are mainly abused by adults (users) and doctors who overprescribe them (their "pushers"), though many drugs do not accomplish their desired effect. Of late, some (especially diazepam) have been used increasingly by adolescents with or without alcohol to achieve a unique type of "high," a dully "stoned" feeling, not entirely pleasant. Much stricter controls, and more judicious prescriptions, are in order.

POTENTIAL DELETERIOUS EFFECTS OF INJUDICIOUS DRUG USE AND USER
TERMINOLOGY

Bad trip refers to a sense of personal discomfort—fear, anxiety, depression, mild confusion, and so forth—while under the influence of drugs. Calm but firm guidance in a quiet room along with minor tranquilizers can usually "bring the tripper down."

Freak out refers to varying degrees of psychological decompensation, which may unleash an acute psychosis with its attendant loose cognitive associations, inappropriate affect (often panic), feelings of derealization and depersonalization, lack of insight, poor judgment, disorientation. There is a continuum ranging from moderate confusion all the way to an acute brain syndrome. Hospitalization may be necessary, and psychotropic medication is indicated, but the exact drug taken must be known as the wrong medication may prove harmful. Determination of the drug ingested is sometimes complicated, since street samples are frequently adulterated with other chemicals. The emergency use of chlorpromazine in youngsters with drug-induced psychoses is contraindicated, since the combination of PCP and chlorpromazine can dramatically depress the blood pressure, causing cardiovascular collapse and even death. Haloperidol is the drug of choice for such youngsters who cannot be talked down.

Each drug has its own roster of specific *side effects.* Further, addiction and/or long-term use can cause specific damage to various body systems (Blum et al. 1969; Cohen 1981; Lowinson and Ruiz 1981).

The term *habituation* connotes psychic dependency on a particular drug. Because of personality or neurotic needs, the individual becomes reliant on the drug to diminish anxiety and unpleasant feelings and to suppress and avoid the intrapsychic and/or environmental sources of difficulty.

Addiction to narcotics, barbiturates, and alcohol means very specifically all of the following:

1. Physiological dependency results. Body cells develop a chemical "need" for the drug and a subjective feeling of "craving" for it on withdrawal.
2. Physical tolerance develops—increasing doses are needed to satisfy.
3. Potentially dangerous withdrawal symptoms (the abstinence syndrome) develop when the drug is suddenly removed from the user's system.

Social Consequences and Their Management

Frequently, even when there is no addiction or habituation, even minimal drug use can precipitate a major family crisis. Parents confronted with evidence of their teenager's use of drugs often feel shocked, disappointed, confused, frightened, and betrayed. The youngster often feels shame, confusion, embarrassment, and guilt. Some youngsters defensively mask these reactions by a display of hostility, aggressive behavior, or bravado. The family equilibrium is upset, and all members of the household may be affected. Like most family crises, such situations need not prove destructive eventually but can often provide an opportunity for clarification of issues, mobilization of resources, and problem resolution that can ultimately lead to increased individual growth and family cohesion (see chapter 20). The drug use, more often than not, turns out to be a relatively minor issue. In the long run, the drug-centered crisis can prove valuable if it allows the "real" sources of tension or conflict to be addressed and resolved.

MANAGEMENT

Following clarification of the total situation, management might proceed in a number of directions. At times, reassurance and education may be all that are needed. If a relatively minor problem is being escalated by excessive parental anxiety, the physician can provide a badly needed balance by clarifying the issues and putting them in perspective. For other

433

families, their clergyman, a respected friend, a drop-in center, free clinic, and so forth, might provide the support and guidance that are required. Psychiatric consultation should be considered when the young person is obviously disturbed, when violent arguments and chronic tensions continue to upset and divide the family, or when other attempts to resolve the crisis have been tried and failed. When clear abuse of drugs coexists with or complicates severe psychologial or family problems, the drug abuse may be untreatable as long as the psychological or family situation remains unchanged.

Onset of Adult Psychosis During Adolescence

SCHIZOPHRENIC DISORDER, ADULT TYPE

Schizophrenia is an important consideration in adolescent psychiatry. It rapidly increases in incidence during middle adolescence (age fifteen), reaches a peak during late adolescence and young adulthood, and levels off by the end of the twenties.

Diagnosis of this syndrome is difficult during adolescence. Only about one-third of schizophrenic adolescents initially present with the classical pathognomonic signs and symptoms of adult schizophrenia and show the characteristic difficulties in cognition, integration, perception, appropriateness of affect, and interpersonal functioning. The remaining two-thirds present with problems or complaints that mask or precede the appearance of the classical features and therefore distract and mislead the clinician (Bunney 1977). Some schizophrenic adolescents first appear severely depressed, hopeless, lacking in all energy and interest, and preoccupied with suicidal thoughts (some having made one or more attempts). Others present with conduct disorders, deteriorating school performance, substance abuse, truancy, lying, fighting, stealing, or running away. Very often it is only after a prolonged passage of time, together with careful and repeated observation, that the underlying schizophrenic features become clear and the initially presented symptoms or behavioral problems lose their prominence.

While each adolescent who eventually demonstrates a clearly defined schizophrenic illness presents features that are unique and idiosyncratic, it is useful to divide the clinical course into three phases: that of acute disorganization, that of integration, and the postpsychotic phase (Feinstein and Miller, 1977).

During the phase of acute disorganization the youngster often appears agitated, assaultive, chaotic in behavior, and withdrawn from social relationships. Mature ego defenses are abandoned in favor of primitive ones such as denial and splitting, causing others to be viewed as either all good or all bad, all powerful or impotent. The schizophrenic teenager frequently appears either excessively frightened by other people (and therefore withdrawn or attacking) or excessively dependent, projecting omnipotent powers onto others.

In the integration phase, anxiety decreases and the youngster regains some ability to relate with some trust and discrimination. Ego boundaries are partially restored and more sophisticated defenses such as rationalization and intellectualization reappear. Reconstitution of the personality is aided by social support offered by a therapeutic milieu, by medication, and by supportive psychotherapy. Therapy aims to enhance the capacity for reality testing, to clarify perceptions, and to reduce precipitating conflictual stress.

The postpsychotic phase is the period ranging from three to eighteen months following the acute psychotic episode. There is a great variation as to the speed and extent of remission. While cognition, appropriateness of affect, and interpersonal relatedness gradually improve, deficits often remain, requiring significant readjustment by the adolescent as well as by the family, friends, and teachers. The adolescent does not quickly become the person he or she was before the illness. Alterations in memory, judgment, ability to concentrate, self-esteem, and intellectual functioning tend to persist. During this phase schizophrenic adolescents often show a diminished capacity for empathy, poorer school performance, faulty judgment with defective problem solving, and affective distortions. Feelings of depersonalization or derealization are frequent, as is a persistent decrease in psychic energy.

Follow-up studies of hospitalized schizophrenic adolescents indicate that 25 percent recover, 25 percent improve but continue to demonstrate residual deficits and occasional relapses, while 50 percent show little improvement (Hudgens 1974). No good data are available regarding the prognosis for nonhospitalized schizophrenic adolescents, although clinical impressions suggest a better prognosis for cases that have an acute onset, respond quickly to treatment, and can be managed entirely on an outpatient basis (Praedor and Wolpert 1979).

MANIC–DEPRESSIVE ILLNESS IN ADOLESCENCE

Elusive and rapid fluctuations in mood and self-esteem are typical of the early phases of the manic-depressive disorder before frank psychotic episodes become obvious and may be confused or confounded by the usual psychological fluctuations of the adolescent developmental process.

Clinical and research evidence indicates that between one-fifth and one-third of diagnosed adult manic-depressives give histories dating the onset of their illness back to adolescence (Weiner 1980). Diagnosis is difficult during adolescence because (1) the adult form of the illness is not yet clearly established, (2) adolescents tend to demonstrate changes in affect through changes in behavior rather than by expressing their feelings through words, and (3) adolescent personality structure is vulnerable, due to normal developmental changes. Either phase of the illness may initiate an exaggerated decompensation of the personality organization during adolescence, often resulting in a confusing, erratic, disorganized clinical presentation.

Descriptions of mania and depression emphasize differences observed in the level of cognitive, emotional, motor, and social activation. Bunney (1977) has described the clinical features as "increased versus decreased intellectual activity, such as flight of ideas versus poverty of ideas, insomnia versus hypersomnia; hyperactivity versus retardation; impulsivity versus immobility; intrusiveness versus withdrawal; increased libido versus decreased libido; pressure of speech versus mutism; and emotional lability versus emotional blunting."

When manic-depressive illness is a possible diagnosis, a trial of lithium carbonate is indicated (Campbell, Schulman, and Rapoport 1978*b*; Steinberg 1980). It is reportedly a relatively safe drug provided there are no medical contraindications and it is monitored by regular serum level assays. If the patient responds, the therapeutic effects are dramatic. Adjunctive psychotherapy is also indicated in order to modify predisposing and precipitating stress factors. Entering dependent, trusting relationships with adults in authority is frequently very difficult for adolescents, who most often need help in understanding the necessity for taking medication and in accepting the support and guidance that are offered. Once the symptoms related to the manic-depressive illness are controlled, attention should be directed toward concomitant characterological or neurotic problems that might precipitate further exacerbations.

PSYCHODYNAMIC CONSIDERATIONS

Adolescence has been considered a second period of separation-individuation, during which considerable remodeling of personality structure can take place (Blos 1963). As a new and distinctive psychosocial identity is sought, many old values, beliefs, and ideals are extruded while new identifications are internalized. During this normal psychological process, the boundaries of the personality are weakened as the adolescent is subjected to considerable stress resulting from rapid physiological change and shifting social pressures and expectations (Wolpert 1975).

While most adolescents do not experience a period of excessive turmoil, most do show evidence of increased moodiness together with frequent fluctuations of mood. Alteration of defense mechanisms is common, and temporary regressions to earlier defense patterns are widely observed.

Given this backdrop of normally changing psychological processes, adolescence may reasonably be viewed as a vulnerable stage in the human life cycle. Teenagers predisposed to adult psychosis via genetic vulnerability, a family history of psychotic reactions, and/or serious and prolonged childhood traumata have greater difficulty negotiating the developmental tasks of adolescence and may therefore decompensate more readily. In the early stages, schizophrenic or manic-depressive illness may mimic normal adolescent psychological changes, and this is possibly why the initial presentation of these syndromes frequently resembles conduct disorders or variations of an adolescent identity disorder. The vicissitudes of the developmental processes of adolescence themselves may obscure, at least initially, recognition of the characteristic phenomenology of the underlying psychosis, making diagnosis exceedingly difficult. All health professionals must be careful not to diagnose psychosis prematurely because of the serious implications this carries, but they must remain willing to do so and to initiate the necessary treatment as the diagnosis progressively becomes clearer.

SUGGESTIONS FOR FURTHER READING

ANDRULONIS, P. A. et al. 1980. Organic brain dysfunction and the borderline syndrome. *Psychiat. Clin. N. Am.* 4(1):47–66.
A preliminary report on research seeking to define specific etiologic factors for the different organic subcategories of borderline patients.

BRUCH, H. 1973. *Eating disorders,* New York: Basic Books.
Almost ten years old, this still-useful book is the fullest statement of Bruch's formulation of the biological, cognitive, and psychodynamic factors contributing to eating disorders. The discussion of the evolution of a psychotherapeutic approach is must reading for those treating anorexics.

———. 1977. Psychotherapy in eating disorders. *Can. J. Psychiat.* 22:102–108.
Describes the similarities and differences of obesity and anorexia. Various parameters and modalities of treatment are discussed based on Bruch's long-term experience with a large number of patients.

CRISP, A. H., 1981. Therapeutic outcome in anorexia nervosa *Can. J. Psychiat.* 26:232–235.
A recent study evaluating treatment in terms of strict criteria for good outcome. Findings suggest that 20 to 30 percent of the population who would not otherwise have done so can be helped through altering the long-term cause of the disorder and some deaths can be prevented.

COHEN, S. 1981. *The drug abuse problems.* New York: Haworth Press.
A valuable, comprehensive, highly readable review of particularly the social causes and implications of substance abuse problems.

FEINSTEIN, S. C., AND MILLER, D. 1979. Psychoses of adolescence. In *Basic handbook of child psychiatry,* vol. 2, ed. J. D. Noshpitz, pp. 708–722. New York: Basic Books.
A good, basic review of adolescent psychosis.

GARFINKEL, P. E.; MOLDOFSKY, H.; AND GARNER, D. M. 1980. The heterogeneity of anorexia nervosa: Bulimia as a distinct subgroup. *Arch. Gen. Psychiat.* 37:1036–1040.
A study of anorexia nervosa patients seen over eight years. Suggests that those with bulimia constitute a distinct subgroup with a higher incidence of premorbid obesity, impulsive and self-destructive behaviors, and a poorer prognosis.

GARNER, D. M.; GARFINKEL, P. E.; AND BEMIS, K. M. 1982. A multidimensional psychotherapy for anorexia nervosa. *Int. J. Eat. Disord.* 1:3–46.
A comprehensive multidimensional psychotherapeutic approach to the underlying pathology in anorexia nervosa.

HALMI, K. A., AND FALK, J. R. 1981. Common physiological changes in anorexia nervosa. *Int. J. Eat. Disord.* 15(1):16–27.
Forty anorexic patients were studied for physiological aberrations when they entered a treatment study in the emaciated state and again after nutritional rehabilitation. Article discusses all those metabolic aberrations that revert to normal with nutritional rehabilitation and those aberrations that occur in the course of weight gain.

HSU, L. K. G. 1980. Outcome of anorexia nervosa: A review of the literature (1954–1978). *Arch. Gen. Psychiat.* 37:1041–1046.
An overview of research on the outcome of anorexia nervosa in the last twenty-five years. Findings in the area of mortality, nutritional states, eating difficulties, menstrual function, psychiatric states, psychosexual and psychosocial adjustment, and treatment effects are discussed.

LEVINE, S. V. 1979. Adolescents, believing and belonging. *Ann. Adol. Psychiat.* 7:41–53.
A social and psychological demonstration that many behaviors of adolescents, both constructive and destructive, are in large part due to the intensity of the belief system and the pressure of the group.

MASTERSON, J. F. 1980. *From borderline adolescent to functioning adult: The test of time.* New York: Brunner/Mazel.
Attempts to integrate four theoretical perspectives—the developmental, ego psychology, object relations, and classical instinctual theory—into an integrated developmental perspective on the borderline syndrome.

PRAEDOR, D., AND WOLPERT, E. A. 1979. Manic depressive illness in adolescence. *J. Youth/Adol.* 8(2):111–130.
Obstacles to timely diagnosis are reviewed. Case studies demonstrate the usefulness of conceiving of the illness in terms of its physiological basis.

RINSLEY, D. B. 1981. Dynamic and developmental issues in borderline and related "Spectrum" disorders. *Psychiat. Clin. N. Am.* 4(1):124–128.
A good but complex formulation of the psychodynamic and developmental issues contributing to borderline psychopathology. Core symptomatology and the relationship of the disorder to a failure of self/other differentiation are discussed.

RUTTER, M.; GRAHAM, P.; AND CHADWICK, O. 1976. Adolescent turmoil—Fact or fiction? *J. Child. Psychol. & Psychiat.* 17:35–76.
Concept of adolescent turmoil is considered in the context of findings from a total population epidemiological study of fourteen- to fifteen-year-olds on the Isle of Wight. The authors conclude that adolescent turmoil is a fact, not a fiction, but its psychiatric importance may have been overestimated in the past.

WEINER, I. B. 1980. Psychopathology in adolescence. In *Handbook of adolescent psychology,* ed. J. Adelson, pp. 447–71 New York: Wiley Interscience.
Focuses on frequent psychological disturbances among adolescents or those bearing special relationship to the developmental tasks of the teenage years. Reviews epidemiological data on adolescent psychopathology, indicating the limitations of both traditional diagnostic categories and problem-oriented classification within this age group.

PART IV

*Psychological Crises
for Child and Family*

20

Paul D. Steinhauer and
David L. Dickman

Psychological Crises in
the Child and Family

Definition and Introduction

A crisis is a state of psychological and/or social disequilibrium experienced
by a person or family confronting a hazardous circumstance that leaves
them feeling helpless and overwhelmed, since they can neither escape nor
solve it with their customary problem-solving resources (Kantor 1980).
The results of the disequilibrium include psychophysiologic symptoms
and disrupted social relationships (Khan 1979; Mattsson, Seese, and Hawkins 1969).*

The definitive work in crisis theory and crisis intervention is that of
Gerald Caplan (1964), who drew upon the observations and basic principles of sociology, social work, psychology, psychiatry, and preventive
medicine to arrive at his conceptual model of a crisis. Caplan suggests that
to understand a given crisis, it must be viewed simultaneously from the
longitudinal as well as the short-term point of view.

From the longitudinal perspective, the ongoing factors that throughout
the years have molded the personality of the individual and the structure
of the family, predisposing them to break down in crisis in response to
(for them) overwhelming stress, must be understood. From the short-term
point of view, the meaning (to child and family) of a particular crisis or
the pattern of repeated crises, each resulting in sudden changes in habitual
behavior patterns, should be learned.

---

*This formulation was derived by combining key elements from the definitions of crisis
found in Caplan (1964), Khan (1979), and Mattsson, Seese, and Hawkins (1969).

Caplan's model assumes that to avoid becoming mentally disorganized, a person needs continual "supplies," that is, adequate sources of incoming gratification. These supplies may be physical, social, or psychological.

An example of physical supplies is the cuddling of a young child or an affectionate embrace between husband and wife. Social supplies are a mother indicating her approval of a child's good behavior or satisfactory school achievement; the admiration of the peer group for a child's athletic ability, physical appearance, or pleasing personality; the respect of one's business or professional colleagues or fellow workers; and so forth. Examples of psychological supplies are the young child's feeling that he has been a good boy; the satisfaction of an older girl with how she has handled a situation, a relationship, or better still, life in general.

The nature and amount of gratification each person needs at any given time will vary with a number of factors, including:

1. *Age.* The infant depends almost entirely on physical supplies to maintain a sense of well-being. With increasing age, first social supplies (the approval of the mother and others) and later psychological supplies (private, internal sense of self-appreciation) become increasingly important.
2. *Stage of development.* Mature fourteen-year-olds will meet many of their own needs through psychological supplies while a chronological fourteen-year-old emotionally blocked at the level of a five-year-old will depend excessively on social supplies (constant approval from others) to maintain a sense of well-being.
3. *Feelings of deprivation.* The more deprived someone feels, the more intense and compelling will be that person's need for gratification and intolerance for frustration (Henderson 1982). While constitutional differences in basic needs do exist, need intensity can be inflated by having experienced past deprivation, marked overindulgence, or inconsistently alternating periods of each. Of concern here is not just the quality of supplies (e.g., the amount of time spent with parents) but even more the quality of the contact (e.g., the ability of the parents to perceive and to respond appropriately to the child's needs).
4. *Basic character structure.* By the end of latency, the child's basic character structure is usually fairly well established, resulting in a characteristic balance between how much gratification the child will continue to demand and how much of others' demands for control and renunciation of needs can be tolerated.
5. *The number and extent of external pressures present at any given time.* Failure in school, marital dissatisfaction or divorce, the stress of final examinations or business failure, separation from attachment figures through physical distance or emotional withdrawal—any of these may temporarily increase a person's need for supplies, if self-esteem and sense of well-being are to be maintained.
6. *Source of gratification available.* The same factor that may provide gratification (supplies) for some people may, for others, be a source of stress and frustration. Work, marriage, and parenting are examples in adults, while school and relationships with peers and parents can cause either gratification or frustration for children.
7. *Variety and effectiveness of defenses and coping mechanisms available.* Everyone periodically experiences times of intense frustration, stress, and conflict. The greater the variety and effectiveness of the defenses and coping mechanisms one can call into play, the less likely one's reservoir of supplies is to become so depleted as to endanger one's well-being and capacity for effective functioning.

Rutter and his colleagues have demonstrated the cumulative effect of environmental stresses in the development of psychiatric disorder in children. They have shown not only that the more stresses operate simultaneously, the greater the resulting stress, but that the total effect of several interacting stresses is greater than the sum of the effects of the same stresses occurring individually (Rutter 1979). Most crises occur in response not to a single overwhelming stress but to the cumulative effect of a number of simultaneously acting ones, some of which (e.g., such predisposing factors as chronic family tensions, a difficult temperament, a family's recurrent inability to identify and resolve sources of tension repeatedly generated in the course of daily living) may have been operative for years. Superimposed on these may be one or more *precipitating* factors such as a school failure, a suicidal attempt, being caught stealing. Any such precipitating factor may serve as the straw that breaks the camel's back, disrupting the family's previously maintained equilibrium and overwhelming its ability to cope. Thus it is often the cumulative effect of simultaneously occurring stresses more than the result of any single intolerable precipitant that tips the balance, precipitating a crisis. A corollary to this is that even when all environmental stresses contributing to or perpetuating crisis cannot be eliminated, by decreasing the number of simultaneously acting stresses by even one or two (e.g., from four to three) the number of children who develop signs of a psychiatric disorder can be decreased by about two-thirds (Rutter 1979).

The concept of the need for adequate supplies can be extended from the individual to the family. Thus the more effectively a family functions (i.e., the more the needs of each family member are being met), the greater the resilience and ability of that family to deal with stress without precipitating a crisis. Thus the pleasure parents take in the development and accomplishments of their children, the reassurance children get from the love and responsiveness of their parents, the pleasure a husband or wife receives from the love and loyalty of the marital partner, or the feeling of achievement that comes from having handled successfully an upsetting and potentially disruptive situation are all sources of supplies available within the well-functioning family system. The greater a family's ability to generate supplies in response to need, the greater its potential for sustaining even severe and continuing stress without being overwhelmed or plunged into a decompensating disequilibrium. In this regard, one specific aspect of family functioning must be considered—the capacity for modifying typical patterns of response in order to deal more effectively with changed or increased stress or demands (Whitaker and Keith 1981).

In chapter 3 the concept of the family as a system in equilibrium was introduced and developed. When a family's equilibrium is stable, the individual members and the family as a unit operate predictably and effectively with minimal self-questioning or sense of strain. The family's capacity for adaptation will be tested if it is faced with any stress or problem

443

demanding a shift in the characteristic pattern of functioning. If, for example, the wife in a traditional marriage beings to redefine her role, the resulting strain on the existing equilibrium will constitute a demand for adaptation. If the husband can and will make the necessary shifts in redefining his role, a new equilibrium will be established. If not, the couple will be faced with either a continuing disequilibrium or a breakdown of the system.

The essential factor in determining whether a crisis will occur is the balance among the cumulative effect of the stresses faced by child and family, the adequacy of the supplies, external sources of support (e.g., the encouragement and help of friends, relatives, or professional counselors), and each individual's internal (psychological) defenses. Together these constitute the resources the family has available to it to offset the combined stresses. Should the stress level at any given time exceed the family's capacity to cope, the existing coping mechanisms will be overwhelmed and the family's equilibrium will be disrupted. When a new equilibrium is eventually achieved, it may differ significantly from the previous one. For many people, lasting and significant shifts in personality development, coping mechanisms, and overall functioning seem to occur during time-limited periods of crisis.

Etiology of Crisis

Caplan has defined a crisis as an "upset in the steady state," meaning a marked change in the person's—or family's—habitual pattern of behavior. But normal development consists of a series of phases, each qualitatively different from those before and after it. Between these are transitional periods, termed "developmental crises" by Erikson (1959), of behavior often temporarily characterized by cognitive and affective upsets. Thus each new developmental advance may cause additional stress that can, at first, upset the balance, causing a temporary period of disorganization and disequilibrium. Generally the child, with the help of the family, soon develops newer, more effective ways of coping with the stress and establishes a new equilibrium at a more advanced developmental level. Similar periods of psychological and behavioral upset can be precipitated in adults by life hazards producing a sudden loss of supplies. Examples would include failure to receive an expected promotion or a couple's suddenly realizing that their marriage is not providing the satisfaction they had hoped for.

While some authors suggest that only certain specific syndromes present bona fide crises (e.g., psychosis, school refusal, etc.), the authors of this chapter consider that for all practical purposes, a crisis is any situation, actual or anticipated, that the family or community respond to as such. Note that real external stress is not needed to precipitate a crisis; mere apprehension regarding what might happen can be quite enough. Thus the mere anticipation of a school or business failure, or the fear that parents have lost control over a child, may have as catastrophic an effect as if the failure or loss of control had actually occurred. Studies attempting to group crises according to precipitating symptoms or major diagnostic categories show such a wide variation that they probably tell as much or more about local gaps in service delivery and the diagnostic bias of the psychiatrists making the diagnosis as they do about the population being studied (Mattsson, Seese, and Hawkins 1969; Morrison 1969; Steinhauer, Levine, and DaCosta 1971). In two studies that even attempted to provide a psychiatric diagnosis (Mattsson, Seese, and Hawkins 1969; Steinhauer, Levine, and DaCosta 1971), the number of cases diagnosed psychotic was identical (9 percent) while those diagnosed psychoneurotic were almost the same (26 percent compared to 27 percent). In all other diagnostic categories, however, and in the frequency of precipitating factors, discrepancies were so great that no valid conclusions could be drawn (e.g., Mattsson and associates diagnosed suicidal behavior in 44 percent, while Steinhauer and colleagues reported suicidal attempts in only 15 percent).

While certain forms of behavior (stealing, running away from home, sexual promiscuity, drug use, etc.) are more likely than others to precipitate crises, it is the family or communal reaction rather than the behavior per se that determines whether or not a crisis will develop. Thus one family may be plunged into crisis on learning that a seventeen-year-old who is doing well in every way has experimented with marijuana, while another may show no apparent response to even a longstanding pattern of known drug abuse. It is not the precipitating event—nor is it the importance that we professionals give that precipitating event—that constitutes the crisis. Rather it is the nature and extent of the perception of and response to that event which determines whether a crisis exists or not.

Classification of Child-Centered Crises

There have been numerous overlapping attempts to classify child-centered crises in terms of the form of intervention required, whether they are generic (i.e., the cause and course are predictable and likely to occur in any individual or family under similar circumstances) or individual (i.e., determined by the unique dynamics of the individual in a particular situation (Jacobsen, Strickler, and Morley 1968), or whether they are developmental (maturational or transitional) or situational (i.e., in response to external situations) (Aguilera and Messick 1974; Baldwin 1978; Morrice 1976; Schneidman 1973). The authors prefer to classify child-centered crises in three main groups: psychopathological syndromes, developmental crises, and situational crises.

THE PSYCHOPATHOLOGICAL SYNDROMES

Although in this group the psychopathology of the child is the most striking feature, a psychosocial crisis rather than a disease entity is nevertheless what is being dealt with.

> Jenny, age eight, was a premature infant. She had mixed developmental delays and suffers from a seizure disorder. She has never related well to her healthy six-year-old brother, John. After John broke a leg and was nursed in the family living room, Jenny had several explosive temper tantrums and repeatedly threatened to leave home. This so upset her parents that they brought her to a hospital emergency room demanding that something be done to change her behavior that was "ruining the family's life together."

Almost any child psychiatric syndrome may precipitate a crisis in a vulnerable family. Other families will tolerate that same illness without significant loss of equilibrium. One study of 109 consecutive emergencies suggested that over two-thirds of what were originally presented as child-centered crises could be described more accurately as social or family crises (Steinhauer, Levine, and DaCosta 1971).

DEVELOPMENTAL CRISES

Reference has already been made to those transitional periods of stress and disequilibrium termed "developmental crises" by Erikson. These may arise suddenly from increases in environmental demands occurring routinely in the course of development, such as the demand that a child be toilet-trained, that she separate from mother to attend school, that he learn to read in the first grade, and so forth. Alternatively, they may originate from a child's difficulty in controlling normal increases in internal (biological) drives, for example, the physiological increase in sexuality and aggressiveness following puberty.

SITUATIONAL CRISES

In a situational crisis, what is presented as a single crisis in the child turns out on examination to be a basically healthy child's response to a seriously aberrant or disrupted family or social situation.

> For the past few weeks Sean, age fourteen, had seldom been on time for dinner. His mother noted that he had also lost interest in his model planes. The day before his parents brought him to the emergency room, he was caught

with two friends while breaking into a school. His father, a seaman, had been unemployed these past months. He had been irritable and moody, drinking at home, and there had been multiple arguments and threats of separation by both parents.

Similarly, internal conflicts against which the child had successfully defended previously may be temporarily activated by a deterioration in the family or social situation. Events that can precipitate situational crises include: parental illness, physical or emotional; parental loss, through death, divorce, or imprisonment; marital maladjustment; the addition of a new member (e.g., stepparent or sibling) to the family; relocation or financial crises; examinations; and hospitalization.

Even in the absence of overt conflict between the parents, marital maladjustment should be considered in any family seeking help for a crisis centering around a disturbed child. Any child-centered crisis, regardless of the presenting symptoms or the manner of presentation, can either reflect or mask chronic disturbance within the family or community. Should a situational crisis coincide with a normal developmental crisis, the combination may cause a crisis of major proportions leaving long-lasting effects.

Natural History of a Crisis

While a number of authors subdivide the stages of a crisis in different though overlapping ways (Hirschowitz 1973; Lindemann 1944; Tyhurst 1957), the authors find Caplan's description of the natural history of a crisis most useful clinically. Caplan (1964) sees the typical crisis as consisting of four overlapping phases:

Phase 1: Tension increases as individual or family seeks to solve the problem in old ways.
Phase 2: As old methods fail to bring a solution or relief, tensions continue to mount.
Phase 3: This escalating tension leads to the mobilization of emergency problem-solving methods, as child and family seek new ways to define the problem, to relate it to previous experience, and to resolve it. These may include focusing on previously neglected aspects of the problem, setting aside others as irrelevant or unmanageable, trial and error (in thought or in action), or active resignation and giving up. These may or may not lead to resolution of the crisis and reestablishment of the previous or a modified and possibly much improved level of equilibrium.
Phase 4: Should the problem remain unresolved, however, tensions continue to mount beyond the limit of tolerance. Unless relief is available at this critical point, there is real danger of major and perhaps lasting disorganization in child and family.

447

Thus a crisis can be viewed as a transitional period presenting child and family with, on one hand, an opportunity for growth and redirection or, on the other hand, a risk of adverse effects resulting in a permanently increased vulnerability to subsequent stress (Brandon 1970).

How do we assess childhood crises in order to derive the understanding that will point to appropriate intervention?

Approach to the Crisis

APPROPRIATE TIMING

Crises are complex situations generating tremendous anxiety, relief of which is sought urgently and immediately. The anxiety may be highest in the person making the referral, such as the school principal, public health nurse, parents or relatives (Mattsson, Seese, and Hawkins 1969). Those who assume primary responsibility for dealing with a crisis must respond promptly but not allow themselves to be stampeded into premature and possibly inappropriate action. Thus crisis intervention begins with an initial assessment conducted when and where the assessor can devote the time and attention the case requires. Much needless anger and frustration are generated when a hurried professional tries to deal with a crisis while under mounting pressure from other sources or service demands. Unless time is set aside, the anxiety generated by the crisis will be aggravated by the competing demands of a waiting room full of other patients or by delayed social commitments. Some practitioners handle this by leaving free a particular time, often at the beginning or end of the working day, to be used when necessary to see families in crisis. If the family has to wait for an extended period, provision of a separate room, coffee, and so forth, is helpful. Waiting in a busy public emergency section often increases tension both in the family in crisis and in other patients or clients waiting to be seen.

HANDLING THE TELEPHONE REFERRAL

Very often, by the time a report of a family crisis reaches the doctor or mental health worker, it has been magnified and distorted by anxious intermediaries. Frequent calls or messages should warn of a mounting crisis. Advice should not be given over the telephone under pressure. An agreement to return the call within a short time and with the prospect of fuller discussion allows the doctor or counselor both time to think and an opportunity to consider alternative actions under less harassed circumstances. Just giving the referring person or family a definite time at which they will be seen—even if it is not immediately—often considerably reduces the anxiety, which is usually greater in adults than in the child.

MOBILIZING SUPPORT FOR THE CRISIS

Doctors or workers themselves often need support in handling crises. If possible, community workers, case aides, and interpreters should be involved, especially if they have worked with the family previously. Their assistance may help decrease the pressure on the professional, thus facilitating a more adequate assessment and deposition.

Identification of Contributing and Precipitating Causes

Nearly always, the designated patient and the parents (or foster parents and social worker for wards of a child welfare association or children's aid society) should be seen as part of the emergency assessment. It is always dangerous to accept as the whole truth any one participant's description of a crisis. All husbands and wives, parents and children, tell the truth as they see it. Without even realizing it, they may try to manipulate their doctor or counselor into taking sides in a family conflict, unconsciously selecting or slanting what they report to gain the professional as an ally against other family members with whom they are in conflict. Professionals who side with a teenager against the parents or with the parents against their child risk losing their potential helpfulness (McPherson, Brocklemanns, and Newman 1974). To avoid this, an increasing number of primary physicians and mental health workers are learning to assess family crises by interviewing the family as a unit. The techniques of family diagnostic interviewing go beyond the scope of this chapter but can be mastered by the primary physician or mental health professional. Once learned, they should prove invaluable diagnostic and therapeutic adjuncts (Barten and Barten 1973; Farley, Eckhardt, and Hebert 1979; Khan 1979).

Families frequently identify a crisis as a normal response to a child's symptomatic behavior. If they confine their investigation to the child and fail to determine whether that child's behavior is secondary to (i.e., a symptom of) significant family pathology and distress, they are in danger of misinterpreting the situation and responding inappropriately. A framework is necessary to clarify the often confused and confusing situation. Inquiry should focus on the following five areas.

THE CHILD AND HIS OR HER OVERALL ADJUSTMENT

The first thing professionals must determine is to what extent psychopathology in the child is a contributing factor. With what pressures, either psychological or interpersonal, is the child trying to cope through the symptoms? Beyond exploring the nature of the presenting symptom, the child's overall adjustment must be assessed. How does she function within the family? Are there academic or behavioral difficulties at school? Can she make and keep friends? Can he appropriately express his feelings? Are there other signs of disturbance that either child or parents recognize? Does the precipitating behavior seem an isolated event or just one more example of what appears a fixed or habitual pattern of behavior?

> As an infant, Adrian, age eight, was difficult to calm and cuddle. He remained distractible and impulsive. His sleep pattern and appetite were irregular. He became uncontrollably silly at a birthday party. When his school was being renovated, Adrian and his class were moved to a portable schoolroom. While the others in the class had no trouble adjusting to their new surroundings, soon after Adrian was sent home after breaking a fellow student's glasses and, the next day, for fighting in the schoolyard.

These questions cannot be answered solely from the nature of the presenting complaint, but this situation is not unique to psychiatry. A patient with a persistent cough could have any one of a number of related or diverse pathological conditions, all of which could cause the coughing. Just as professionals cannot intelligently treat a cough without understanding the pathology producing it, they cannot manage appropriately a behavioral symptom or crisis without first understanding the psychopathology of child and family that are contributing to it. Thus the more professionals understand the meaning to child and family of the symptomatic behavior, the more accurately they can focus intervention. Various causative factors may, of course, overlap. A child's classroom behavior may suddenly deteriorate rapidly for a number of reasons. The more clearly the various educational, social, familial, and psychological factors contributing to the deterioration are understood, the better the chance of helping the situation.

THE FAMILY

How does the crisis reflect—and in what way is it affecting—the day-to-day functioning of the family? (See chapter 3.) What, if any, family pressures are contributing to symptoms in the child the family considers to be the patient? How are the family members, as individuals and as a unit, affected by the symptomatic behavior of the identified patient?

Some crises seem clearly related to such obvious family threats as serious physical or emotional illness, marital separation, loss of job or financial security, and so forth. In others the precipitating factors, while more obscure, may be no less important. When the professional asks "why now?" and cannot find an answer, the possibility that essential information is being withheld, either deliberately or because it is not considered relevant to the problem at hand, should be considered. For example, parents may fail to mention a serious marital problem either out of deliberate or unrecognized defensiveness or because they never connected it with their child's beginning to steal. If, however, the stealing was, in fact, their child's way of handling distress at the marital conflict, the key to understanding could come from identifying what had changed in the family to disrupt a previously tolerable equilibrium.

THE COMMUNITY

Stress from community pressures and expectations may precipitate the breakdown of an already fragile family situation. These pressures may stem from family moves, from changes in community tolerance of certain types of behavior, or from confrontation between school system or police and the child or family. Peer group pressure on children from a middle-class family now living in public housing may be a source of extreme pressure, as indeed may the economic changes that have led to the move. The effect of crowded apartment living on a rural family lately moved to the city and the loss of social supports (e.g., church, extended family, friends, and neighbors) may be other important factors contributing to crisis generation.

> Tom, age fifteen, grew up in the Canadian Far North. Although boisterous and reckless, Tom was accepted because of the deep respect his grandfather commanded in the village. Tom himself was also valued as a skilled young hunter.
> Forced to move to an urban center because of a mining development, Tom was placed in a large urban high school. He was soon in trouble. Although very popular at school, he had taken to truanting and was caught after taking the vice-principal's car for a joy-ride.

THE CHILD'S DEVELOPMENT

How is the crisis related to—and how does it affect—the child's ongoing development? Is this what has been defined earlier as a developmental crisis, or has there been enough internalization of the disturbance to suggest the presence of a diagnosible syndrome requiring ongoing treatment?

It should not be forgotten that parents as well as children continue to develop and that crises in adult development may change marital and parent-child relationships significantly, precipitating crises in the family unit.

451

THE PRECIPITATING FACTOR

What change or event has disrupted the family's customary equilibrium and precipitated the crisis? An understanding of the precipitating event and its meaning is always an important part of a crisis assessment.

Intervention

Families may be particularly accessible to intervention during the period of disorganization and suggestibility at the height of crisis (Farley, Eckhardt, and Hebert 1979). Many recent writers are emphasizing the potential for growth and the possibility of individual or family reintegration at a newer and higher level of equilibrium that can result from prompt and effective crisis intervention (Alexander and Parsons 1974; Davanloo 1978; Farley, Eckhardt, and Hebert 1979; Morrice 1976). Excessive haste or delay are to be avoided. Generally, frequent support is needed. The family may need their doctor, the primary worker, or an associate available at least by telephone until the crisis settles. For some families the need for support may activate a fear that to accept help is to acknowledge intolerable weakness and dependency. In such cases, too much help—or help given in a way that intensifies the parents' fears of dependency and feelings of inadequacy—may itself be an additional stress and as harmful as too little.

Intervention involves a continuing reassessment, analysis, and treatment of the factors contributing to the crisis. The main causes—and the precipitating factor may either be one of these or merely the straw that broke the camel's back—must be identified, sorted, and, if possible, resolved. Not all of the causative factors will prove equally accessible to intervention. The professional must be concerned not just with areas of weakness but with the family's strengths and with which factors most need modification, which are most accessible to intervention, and how this can best be undertaken to ensure family cooperation while minimizing the threat of further decompensation. Adequate short- and long-term follow-up should be a regular part of the protocol to assess realistically its effectiveness. What follows is a description of some of the methods used.

METHODS OF MANAGEMENT

Review and Return

When, following an adequate assessment, a developmental crisis is diagnosed in a basically normal child, a wait-and-see attitude on the part of the professional is justified. In time, many such children find more successful ways of dealing with the temporarily increased tension level. However, professionals should avoid giving unqualified reassurance, since not all such children go on to develop more successful ways of dealing with the stress. Some instead rely increasingly on their neurotic or behavioral defenses so that what was once a transient response to unaccustomed stress becomes in time a fixed and habitual behavior pattern that shapes the child's character and dominates his or her behavior and relationships. When such pathological responses have become automatic and internalized, implying significant entrenched psychopathology, definite psychotherapeutic intervention is indicated. The aim of psychotherapy in such cases is the resolution of the child's internal conflict, thus freeing him or her to live more fully, more productively, and more comfortably.

Reassurance

There are undoubtedly times at which, having understood the child's behavior in the family and developmental context, the professional can safely say, "She'll grow out of it." Helping overconcerned parents regain their perspective in such situations may be invaluable. But, at other times, anxious parents attempt to minimize their anxiety by a seemingly casual request for reassurance in a situation that, if all the facts were known, would demand further investigation. Premature, inappropriate, or unqualified reassurance may be damaging if it postpones dealing with a problem that is still reactive to external events and has not yet become a habitual (i.e., internalized) pattern of response. For example, while it is true that most boys at some point steal, professionals should avoid categorically reassuring a mother that her son's stealing is normal until the extent of the pattern and its determinants are sufficiently understood to rule out the possibility that this particular child's stealing is a symptom of significant underlying disturbance. Similarly, to respond to a fourteen-year-old's anxiety about a homosexual experience with light reassurance that such things are normal for teenagers may do more to relieve the professional's embarrassment than to address the boy's need, which, if the extent and duration of the homosexual behavior and the degree of the associated anxiety were understood, might be recognized as a serious problem with which he was struggling.

Symptomatic Treatment

When, based on an adequate assessment, the professional is confident that there are no major underlying problems in either child or family, symptomatic treatment (e.g., imipramine for enuresis or a change of living arrangements for a teenager in conflict with her parents) is indicated. Here again, the situation is analogous to that in other areas of medicine. A physician would not, for example, suppress a cough symptomatically before ruling out the presence of a serious condition requiring direct treatment.

453

Indeed, suppression of a cough could prove harmful if it led to the neglect of an underlying inflammatory, obstructive, or neoplastic disease. Similarly, the family may be preoccupied with their child's presenting symptom (e.g., hyperactivity), focusing on it in a way that interferes with their recognizing and dealing with other disorders (e.g., serious family problems, learning problems, or a conduct disorder). To concentrate management on the relief of the current symptom (e.g., through treating the hyperactivity with methylphenidate) while ignoring the other serious and associated problems requiring prompt and appropriate intervention would be an equally serious error in management. To offer only symptomatic treatment in such a situation would be to risk ignoring and possibly aggravating significant and often treatable sources of distress.

Brief Therapy

The family physician or some other worker with whom the family was previously involved is often the first to whom families turn for advice and help. If the professional has known and treated the family for some time, their confidence and trust in him or her will provide an unequalled opportunity for helping at the point of crisis.

Wherever possible, the aim of intervention should extend beyond just relieving presenting symptoms to using the crisis as an opportunity to improve the coping and functioning capacities of child and family. Viewed this way, crises provide useful opportunities for relatively brief intervention. (Langsley and Kaplan 1968) They allow families to examine patterns of maladaptive behavior and to increase their ability to manage stress. This is done by encouraging the ventilation of pent-up negative feelings, with the doctor or worker providing a measure of safety, clarity, and encouragement. The professional can serve as a catalyst, improving communication that has broken down and helping each family member understand the other's position, thus providing a basis for problem solving and badly needed negotiations. The professional can also help clarify and identify important areas of conflict and distress by eliciting possible directions of action and by supporting those most appropriate (Eisler and Hersen 1973; Keith 1974). Physicians or workers cannot provide a solution for all the family's mental health problems, even though the family, drawing on the medical model, may demand that they do so. But a crisis allows an opening for the alert and concerned professional to help child and family not just weather the current crisis but learn from it to avoid—or, at least, deal more successfully with—similar situations in the future.

Successful brief therapy requires the professional to intervene at a conscious problem-solving level using actions derived from a deeper understanding of the factors causing and maintaining the crisis. Therapist and family agree on a series of short-term goals toward which they contract to work for a predetermined number of sessions. The agenda should be followed closely and temptation to allow the therapeutic goals to become diffused resisted. At the end of the agreed-on number of sessions, therapist and family can always recontract to work together for an additional period toward a new set of goals, if required (Davanloo 1978).

Role of Medication

Occasionally a child's behavior may be so out of control and the anxiety level so high that medication may be indicated temporarily. At best, this can only be part of the total treatment, and professionals should be cautious since an overmedicated person, child or adult, cannot utilize the opportunities for adaptive change presented by crisis intervention. Details of drug use will be found in chapter 29.

Referral

This brings us to a discussion of referral for psychiatric and specific mental health consultations. The professional is advised to seek psychiatric or mental health consultation for the family if:

1. The family situation continues to deteriorate in spite of his or her best efforts.
2. Following assessment, he or she remains unaware of the nature of the problem to be dealt with.
3. While attempting to help the family resolve the crisis, the professional finds that the case demands more time than he or she has to give.
4. The ongoing management of the family in crisis is producing personal discomfort in the worker or doctor that is interfering with management of the case or carrying over into his or her personal life.

When in doubt, it is wiser to seek consultation than to wait too long, allowing the situation to deteriorate.

The factors governing the timing and the process of referral for psychiatric or mental health consultation, often crucial to the usefulness of the referral, are discussed in detail in chapter 30. Every primary physician, social worker, or counselor in private practice would be wise to develop a working relationship with a few psychiatrists and mental health facilities to have available sources of consultation and backup when necessary according to the criteria just listed.

SUGGESTIONS FOR FURTHER READING

BALDWIN, B.A. 1977. Crisis intervention in professional practice: Implications for clinical training. *Amer. J. Orthopsychiat.* 47(4):659–670.
Crisis intervention is currently defined in a body of principles that provides an effective framework for professional practice. Strategies toward the development of an effective training model for crisis therapists are suggested.

———. 1978. A paradigm for the classification of emotional crises: Implications for crisis intervention. *Am. J. Orthopsychiat.* 48 (3):538–551.

Baldwin distinguishes six general types of crises frequently encountered, with defining characteristics, intervention strategy, and a case example given for each.

CAPLAN, G. 1964. *Principles of preventive psychiatry.* New York: Basic Books.

Presents Caplan's basic conceptual model and a guide to assessment.

CONROE, R. M., et al. 1978. A Systematic Approach to Brief Psychological Intervention That Can Be Used by the Primary Care Physician. *J. Fam. Prac.* 7(6):1137–1142.

Presents a systematic approach to brief psychological interventions for the primary-care physician. Four types of interventions are discussed: short-term therapy, structured assessment, crisis intervention, and referral.

DOYLE, A. M., AND DORLAC, C. 1978. Treating chronic crisis bearers and their families. *J. Marr. & Fam. Counsel.* 4(3):37–42.

Presents a method for family crisis intervention. The goal is extended from restoring the crisis-bearing unit to its precrisis level of coping to a basic restructuring of maladaptive precrisis behaviors. The method minimizes the tendency to identify one member of the family as the patient without considering the impact of the other members.

FARLEY, G. K.; ECKHARDT, L. O.; AND HEBERT, F. B. 1979. *Handbook of child and adolescent psychiatric emergencies.* New York: Medical Examination Publishing Co.

A thorough, well-written book including (1) general principles of evaluation of psychiatric emergencies; (2) reasons for referral to the emergency room; (3) child and adolescent psychiatric syndromes; (4) child and adolescent psychopharmacology.

KANTOR, D. 1980. Critical Identity Image: A Concept Linking Individual, Couple and Family Development. In *Family therapy: Combining psychodynamic and family systems approaches,* ed. J. K. Pearce and L. J. Friedman, pp. 137–167. New York: Grune & Stratton.

Introduces the concept of the developmental crisis that occurs after a breakdown in adapatation leads to the family getting stuck in habitual and inflexible behavior. Clinical implications for family therapists are presented with a case example illustrating the treatment process.

KHAN, A. U. 1979. *Psychiatric emergencies in pediatrics.* Chicago: Year Book Medical Publishers Ltd.

A highly recommended handbook for physicians and mental health professionals who encounter psychological crises in children and their families.

LANGSLEY, D. G. 1978. Three models of family therapy: Prevention, crisis treatment or rehabilitation. *J. Clin. Psychiat.* 39(11):792–796.

Describes models of intervention at a family level as preventive, crisis intervention, or rehabilitative. Review of data suggests that early intervention with children has produced the most promising results.

———, and KAPLAN, D. M. 1968. *The treatment of families in crisis.* New York: Grune & Stratton.

A guide to understanding and managing the family in crisis.

MORRISON, G. C. 1969. Therapeutic intervention in a child psychiatry emergency service. *J. Amer. Acad. Child Psychiat.* 8:542–558.

Provides a good description of a child-oriented crisis intervention clinic. Stresses the importance of prompt but flexible intervention. Bibliography up to the date of publication is excellent.

———. 1975. *Emergencies in child psychiatry: Emotional crises of children, youth and their families.* Springfield, Ill.: Charles C Thomas.

An important work by an authority in the field of psychological crises.

———, and COLLIER, J. G. 1969. Family treatment approaches to suicidal children and adolescents. *J. Am. Acad. Child Psychiat.* 8:140–153.

Suggests that attempted or threatened suicide is frequently symptomatic not only of acute emotional distress in the individual but also of disruption in the family. Reports clinical experience of a child psychiatric emergency service working with families of suicidal children.

21 Paul D. Steinhauer, David N. Mushin, and Quentin Rae-Grant

Psychological Aspects of Chronic Illness

When parents bring a sick child to a physician, they come with a number of questions: What is the matter with my child? What has caused it? What can the doctor do to help? What can we, as parents, do? How long will it last? Will my child be completely cured? But their overriding request and hope is that somehow, by medicine or by magic, the child will be rapidly and completely returned to former health. However, this is frequently asking more than the physician can deliver.

With improvements in treating infectious diseases and a growing ability to sustain life even when health cannot be restored, pediatricians are increasingly required to aid in managing children who are severely and chronically ill. Here, contrary to parental expectations, they cannot cure. But there are a number of things, all important, that they can do. They may be able to control the rate of progress or the frequency and severity of complications of the disease. They may do much to help children compensate for some of the more destructive effects of their illness. Finally, and equally important, they may be able to help child and family face the limitations, anxieties, and discouragement generated by the disease, develop a plan of management that can help them counteract feelings of helplessness and rise above the resentment and despair that threaten to overwhelm them (Garrard and Richmond 1963; Pakes 1974). Any severe illness in a child represents a crisis for the family (Pless and Pinkerton 1975). How this crisis is sustained or resolved will depend on the answers to the preceding questions as well as on the preexisting strengths of the family. Even an acute and rapidly responsive illness can cause decompensation in a family whose adjustment is already precarious. On the other hand, great strength, stability, and support are required to sustain a family through a severe chronic illness in one of its members (Meyerowitz and Kaplan 1967). (See table 21.1.)

Since children are still developing and have different needs and capacities depending on their stage of development, the nature and extent of disruption accompanying an illness will vary according to the age at which it occurs (Kluger 1979; Lowit 1973; Maddison and Raphael 1971; Sperling 1978). Either the illness itself or restrictions imposed by its management may interfere with functioning and disrupt development and normal living. By and large, the common acute illnesses of childhood leave few major or lasting emotional sequelae. Although their behavior while in the hospital may present problems, few children have residual effects following short-term hospitalization, unless they were previously maladjusted (Vernon, Schulman, and Foley 1966).

Chronic illness, however, is frequently associated with ongoing problems (Pless and Roghmann 1971; Rutter 1970). The prolonged disruption of children's lives can have lasting effects on their cognitive and emotional development. To manage chronically ill children and their families, physicians must understand the child's premorbid personality and needs, their stage of development and its vulnerabilities, the child's perception of the illness and its management, the nature of the illness and its potential effects on child and family, the nature of management procedures, and the potential for support of the child by family and medical staff (Seligman 1974).

Premorbid Personality and Needs

A child's development and adjustment prior to becoming ill will affect that child's response to illness. The child who has had difficulty separating from parents may have problems coping with hospitalization. The previously phobic child is likely to develop excessive fears of minor procedures, while the hyperactive child will have difficulty tolerating forced immobilization. The child who already fears and resents authority will probably rebel against doctors and nurses, whereas a previously shy and withdrawn child whose illness produces deformity may become so self-conscious as to seriously undermine social adjustment. A child from a depriving environment may, through the demand for enforced isolation, fall even further behind intellectually.

Circumstances at the onset of illness may influence the child's adjust-

TABLE 21.1

Emotional Responses to Acute and Chronic Illness

	Acute Illness	Chronic Illness
Onset	Sudden	Sudden or insidious
Duration of illness	Brief	Prolonged
Treatment	Often effective	Palliative or none
Outlook	Frequently excellent	Generally poor
Crisis identity	High	High
Crisis duration	Brief	Prolonged
Family reactions	Anxiety	Denial and disbelief, anxiety, depression, guilt and responsibility, resentment
Physician's reactions	Relief	?

ment to the disease. Thus a young child severely burned during a phase of jealousy following the birth of a sibling might ascribe infrequent parental visits to their being more interested in the new sibling than in him. Such a child might interpret the burn as punishment for hostile and rivalrous feelings toward the sibling. Most independent, secure children cope better with a chronic illness than ones who are immature, insecure, and inhibited. At least in acute illness, some children's emotional adjustment may actually be improved with successful handling of their disease.

Nature of the Illness and Management and Potential Effects on the Child

The child's adjustment will be affected by a number of factors that, separately or together, may occur during the course of an illness.

SEPARATION FROM PARENTS

Several authors have suggested that even life-threatening diseases and ugly deformities are less shattering to children than the separation from family that chronic illness necessitates (Burton 1975; Hollenbeck et al. 1980; Travis 1976). Separation is particularly upsetting for children between six months and four years, but it may also be stressful for older children who have had prior separations. Bowlby's description of the three stages of children's reactions to separation (i.e., protest, despair, detachment) are discussed in chapter 4. While the stages of protest and despair are reversible on reunion with parents under appropriate circumstances, persistent defects in the capacity for relationships and development may result if the third stage, detachment, is reached. The child who is institutionalized for long periods is particularly vulnerable to these complications of separation. Repeated actual or threatened separations may produce frequent and irrational anger and anxiety which, in turn, cause difficulty in management (Linde et al. 1979).

Separation problems can be minimized by regular, predictable visiting or rooming-in by the parents (Barowsky 1978; Wallinga 1979), and by ensuring that the child is cared for by a small number of familiar staff. Infrequent or sporadic visiting by parents and care from many adults with whom there is no regular contact increase the damaging effects of separation (Burton 1975).

RESTRICTION, SENSORY IMPAIRMENT, AND ISOLATION

Some illnesses require periods of restricted mobility or isolation from familiar people and surroundings. In addition, certain illnesses such as blindness, deafness, and the decreased tactile stimulation that accompanies the treatment of the burned child can impose sensory restrictions. (See chapter 22 for more specific discussion of the blind and deaf child.) Cognitive development, particularly in young children, requires physical exploration of the environment. All children need environmental stimulation and must be free to respond to such stimulation. Restrictions on play may remove the safety valve a child needs to deal with anxiety, apprehension, and resentment, while sensory impairment may make it difficult to explain procedures to the child, as well as disrupting relationships with parents and medical staff. When such avenues are blocked, children may withdraw into excessive fantasy as a means of coping, this tendency being enhanced by isolation. This may lead to an escalation of fears and unrealistic expectations regarding the illness and management.

DEPENDENCY AND LACK OF CONSISTENCY

Adults dealing with sick children tend to gratify dependency needs to help the child feel more secure and to provide comfort. While to some extent this may be needed, prolonged and excessive gratification of these needs may be so satisfying that the child may resist giving it up (Sigal et al. 1973). This, then, interferes with the normal striving toward independence, blocking the development of self-confidence and initiative (Mattsson 1972). Such tendencies are more marked in children who for any reason (including congenital illnesses, where parental guilt fosters overprotection) have prior dependency problems. Rehabilitation and the maintenance of maximal functioning in spite of residual physical problems may be impeded. The aim of management is to strike a balance between allowing dependence during the acute phase and gradual encouragement toward independence whenever possible.

PAIN AND DEFORMITY

A child's response to pain varies with how that pain is perceived as well as with the amount of pain accountable for on a physiologic basis (Freud 1952; Nover 1973). Pain interpreted as punishment or maltreatment (e.g., reaction to injections) may be intensified by the accompanying anxiety (Mattsson 1972). Those children who perceive pain as pleasurable may become pathologically submissive to the medical staff who inflict it (Freud 1952; Raimbault 1973). The young child who fantasies adults as all-powerful and able to remove all pain may interpret their not doing so as an expression of anger. This may be reinforced if the adults become angry at the child's persistent complaints or apprehensions regarding procedures. During the late preschool and early adolescent years, the threat of surgery and deformity is greatest (Geist 1979; Gluck 1977; Kaplan and De-Nour 1979). Toddlers see surgery as a punishment with potentially dire consequences, for at this age the least scratch is often blown up to the proportions of a major wound. Fears of mutilation and deformity are exaggerated by the adolescent's typically increased concern with body image, need to be the same as peers, and fears of being a defective, and hence inadequate, person.

THREAT OF DEATH

Should the illness be one that is potentially fatal, the possibility or approach of death will have major effects on the sick child, that child's family, the caregivers, and their relationships with each other. A discussion of the process by which child, family, and caregivers cope with impending death and issues related to how each deals with the feelings this arouses will be found in chapter 24. (See also Friedman 1967; Green 1976; Heagarty 1978.)

MEDICATION

Certain forms of medication may affect the child's alertness (e.g., barbiturates) and behavior (e.g., corticosteroids). Such effects should be considered in prescribing these drugs. Drugs having physical side effects (e.g., cytotoxic drugs) can cause anxiety through disturbance of body image. Prolonged and regular use of drugs (e.g., insulin) or diets may be tolerated at younger ages but rebelled against as an imposition by authority figures in early adolescence. Adolescents may see acceptance of such regimens as a sign of weakness, a constant reminder of the illness and a symbol of dependence and inadequacy that they would rather forget (Burton 1974*b*, 1975; Kaplan and De-Nour 1979; Pless and Pinkerton 1975).

461

Multiple absences may lead to the child's falling behind in school and seriously interfere with peer relationships that may be extremely important to the older child or adolescent. Relaxed visiting privileges and provision for continuing schooling while in the hospital or at home may minimize these potential complications.

Problems Specific to Certain Illnesses

Certain illnesses may directly influence behavior and cognitive development. Some forms of brain damage may be associated with hyperactivity, poor impulse control, and poor attention span and/or mental retardation. These may affect perception and thus learning in a child with normal intelligence (see chapter 17). Children with temporal lobe epilepsy may exhibit a wide range of psychological problems ranging from behavior disorder to episodes of depersonalization to hallucinations (see chapter 11). Some psychoses in children, for example, types of autism, have at least in part a physiologic basis (see chapter 15). In such conditions the specific effects of the illness interact with the general problems already described.

The Effect of the Illness on Development

Illness may interfere with the child's achieving the tasks of normal development (McCollum and Gibson 1970; Travis 1976). Thus the progress a toddler who is learning to walk and to develop bowel control has already made will be disrupted by forced confinement to bed and chronic diarrhea. Such a child, requiring mother's help during the illness, may substitute the gratification this provides for the advantages of autonomy. If the confinement is prolonged or repeated, there is danger that, at a later age, some such children will remain overly dependent rather than learning to rely on their own resources. Unresolved problems from an earlier stage of development (e.g., separation problems) can interfere with development at a later stage (e.g., acquisition of an independent identity as an adolescent) (Sigal et al. 1973). In addition, the immobility and isolation imposed by chronic illness and hospitalization can impede the development of the relationship skills crucial to social success in adolescence (Geist 1979; Maddison and Raphael 1971; Seidl and Altshuler 1979).

Family Reactions to Chronic Illness

Severe and chronic illness in a child confronts the entire family with tensions and demands that will tax relationships both within and beyond the family unit. Recent writers suggest that it is during the initial period that the stress is maximal so that psychological assistance may be required (Geist 1979; Leaverton 1979). The degree and nature of the stress will vary as will a particular family's ability to meet it (McKey 1973). One common pattern is for the father to abdicate family responsibility, using overinvolvement in work or other social activities to distance himself from emotional involvement with the sick child, leaving the major physical and emotional burden of caring for the child with the mother, who then becomes enmeshed and overprotective to an extent that is destructive to all (Khan 1979; Minuchin et al. 1978). A number of factors influence the family's response to the illness.

ILLNESS SEVERITY, LIKELY PROGNOSIS, AND AVAILABILITY OF EFFECTIVE TREATMENT

Generally speaking, the more debilitating the illness and the poorer the prognosis, the greater the stress on the family. Recent reports have indicated that the severity of the illness—measured in terms of physical impairment, visibility of physical residua, and functional limitations—is not directly related to psychosocial adjustment (Drotar 1981; O'Malley et al. 1980). This is probably due to the simultaneous influence of other factors (e.g., family's ability to cope with stress, etc.), but it is safe to say that a serious chronic illness, especially if the clinical course is one of relentless progression, is bound to produce terrible stress—though not necessarily maladjustment—in the family. In such cases the parents face the constant threat of losing their child. The resulting strain is intensified if sudden death at any time is a possibility (e.g., some forms of congenital heart disease, Riley-Day syndrome, severe asthma) (Freedman et al. 1957; McKey 1973).

WHETHER THE DISEASE IS CONGENITAL OR ACQUIRED

Illnesses in which congenital factors have been implicated (e.g., fibrocystic disease, the muscular dystrophies, congenital heart disease, some

463

forms of mental retardation) are likely to intensify parental feelings of guilt and responsibility (Burton 1975; Khan, 1979; Travis 1976).

AGE OF ONSET OF ILLNESS AND DIAGNOSIS

If the diagnosis is made at birth, the family will never have experienced the child as normal. Their concept of the child will always have included expectations altered because of the illness. If, however, the illness appears or is diagnosed after the child's personality has developed and his or her place in the family is established, family members will think of the child as normal and will experience an even greater sense of loss and depression when they are forced by the illness to scale down their hopes and expectations. Chronic illness occurring first in adolescence is resented by both child and family as a particularly painful cheating of someone about to experience all the supposed freedoms and opportunities that go with adult status.

The effects of parents' expectations on ongoing development must also be considered. The more the child is seen and treated like a normal child, the less development will be interfered with. However, the earlier the diagnosis is made—and the more parents see the child as fragile, handicapped, or limited—the more likely parents are to grossly overprotect and overindulge the child, thus distorting the parent-child relationship and the normal developmental process.

PREEXISTING STABILITY AND STRENGTH OF THE MARITAL
AND FAMILY UNIT

The greatest psychological or social problems usually develop when serious chronic illness strikes a child in an already disturbed family. While the entire family will inevitably affect—and be affected by—severe chronic illness in any member, disease poses a particular threat in two situations. The first is when chronic illness develops in a child with whom relationships are already disturbed. The second is when, even before, the parents' marriage was already strained almost to the limit of tolerance. A strong network of extended family and friends may ease the physical and emotional burden of day-to-day care of the chronically ill or handicapped child.

THE NATURE AND EFFECTS OF THE ILLNESS ITSELF

Pain or malaise caused by the child's illness or a resented treatment program may produce a child who is cranky, irritable, unpleasant, or demanding. These same traits will present additional pressures and evoke resentment, guilt, and feelings of inadequacy in the parents. If the illness is clearly visible and frequently elicits reactions of disgust or aversion from others (e.g., congenital amputations or deformities, severe scarring from burns, conspicuous mental retardation), the continued confrontation with the discomfort of others may prove a serious blow to the normal parental wish to have an attractive, healthy child who reflects well on them. This may also be the case if failure to thrive secondary to the disease rather than a more obvious deformity deprives the parents of the beautiful, healthy child they long for (Maddison and Raphael 1971).

EFFECTS OF HOME MANAGEMENT PROGRAM AND RESTRICTIONS ON
FAMILY LIFE

Some illnesses require a demanding program of home management and restrictions, such as fibrocystic disease with its daily regimen of inhalations, postural drainage, and frequent medications, or juvenile diabetes with its dietary restrictions, regular testing, and daily insulin injections. These demands, despite their absolute medical necessity, may be resented and vigorously resisted by children. Even appropriate explanations of the purpose and importance of the treatment may not persuade the child to accept willingly the unpleasant restrictions or procedures (Burton 1975). Indeed, excessive compliance by the child is more likely to indicate pathologic passivity and depression than mental health (Mattsson 1972). Even normal resistance, however, will cause additional work and emotional strain for parents who are struggling to administer the prescribed regimen. If they respond with excessive impatience, resentment, and guilt—or, alternatively, if they back off and provide only inconsistent care—both physical health and emotional relationships will suffer (Burton 1974*b*; Mannino and Shore 1974).

Moderate self-assertion and some opposition to parental authority are essential features of the normal child's progress toward independence (Lowit 1973). In the chronically ill child, this opposition may become concentrated on opposing the unwanted treatment regimen, which then becomes a daily battleground (Kaplan and De-Nour 1979; Zeidel 1973). Many authors comment on the frequency with which chronically ill older children and adolescents behave in ways they know is harmful to their health—consider the hemophiliac who gets into fights or the diabetic who stays up all night drinking beer at a party (Leaverton 1979; Mattsson 1966; Schowalter 1979). Such behavior may be seen in part as typical adolescent rebellion against parents (and in this case, medical authorities) but also as an attempt to be like healthy peers and to deny the disease (Sperling 1978). The danger, over and above any potential risks in the behavior itself, is that the acting-out and the parental response to it may cause developmental distortions, resentment, and guilt in both parents and child that may seriously undermine not only their relationship but the emotional life of the family as a whole.

PRESENCE OR ABSENCE OF OTHER AFFECTED SIBLINGS

The parental reaction may be affected by whether or not more than one child has the illness. The presence of other healthy children— especially if a congenital factor has been demonstrated—may mitigate parental feelings of inadequacy and distress (Lefebvre and Munro 1978). Alternatively, parents with more than one afflicted child will frequently have even more than usual guilt in response to the illness of a subsequent affected child (Atkin 1974), even if they had no prior knowledge of carrier status or if the diagnosis of the older child came too late to avoid the risk of a subsequent pregnancy (Burton 1975; Travis 1976).

REPEATED HOSPITALIZATIONS AND SURGICAL PROCEDURES

Diseases requiring frequent hospitalizations, painful treatments, or repeated surgery (e.g., renal failure, severe burns) present particular difficulties for both child and parents (Aisenberg et al. 1973; Cline and Rothenberg 1974). Children, especially toddlers, are often upset by going into the hospital and may not understand why they must leave the family or submit to frightening or painful procedures Barowsky 1978; (Danilowicz and Gabriel 1971; Simeonsson et al. 1979; Wallinga 1979). As a result, they often feel punished or abandoned by their parents, whose uncertainty and guilt may be intensified by the child's unhappiness and resentment (Rosberg 1971). At times parents are unable to comfort their suffering child, as in the case of a severely burned child. Even worse, they may be forced to make decisions that can literally determine whether their child lives or dies, without any assurance that they are deciding correctly, as when the parents of a child with congenital heart disease must decide for or against an operation.

RELIGIOUS AFFILIATIONS AND ACTIVE CAREERS OF PARENTS

While religious affiliations and parents' careers are usually positive resources, they may interfere with the acceptance of chronic illness or disability. Traditionally some religious denominations (e.g., Quakers) are more accepting of disabled individuals than others that view disability as a punishment for past sins. Professionals must consider the family's beliefs when counseling (e.g., attitudes about avoiding or terminating future pregnancies) or in preparing for surgery, since some groups (e.g., Jehovah's Witnesses) do not permit blood transfusions. Upward mobility in work, often a major source of self-esteem, may require frequent transfers, late hours, and so forth, which can be seriously limited by the care needed by a chronically ill or a handicapped child.

COST OF THE ILLNESS

In estimating the costs of an illness, even in state-underwritten systems, the hidden dollars-and-cents cost must be considered (e.g., doctor and hospital bills, medications, special diets, needed equipment and appliances, etc.) (Kalnins et al. 1980; Lansky et al. 1979). For families with limited income, these expenses may be a major source of additional pressure that may necessitate both parents going out to work or even having to take on a second job to make ends meet. Drained and exhausted, the parents then come home to the demands of administering or supervising a demanding and unpopular program of management and restrictions. The cycle is vicious. Emotional needs of both parents and children frequently go unmet and marital stress is aggravated (Crain, Sussman, and Weil 1966; Lansky et al. 1978). The rate of family conflict and/or breakdown in families with severe chronic illness is high (Pakes 1974; Solnit and Green 1959).

SPECIFIC EMOTIONAL REACTIONS

Specific emotional reactions are depicted in figure 21.1.

Denial

To some extent, all parents react with denial to the shock of their child's illness. While denial may help the parents through the initial trauma and

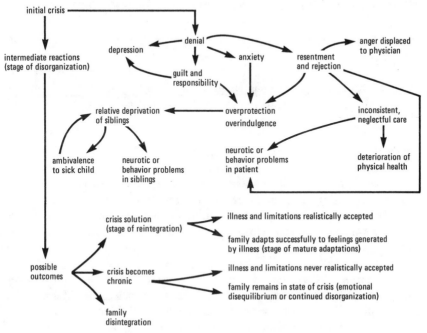

Figure 21.1 Family Reaction to Severe Chronic Illness

subsequent disorganization, normally—but by no means always—the family's use of denial should gradually decrease as the ability to come to grips with the implications of the illness increases. Denial is probably never completely abandoned, certainly not at any single time. Persistent massive denial in the face of obvious illness will interfere with the family's ability to master its initial catastrophic reaction to the illness and to meet successfully the child's needs, thus perpetuating the crisis precipitated by the illness. It is this denial, closely related to their need for hope, that often leads parents to misinterpret what their doctor has said or to shop from doctor to doctor until they find one who will give them the diagnosis and prognosis they want to hear (Mattsson 1972; Raimbault 1973; Schowalter 1979).

Anxiety

All parents of a chronically ill child are more or less anxious about the health—or even the survival—of their child. If their anxiety is excessive, either because of the real threat of sudden death or because of a neurotic overreaction, it may lead to overprotection, overindulgence, and difficulties setting reasonable and consistent limits for the child.

Feelings of Guilt, Responsibility, and Self-Blame

Some parents see their child's illness as a punishment from God, while others feel victimized by Fate. Still others, particularly if the disease is a congenital one, feel that the illness is proof of their personal inadequacy (i.e., their inability to bear a normal child). Although these feelings are totally irrational, attempts to logically argue parents out of them rarely succeed. All of us have our own secret sins and personal inadequacies (e.g., an unwanted pregnancy, an abortion attempt, unacceptable resentment of the sick child), and these may be elaborated on in a way that grinds the depressed parent ever deeper into the rut of despondency.

Depression

Basically the parents are mourning for the child who, but for the illness, might have been. Depression is a stage in their coming to terms with the implications of the child's disease. Some parents learn to accept the illness or handicap and its consequences for their family. Others never do so, and their family's life—and even its continued existence—may be dominated by their unresolved depression.

Resentment and Rejection

The parents' resentment, a reaction to their disappointment and despair, may be converted to bitterness toward each other, family and friends, physicians, the community at large, or the child, who may be overtly or covertly rejected. Covert rejection may lead to inadequate or inconsistent care, to unnecessary demands for hospitalization, or to avoidance of the child through overinvolvement in work or other activities. It may be masked by its opposite, overprotection, resulting in failure to discipline the child appropriately. The resulting misbehavior is then used by the parents to rationalize their rejection. Rejection is more common with visible deformities (e.g., spina bifida) or other congenital malformations (Mattsson 1972; Travis 1976).

Reactions to the Extended Community

Excessive sympathy on the part of parents and others may allow chronically ill children to manipulate, using the illness to get their own way, thereby inhibiting the development of full potential (Mattsson 1972). Shame, embarrassment, or sheer exhaustion may decrease the family's interest and involvement in recreational and other activities, or may cause bitterness and alienation from relatives, friends, or neighbors just when they are more needed for support. Some parents use the burden of a child's illness to justify their own failure to advance vocationally or professionally.

Sibling Reactions

The siblings of a sick child often react with jealousy and resentment toward the child who monopolizes so much of the family's attention and energies (Burton 1975; Lavigne and Ryan 1979). The parents' preoccupation with the sick child and their personal responses to the illness may leave the other children feeling emotionally deprived. Furthermore, many families cannot tolerate expressions of jealousy toward a sick or dying child. If parents cannot allow the other children to openly express their resentment or their feelings of being shortchanged, the guilt the children feel for harboring these feelings will be intensified. This frequently results in the hostility being repressed, only to be expressed covertly by pathological withdrawal, underachievement in school, behavior problems or delinquency, or neurotic reactions. The case of Nina, discussed in chapter 12, illustrates the effect of one severely and chronically ill child on a sibling.

In recent years there has been mounting evidence that the development and adjustment of healthy siblings may be more seriously undermined than those of the chronically ill child. Vance and associates (1980) have demonstrated that siblings of nephrotic children showed more neurotic tendencies, less self-acceptance, diminished social confidence, more inhibition of aggression, and poorer academic performance. Although a minority disagree (Gayton et al. 1977), most of those reporting have found that siblings of chronically ill chilren rate lower in school achievement and/or cognitive level but higher in dropout rates and emotional disturbance (Carandang et al. 1979; Demb and Ruess 1967; Shere and Kastenbaum 1966). In another controlled study, Cairns and colleagues (1979) found more aggressive and conduct disorders but not significantly more psychological disturbance in siblings of chronically ill children. They report that siblings exceed pediatric cancer patients themselves in perceived social isolation, fear of confronting other family members with negative feelings, fear of failure, and a perception of the parents as overindulging and overprotecting the sick child. These results support the authors' earlier findings that siblings of the ill child may, in fact, bear the heaviest burden of stress while receiving less support from the parents (Crain, Sussman, and Weil 1966). Binger (1973), studying children's reactions to the death of a sibling, reported that in over half the families, siblings showed later psychiatric difficulties even when they had previously appeared well adjusted. And it was not just siblings who had the same disease who were affected, as even healthy siblings were preoccupied with fantasies about the death, demonstrated feelings of contamination and fears that they would be next, and resentment of the parents for allowing the child to become ill and die or for spending too much time with the sick child (see also chapter 24).

Cain, Fast, and Erickson (1964) studied children's disturbed reactions to the death of a sibling. They found the reactions related to factors such as the nature of the death, the child's preexisting relationship with the dead sibling, the immediate and the long-term impact of the death on the parents, the child's cognitive ability to understand death, the parents' handling of the immediate impact of death on the surviving child, and the impact of the death on the whole family. Pathologic reactions, when they occurred, took the form of excessive and prolonged guilt reactions; depressions; blaming the parents for the death of the sibling; distorted concepts of illness and death; disturbed attitudes toward doctors, hospitals, and religion; death phobias; and identification with the dead child. The need to recognize the impact of a child's death on the surviving siblings cannot be overstressed if these disturbed reactions are to be avoided.

PHYSICIAN'S REACTIONS TO CHRONIC ILLNESS

Physicians and other attending staff may react emotionally to chronic or fatal illness in a child (Geist 1979; Khan 1979). The physician who cannot tolerate being unable to provide a cure may feel increasingly helpless, hopeless, and guilty. This often leads to withdrawal from patient and family, leaving them to face the stress of the disease without support. Professionals who overidentify with the parents may say too much too soon, that is, before they have overcome their initial shock and denial enough to hear what they are being told. Physicians may resent parents, sometimes in response to parental hostility but at other times in reaction to parental dependence, which merely underlines their own feelings of helplessness. Garrard and Richmond (1963), while recognizing how difficult this may prove, have stressed the need for doctors to maintain an awareness of their own separateness from the family in order to relate with "empathy, not sympathy; detachment rather than avoidance." Pakes (1974) suggested that physicians' reactions to their chronically ill patients often parallel those of the parents.

Management

Successful management of the emotional aspects of chronic illness is based on a recognition that illness in one child will have major implications on mental health, relationships, and possibly even the continued existence of the family. The more family members (especially parents) have resolved their anxiety, depression, feelings of responsibility, and resentment stirred up by the illness, the better they will be able to meet the physical and emotional needs of the child and to deal successfully with the additional strains imposed by illness with minimal damage and disruption to the family as a whole. On the other hand, failure to resolve the emotional responses to the illness will decrease the family's ability to satisfy the emotional needs of all its members, thus increasing the likelihood of severe ongoing family tension and possible breakdown. Only when parents have received a clear and definitive diagnosis can they begin to deal first with the necessary practical planning and later with the arduous but no less important task of emotionally accepting the inevitable.

The diagnosis of a severe chronic illness will precipitate a crisis in the family. The physician or other professional who recognizes the potential for disorganization that this will inevitably produce can do much to minimize the destructive effects and to aid in the reintegration and adaptation of the family as a whole. The family's past history of dealing with stress will often allow professionals to anticipate the nature of potential difficulties. Therefore an assessment of previous family responses to stress is helpful. If marital tensions are noted, professionals should be particularly careful to communicate with both parents to help them face problems together. Prior peer, school, and behavior problems may suggest possible difficulties for child and staff during management. Observed interaction between child and parents is a guide to possible reactions to medical staff.

The attending physician must recognize that what the family members *hear* and *understand* may differ considerably from what they have been told. Parents can assimilate only what they are emotionally ready for; in distress, they may hear only what they want to hear, selecting or distorting what was actually said either to obtain false reassurance or to confirm their worst fears. They need honest and repeated explanations of their child's diagnosis, progress, and prognosis, and time to digest this information. All professionals must be simple and direct, avoiding unwarranted optimism or excessive pessimism. Timing may be important. While saying too much too soon may cause unnecessary anxiety, more commonly too little is said too late and in too ambiguous a manner. One important reason for physicians' maintaining regular contact with the family is to explore what they have heard regarding diagnosis, prognosis, and management and how they are coping, in terms of both day-to-day management and emotional adjustment.

Physicians should periodically review with the parents of chronically ill children their understanding of the overall management of the child. Severe overprotection and unnecessary restrictions on activity, failure to provide age-appropriate expectations and to supply reasonable discipline, the presence of obvious behavior or academic problems in a sibling or mounting tension within the marriage, and a major and continuing discrepancy between physician and parents around what the child can do may be as serious an indication that the family is in trouble as inadequate or inconsistent care.

Similarly, ongoing contacts with the child allow various professionals to explore the child's understanding of the illness and help deal with emotional reactions to it. By asking how the child sees him- or herself and the illness, the child can be encouraged to raise concerns. Often parents are too anxious to allow children, including the sick child, to discuss openly any of their fears. Those parents who understand and perceive accurately the nature of the disease, its symptoms and prognosis, and who can discuss these directly with their family will greatly safeguard the family's adjustment. Traditionally parents and health professionals have discouraged chronically ill patients from discussing their illness for fear of upsetting or depressing them. However, recently an increasing number of authors*️ are supporting discussion of even the most painful feelings related to the illness. It has been shown that those pediatric cancer patients who talked most about their illness were the ones where were least depressed (Kellerman et al. 1977).

Helping parents overcome their own anxieties so that they can tolerate and deal with the children's concerns plays a crucial part in minimizing serious and long-lasting emotional damage. What is openly acknowledged is generally less threatening than that which is known but not discussed. The conspiracy of silence that leads to avoiding any mention of consequences of the illness—including hospitalizations, operations (especially when they involve mutilations, such as amputations), or approaching death—is usually a pretense, trying for all, but especially for the child who is the central character. This is discussed in more detail by Bluebond-Langer (1978), Burton (1974a), Cain, Fast, and Erickson (1964), Kubler-Ross (1974), and Patterson, Denning, and Kutscher (1973).

School and peer relationships are an extremely important part of children's lives. The chronically ill child may miss a great deal of school and may need tutoring during hospitalization. The cooperation of the child's teacher should be sought to coordinate schooling. Throughout hospitalization, the child should be encouraged to keep in contact with friends, either

---

*See Alby and Alby 1973; Burton 1974a; Geist 1979; Gogan et al. 1978; Spinetta 1977; and Vernick 1973.

through visits or by mail. Embarrassment or shame because of the illness and deformity, fear of exclusion or teasing may contribute to an alienation from peers who, given proper encouragement, could be a major source of support for the child. Hospitals should encourage chronically ill older children and adolescents to meet in groups to discuss their feelings and concerns about how their illness has affected their lives, their family relationships, their involvement with friends, and so forth. Alertness of medical staff to a refusal by an older child to contact friends may help them discuss with the child fears of growing isolation and alienation. Physicians and hospital staff are frequently the undeserving objects of hostility. This is not meant, and should not be taken, as an attack on them personally, even when expressed in very personal terms. Rather it is a displacement of the parents' resentment that the illness has occurred and a reaction against those whose job it was to confront them with realities they would rather not hear. If the physician or staff members respond with hostility or by withdrawing from or rejecting the family, an opportunity to provide much-needed support at the time of maximal distress will be lost. If the feelings are too intense to be resolved right at the moment, it is best to have the parents back in the near future, to discuss the situation again. Some parents need a chance to vent their frustrations before they can listen, make the necessary decisions, or cooperate regarding management. Physicians and hospital staff who continue to approach the parents with empathy and objectivity may be able to help them focus and resolve their distress more appropriately, leaving them free to move on to the issues of practical management. Most parents require repeated opportunities to ask their child's doctor what could have caused or prevented the illness or the defect, whether or not they are responsible, and, if there is an inherited condition, what their chances are of having another affected child. The opportunity to go over these questions *again* and *again* with a trusted advisor is an important part of the process of learning to accept the disappointment. While specialists (e.g., a genetic counselor) may be needed to answer specific questions, no one is more important to the parents than the reliable, responsible, humane physician who continues to care even when unable to cure and who is willing to take the time to listen to the parents and to sustain them through periods of discouragement and frustration.

The management of the chronically ill child and family requires the resources of a team of professionals. Adequate communication must be maintained between team members for coordination of management. A frustrating family, by increasing demands and creating tension between team members, may cause friction and invite breakdown of team coordination. Disagreements among team members may be unwittingly taken out on the patient. Under such circumstances, regular team meetings can help keep problems in perspective, avoiding unnecessary and potentially harmful splits among team members and allowing them to support each other in times of stress (Pakes 1974).

Restrictions on the ill child's activity are often inevitable. While pre-schoolers generally limit their own activities, older children who need to confirm and prove their social adequacy may tend to overtax themselves. Physicians may help by defining and explaining necessary activity restrictions as well as by arbitrating between parent and child when conflicts arise because the child rebels. Realistic restrictions required by the illness, however irritating, may be less crippling than those constructed or fantasied by parent or child. By emphasizing areas of satisfactory function and potential strengths, physicians may do much to help the family achieve a balanced acceptance of the child's strengths and limitations.

Children need and use play as an outlet for their feelings and as one method of resolving conflicts (Crocker 1978; Linde et al. 1979). Puppets, paints, and toy medical equipment can be used for this purpose. Such play also provides the immobilized child with an outlet for activity and an opportunity for independence. Occupational therapists can be extremely helpful in involving children in play activities appropriate to their needs.

Any major decision (regarding hospitalization or surgical intervention) or any necessary but disappointing statement regarding prognosis may precipitate emotional upset or be greeted with docile passivity. In either case, physicians and other staff members should realize that how the parents behave may be very different from what they are feeling. Some parents may need active encouragement to express feelings that have been held in but are tearing them and their family apart. In making important decisions, some families need help to recognize and weigh the facts of the situation, and reassurance and encouragement once a decision has been made.

Physicians differ in their ability to help families cope with their emotional reactions to chronic illness. While each family needs someone to help them deal with their emotional responses to the illness, this might or might not be their physician. Should the demands of meeting the emotional needs of families of chronically ill patients exceed what the physician can tolerate or provide, the family can always be referred to an allied professional prepared to help them deal with the emotional sequelae of the illness. A child psychiatrist, a social worker, a pastoral counselor, or an association of parents who have experienced a similar problem can be extremely helpful to the family and to the physician. Before making such a referral, physicians should be clear on whether they themselves are prepared to continue to assume a major role in helping the family with its emotional difficulties and are seeking a consultation or whether they prefer to have the referral agent take over the management of the psychological and social aspects of the case.

Episodes of hospitalization may precipitate acute or chronic crises. When hospitalization is necessary, hospital staff may be at the receiving end of parental criticism or overinvolvement. Parents may be demanding, critical, and competitive with nursing staff. But hospital staff may need reminding that *their* patient is *still* the parents' child and that the parents' reactions are an expression of their anxiety and a displacement of their resentment at having a seriously ill child. Remembering this may help hospital staff maintain some understanding and empathy even for difficult parents, instead of responding with hostility and rejection, which will only aggravate the parental distress and increase friction and antagonism between parents and hospital staff. By anticipating, recognizing, and mediating such conflicts as they appear to arise, the physician may help all avoid or break the vicious circle of recrimination.

SUGGESTIONS FOR FURTHER READING

ANTHONY, E. J., AND KOUPERNIK, C., eds. 1973. *The child in his family, vol. 2: The impact of disease and death.* New York: John Wiley & Sons.
    A highly recommended collection of papers dealing with the reactions of children and parents to disease, death, and mourning.

BINGER, C. M. 1973. Childhood leukemia: Emotional impact on siblings. In *The child in his family, vol. 2: The impact of disease and death,* ed. E. J. Anthony and C. Koupernik, pp. 195–209. New York: John Wiley & Sons.
    Illustrates with a case history the short- and long-term reactions of siblings to the death of a leukemic child.

BURTON, L. 1975. *The family life of sick children.* London: Routledge & Kegan Paul.
    A controlled study of fifty-three families in Northern Ireland, each with a child with cystic fibrosis. Examines problems of chronic illness as well as adaptive and maladaptive ways of coping with stress.

CAIRNS, N., et al. 1979. Adaptation of siblings to childhood malignancy. *Pediatrics* 95(3):484–487.
    Siblings experience as much as or more stress than pediatric patients themselves when confronted with chronic, life-threatening illness such as cancer.

FRIEDRICH, W. M. 1977. Ameliorating the psychological impact of chronic physical disease on the child and family. *J. Pediat. Psychol.* 2(1):26–31.
    Reviews previous research demonstrating the deleterious effects of a child's chronic illness on siblings and parents as well as on the patient. Suggests total family intervention and presents a sample Goal Attainment Scale to evaluate this.

FRYDMAN, M. I. 1980. Perception of illness severity and psychiatric symptoms in parents of chronically ill children. *J. Psychosom. Res.* 24(6):361–369.
    Two hundred twenty parents of children with cystic fibrosis or leukemia were identified as either overestimators, underestimators, and accurate perceivers of the severity of their child's illness. An association was found between how much parents distort symptom severity and prognosis and parental psychiatric symptoms. Processes by which distortion might arise and association with parental psychiatric morbidity are discussed.

GAYTON, W. F., et al. 1977. Children with cystic fibrosis: I. Psychological test findings of patients, siblings and parents. *Pediatrics* 59(6):888–894.
    Psychological evaluation of forty-three families of children with cystic fibrosis does not show increased emotional disturbances in patients or siblings.

GEIST, R. A. 1979. Onset of chronic illness in children and adolescents: Psychotherapeutic and consultative intervention. *Am. J. Orthopsychiat.* 49(1):4–23.

Children with different chronic illnesses exhibit both similar and specific reactions during onset phase. Psychological intervention during the initial stages of illness is stressed and recommendations for psychotherapeutic and consultative management of the patient are made. Examines the effects of intervention on both child and psychotherapist.

GREY, M. J.; GENEL, M.; AND TAMBORLANE, W. V. 1980. Psychosocial adjustment of latency-aged diabetics: Determinants and relationship to control. *Pediatrics* 65(1):69–73.
Psychosocial adjustment problems frequently occur in latency-age diabetic children and are associated with poorer chemical control and require a family-centered approach to intervention and management.

HOLLENBECK, A. R., et al. 1980. Children with serious illness: Behavioral correlates of separation and isolation. *Child Psychiat. & Hum. Dev.,* 11(1):3–11.
Preschool children receiving chemotherapy for cancer showed agitation followed by behavioral depression. Findings underscore the seriousness of parent-child separation and the need to ameliorate these deleterious effects for ill and hospitalized children.

JOHNSON, M. R.; SOURKES B.; AND SPINETTA, J. J. 1979. Mental health interventions with medically ill children: A review of the literature, 1970–1977. *J. Pediat. Psychol.* 4(2):147–162.
Reviews the literature on the psychological impact of chronic illness on the child, identifying six broad goals for therapy: amelioration of disease-related stress, treatment of personality problems arising from illness, preparing children for medical experiences, helping them cope with impending death, behavior management and rehabilitation.

KAGEN-GOODHEART, L. 1977. Re-entry: Living with childhood cancer. *Am. J. Orthopsychiat.* 47(4):651–658.
Discusses problems of child with cancer returning to the community while still undergoing medical treatment and how the mental health professional can facilitate the resumption of normal activities and productive coping patterns.

KALNINS, I. V.; CHURCHILL, M. P.; AND TERRY, G. E. 1980. Concurrent stresses in families with a leukemic child. *J. Pediat. Psychol.* 5(1):81–92.
The majority of forty-five families of leukemic children had to cope with other stresses over and above those of dealing with chronic illness (e.g., financial worries, death in the family, occupational changes). They may need assistance for coping with these problems along with disease-related anxiety.

KAPLAN D. M. AND DE NOUR, A. K. 1979. Adolescents' adjustment to chronic hemodialysis. *Am. J. Psychiat.* 136:430–433.
Compares the adjustment of eighteen adolescents to sixty-three adult patients on chronic hemodialysis. The author suggests that chronic illness is especially different for this age group (e.g., body image, restriction on social activity, medical regimen).

KHAN, A. U. 1979. Coping with chronic illness *and* Facing a dying child and his family. In *Psychiatric emergencies in pediatrics,* ed. A. U. Khan, pp. 53–65; 195–208. Chicago: Year Book Medical Pubs. Ltd.
Two well-written and sensitive chapters about psychological aspects of chronic and fatal illness. Discusses the role of the mental health professional in facilitating family coping with the stress imposed by childhood disease.

LANSKY, S. B., et al. 1978. Childhood cancer: Parental discord and divorce. *Pediatrics* 62(2):184–188.
Parents of 191 pediatric cancer patients had greater marital stress but not a higher divorce rate than the general population.

LAVIGNE, J. V., AND RYAN, M. 1979. Psychologic adjustment of siblings of children with chronic illness. *Pediatrics* 63(4):616–627.
A controlled study comparing the adjustment of siblings of chronically ill children to those of healthy children, finding increased irritability and social withdrawal among the former.

MANNINO, F. V., AND SHORE, M. F. 1974. Family structure, aftercare, and post-hospital adjustment. *Am. J. Orthopsychiat.* 44:76–85.
Confirms the important effect of family variables on posthospital adjustment and treatment outcome in an after-care program. Has important implications for program planning.

MATTSSON, A. 1972. Long-term physical illness in childhood: A challenge to psychosocial adaptation. *Pediatrics* 50(5):801–811.

Reviews psychologic stresses and the related adaptational techniques used by child and parents to master the distressing feelings resulting from chronic illnesses in childhood.

NOVER, R. A. 1973. Pain and the burned child. *J. Am. Acad. Child Psychiat.* 12:499–505.

Discusses pain as a central factor influencing the behavior of the burned child. Relates the child's experience of pain to the degree to which the pain is charged with psychic meaning.

PLESS, I. B., AND PINKERTON, P. 1975. *Chronic childhood disorder: Promoting patterns of adjustment.* London: Henry Kimpton Publishers.

A thorough summary and interpretation of previous research on chronic illness in childhood, stressing adaptive methods of coping.

SEIDL, A. H., AND ALTSHULER, A. 1979. Interventions for adolescents who are chronically ill. *Children Today,* Nov./Dec., pp. 16–19.

Offers suggestions for mental health professionals who work with chronically ill adolescents to help facilitate individual maturation with specific reference to Erikson's "developmental tasks."

SOLNIT, A. J., ed. 1977. *An anthology of "The psychoanalytic study of the child": Physical illness and handicap in childhood.* New Haven, Conn.: Yale University Press.

Contains articles under three basic headings: hospitalization, physical illness, and physical defectiveness.

SOURKES, B. 1977. Facilitating family coping with childhood cancer. *J. Pediat. Psychol.* 2(2):65–67.

Four specific types of interventions are discussed, including: the facilitation of communication; being available on an ongoing basis; "giving permission" to the parents to use that availability; modeling skills for parents to use with their children.

SPINETTA, J. J. 1977. Adjustment in children with cancer. *J. Pediat. Psycho.,* 2(2):49–51.

Parents' four assumptions expressing the basic values of professionals dealing with children with cancer: that the quality of life is enhanced by maximal efforts devoted to living; that preparation for necessary painful procedures should be provided; that communication of even the child's painful thoughts is healthy; that the child's life style prior to illness is the main baseline against which to evaluate change.

TRAVIS, G. 1976. *Chronic illness in children: Its impact on child and family.* Stanford, Calif.: Stanford University Press.

A comprehensive and sensitive book that examines, using a developmental approach, prevalent long-term illnesses of childhood and describes their effects on children and their families. Stresses the social component.

VANCE, J. C., et al. 1980. Effects of nephrotic syndrome on the family: A controlled study. *Pediatrics,* 65(5):948–955.

Although few striking differences were found, findings suggest several areas of increased vulnerability to psychosocial problems among parents and siblings of nephrotic children.

22

Arlette Lefebvre

The Child with Physical Handicaps

Introduction

Only twenty-five years ago few handicapped children were expected to survive into adulthood. Since then improved neonatal care and advances in diagnostic, medical, and surgical techniques have dramatically improved the prognosis and prolonged the lifespan of many. Yet only in the last decade have physicians and mental health workers seriously begun considering the quality of the lives that medicine has prolonged.

This chapter will review common emotional and social problems of children with major physical disabilities, describing common adjustment patterns shown by the children and their families. It will then consider the medical, surgical, educational, and psychosocial needs of handicapped children, suggesting guidelines for rehabilitation programs designed to meet these needs.

Definitions and Incidence

The United Nations Declaration on the Rights of Disabled Persons (Health and Welfare Canada 1981) defines a disabled person as "any person unable to ensure by himself or herself wholly or partly the necessities of a normal

478

individual and/or social life, as a result of a deficiency, either congenital or not, in his or her physical or mental capabilities." Even within this definition, there is little agreement about which conditions to consider handicapping or disabling. Some surveys include congenital heart disease (Hirsch 1979), diabetes, epilepsy, dialysis, or hemophilia (Diller 1972; Schlesinger 1979), while others consider them in the chronic illness category only. In some cases (e.g., rheumatoid arthritis) the distinction is even less clear, as disability can result from chronic illness.

This chapter will confine itself to major physical disabilities, excluding mental retardation, which is discussed in chapter 18, and chronic illness, reviewed in chapter 21. The terms limitation, disability, handicap, and management will be used as follows:

Limitation—a minor physical impairment requiring some adaptation but not significantly impairing life style or adjustment (e.g., poor vision, requiring glasses).

Disability—the partial or total loss of a physical structure or function (e.g., loss of vision, hearing, or use of a limb).

Handicap—the social and psychological consequences of a disability.

Management—the efforts of "helping persons" including doctors, educators, and employers to facilitate optimal development of the child.

However, as the number of people considered disabled varies depending on how the term *disabled* is defined, how the data are collected, and the purpose and interpretation of the data, it is impossible to obtain accurate figures on the prevalence of physical handicap in the general population. Rates ranging from 8.5 percent in Great Britain (Weale and Bradshaw 1980) to 9.5 percent in Canada (Health and Welfare Canada 1981) have been reported. American figures quoted range from 8 to 10 percent (Pless and Douglas 1971). These undoubtedly contain many who, while not physically disabled, are chronically ill or functionally impaired, as they include all those requiring special educational, medical, or transportation services, many of whom have learning or mental disabilities but no physical handicap. Prevalence figures for children under sixteen vary between 7 and 10 percent (Sperling 1978) although again, the definition is more inclusive than that used in this chapter. As the prevalence of physical handicap has increased, there has been a corresponding rise in social awareness of physical handicap. The polio epidemic of the early 1950s, the Thalidomide tragedy of the 1960s, the return of thousands of disabled veterans from Vietnam, the greater sensitivity across North America to the rights of all minorities, and the emergence of effective and articulate groups of handicapped persons demanding social recognition of their problems and community action in solving them have profoundly influenced public attitudes toward the rights, needs, and rehabilitation of the handicapped.

Classification

There are two groups of handicapped children: those who are congenitally handicapped and those who become handicapped at some point after birth. Types and/or causes of congenital handicaps include blindness, deafness or severe hearing impairment, cerebral palsy, spina bifida, facial deformities, mental retardation (see chapter 18), and congenital amputations (see pages 465, 480, 504).

Handicaps occurring postnatally fall into two categories: (1) *those caused by acute or chronic illness,* such as eye problems, tumor, retinoblastoma, retinitis pigmentosa; hearing impairments secondary to middle and inner ear infections; neurological and mental deterioration secondary to encephalitis (e.g., from measles), meningitis, or virus; disorders of mobility, for example, muscular dystrophy, Friedrich's ataxia, rheumatoid arthritis, osteogenesis imperfecta; and (2) *those caused by sudden injury,* such as burns and amputations secondary to trauma or surgery for malignant growth.

General Considerations

PSYCHOLOGICAL IMPACT ON THE CHILD

Most disabled children resemble normal children more than they differ from them. They are just as likely to dream of becoming a superstar in hockey or baseball or a beautiful actress, despite a missing limb or ear, confinement to a wheelchair, or gross disfigurement. As they grow older, however, their growing recognition that their disability will make the fulfillment of these dreams impossible often evokes increasing resentment and depression. While as a group disabled children are more prone to emotional and social problems, the severity of these in any given child may vary from severe to nonexistent (Sperling 1978).

The biggest obstacle for the disabled child is the fear and curiosity of other people. Because they look different, disabled children make others feel uncomfortable, stare, or look away (Freeman 1967). Children frequently ask questions about or make fun of the disability, while adults typically mask their discomfort behind an overpolite or overprotective attitude. The net result is a strained relationship with strangers who seldom talk to or treat the child spontaneously, thus making the youngster feel "different," an "outsider," or a "freak" (Bender 1980; Bernstein 1976).

COPING STYLES

Handicapped children have few alternatives for coping with such universal rejection. They can pretend not to see the stares or whispers, not to feel different, or, at least, they can hope that some day a magic operation or pill will make them just like everyone else. The opposite of this defense through denial is overawareness and preoccupation with the disability even when others are not reacting to it. Examples would include the child who hides her scarred face behind a book even in an empty waiting room, who refuses to appear even in family pictures, or who believes that no one could ever genuinely care for someone so ugly.

These extremes of feeling in response to social rejection are often mirrored by extremes of behavior. The disabled child who is accepted at home usually approaches peers in kindergarten eagerly, often with the encouragement of teachers who marvel at the lack of shame or self-doubt (Bernstein 1976; Diller 1972). The disabled teenager who constantly needs to prove that he is smarter, funnier, and harder working than normal peers (Wright 1960) will go out of his way to pick the most difficult project, to be the most gregarious, fun-loving, reliable friend. Such children may be too ambitious, setting life goals beyond their capacities but often making many friends in the process. On the other hand, the constantly self-conscious, anxious child soon learns to avoid potentially embarrassing social situations, to choose only solitary hobbies, and to feign disinterest in sports, shopping excursions, sexual encounters, or any other challenge that involves possible failure or embarrassment. The resulting shyness and awkwardness are often misinterpreted as evidence of suspiciousness, intellectual dullness, or emotional disturbance. Rigidity, social isolation, and overdependence on the family are common sequelae.

No single coping style or defense mechanism is "normal" or "ideal" for all situations. Handicapped children who underestimate their limitations usually take on too many impossible challenges, only to meet repeated frustration. Those who overestimate their disability excessively restrict their interest, activities, friendships, and career goals, soon losing faith in themselves and in their potential for being loved or accepted as worthwhile.

Figure 22.1 illustrates the dynamic interplay between opposing defense mechanisms.

FACTORS AFFECTING OUTCOME

In general, children with chronic ailments (illness or disability) have a higher rate of maladjustment than comparable peers (Adams 1980). Seidel, Chadwick, and Rutter (1975) found psychiatric disorder more than twice as common in handicapped children of normal intelligence than in

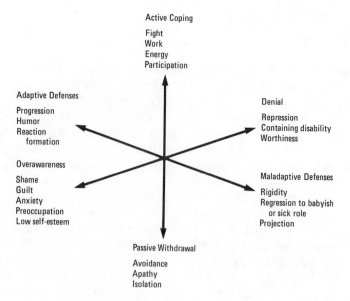

Figure 22.1 Dynamic Interplay of Opposing Defenses

healthy five- to fifteen-year-olds (17 percent vs. 7 percent). Particularly at risk were children whose disability was caused by disease of the central nervous system.

Nature of Disability

The nature of the disability is often a poor predictor of emotional problems. The child's age, personality strengths, and family relationships are much more likely to predict emotional disturbance in younger children (Pringle and Fiddes 1970). In teenagers and adults, however, visibility of handicap correlates highly with social maladjustment (Bernstein 1976; Freeman 1967; Goffman 1963), though some researchers contradict this (Spiegel 1959), while others (Minde 1978; Minde et al. 1972) state that invisible handicaps are often treated as guilty secrets.

The Severity of Disability*

The severity of the disability does not directly parallel the degree of psychological handicap. In some conditions such as rheumatoid arthritis (McAnarney et al. 1974) and facial deformities (Lefebvre and Munro 1978; Lefebvre and Barclay 1980; Olshansky 1962), children with minimal dis-

---

*The terms severity and visibility overlap but are not identical. For example, a third-degree burn covering 10 percent of the body surface may be much more severe (in terms of functional impairment) if it involves the hands and more visible (if located on the face) than even a 30 to 40 percent burn on normally covered areas of the body. This overlap probably contributes to many of the discrepancies and much of the confusion that results from a survey of the literature in either of these areas.

ability appear at greater risk psychologically. This could be because the severely handicapped child has a readily available and obvious excuse for the failure to compete with normal children. Also, in some cases (e.g., total as opposed to partial deafness) the more severe disability leads to the child being raised in an institution, exposing the child to less frustration and social stigma than the significantly but less disabled child who is struggling to cope and compete with normal peers in the community.

Age of Onset

At first, children with congenital handicaps are likely to deny their deformity or the severity of their disability (MacGregor 1979). However, because congenital disabilities are generally more severe than acquired ones and because they interfere with normal development from birth or even earlier, they usually cause greater psychosocial handicaps in later years (Travis 1976; Woods 1975).

The child who becomes disabled during early or middle childhood may interpret the disability as punishment for "being bad," thus accentuating secret guilt and shame (Kutner 1980; Mattsson 1972). Secretiveness by parents and hospital staff about diagnosis or medical and surgical procedures may heighten this sense of guilt.

The older child who was normal until being disabled in late childhood or adolescence is most vulnerable to a sudden crushing loss of self-esteem and despair about the future (Richardson 1963; Richman and Harper 1980). Such children, who only yesterday considered acne or short stature major disasters, find it extremely difficult to adjust to the much greater disability involved in a severe burn or an amputated limb.

Interplay Between Disability and Normal Development

Major physical disabilities such as blindness, deafness, and cerebral palsy obviously interfere with a child's seeing, hearing, and motor performance respectively. However, most major disabilities also affect other aspects of development in addition to those functions directly affected by the disability itself. For example, the blind child usually walks later than average, the deaf child is usually impulsive and socially immature, and even the bright cerebral palsy child is more likely to underachieve in school. Specific developmental implications will be described for each condition later in this chapter.

But if disability affects development, the converse is also true. Children's understanding of and reaction to their disabilities follows a typical developmental pattern. They recognize early their physical difference from others. As preschoolers, children's self-esteem and their opinion of their physical competence are based largely on the relationship with the parents. The young handicapped child whose parents can take pride in her personality and developmental accomplishments will approach school with the self-confidence and eagerness of physically normal children (Nelson 1975).

483

If the child lives in a small community so that classmates in kindergarten and first grade are long-time neighborhood friends, teasing, questioning, and name-calling may not be experienced for several years (Lefebvre and Barclay 1980).

But many handicapped children live in large communities, closer to the medical or surgical care they need. For them, the beginning of school is often their first exposure to social rejection and cruelty (Anastasiow 1981). While their initial response is typically tears and anger, children soon learn to use denial to overcome even the cruelest teasing. Those who feel valued at home usually ignore or walk away from their tormentors, dismissing them as "stupid" or "crazy" or muttering "nobody is perfect" as the parents have taught them to respond. Denial is also used in clinical situations, as when the child tells medical personnel that "everything is fine," that "I have lots of friends," or that "I just ignore the teasing." In time, the repeated use of denial drains off valuable energy badly needed for learning and socializing. Eventually the defense loses its effectiveness, and the repeated harassment undermines the child's self-esteem and trust in others. Unless the child is unusually smart, witty, talented, popular, or entertaining, his circle of friends and activities gradually narrows during middle childhood, as he increasingly withdraws and turns to the family for security and companionship.

With adolescence, the peer group becomes the major judge of social competence. The disabled adolescent's physical inadequacies, restricted career and athletic activities, and limited sexual appeal all seem insurmountable obstacles. At the same time sexual urges and emotional lability increase the adolescent's vulnerability to rejection (Berscheid and Walster 1972) and loss of self-control, often precipitating sudden and devastating depression. Although teenagers have known about the disability and its associated physical limitations for years, only in adolescence do they grasp the full impact of its social implications (Anastasiow 1981). Some handicapped adolescents respond by giving up, quitting school, discontinuing treatment, or retreating into a wheelchair or behind a television set. Others continue to compete with nonhandicapped peers in an attempt to salvage as much of a normal life as possible, although this inevitably means much loneliness, defeat, and rejection. The only other alternative is to restrict their contacts to "safe," nonthreatening peers (i.e., handicapped groups) or activities (such as pen pal clubs, high school newspapers, solitary hobbies).

Overall adjustment is shaped not only by the child's intelligence or the nature, severity, and prognosis of the disability but also by the individual child's character structure, defenses, strength of determination to live as full a life as possible, and the closeness and support of the family (Harvey and Greenway 1982). For example, a recent television documentary contrasted the persistence of an armless Thalidomine baby, now a mother, who feeds her own baby by holding the bottle between her feet, with the despair and withdrawal of a brilliant, handsome twenty-year-old paraplegic who has become a bitter recluse since his car accident.

General Factors

No crisis can be more devastating to a family than the birth of a defective or deformed child (Hirsch 1979). Especially if the imperfect baby is their first, parents react with grief as acute as if the ideal child whom they had dreamed about for nine months was stillborn (Solnit and Stark 1961).

Parents whose normal child is suddenly disabled in later childhood experience a different shock: they are more likely to react with anger or guilt over an accident or twist of fate. However, both congenital and acquired disabilities may vary widely.

Congenital defects may be as minor as a small hemangioma or as shocking as missing limbs or a grossly distorted face. Acquired or late-diagnosed disabilities can vary from a mild hearing impairment to a sudden paraplegia. The condition may or may not imply a shortened life span, may or may not be surgically repairable or medically treatable, may or may not imply serious lifelong mental or physical deficiency, may or may not require prolonged dependency on the family, and may or may not be linked to a hereditary pattern.

Responses of families whose child has a severe disability may vary as much as those of the children. Some derive strength from the satisfactions of their career, marriage, or the religious faith that allows them to accept the birth of a defective child as God's will. Others spend a lifetime trying to prove doctors wrong, refusing to accept the diagnosis. Hirsch (1979) speaks of three typical phases that parents go through in coming to terms with reality.

In the discovery phase, the parents are usually shocked and overwhelmed. Fears and feelings of disbelief may be converted into anger and displaced onto medical personnel, either for predicting a gloomy prognosis or, conversely, for not having diagnosed the problem earlier. Their feelings for the child swing from extremes of hatred ("this can't be mine") to overidentification ("you and me against the world"), either of which at this stage is a normal attempt to reconstitute shattered self-esteem rather than experience the disbility as evidence of personal inadequacy. Unfortunately, this is often the time of maximum pressure to decide about surgery and to choose between placement or home care.

Regarding early life care, many handicapped children require repeated medical and surgical interventions during infancy and early childhood. Some parents see these as positive, corrective procedures. If viewed this way, the interventions may attenuate the parents' grief and give hope for a nearly normal future (as in a child with cleft lip and palate) (Hirsch 1979).

In other conditions such as cerebral palsy, each new developmental stage may uncover unsuspected mental or physical disabilities that may or may not respond to treatment. For still other children (e.g., those with muscular dystrophy), the disabilities increase as the disease progresses. Thus each advance in the level of disability (e.g., walking with braces, walking with crutches, using a wheelchair, using an electric wheelchair) is a grim reminder of the inevitable outcome.

Concerning long-range planning, it should be recognized that most seriously disabled children grow up to become disabled and handicapped adults who will remain more or less dependent on their families and society for survival. Many parents who already had to nurture their child through a precarious early development, help her over school hurdles, sustain her through the disappointments of a lonely adolescence, now find themselves emotionally drained and fearful of the future once they are gone. Children who have been sheltered are usually unprepared to cope in a competitive world; will they become a burden for brothers or sisters to care for or will they eventually require institutionalization, the avoidance of which has been the main reason for years of effort and self-sacrifice?

These three phases do not necessarily follow in sequence. For most families denial and despair, anger and "bargaining" go hand in hand so that hope and fear, optimism and realism alternate throughout the child's life (Cohen 1962; Gath 1977).

Sibling Reactions to the Handicapped Child

Recent studies of the impact of physical and mental handicaps suggest that the siblings of handicapped children are often the forgotten members of the family. Shere and Kastenbaum (1966) have found that the nonaffected sibling of a handicapped twin is emotionally disturbed more frequently than the affected twin, given similar genetic endowment.

The nonaffected sibling, if older, is often given additional household responsibilities, expected to be an outstanding student to compensate the parents for the handicapped child's shortcomings, and to be a patient and understanding companion to the "special" (i.e., disabled) sibling. This means masking any resentment or jealousy even when the handicapped child monopolizes the parents' time and energy or elicits depreciating or hostile comments from classmates (Balikov and Feinstein 1979; Goffman 1963). Siblings of handicapped children show more irritability and social withdrawal during preschool years than do siblings of children who are chronically ill but not deformed (Lavigne and Ryan 1979). Teenagers with disabled siblings, especially boys, are also vulnerable to emotional and behavioral problems. In one study children with cleft lip and palate were more likely than the national average to complete their education while their siblings were more vulnerable to early school dropout (Demb and Ruess 1967).

Social Aspects of Handicaps

HISTORICAL PERSPECTIVE

In primitive cultures, society rejects its abnormal members, allowing only the fittest to survive (Marinelli and Kelz 1975). In "modern" civilizations, painters, poets, and minstrels have traditionally linked disability to evil, portraying the handicapped person as someone to be persecuted or at least avoided, someone punished by God for personal or ancestral sins or as the carrier of a satanic curse. Fairy tales and nursery rhymes have reinforced the prototypes of the ugly witch, the grotesque monster, the evil Captain Hook, and so forth. In view of this cultural bias, it is not surprising that even today physicians often assure parents that handicapped children will also be severely retarded, even though there is little evidence to support this generalization (MacGregor 1979).

If they are to gain acceptance, disabled children must struggle to overcome deep-seated prejudices and stigma in order to break through the initial rejection based on stereotypes. Handicapped children are constantly bombarded with commercials, magazine articles, and television programs that reinforce the belief that physical strength or beauty is essential for success and happiness. A 1980 study of prime-time television programming concluded that the handicapped are still rarely portrayed in television shows and when they are, they are more likely to be portrayed in a negative than in a positive role (Donaldson 1981). Similar stereotyping in comic strips had been demonstrated previously (Weinberg and Santana 1978). There is a major need for public portrayal of disabled persons who are capable and successful in spite of handicaps to serve as role models for the disabled (Donaldson 1981).

SPECIFIC FACTORS AFFECTING SOCIAL RESPONSE

Community Size and Number of Moves:

The smaller the disabled child's hometown, the greater the chance of the child being accepted as a "regular" person and adjusting to the handicap (Warnick 1969). However, each move to a new neighborhood or community is likely to initiate a new barrage of stares, questions, and cruel comments (Lefebvre and Barclay 1980). Moves are particularly traumatic during the first two or three school grades, when teasing reaches a peak (Lefebvre and Munro 1978), or during early adolescence, when self-consciousness about being different from peers is at its height.

Family Size and Support

A large or extended family or network of family friends or supportive classmates may act as a buffer to defend the handicapped child against the cruelty of bullies.

Sex of the Disabled Child

Functional disabilities are generally more incapacitating for a boy who cannot live up to the expectation of being a successful athlete, while cosmetic defects, especially facial disfigurement, are harder to accept in girls (Lefebvre and Munro 1978; MacGregor 1979). This may explain why boys with orthopedic impairments more frequently develop emotional problems, while girls are more likely to become depressed even after correction of cleft lip and palate (Lefebvre and Barclay 1980).

Politics

Government services and municipal by-laws can greatly affect the scope and comfort of disabled people's lives by providing or withholding easy access to public transportation, shopping centers, and public washrooms. Community sensitivity also affects the attitudes of the nonhandicapped majority toward the disabled minority. In Sweden, where the state has underwritten the education and financial security of handicapped children for years, disabled children are treated with more respect and warmth (Health and Welfare Canada 1981). In countries with minimal or no government assistance, the care of a disabled member constitutes a major financial burden to a family, while in all countries having a handicapped member may threaten the family's chances for social and economic improvement through lost promotion opportunities, time off work for hospital visits, and social restrictions necessary for the care of the disabled members.

Reactions of Helping Professionals

Doctors who are trained to treat and cure illness often feel helpless when faced with an uncorrectable disability. This feeling of impotence, coupled with a fear of unnecessarily alarming parents, often causes them to minimize or ignore early signs of developmental delay. Instead of realistically presenting the facts, they often reassure mothers that the child will "grow out of it" and label normal parental concerns as overanxiety that can only make things worse. Such a "wait-and-see" approach works well for children who are only immature; however, it may delay the early diagnosis of hearing impairment, speech delay, organic brain damage, or other conditions that could have been corrected or at least partially compensated for earlier. By the time the disability is recognized by teachers in kindergarten or first grade, the child may already have developed a secondary behavior problem while the parents, understandably angry that their earlier concerns were disregarded, blame the original doctor for any later failures of treatment or remedial help.

Doctors or other health-care givers, even specialists in the field of disability, are not immune from anxiety and depression in response to disability. Doctors and nurses frequently deal with their anxieties first by repressing them and then by assuming one of two defensive attitudes. Some adopt a rigid professional stance, focusing on the technical aspects of management and ordering a multitude of tests and consultations in an aggressive attempt to correct and cure the child. This is encouraging for parents who also keep hoping for a cure but, if unrealistic, may cause unnecessary suffering for the child. It may also interfere with the parents' facing the irreversible aspects of their child's disability. Other medical staff may fall into the other trap of overidentifying with the child and feeling that only they, the sensitive, knowledgeable, understanding physician, nurse, or teacher, can rescue the child from psychological and social handicaps. Such an overidentification can cause insensitivity to the parents' needs and frustrations, competition with the parents, and criticism of real or supposed shortcomings (Weinberg and Santana 1978). The teacher of handicapped children has the particularly difficult task of dealing daily and often on a one-to-one basis with children of uneven developmental levels and ability, each with different capacities and limitations. Teachers are more likely than doctors to overestimate a child's intellectual potential or to have excessively high hopes of normalizing academic achievements, only to see them deflated again and again. The teacher who is overworked and whose dedication is not recognized by superiors, parents, or physicians may "burn out" (Weinberg and Santana 1978), carrying out the job in a routine, automatic manner with diminished sensitivity toward the needs of the individual child, or may leave the field altogether, thereby contributing to the high turnover of special education teachers. Physicians, nurses, and social workers may also "burn out," with serious repercussions both on their personal satisfaction and adjustment and on the quality of the care that they provide.

Management

Treatment implies correction of a deficiency or illness. Management includes both treatment and the broader goals of promoting normal growth, development, and adaptive functioning of the child and family. Management principles will be considered under three theoretically distinct but often overlapping phases of primary, secondary, and tertiary prevention (see chapter 27). *Primary prevention* aims at eradicating future occurrence of a disability; *secondary prevention* deals with early identification and medical treatment of a disability; while *tertiary prevention* has as its goal the physical and mental rehabilitation of the individual into society (Health and Welfare Canada 1981).

PRIMARY PREVENTION

General Education

Anastasiow (1981) recommends more teaching of parenting skills, child development, family planning, and birth control in order to prepare teenagers for the responsibilities of parenthood.

Early identification and genetic counseling of young couples with family histories of birth defects or genetically transmitted diseases allows them to make informed decisions about having children and to detect and begin correcting defects early. Tests are now available to detect carriers of spina bifida, chromosomal translocations (Down's syndrome), cystic fibrosis, Tay-Sachs disease, and so forth. Amniocentesis permits prenatal diagnosis of congenital defects in genetically vulnerable infants, allowing sufficient time for therapeutic termination of pregnancy when indicated. Prenatal and neonatal education of prospective parents and physicians could further reduce the incidence of cerebral palsy related to fetal anoxia.

Finally, many fires and accidents that kill or disable young children can be prevented. Accidental injury is the primary cause of death and disability for people under age twenty-five (Health and Welfare Canada 1981). Government regulations insisting on the use of seat belts for vehicles and controlling the temperature of water heaters, flammability of children's clothes, and safety of toys and recreational equipment could decrease the accident rate, as can the use of media and school demonstrations to alert children and parents to common safety hazards.

SECONDARY PREVENTION

Early Identification

Early identification may start prenatally with amniocentesis but usually occurs at the time of pediatric checkups or school entry when the child presents either with a specific somatic symptom or developmental delay or shows early learning disabilities.

Anastasiow (1981) recommends establishing family centers to provide ongoing health counseling of parents. Prenatal classes, well-baby checkups, and immunization schedules are all recommended, as well as preschool assessment groups of children monitored by physicians, psychologists, teachers, and social workers (Berscheid and Walster 1972). In this ideal framework, disability could be identified and treated before psychological and social handicap had a chance to develop.

Direct Treatment

More commonly, however, a specialist in one particular area becomes involved in treating only one aspect of a child's disability. Family moves, changes of schools, referrals to different hospitals for consultation, speech therapy, or physiotherapy often add to the confusion of multiple uncoordinated approaches. The single most crucial ingredient of good management is a trusting, ongoing relationship with one primary caregiving person, often but not necessarily the family physician. This central figure should be available to review the diagnosis, progress, management, and prognosis as often as the family request or seem to need it; to suggest, refer for, and coordinate such specialized investigation and treatment as are necessary; to listen to the parents' concerns, accepting their discouragement and anger while still providing enough realistic optimism to support them in the face of all the difficulties involved in raising a handicapped child. Only when the parents are fully involved as auxiliary therapists can they direct their child's optimal development, build up self-esteem, and become effective agents for social change as well as knowledgeable consumers of services available for the handicapped.

TERTIARY PREVENTION

Tertiary prevention—that is, providing disabled children every possible opportunity for normal growth and development—begins with the diagnosis and hinges on the quality of the relationship between family and health team. Parents can be helped to become as knowledgeable and comfortable as possible in dealing with the handicap and its consequences, accepting real limitations where necessary but setting realistic expectations when required. Specific issues in tertiary prevention arise in the areas of education, employment, housing, leisure, and communication.

Education

Currently the move is away from segregating handicapped children and toward integrating them within the usual educational stream. Integration offers many new opportunities for handicapped students but also carries the risk of exposing them to further social segregation (Hobben 1980; Johnson and Johnson 1980). To minimize the social stimatization and rejection of disabled students, physical integration must go hand in hand with systematic sensitization of healthy students to the needs and potential of their handicapped peers.

Mental health professionals specifically recommend structuring cooperative, noncompetitive learning experiences for mixed groups of handicapped and nonhandicapped students (Handlers and Austin 1980); setting up simulation experiments and personal interviews with handicapped adults (Johnson and Johnson 1980); and ensuring collaboration between special education and regular classroom teachers.

Employment

Because of a lack of career opportunities for even the capable and competent handicapped adult, disabled persons are unemployed and underemployed far more than the normal adult population. This has major effects in undermining both their ability to support themselves and their feelings of self-worth (Health and Welfare Canada 1981; Sitlington 1981). Since employment is an issue primarily for older adolescents or adults, it will not be dealt herein. Those interested in pursuing the topic should refer to the Suggestions for Further Reading following this chapter.

Housing

Efforts to close down large residential institutions for the severely mentally and physically disabled have often been undertaken without adequate preparation of alternate resources in the community. Almost nothing has provoked more fear and prejudice against handicapped minorities than efforts to establish group homes in "nice" residential areas (Health and Welfare Canada 1981). The consumer movement, and particularly self-help organizations for the disabled, are slowly providing effective advocacy for the disabled.

Leisure, Sports, Art, and Culture

Disabled children have fewer opportunities for active involvement in recreation and sports necessary for healthy development and self-esteem. The success of organizations such as the Olympics for the Disabled and War Amputee Artists shows how much can be done to improve recreational opportunities. However, for many disabled people who cannot use public transit, the absence of readily available transportation remains a major and costly barrier, discouraging and preventing their participation in community activities. Government-supported public/private transit systems are part of the new conceptual approaches planned for the 1980s.

Technology and the Quality of Life

The increased use of electronic information storage, bioengineering, and language synthesizers is broadening the horizons of many disabled persons. Telephones and television programs with captions for the hearing impaired and improved prostheses for the amputee are examples of such technical progress. However, indiscriminate substitution of technological aids for human contacts can encourage some disabled persons to remain homebound and aggravate their personal isolation and social handicap, as in the case of the homebound ham-radio operator.

Specific Considerations of Congenital Handicaps

THE BLIND CHILD

Definition. Legal blindness is defined as central visual acuity of 20/200 or less in the better eye with correction, or a field of vision of no greater than twenty degrees.

Prevalence. The prevalence of blindness in children under age sixteen is 0.4 per 1,000 (Weale and Bradshaw 1980). From 1968 to 1978, it is estimated that more than 20,000 blind students were enrolled in schools in the United States.

Age of Onset. Congenital causes account for two-thirds of blind children, but for more than three-quarters of affected children the age of onset is under one year of age, since many conditions that begin prior to birth (e.g., retinoblastoma) only become manifest some months later.

Clinical Picture. The development of the blind infant is so distinctly different that it has been the subject of numerous studies and excellent reviews (Adams 1980; Froyd 1973). Some of the salient points made include the following.

1. Blind infants do not establish eye contact and have a weak or rare social smile. They usually exhibit a blank facial expression and maintain a state of passive immobility, especially when acutely attentive to sounds or tactile sensations. These features may convey a sense of nonresponsiveness to the mother and

TABLE 22.1
Common Causes of Blindness in Children

	Total %	%
Prenatal influences resulting from hereditary conditions (cataracts, optic atrophy, retinoblastoma, retinitis pigmentosa, etc.)	50	41
Other congenital reasons (e.g., rubella)		9
Retrolental fibroplasia	24	
Due to excess oxygen administration in neonatal period		6
Without established history of oxygen excess		18
Accidental injury	26	

inhibit (a) her bonding to the baby; (b) the likelihood of her stimulating the child by talking, smiling, offering food or cuddling (Fraiberg 1968).

2. The motor development of blind children is usually delayed. They start reaching toward and grasping objects at nine months instead of three to four months. They take longer to crawl and may not walk until after their second birthday. As toddlers, they are usually less adventurous, remaining much more dependent on adults to explore environments. Because of their helplessness, they rarely fight back, for example, when toys are taken from them.

3. Language development occurs at a normal rate but differs in quality. The blind child uses language to keep in touch with people, asking many repetitive questions in a constant stream of talk (Adams 1980; Lowenfeld 1977).

4. Regarding social development, blind children are slower to develop mental images of mother and prone to panic when she leaves the room. Their ability to distinguish between self and environment and, later on, between their own ideas and those of others is impaired. The struggle between the wish to be independent and the need to remain dependent is prolonged because of the lifelong difficulty in traveling and in orientating themselves in new surroundings.

5. In terms of behavioral patterns, "blindisms"—repetitive actions such as body swaying, eye rubbing, and head knocking—are commonly found. These forms of tension discharge are occasionally so pronounced during the preschool years that a picture of pseudoautism occurs (Balikov and Feinstein 1979; Lowenfeld 1977). (See chapter 15 for description of autism.)

THE DEAF CHILD

Definition. Deafness is a hearing loss present from birth or early childhood that prevents the child from making effective, meaningful auditory contact with the environment.

Prevalence. Total hearing loss is rare. Severe (51 to 80 decibels) and profound (81 to 100) hearing losses occur in 1.4 per 1,000 children under sixteen years of age (Weale and Bradshaw 1980). Moderate (31 to 50 decibels) and mild (15 to 30 decibels) hearing losses are three to four times as common. Prevalence rates vary widely from country to country according to screening programs. It is estimated that 8.5 school children per 10,000 in Britain require special educational help because of hearing impairments (Schlesinger 1979).

Etiology. Prenatal (rubella) and postnatal (otitis) infections and trauma account for over two-thirds of cases of severe hearing impairment. Genetic inheritance causes the most profound congenital cases.

Clinical Picture. The symptoms produced in infants by deafness include the following.

1. Delayed speech and inattentiveness are common and often confused with other disorders, such as developmental lags. Since most parents of deaf children can hear, they do not suspect deafness until the child fails to talk at an appropriate age. Deaf parents, on the other hand, expect the diagnosis and by verifying it at an earlier age are usually more able to help the child deal with this disability.

2. The "typical" deaf child is likely to be academically and linguistically retarded, despite normal intelligence (Schlesinger 1979).

3. Deaf children are significantly less accurate in their self-perception than hearing children (Woods 1975). Their self-esteem is usually above average in early childhood but drops dramatically when they enter school. Their body image is likely to overemphasize hands and fingers, especially if they attend a residential school that teaches sign language. Deaf children in schools that stress oral communication emphasize the mouth and lips in self-portraits and are likely to be inhibited in hand gestures. Very few children are totally deaf, and residual hearing can be used to encourage both lip reading and understanding of language. The traditional approach to partially deaf children advocated verbal communication exclusively, discouraging all use of sign language (Schlesinger 1979; Woods 1975). However, it is now well established that early signing in deaf preschoolers actually facilitates lip reading and speech acquisition besides decreasing communicative frustration and improving esteem (Schlesinger 1979). Parents of deaf children advised to insist exclusively on verbalization often run into power struggles with frustrated, angry children who refuse to try to talk. At the other extreme is a group of children who are overly compliant and too obedient for their own good (Diller 1972). The deaf adolescent is often extremely isolated, with an underdeveloped capacity for abstact thinking, limited interpersonal relationships, and a narrow outlook on life (Lesser and Easser 1972; Schlesinger 1979). Thus hearing and speaking seem more essential to our mental development than seeing.

THE CHILD WITH CEREBRAL PALSY

The term cerebral palsy covers a variety of neurological disorders characterized by weakness, paralysis, poor coordination, spasticity, and multiple involuntary movements. Discussed in more detail in chapter 11, it is included here because of the severe psychological and social handicaps that frequently complicate the neurological condition. Children with cerebral palsy typically present with multiple handicaps. For example, sixty percent usually have defective vision. Fifty percent usually have borderline or below-average intelligence (this is especially common in spastic children). Forty percent typically present with deafness, speech, and other associated impairments, including poor articulation, open mouth and breathless speech, difficulty chewing and swallowing, and excessive drooling. (These last three impairments are especially common in athetoid children.)

The child with cerebral palsy learns to crawl after the second birthday (instead of before the first) and does not use single words until well into the third year (instead of early in the second year). Minde (1978; Minde et al. 1972) has described two psychological crises usually experienced by cerebral palsy children. When the children first enter school, they are first exposed to teasing, stares, exclusion from sports and games, and academic difficulties. In early adolescence the children, fully understanding for the first time the permanence and social implications of the handicap, frequently become discouraged, give up, stop trying academically, and withdraw socially. Minde confirmed Seidel, Chadwick, and Rutter's earlier findings that even cerebral palsy children with normal intelligence are more vulnerable to psychiatric problems than nondisabled children. For cerebral palsy victims with a brain damage syndrome, the risk of psychiatric morbidity is even greater (three times the average) (Seidel, Chadwick, and Rutter 1975).

The parents of cerebral palsy children typically experience three different stages of worry and anxiety. First they worry over developmental milestones and zealously adhere to therapeutic programs, hoping to prove the doctors wrong. Then they worry over poor academic performance, become angry at social rejection, and determine to ensure their child a fair chance to fully develop his or her capacities. Finally they worry about the future of their handicapped child once they are gone, having given up on their dream of a normal life for the child and resigned themselves to encouraging the child's association with the "handicapped community" to ensure at least physical and financial security.

THE CHILD WITH SPINA BIFIDA

Definition. Spina bifida results from incomplete closure of the vertebral column over the spinal cord. In its most severe form, anencephaly, the contents of the brain exude through the back of the head; such children are usually stillborn or die soon after birth. The most benign form, spina bifida occulta, is extremely common, occurring in 20 to 58 percent of all children (Nelson 1975; Seidel, Chadwick, and Rutter 1975). It has no clinical significance and is usually unnoticed except for a dimple or tuft of hair over the lumbosacral region (Pringle and Fiddes 1970).

Generally speaking, the term spina bifida is reserved for those cases where there is an associated myelomeningocele, that is, a protrusion of the meninges and nerve tissue with corresponding neurological deficits.

Incidence. Spina bifida has now replaced poliomyelitis as the major cause of paraplegia in young children. It occurs in between 1 and 10 per 1,000 live births, and only 50 percent of those afflicted live a full year. Its prevalence is 1.1 per 1,000 in children under sixteen years. Parents who already have an affected child have a 1 in 12 to 1 in 33 chance of having a subsequent child affected.

Clinical Picture: Neurological Impairment. In addition to loss of sensation and/or paralysis of the lower limbs, two-thirds of affected children are either born with or develop hydrocephalus after birth. The hydrocephalic children score an average 10 points lower on intelligence tests than affected children without hydrocephalus, whose intelligence is normal. Many of these children are incontinent, and their constant dribbling requires diapers or plastic pants with disposable liners. Bowel incontinence is managed with laxatives and enemas, but the smell of urine surrounding many of these children often makes them social outcasts. Because of inactivity and lack of exercise many become obese, and power struggles over food create problems with parents. These children find schooling particularly difficult. Because of their multiple handicaps, they are often placed in classes for retarded children. The resulting lack of stimulation and structure, especially for those with normal intelligence, contributes to feelings of inferiority and lack of motivation, which are additional handicaps. Missing an average of two months out of every school year because of hospitalizations and investigations only compounds their academic difficulties.

Personality Features. Toddlers with spina bifida, particularly those with hydrocephalus, are often described as having an attractive "chatterbox quality" due to their accelerated speech development and rapid verbal output. Unfortunately, this incessant chattering is less appealing in older children. Their adolescence is particularly difficult because of urological and sexual difficulties; they have normal sexual drives but impotence, frequent incontinence, and paraplegia make normal sexual relationships difficult or impossible. The resulting frustration may be expressed as resentment, bravado, or neglect of personal grooming and physical deterioration. Frequently the young adult with myelomeningocele is both emotionally immature and physically dependent on family and community. Few achieve independent living. Total care must include provision for eventual permanent out-of-home care (Seidel, Chadwick, and Rutter, 1975).

Family Reactions. Spina bifida is one of those human tragedies that strengthens good marriages and destroys weak ones (Hare et al. 1966). The multiple handicaps, uncertain prognosis, and constant monitoring of neurological signs require enormous physical and emotional energy from parents. Some fathers are extraordinarily involved in parenting, forming a close bond with the affected child,* while others abdicate all responsibility, rejecting the child. Mothers are frequently chronically depressed and anxious (Hare et al. 1966; Seidel, Chadwick, and Rutter, 1975).

THE CHILD WITH CRANIOFACIAL DEFORMITIES

Definition. The term craniofacial deformities covers a wide variety of conditions involving facial disfigurement with or without accompanying body deformities. Children may become disfigured at any age as a result of injury, burns, or a late-appearing gentically inherited tumor such as neurofibromatosis (which afflicted the "Elephant Man") that typically becomes manifest around age five. Since most facial deformities are present at birth, this section will deal only with congenital disorders.

Classification. *Cleft lip and palate* ("hare lip") is the least severe and most easily correctable defect. It is inherited as an autosomal recessive gene with a 25 percent risk from a carrier parent.

Crouzon's disease and *Apert's syndrome* both involve premature fusion of the cranial sutures, with a flattened, underdeveloped middle face and bulging eyeballs. Apert's syndrome also results in fusion of the fingers and toes (syndactyly).

*G. Byrne, personal communication, 1981.

Treacher-Collins syndrome has been described as producing "antimongoloid" features (downward sloping eyes with flattened cheeks, a small chin, and deformed or absent ears with accompanying hearing loss).

Hypertelorism refers to abnormally wide spacing of the eyes, with or without a bulging of the meninges and brain in a nasal protrusion (encephalocele). Crouzon's, Apert's, and Treacher-Collins syndromes and hypertelorism usually occur as spontaneous mutations in infants born to healthy young mothers without any genetic or prenatal morbidity. However, they are autosomal dominants, in that patients affected have a 50 percent chance of passing on the disability to their offspring. Incidence figures are not available.

The following four conditions have only been identified in the past ten years and their genetic implications are largely unknown.

Both *Goldenhar's syndrome* and *lateral facial dysplasia* produce striking facial symmetries, sometimes accompanied by a deformed ear and hearing loss. Goldenhar's is the more severe, also involving the upper face.

Moebius syndrome is a congenital paralysis of the facial nerves that prevents all mobility and expressiveness, leaving the patient's face with a flat, fixed expression.

Binder's syndrome is commonly referred to by plastic surgeons as the "boxer face" in that the nose and cheeks look as if they had been pounded in.

Clinical Picture. Little is known about the typical personality, prognosis, and treatment of most children with facial deformities, except for those with cleft lip and palate. Even with these there is considerable disagreement as to their average intelligence, personality traits, and academic, occupational, and social outcome (Bernstein 1976; Lefebvre and Barclay 1980). Revolutionary new techniques of reconstructive facial surgery have renewed clinical interest in conditions formerly regarded as hopeless. It has so far been established that:

1. Most children with severe craniofacial deformities have normal intelligence. Their parents, however, are often given sweeping and incorrect statements about the deformed child at birth (e.g., he will never walk, talk, etc.).
2. Craniofacial deformities accompanied by premature fusion of the cranial sutures will cause permanent neurological and secondary intellectual damage unless corrected in infancy to allow normal brain growth.
3. Each craniofacial deformity has specific medical and functional complications associated with it. (See table 22.2.)

Facial deformities profoundly affect psychological development (Adams and Lindemann 1974; Lefebvre and Munro 1978). Disfigured toddlers become aware of their deformities and are anxious on meeting strangers. In primary school they are teased mercilessly, ostracized, rarely called on to speak in class, and expected by teachers and classmates to be retarded. Yet in spite of the repeated harassment and rejection, which

TABLE 22.2

Complications of Craniofacial Deformities

Crouzon's Disease	Risk of blindness due to extrusion of the eyeballs, (exophthalmos)
Apert's Syndrome	Breathing difficulties Motor coordination problems Hyperactivity and learning problems
Treacher-Collins Syndrome	Hearing impairments and speech defects
Hypertelorism	Risk of blindness Risk of brain infection or trauma if an associated encephalocele
Goldenhar's Syndrome and Lateral Facial Dysplasia	Hearing impairments and/or speech defects
Moebius Syndrome	Hearing impairments and/or speech defects Nystagmus Drooling

usually peaks in second or third grade, they generally maintain adequate academic performance and self-esteem provided they have the support and confidence of their families. They do this by denying their deformity (rating their appearance as perfect or almost perfect) and by avoiding situations or people that arouse discomfort. Paradoxically, this protective denial seems more effective with major than minor or more ambiguous deformities. Life in a small community with few changes of residence or school is an important protective factor for the facially deformed. The breakdown of the defenses of avoidance and denial during adolescence as described earlier leads to marked deterioration in these children's ratings of their appearance and of self-esteem, as well as narrowing their career choices to exclude ones involving public contact. Unless they retreat to the safety of a handicapped community for companionship and support, they become increasingly isolated and despairing and may even contemplate suicide. New techniques in reconstructive surgery offer many of these children a chance of approaching normalcy. The timing of the surgery is crucial; an early intervention before school entry will minimize social problems but may increase surgical risks and will almost always have to be repeated as the child's face grows. Surgery during adolescence is less risky and offers more permanent results, besides allowing the teenager to participate in the decision-making process. There is danger, however, that a depressed, socially isolated, academically delayed teenager may expect the operation to solve, magically, all these problems, not just the cosmetic ones. Such unrealistic expectations always lead to disappointment and even deeper depression (Lefebvre and Barclay 1980).

Specific Considerations of Postnatal Handicaps

HANDICAPS CAUSED BY ACUTE OR CHRONIC ILLNESS

The problems of children who become partially deaf or blind will not be discussed as they are similar to those discussed under congenital blindness and deafness, though less extensive and less likely to interfere with ongoing development. Regarding acquired neurological impairments secondary to encephalitis or meningitis and traumatic injuries, the reader is referred to the chapters on neurological disorders (chapter 11) and mental retardation (chapter 18). This chapter will focus on three specific types of acquired handicaps: disorders of motility, burns, and amputations.

Disorders of Motility

The Degenerative Dystrophies. The *muscular dystrophies* are a group of disorders characterized by a progressive, genetically determined primary degenerative myopathy. The most common form, Duchenne muscular dystrophy, affects approximately 1 in 4,000 boys and is usually inherited as an X-linked recessive trait. Thus sons of carriers have a 50 percent chance of developing the disease, while daughters have an equal chance of being a carrier. Some cases, however, occur from mutations in the ovum of a genetically normal mother. Muscular dystrophy affects 1 in 6,000 school-age children (i.e., 0.14 per 1,000) (Nelson 1975; VanLeeuwen 1979). The disorder usually becomes apparent in the second to fourth year of life, by which time a second affected child may have been conceived. Most children require a wheelchair by midadolescence and die in early adulthood.

Friedrich's ataxia, inherited as an autosomal recessive gene, involves progressive deterioration of the posterior columns of the spinal cord. *Pes cavus* (arched foot) is the first sign. Ataxia and muscle atrophy increase during late childhood. The child becomes wheelchairbound during adolescence, and death, usually from heart atrophy or diabetes, occurs between twenty and fifty years.

Clinical Picture. Both of these conditions cause a progressive loss of muscular strength and increasing weakness until the child dies from respiratory or cardiac failure during late adolescence or early adulthood.

Medical treatment is essentially palliative, consisting largely of exercises to maintain as much as possible of the child's ability to care for self and to prevent deformities. The progressive nature of the disease and the inevitability of a premature death cause severe emotional difficulties for both child and family, eliciting uncontained hostility and aggression in some children and total passivity with loss of any personal ambition or interest in others. Although one-fourth to one-third of those with muscular dystrophy are retarded, most affected children have normal intelligence. It is important for their morale that they carry on in a normal school at their level of ability until the disease confines them to a wheelchair, at which point the move to a special school can no longer be avoided. Their tragic prognosis elicits either fierce denial or overwhelming anxiety, guilt, and depression in the parents.

As the child's range of movement and capacity for self-care progressively decrease, each new limitation of functioning may elicit fresh anxiety, depression, and resentment in both child and parents. As the disease progresses, the child becomes increasingly dependent on the parents to the point where even feeding, elimination, or changing positions to avoid pressure sores require their assistance. As this stage is usually reached during adolescence, a time when the progression toward independence is normally at its peak, the extreme dependence is often a source of major depression (grieving for missed opportunities), frustration, and guilt in the youngsters as well as a major physical and emotional drain on the parents. The move to institutional care, eventually precipitated by some combination of continued deterioration in the patient and exhaustion in the parents, often results in a period of intense anxiety and guilt for both parents and adolescent. At this time they badly need a realistic but concerned physician who is prepared to remain involved and to help them make the decisions necessary for the care of the affected child, to direct them to appropriate sources of relief and support, and to help them achieve as close to normal a life style as is possible considering the additional burden caused by the illness.

Juvenile Rheumatoid Arthritis

Definition. Juvenile rheumatoid arthritis refers to a number of different syndromes that all involve inflammation of one or more joints that persists for at least six consecutive weeks and is not related to other known causes of childhood arthritis. Three subtypes of the disease are defined by the type of onset: (1) systemic, (2) pauciarticular (i.e., few joints involved), and (3) polyarticular (i.e., many joints involved) (McAnarney et al. 1974; Mikkelson 1981).

Incidence. The incidence remains unclear, because there is still widespread disagreement whether or not to include conditions such as Reiter's syndrome, that are difficult to diagnose early in the disease.

Clinical Picture. The overall prognosis for juvenile rheumatoid arthritis is usually reasonably good. However, long-term follow-up studies still show a significant number of disabled patients.

Patients with a systemic onset have a 25 percent chance of developing destructive arthritis. The risk of joint deformities may be as high as 40 percent in the minority of children who are rheumatoid-factor positive. Wrists, feet, knees, and hips are the most commonly deformed joints.

In contrast with the adult form of the disease, pain is not prominent in juvenile rheumatoid arthritis. Mortality estimates vary from 0.65 percent to 4.2 percent.

Psychosocial Factors. Very few studies have specifically looked at the psychosocial aspect of juvenile rheumatoid arthritis. Two studies report a high incidence of emotional conflicts and frequently disturbed family relationships at the onset of illness (37 percent) (Henoch, Batson, and Baum 1978; Rimon et al. 1977). One suggests that adolescents with juvenile rheumatoid arthritis are in need of sexual counseling (Herstein 1977).

Because juvenile rheumatoid arthritis has been recognized only recently, there are no prospective studies dealing with the psychosocial impact of its disabilities in adolescents and young adults, even though it is adolescents who are most likely to need orthopedic procedures and to resent strenuous physiotherapy and disfiguring steroid treatment.

Osteogenesis Imperfecta

Definition. Osteogenesis imperfecta is characterized by brittle bones that break easily due to a collagen deficiency. It is inherited as an autosomal dominant gene with variable penetrance (Sillence, Senn, and Dansk 1979). *Incidence.* Figures for incidence vary between 0.01 and 0.05 per 1,000 live births.

Clinical Picture. Fractures occur so easily in children with this condition that even hugging the child may be hazardous. The skull is large, soft, and flattened. The child is often dwarfed even without fractures. These children may be unable to walk but may have normal or above-normal intelligence. Deafness may develop in early adult life, and the children usually die in adulthood although newer orthopedic techniques may improve the prognosis. The few scattered reports describe their personalities as sensitive, dependent, and greatly overprotected. Every effort should be made to keep them in regular schools, since fractures are as likely to occur among a group of uncoordinated and handicapped children as among normal children.

THE SEVERELY BURNED CHILD

Definition. There are many different types of burns—electrical, chemical, hot-water scalding, and flame burns—and three degrees of burn severity of which the most severe (third degree) requires grafting. Burns involving over 50 percent of the body surface are life threatening, with only 50 percent of children thus affected surviving the risk of infection.

Incidence. There are no incidence figures for severe burns in children. At least 12,000 people die annually of burns in the United States and 1,000 to 2,000 in Canada (Bernstein 1979; Health and Welfare Canada 1981). Many of these victims are children. Most fires are accidental, but an increasing proportion is related to arson (Health and Welfare Canada 1981).

Clinical Picture. All severe burns have a catastrophic impact on the child and family (Bernstein 1976), especially if the face or hands are affected. A previously healthy child suddenly becomes critically ill and may die. Bernstein (1976) has divided management and clinical picture into three phases: the acute phase, the late-hospitalization phase, and the rehabilitation phase.

In *the acute phase,* the child is usually in shock, both physically and emotionally. This partially dulls the diffuse pain. For the first two weeks disorientation, confusion, hallucinations, fears of abandonment and fire in the room are common, probably due to a combination of neurological dysfunction (toxemia, electrolyte depletion) and the complete isolation to which the patient is confined to minimize the risk of infection. Although the family is customarily overwhelmed by anxiety and/or guilt during this stage, their feelings and presence are often ignored due to the medical staff's preoccupation with providing intensive care for the child.

In the *late-hospitalization phase,* the child is frequently taken to the operating room for débridement (removal of dead skin), grafting, or amputation. Daily sessions of physical therapy and tank tub débridement are extremely painful: the lack of effective pain relief can cause extremely upsetting screaming sessions between patient and staff. Symptoms of toxic psychosis are replaced by flashbacks of the actual accident, weepiness, extreme anxiety, anger, and feelings of guilt related to causing or surviving the accident (especially if someone close perished). "Coming out" of isolation is a major step that allows the child to have unrestricted visitors but also exposes him or her to the shame of being stared at by friends or in hallways and elevators.

In the *rehabilitation phase,* discharge from hospital is only one step in a long series of therapeutic interventions. The burned child must return to the hospital for regular physiotherapy sessions and, frequently, for surgical release of scar tissue and adjustment of splints and body-suits (jobsts). The latter are particularly uncomfortable, tight-fitting elastic garments that must be worn day and night for up to a year to minimize raised scar tissue. Continuing discomfort and/or frequent nightmares may interfere with sleep. But by far the greatest battle for the burned child is that of renewal of contacts with friends and teachers, resuming normal physical activities, schoolwork, and outings to public places where stares and questions will unavoidably occur. This is the stage during which family and community support, as well as intelligence and humor, are vital to rehabilitation. School visits by a public health nurse prior to discharge to prepare the class for the child's appearance, body-suits, and masks, as well as group meetings with members of a burn survivors' association, can facilitate the arduous task of reentering the real world.

The long-term prognosis of severely burned children is poor (Nover 1973; Sawyer 1980; Seligman 1974). Over 80 percent are described by their parents as emotionally disturbed one year after the accident. For many with facial or hand scars, adolescence is a time of anguish, social withdrawal, and "a closeted avoidance of public exposure" (Nelson 1975). In adult life their academic and social performance are usually below average, and many will struggle with depression for the rest of their lives.

Bernstein (1976) has described two general patterns of family response: the intact middle-class family is typically overwhelmed by guilt over the accident but responds compliantly to all treatment requests, involving itself with community prevention groups; multiproblem families (in which burns are more likely to occur) are more likely to deny the severity, permanence, or social impact of the burns. In these families parents are less often involved in treatment and have magical expectations of doctors and nurses, responding with resentment and antagonism when the expected miracles are not produced.

THE CHILD AMPUTEE

Definition. There are two types of childhood amputation: congenital and acquired. Most children with limb deformities or amputations are born that way. These deformities are usually genetically linked and consist either of the absence of a limb or part of a limb or of a deep circular constriction around an arm or leg. They may also be caused by the ingestion of various agents by the mother during pregnancy (such as Thalidomide or alcohol) or by her exposure to excess radiation.

The most common causes of acquired amputations are, in order of decreasing frequency: trauma, burns, tumors, infection, and vascular accidents.

Incidence. There are 25,000 juvenile amputees in the United States.

Clinical Picture. Since amputations occur much more frequently in adults, there is relatively little data regarding the psychological problems specific to the child amputee. Most reports agree that congenital amputees, as a rule, demonstrate, less psychological disturbance than children experiencing traumatic or surgical amputations (Diller 1972). For instance, "phantom limb" sensations do not occur in congenital amputees and are relatively painless in traumatic child, as compared to adult, amputations (Ritchie 1977; Schechter and Holter 1979). However, arm, hand, and finger amputations in very young children may limit range of movement and environmental manipulation, thus interfering with the child's personality development and fostering the passive-dependent or passive-aggressive coping style seen in many congenital amputees (Diller 1972). During the early school years, denial of the amputation may lead to hyperactive or antisocial behavior that masks an underlying depression (Schechter and Holter 1979). Adolescence forces the child to give up any fantasies of magical limb replacement. As peers progress to sexual or athletic activities from which the child is or feels excluded, a sense of pervasive helplessness develops. Teenage amputees may blame themselves for having brought on the amputation as punishment for imagined or real misdeeds or unacceptable thoughts or sexual or aggressive feelings (Schechter and Holter 1979). A masochistic personality structure then ensues. The most common coping style is that of an "identification with the aggressor," for instance, a wish to become a surgeon in order to do unto others what was done to the child.

The Management Issue

The child psychiatrist may be called upon to help the child mourn for the absent limb (Ritchie 1977), to limit regression to infantile levels of behavior, or to broaden the scope of interpersonal relationships. But often the most crucial aspect of psychiatric treatment is to reduce guilt in the parents or other relatives: the mother who feels inadequate because she gave birth to a monster, the father who left his son unattended near the lawn mower, the grandparent who hides feelings of disgust with an overprotective, oversolicitous concern. All of these people quickly convey their sense of shame or guilt to the child, whether the amputation is congenital or accidental. For the impact of cancer-related amputations, the reader is referred to chapter 24.

SUGGESTIONS FOR FURTHER READING

Handicap and Disabilities

ADAMS, J. E., AND LINDEMANN, E. 1974. Coping with long-term disability. In *Coping and adaptation,* ed. G. V. Coelho, D. A. Hamburg, and J. E. Adams, pp. 127–138. New York: Basic Books. Dramatically illustrates the interplay between disability and coping styles by comparing two young men with traumatic quadriplegia, one of whom never accepted the disability and the other who faced and overcame its social consequences.

ANASTASIOW, N. 1981. Early childhood education for the handicapped in the 1980's: Recommendations. *Except. Child.* 47(4):277–282.
Reviews recommendations of thirteen specialists in early childhood education for the handicapped. These include more emphasis on development, on working with parents, on multidisciplinary training, the broad-base screening of infants, family centers for prenatal care, stress on child rearing in high school, and legal advocates for impaired individuals.

DEMB, N., AND RUESS, A. L. 1967. High school drop-out rates for cleft palate children and their siblings. *Cleft Palate J.* 4:327–333.
Although the national (American) average rate of high school dropouts is 30 percent, the rate for children with "clefts" (lip and/or palate) is 25 percent, while the rate for their siblings is 42 percent.

DILLER, L. 1972. Psychological aspects of physically handicapped children. In *Handbook of child therapy,* ed. B. B. Wolman, pp. 591–623. New York: McGraw-Hill.
Excellent, practical review of terms and common management problems for all handicapped children. Little attention given to specific conditions.

GATH, A. 1972. The mental health of siblings of congenitally abnormal children. *J. Child Psychol. Psychiat.* 13:211–218.
Investigates evidence that a congenitally abnormal child may adversely affect the mental

health of siblings. Discusses the serious problems a handicapped child living at home may present to the family.

HANDLERS, A., AND AUSTIN, K. 1980. Improving attitudes of high school students toward their handicapped peers. *Except. Child.* 47(3):228–229.

Compares several ways of increasing high school students' knowledge of and sensitivity toward handicapped people. A personal interview with a handicapped student did more to create positive attitudes than did discussions, research, films, or simulation activities. Eighty-two percent reported a more positive attitude.

HEALTH AND WELFARE CANADA. 1981. *Disabled persons in Canada.* Ottawa: Ministry of National Health and Welfare.

A comprehensive overview of the current definition and epidemiology of disability and handicap in 1980. Also reviews some of the social, educational, and occupational problems met by handicapped, and lists current management principles and ongoing research in the field.

HIRSCH, J. G. 1979. Helping the family whose child has a birth defect. In *Basic handbook of child psychiatry,* ed. J. D. Noshpitz, vol. 4, pp. 121–128. New York: Basic Books.

A review of the psychiatric and social literature on family reactions to congenital abnormalities.

JOHNSON, D., AND JOHNSON, R. 1980. Integrating handicapped children into the mainstream. *Except. Child.* 47(2):90–98.

Discusses the trend toward integrating handicapped students into the mainstream of a nonhandicapped classroom. This can widen the handicapped's horizon but carries the risk of making things worse if handicapped students are stigmatized, ignored, or treated paternalistically.

KENNY, T., AND LENTZ, G. 1978. Management of the handicapped child. In *Psychiatric problems in medical practice,* ed. G. Balis, et al., pp. 415–426. New York: Butterworth Publications.

An excellent review of definitions of the terms handicap and disability. Considers speech impairments as the most frequent emotional and social impairments as second largest group of the estimated 8 million handicapped Americans.

LAVIGNE, J. V., AND RYAN, M. 1979. Psychological adjustment of siblings of children with chronic illness. *Pediatrics* 63(4):616–627.

Compares the adjustment of three- to thirteen-year-old siblings of pediatric hematology (N 62), cardiology (N 57), and plastic surgery (N 37) patients with that of children with healthy siblings. Significant interactions between sex and age relationship to the child were noted on scales of social withdrawal, inhibitions, immaturity, and irritability.

LIPPMAN, L. 1972. *Attitudes toward the handicapped: A comparison between Europe and the United States.* Springfield, Ill.: Charles C Thomas.

The author praises the European attitudes toward the handicapped, relates his observations, and gives suggestions as to how a similar situation can be achieved in the United States.

MATTSSON, A. 1972. Long-term physical illness in childhood: A challenge to psychosocial adaptation. *Pediatrics* 50:801–811.

This highly recommended article reviews chronic illnesses from the standpoint of the attendant psychologic stresses and the related adaptational techniques used by child and parents to master negative and distressing emotions.

MOORE, C. B., AND NORTON, K. G. 1979. *A reader's guide for parents of children with mental, physical or emotional disabilities.* Rockville, Md.: U.S. Dept. of Health, Education and Welfare.

An annotated bibliography written by parents of children with disabilities who believe that reading about others' experiences, learning about sources of help, and becoming familiar with what professionals are advising will make the job of raising a handicapped child more successful and satisfying.

OLSHANSKY, S. 1962. Chronic sorrow: A response to having a mentally defective child. *Social Casework* 43:191–193.

Classic paper that describes "chronic sorrow" as a normal parental reaction to their child's handicap.

PLESS, I. B., AND ROGHMANN, K. J. 1971. Chronic illness and its consequences: Observations based on 3 epidemiological surveys. *J. Ped.* 79:351–359.

Classic review of the psychological and social impact of chronic illness as defined in three surveys conducted during the 1960s in the United States.

Sims, B., and Manley, S. 1982. Keeping the disabled out of the employment market: Financial disincentives. In *Disabled people as second-class citizens,* ed. M. G. Eisenberg, C. Griggins, and R. Duval, pp. 123–136. New York: Springer Publishing Co.

Since substantial disability benefits are terminated once a disabled person becomes employed, many persons who suffered spinal cord and other traumatic injuries have no incentive to return to the work force.

Sitlington, P. L. 1981. Vocational and special education in career programming for the mildly handicapped adolescent. *Except. Child.* 47(8):592–598.

American employment statistics reveal that only 40 percent of the adult handicapped population is employed compared to 74 percent of the nonhandicapped population and that 52 percent of the handicapped earn less than $2,000 a year. Proposes a career programming continuum integrating special education and vocational planning at the elementary school level.

Solnit, A. J., and Stark, M. H. 1961. Mourning and the birth of a defective child. Psychoanal. Stud. Child. 16: 523–37.

Describes the developmental task of motherhood as working out the discrepancy between the image of the expected baby and that of the actual child, and becoming attached to the real child.

Sperling, E. 1978. Psychological issues in chronic illness and handicap. In *Psychosocial aspects of pediatric care,* ed. pp. 51–63. New York: Grune & Stratton.

An excellent review of the developmental stress imposed by handicapping illnesses, although the author does not differentiate between congenital and acquired disability or between medical and nonmedical handicaps. Stresses the social hierarchy of disability, with crutches eliciting the most sympathy and facial deformity and obesity the most rejection.

Weale, T., and Bradshaw, J. 1980 Prevalence and characteristics of disabled children: Findings from the 1974 general household survey. *J. Epidem. & Comm. H.* 34:111–118.

A 1974 British prevalence study based on a survey of disability per 1,000 live births. Disability is defined broadly to include many forms of chronic illness, such as asthma.

Wehman, P., and Hill, J. 1981. Competitive employment for moderately and severely handicapped individuals. *Except. Child.* 47(5):338–345.

Describes a model program with a trainer-advocacy approach to open competitive job placements to handicapped adults.

Weiskopf, P. E. 1980. Burnout among teachers of exceptional children. *Except. Child.* 47(1):18–23.

Special education teachers are subjected to varying degrees of occupational stress that can cause burnout. Suggestions are given to prevent burnout.

Woods, G. 1975. *The handicapped child: Assessment and management.* Philadelphia: Blackwell Scientific Publications.

An etiological review of the conditions associated with both congenital and acquired handicaps. Detailed classifications are provided under each heading. No psychosocial discussions.

Specific Disabilities

Balikov, H., and Feinstein, C. B. 1980. The blind child. In *Basic handbook of child psychiatry,* vol. 1, ed. J. D. Noshpitz, pp. 413–420. New York: Basic Books.

A superb review of the development, family relationships, psychopathology, and treatment of blind children. No etiological classification and little reference to education.

Bernstein, N. R. 1976. *Emotional care of the facially burned and disfigured.* Boston: Little, Brown & Co.

Excellent reference. Reviews the literature on body image and how it is altered by disfigurement, as well as the field of social stereotyping of disabled and disfigured individuals. Pictures, charts, and fascinating vignettes make this instructive and interesting reading.

Diller, L. 1972. Psychological aspects of physically handicapped children. In *Handbook of child therapy,* ed. B. B. Wolman, pp. 591–623. New York: McGraw-Hill.

A concise but pertinent review of the most common psychological problems encountered by children with spina bifida.

MINDE, K. 1978. Coping styles of 34 adolescents with cerebral palsy. *Am. J. Psychiat.* 135(11):1344–1349.

A follow-up of thirty-four children with cerebral palsy studied by informal interviews and parent and teaching ratings showed that adolescents with cerebral palsy continue to show increased psychological difficulties and often slip into a passive, stereotyped role.

RITCHIE, J. A. 1977. Children's adjustive and affective responses in the process of reformulating a body image following limb amputation. II*Mat-Child Nurs. J.* Spring, pp. 125–135.

Reviews the literature on the mourning undergone by children between three and sixteen years of age after amputations. From a study of only five patients, the author found that adjustment to an altered body image is a continuous process that begins before surgery and proceeds from global to specific aspects.

SCHECHTER, M. D., AND HOLTER, F. R. 1979. The child amputee. In *Basic handbook of child psychiatry,* vol. 1, ed. J. D. Noshpitz, pp. 427–432. New York: Basic Books.

Reviews the developmental consideration involved in reactions to childhood amputation, giving detailed illustrations of pathological and adaptive coping mechanisms.

SCHLESINGER, H. S. 1979. The deaf child. In *Basic handbook of child psychiatry,* vol. 1, ed. J. D. Noshpitz, pp. 421–427. New York: Basic Books.

Good review of diagnosis, early development, school placement, and psychological problems of deaf children. Nondeaf parents compared to deaf parents are generally more rejecting of their handicapped child. Little discussion of long-range prognosis.

TRAVIS, G. 1976. *Chronic illness in children: Its impact on child and family.* Stanford, Calif.: Stanford University Press,

An excellent review of the pediatric and educational management of children with severe hearing loss, visual impairments, cerebral palsy, and spina bifida.

23
James VanLeeuwen

Hospitalization and Its Meaning to Child and Family

The criteria for the hospitalization of children are not always clear (North 1976). Many children are admitted for observation, laboratory investigations, or minor treatments merely out of custom or for the convenience of the physician or the parents. However, in dealing with families known to offer inadequate child care, which can be hazardous to children with even relatively minor illnesses, hospital admission on social grounds may be the lesser of two evils, even though the disease per se would not ordinarily warrant inpatient care. Whether or not it is valid, hospital treatment offers a sense of security that some physicians need more than others. Styles of medical practice differ; some doctors are more oriented toward office management and more willing to make house calls and utilize home care, while others prefer to admit patients to the hospital.

Not only criteria for admission but also the average duration of hospital stay for identical illnesses varies from hospital to hospital and physician to physician (North 1976; Provence and Lipton 1967). Cultural factors influence how frequently certain procedures such as tonsillectomy and circumcision are carried out (American Academy of Pediatrics 1975; Wolff 1981). Similarly, the dying child is often routinely hospitalized because of what seems to be a cultural intolerance to death taking place at home (Kubler-Ross 1980; Martinson 1978).

While the effect of hospital admission on a child can legitimately be

509

questioned, it must not be forgotten that behavior problems in response to illness are also common in children nursed at home. In general, psychiatrists accept hospitalization when it is clearly indicated but urge that it be taken seriously since it bears a significant risk of emotional stress, especially to certain vulnerable children and families. Many parents do not expect behavioral changes as a result of hospitalization, although such changes have been described for many years (Droske 1978; Jessner, Blom, and Waldfogel 1952; Prugh et al. 1953). Robertson (1958, p. 21) observed that "on return home after even only a few days in hospital there is usually a period of days, weeks, or longer during which the child shows by clinging, temper tantrums, aggression against the mother, and by other forms of insecure behaviour, the effects of the interrupted relationship with his mother." Vernon, Schulman, and Foley (1966), studying a sample 387 children with a mean age of 5.68 years after an average hospital stay of 8.8 days through the use of a questionnaire sent to the parents a week after discharge, found that the combination of illness and hospitalization psychologically upsets children generally, resulting in increase in separation anxiety, sleep anxiety, and aggression toward authority. This was especially so for children between six months and three years, eleven months. Douglas (1975), studying a much larger sample, also found preschoolers most vulnerable, with 22 percent of them showing behavioral deterioration on returning home.

Douglas attempted to determine whether hospital admission in the first five years is associated with disturbed behavior or learning problems in adolescence by studying all children born in Great Britain during the first week of March 1946. For twenty-six years, they were contacted every two years. Among the data collected was a complete account of hospital admissions, details of educational progress, behavior in and out of school, parental attitudes, and home circumstances. This study provides strong evidence that even one admission of more than a week's duration or repeated admissions before age five are associated with an increased risk of behavior disturbance and poor reading in adolescence. The children most vulnerable to early admission are those highly dependent on their mothers or those under stress at home at the time of admission. Quinton and Rutter (1976), replicating Douglas's findings, confirmed that while single hospital admissions lasting a week or less were not associated with later emotional or behavioral disturbance, repeated and long-term admissions were significantly associated with later disturbance. A spectrum of health care facilities can avert unnecessary hospitalization while at the same time reducing the cost of treatment. These include care-by-parent units, ambulatory services, multidisciplinary outpatient programs, surgical day-care units, home care, rehabilitation centers, and educational facilities suitable for chronically ill or handicapped children (*Better Health for Our Children*, 1981; Robinson and Clarke 1980).

The Hospital Environment

A hospital is not a home. It cannot be and does not need to be a home, despite the fact that for some children it must serve as one. Facilities vary, depending on the hospital's size, location, architecture, and orientation toward research, service, or teaching. From the child's point of view, however, the emotional climate or atmosphere is crucial. Furniture, decorations, and play materials can reflect thoughtfulness and relieve the child's apprehension, but a wholesome emotional climate demands more than the mere provision of material things; it depends primarily on the quality of staff-parent-patient relationships (Pearson 1941; Rae 1981; Robertson 1958). These should be responsive to children's reactions to illness and their need for continuing psychosocial development even while in the hospital. If the parents are actively involved in preparing the child for admission, visit regularly, and cooperate easily with ward staff, then children show fewer difficulties in adaptation and fewer severe immediate reactions to hospitalization (Prugh et al. 1953; Stevens 1949). Although hospitals exist primarily to treat disease, the care of children in them should not be limited to the treatment of their illness. While treatment, for example, may require prolonged immobilization, total care demands an active social and educational program to help a child counter boredom, depression, and school failure. Treatment may necessitate a two-year-old's being hospitalized far from home, but total care may require that the child's mother live in the hospital for a short time as well. Treatment may consist of minor surgery performed under local anesthetic, but total care requires preparing children psychologically for the major impact that needles, masks, lights, sounds, and blood may have on them if they are conscious during the operation. If the procedure involves the head, abdominal, or genital area, a child may be particularly threatened by even a relatively minor diagnostic or surgical procedure. Commenting on the child's response to surgery, Anna Freud states, "What the experience means in his life, therefore, does not depend on the type or seriousness of the operation which has actually been performed, but on the type and depth of the fantasies aroused by it" (A. Freud 1952, p. 74). Many clinical examples illustrating children's reactions to medical procedures can be found in the literature (Howells 1976; Jackson et al. 1952).

It has been shown repeatedly that hospital staff need to be aware that they can inadvertently contribute to a disturbing emotional atmosphere in the hospital (De-Nour, Czaczkes, and Lilos 1972; Mason 1965; Moore 1972). Staff tensions and arguments are perceived and responded to by patients much as children at home are made anxious by tension and discord between parents. Doctors and nurses should know that in their child patient's fantasies they may be seen as having unnatural power. This fantasied power can be harmful if it leaves children unable to express fear or anger at frightening or painful aspects of their treatment for fear of retaliation by the doctor or nurse on whose continued goodwill they feel their health and life depend. Hospital staff are often unaware of how much their own frustration, annoyance, anxiety, or feelings of professional impotence may unwittingly affect patient care. The reflection and self-examination that can be an important part of conferences or ward rounds sometimes reveals previously unrecognized attitudes such as hostility toward patients with messy illnesses, competitiveness with parents, avoidance maneuvers to escape difficult parents or patients, and subtle desertion of the dying child that, if not noted and properly controlled, will adversely affect patient care.

The pediatric hospital environment should be designed to meet the needs of infants and adolescents (Provence and Lipton 1967; Robinson and Clarke 1980). Design intervention can support the infant's needs for sensorimotor development in a safe, predictable, and stimulating environment, where parents and nursing staff can feel at ease to allow for intimacy and humanness. Some hospitals admit teenagers to separate adolescent units, others accommodate adolescents and children on the same ward, while still others integrate adolescents with adults as is done in many general hospitals (Schowalter 1971). Each system has its own history, advantages, and problems, but all should provide adolescents a milieu that simultaneously offers structure and freedom, privacy and social stimulation, education and recreation.

The University Hospital

There is a potential conflict between medical students' need for clinical training and the traditional expectation that doctors do all they can to treat disease and to relieve suffering. We need to understand better how to make clinical teaching a reassuring, even positive experience for some patients, while avoiding making it hazardous to the emotional health of others. Children usually tolerate a degree of embarrassment, discomfort, and even pain inflicted in the course of teaching, provided the teaching physician maintains a wholesome relationship with them throughout the session. This has the additional advantage of letting the clinician serve as a model for the students.

Shy, overly anxious, deprived, or homesick children are more vulnerable than those who are happy and well adjusted. The effect of age can be illustrated by the reactions of four children to the same group of medical students: a baby enjoyed the handling; a ten-month-old was frightened and overwhelmed by all the strangers; an inquisitive school-age child enjoyed the challenge and tried to learn as much as possible; a self-conscious teenager spoke of her embarrassment, awkwardness, and self-consciousness during the physical examination in front of a group.

Obviously some children are too ill to be exposed to the stress of teaching. External manifestations of disease are easier to demonstrate than the internal findings that require direct physical examination. Teaching of rectal examinations and genital inspection requires special consideration. Painful examinations need to be restricted in teaching hospitals. Certain illnesses that tend to make patients "interesting cases" or "good teaching material" create emotional hazards implied in the label. Teaching usually calls for a certain amount of repetition, which may lead to recurrent exposure of personal, confidential information or violation of the child's normal modesty through repeated examinations or through the repeated probing of emotionally painful experiences related to sexual problems, body image, hereditary illnesses, neglect, grief, and so forth.

Patients who need long-term or recurring admissions disproportionately bear the brunt of teaching-related problems. This can add to the already massive emotional burden of their chronic illness. In teaching hospitals these patients are exposed to an extraordinary amount of undergraduate and postgraduate turnover, resulting in discontinuity of care, staff confusion, and unwarranted repetition of history taking and physical examinations. The transient nature of these contacts between patients and students may erode the human quality of patient care. The problems of clinical teaching can be reduced, however, by recognition of the patient's vulnerability, by adequate psychological preparation of patient and students prior to teaching sessions, by awareness of patients' emotional needs, and by using good judgment as to what is discussed in the presence of the patient.

The Family's Reaction

The parents whose child is in the hospital are under considerable stress. They have to cope with uncertainty and anxiety about their sick child, their feelings about the hospital and its staff, as well as the additional expenses and inconvenience involved in frequent trips to the hospital. Hospitalization of a child with its attendant problems can constitute a crisis that may result in family consolidation but instead often leads to family disruption. Love and concern for the sick child are often counterbalanced by frustration and resentment due to the trouble caused by the illness, producing psychological conflicts that many parents find difficult to resolve. Siblings of children with chronic illness are at risk for emotional disturbance (Breslau, Weitzman, and Messenger 1981; Lavigne and Ryan 1979), and death of a child frequently disturbs the siblings (Cain, Fast, and Erickson 1964). The impact of hospitalization on siblings is difficult to assess apart from the effect of the illness or the death of the patient. Parents frequently report siblings' sadness, fears, and fantasies concerning the hospitalized patient. Siblings often perceive parental preoccupation with the hospitalized child as favoritism, feel deprived, and express direct or indirect resentment. Parents often find it difficult to divide their loyalties between hospital and home. Although it is not easy for hospitals to open their doors for siblings less than age twelve (Robinson and Clarke 1980), the Committee on Hospital Care of the American Academy of Pediatrics offers the following guideline: "If medically appropriate, siblings should be allowed to visit under parental supervision, provided they have no known infection or recent exposure to a communicable disease (American Academy of Pediatrics 1978, p. 85).

Not infrequently, parents decrease or altogether stop visiting their hospitalized children. Often this is not because of disinterest or rejection but because of an unfortunate combination of omissions and misinterpretations. The following story is typical.

> As parents enter the hospital room to visit their hospitalized child, their child starts to cry. When they prepare to leave, the child cries again, clinging and making a scene. Although this is appropriate behavior under the circumstances, embarrassed parents often interpret it as a sign of weakness in their child and their failure to raise a well-behaved child. A well-meaning staff person reassures them that their child is really quite good and does not cry when they are not around. The parents take this to mean that their visits must, in some way, be upsetting the child. So they stay home, causing even greater distress and turmoil at their next visit, which confirms their belief that their visits are indeed too upsetting, making hospitalization even harder to endure.

Parental failure to visit regularly may indicate that parents are immobilized by their reactions to their child's illness and hospitalization. By recognizing and freeing them from their immobilization, medical and nursing staff can do much to avoid a potentially serious but unnecessary psychological risk.

Reaction of the Child

RESPONSES TO THE DISCOMFORTS OF BEING ILL

The hospitalized child has many fears: fears of symptoms, pain, damage, exposure, and loss of control; fear of strangers, separation, abandonment, and death; fears of the unknown and of his or her own terrible fantasies (Bergmann and Freud 1966; Robertson 1952). A particular child's response will depend on age, previous adjustment, illness, and hospital climate. Children in the hospital normally react at times with sadness, anxiety, refusal to accept unpleasant treatments, and attempts to secure mothering. Unless the hospital environment can accept these, the child may be labeled childish, silly, stubborn, or spoiled. If hospital staff become angry with a child, they may further increase that child's distress and symptomatic behavior, eliciting further rejection. If, on the other hand, the staff's natural tendency to comfort a sad child makes them overly solicitous, they may feed into the child's wish to be taken care of, and unnecessarily regressive behavior such as spoon feeding, wheelchair rides, and other types of babying that encourage the child to function at less advanced developmental levels may emerge. Hospitalization of children in developmental transition increases the risk of the child's losing such newly gained ground as self-care, bowel control, or social skills, in which case pride in achievement turns into a sense of loss or failure.

With so many reasons for children to find hospitalization upsetting, it is sometimes difficult to differentiate between normally expected behavior, and behavior indicating pathological reactions to hospitalization (Danilowicz and Gabriel 1971; Jessner, Blom, and Waldfogel 1952). There are no absolute rules, but workers should be concerned when staff or parents identify behavior different from the child's previous pattern. Such new behaviors might include sucking, rocking, self-injury, food refusal, incontinence, refusal to sleep, extreme fears, inability to play, withdrawal, or absence of crying.

When children's tears and protests are not effective in getting them out of the hospital, some become resigned and apathetic, allowing the staff to do with them as they please. This makes for an "easy" patient. Unfortunately, many such "easy" patients are actually depressed, but they often receive less attention because they are withdrawn and undemonstrative. This, in turn, increases their sense of abandonment.

How stressful a particular child finds hospitalization will depend on that child's vulnerability to separation from the family, the response of child and family to the disease itself, and the quality of hospital care provided (King and Ziegler 1981). While all of these factors are important, for the infant and younger child the experience of separation from mother and family is particularly significant.

HOSPITALIZATION AS A SEPARATION EXPERIENCE

Infants under five months do not yet conceptualize the mother as a person separate from themselves, a concept essential to the "separation anxiety" that peaks in the second year and is typical of toddlers. Nevertheless, infants do show a "global" reaction to hospitalization, including changes in feeding, sleeping, and elimination patterns. These disturbances continue for a few days to several weeks after the infant's return home (Schaffer and Callender 1959; Spitz 1945; Wolff 1981). Soon after six months of age, children begin to be upset when strangers approach or when their mother leaves them in unfamiliar surroundings. A sick child of two, finding him- or herself in hospital without familiar toys and clothes, left to the care of strangers, separated from mother for an extended period of time, frequently shows the characteristic sequence of protest, despair, and detachment described by Robertson and Bowlby (Bowlby 1952; Robertson 1952); (see chapter 4).

In the 1940s, Spitz (1945, 1946) first reported his studies on the effect an emotionally sterile foundling home had on the development of infants placed there at four months of age. He coined the term hospitalism (not to be confused with hospitalization) to characterize physical and psychological disturbance that commonly resulted in developmental retardation, increased susceptibility to infections, apathy, extreme emaciation (i.e., marasmus), and profound sadness (i.e., anaclitic depression), which he attributed to institutional depression. On follow-up after two years, 37 percent of this group were dead. Those who survived showed delayed development, both emotionally and intellectually, and profound disruption in the capacity for social relationships. This study, admittedly of extreme situations that no longer exist, for the first time drew attention to the degree to which failure to meet children's emotional needs can undermine their normal development and threaten life itself.

Later, Robertson and Robertson (1971), studying children placed in good foster homes, found that separation per se need not result in emotional deprivation or produce protest, despair, and detachment as long as the substitute environment provides adequate surrogate parenting. Hospitals will never be perfect in this respect. However, when children are free to bring their own clothes, toys, and family portraits, and when the staff is sensitive and committed to meeting emotional as well as physical needs, the potential adverse effects can be minimized. Branstetter (1969) confirmed that having someone give substitute mothering during most of the waking hours protected a selected group of not very ill toddlers from the distress often seen in children whose parents cannot stay in the hospital with them. This study also demonstrated that a control group of similar toddlers, without special substitute mothering, did experience extreme distress despite the usual nursing care offered in the pediatric unit.

Separation from home is less threatening for the older child, particularly when adequate contact with the family and friends is maintained. The child's favorite television program, foods, music, or hobby can minimize loneliness and unhappiness. Some school-age children, however, become intensely homesick, and their suffering is often aggravated if hospital staff are intolerant or ridicule their distress. Parents and siblings are not the only important visitors to be considered. Separation from one's best friend—which, incidentally, could be the family pet—can be very painful.

One survey showed that more than a quarter of hospitalized adolescents preferred peers to parents as visitors (Schowalter 1977).

LONG-TERM HOSPITALIZATION

A universal problem with long-term hospitalization is the associated risk of serious and cumulative emotional deprivation that predisposes to chronic depression, failure to thrive, delay in development, poor impulse control, or erosion of relationships (Douglas 1975; Schaffer and Callender 1959; World Health Organization 1962).

In contrast to the sudden sharp, traumatic, but time-limited stresses of acute hospitalization, long-term patients are expected to adapt to the peculiar social milieu of a hospital. Their life style will reflect the relationships, attitudes, and priorities they observe among the doctors, nurses, technicians, physiotherapists, students, cleaners, and so forth. Unless the total staff is organized to present a goal-directed, child-centered treatment plan, the hospital will be perceived by the children as disease oriented, undemocratic, disorganized, manipulative, and insensitive, as compared with their own home environment. These perceptions will be reflected in their adaptation in the hospital, which will include similar undesirable methods of handling people, feelings, and situations (Hall and Stacey 1979).

In addition to the behaviors acquired from the hospital atmosphere, long-term patients lose many opportunities for normal development because of being in the hospital. They are deprived of the chance to grow up within their own committed family environment as well as of their freedom and of many social and educational opportunities experienced by other children. Their development of autonomy and responsibility are diminished by all the things that have to be done to them or for them.

A child's feelings of alienation can be exacerbated in a teaching hospital, where there is a distinct possibility that the kind of case presentation and staff conferences that medical students are exposed to repeatedly during training may blunt their inherent sensitivity, leaving them well organized but rather intellectual and disease oriented. Doctors often lapse into medical jargon, at times without noticing it, losing sight of the patient who is going through the intensely threatening experience of illness. For example, a physician might describe the illness of a fifteen-year-old boy with Wilson's disease as follows:

> Wilson's disease is a familial, recessively inherited disorder due to the defective metabolism of copper. As a result, copper is deposited in the liver, cornea, kidneys, and brain. This disease runs a progressive course with periodic exacerbations, leading to cirrhosis, Kayser-Fleischer rings in the cornea, renal failure, and brain damage. If started early, copper-removing agents such as penicillamine are usually effective. This fifteen-year-old boy, unfortunately, started treatment one year after the onset of his symptoms, hence has permanent brain damage with rigidity, spasms, tremors, and a Parkinsonian appearance.

517

The boy involved, however, might describe his experiences from a different perspective and in his own language.

> Here I am in the hospital, hundreds of miles from home and my parents. I've lost my friends and failed my year in school. I'm scared. I can't even move properly any more, and talking is impossible. I must look kind of stupid; that's probably why they sometimes treat me as if I'm stupid. People get frustrated caring for me because I'm so helpless. Why me? I guess my parents should not have married: our whole family seems doomed. I may die just like my two sisters. What have I done wrong? All these lab tests drive me up the wall. Even what they call "therapy" means an awful diet and painful needles. I hate it all. I can't stand not knowing what's going to happen.

Care for this boy consists of more than just penicillamine; he needs understanding and help to become a person who can function despite his handicaps.

There is a growing recognition that treatment for groups of children requiring long-term and intermittent hospitalization for conditions such as hemophilia, diabetes, burns, cerebral palsy, heart disease, fibrocystic disease, leukemia, chronic renal disease, and so forth must meet the child's medical needs while, at the same time, addressing the psychological and social problems associated with the illness (see chapter 21). Many centers try to go beyond mere treatment of the disease to provide comprehensive care for the child by including social workers, psychiatrists, or psychologists as an integral part of the treatment team. These mental health personnel, trained to recognize and respond to psychological and developmental needs of affected children and their families, can assist the team in various ways. They may be particularly helpful in dealing with those children and families in which emotional conflicts are interfering with the child's treatment or undermining developmental progress. Examples would include the diabetic child who manipulates her insulin dosage to control or punish parents, the hemophiliac who repeatedly gets involved in activities he knows cause unnecessary bleeds only to use minor or pretended bleeds to avoid attending school, the fibrocystic child who resists postural drainage or refuses medication, and so on. While medical and nursing staff usually recognize these children as problems, they often lack the time, patience, interest, or training to help child and family resolve these problems, especially if the people involved prove resistant to immediate advice or seem unable to cooperate. In addition to direct counseling of such children and their families, mental health personnel can ensure proper attention to adequate psychological preparation for admission or for potentially frightening or painful procedures and adequate provision for the social and educational experiences chronically ill children so badly need. One or more such person on the treatment team and their regular participation in multidisciplinary treatment planning meetings can minimize the emotional and social difficulties that so often complicate severe chronic illness.

PSYCHOLOGICAL BENEFITS OF HOSPITALIZATION

Despite the possible consequences associated with hospital admission, some children, in addition to medical benefits, derive psychosocial assistance from hospitalization (Jessner, Blom, and Waldfogel 1952; Vernon, Schulman, and Foley 1966). Children differ in their vulnerability to stress. Some who are relatively capable and "invulnerable" seem able to strengthen themselves as they master the stress produced by hospitalization. Certainly other children from relatively depriving families thrive in a hospital where their emotional growth is facilitated. Richer and Gantcheff (1976) reported on fifteen hospitalized young pediatric patients who received comprehensive intervention as well as traditional pediatric care for their developmental needs. Instead of being detrimental, hospitalization improved their competence. Occasionally the family and community resources mobilized by a sick child's admission can help a family achieve a higher level of functioning than that existing prior to admission. Both the Vernon and Douglas studies referred to earlier (Douglas 1975; Vernon, Schulman, and Foley 1966;) also demonstrate that even some preschoolers can show improved behavior on return home. This indicates that hospitalization, despite its potential risks to some children, can be psychologically beneficial for others.

Preventive Intervention

Any attempt to reduce the discomfort and disruption of illness and hospitalization by a carefully planned approach to health care for children and adolescents is not only worthwhile in human terms but also valuable in preventing emotional disorders. Most preventive interventions either reduce risk factors or modify intermediate variables. This can be done by (1) improving the competence of children at risk, focusing either on the child or on the parent-child system; (2) crisis intervention consisting of anticipatory guidance (i.e., preparation programs) and guidance during the crisis; (3) facilitation of support systems (Caplan 1980). In practice these approaches overlap and can exist simultaneously in a single intervention. The following examples of preventive intervention were selected because they pertain to hospital care.

REDUCING RISK FACTORS

Substituting surgical day care for inpatient care is an excellent example of one way to reduce risk factors. This also reduces the risk of cross-infection associated with longer hospital stays while avoiding many psychological sequelae. Additionally, it is as effective as inpatient care in many conditions and less expensive (Evans and Robinson 1980).

IMPROVING COMPETENCE

Three examples, each demonstrating a different way of improving the competence of a child or parent-child system at risk, will be described.

Scarr-Salapatek and Williams (1973) offered a program of visual, tactile, and kinesthetic stimulation to a group of hospitalized infants born at low birth weights to disadvantaged mothers. The nursery staff was instructed to introduce handling, human faces and voices, and patterned visual stimulation, not including the mothers', until the babies were discharged an average of six weeks later. A control group received the then standard pediatric care for low-birth-weight infants. They were maintained in isolettes and fed and changed with minimum disturbance. Tests at four weeks and at one year indicated greater developmental progress for the stimulated children than for the control children. Masi (1979), reviewing a number of premature infant stimulation studies, generally found some benefit to the stimulated infants, ranging from improvement in motor development, weight gain, or cognitive function.

Klaus and Kennell (1970) hypothesized that mother-infant separation during the sensitive period of early bonding could lead to serious difficulties in a mother's later caregiving abilities. They were concerned that the high-risk infant, besides being biologically vulnerable and in need of a controlled environment and intensive care, also suffered from a lack of parent participation in the intensive care nurseries. Their concern was supported by the finding that children born prematurely were overrepresented in the failure-to-thrive and child abuse syndromes (Klein and Stern 1971).

These studies, although questioned by Minde (1980), have at least fostered considerable interest in helping parents to be with their high-risk infants in the hospital. However, visiting alone does not guarantee the establishment of a bond. The condition of the child and the technology essential to his or her survival can be intimidating and distancing to the parents. Minde's studies of the interaction of mothers and nurses with infants in a premature nursery (Minde 1980; Minde et al. 1980a, 1980b) have helped to define criteria for early recognition of particularly vulnerable mother-infant pairs and to develop techniques for enhancing competence in parent-infant bonding. Slade, Reidl, and Mangurten (1977) frequently start before the baby's birth to provide the parents of high-risk infants with guidance on how to take a significant role in caring for their children despite the obstacles of an intensive care nursery.

Haka-Ikse and VanLeeuwen (1976) organized a team consisting of a pediatrician, head nurse, social worker, occupational therapist, physiotherapist, play therapist, public health nurse, and child psychiatrist to plan

520

for the "nonmedical" needs of long-term hospitalized children less than three years of age and their families. This pilot project's approach was based on common sense, developmental principles, and a child advocacy stance. Weekly meetings were held for one year on a twenty-five-bed medical unit in a large pediatric hospital. Forty-five children were discussed repeatedly and followed through their stay in the hospital. Once an area of need was identified, remedial action would be taken by the appropriate team members. Although no firm conclusions could be drawn because of a lack of controls, the results were sufficiently encouraging that the hospital began to institute an automatic review process by multidisciplinary teams of three or more professionals for all children under three hospitalized for more than two weeks.

PREPARATION AND SUPPORT FOR HOSPITAL AND MEDICAL PROCEDURES AND SURGERY

Many popular television programs for children (e.g., *Sesame Street, Mr. Rogers,* etc.) have given viewers considerable information about what being in a hospital is like. Also, most pediatric hospitals offer general information for individuals or groups of children through pamphlets, tours, slide shows, coloring books, puppet shows, and so forth. (Robinson and Clarke 1980; Siegel 1976).

Children usually have an opportunity to make a preadmission visit with their parents to be introduced to the hospital and such routine procedures as examinations and urine and blood collection. For tonsillectomies and other elective procedures, children and parents are often prepared in a group, but on the whole families are prepared individually. Physicians should do the preparation for medical procedures, as they know what is to be done and when it will happen. Preparation not only provides patients and families with information but strengthens the doctor-patient relationship, alleviating anxiety through the trust and confidence it provides (Bergmann and Freud 1966; Visintainer and Wolfer 1975). Although it is essential that physicians communicate with children and parents, they cannot be the only ones to prepare patients. Nurses, technicians, social workers, recreationists, teachers, and psychotherapists can all contribute depending on the situation or condition (Petrillo and Sanger 1980). The following example illustrates an application of the principles of preparing and supporting children and families for hospital, medical, and surgical procedures.

As a consultant to the dialysis-transplantation program at The Hospital for Sick Children in Toronto, the author has participated in preparing children and families for admissions, transfers, medical and surgical procedures, complications, drug effects, and so forth. From this experience he has arrived at a number of generally applicable principles. Significant information should be given in privacy and comfort rather than in the corridors and, where possible, to both parents. Especially when parents or patients are required to follow specific procedures, what matters is not what they are told but what is understood and retained. There is an art to giving information successfully. Unless it is conveyed with empathy, the chances of its not being grasped are considerable. The surest way to confirm people's comprehension is to have patient or family explain what they have been told to another staff member some time after the original explanation. Children and parents should be prepared separately, with the information and delivery tailored to their needs and competence. A well-informed, trusting, participating, and concerned parent can best protect the child against overwhelming anxiety. Children deserve information appropriately timed and put into terms they can assimilate. Obviously the younger the child, the more pictures, puppetry, and play techniques rather than verbal explanations may help.

Helplessness and passivity in the face of a feared or painful event almost universally provokes anxiety. Children love to play doctor with toy medical instruments. The nurses designed a large doll with all the zippered spaces, tubing, and cloth organs needed for the children to enact full-scale operations. Feelings and fantasies were expressed remarkably clearly in play sessions, and important but correctable misconceptions were revealed. The play helps children work out some of their fears and frustrations as they take the part not of passive victims but of powerful adults with a sense of freedom and mastery.

Many school-age children achieve a similar sense of mastery by presenting a dialysis-transplantation project at school. Successful and experienced patients and families are invited to instruct and guide the new and anxious patients and families through frightening experiences. A loose-leaf manual explaining all aspects of dialysis-transplantation in simple terms has been very helpful in providing information and security for families in their relation to the hospital.

In the program, there may be unanticipated technical problems, seizures, cardiac arrests, or surgical complications that are stressful not only for the patient involved but also for the patients sharing the room or the dialysis unit who witness the crisis. The successful mastery of such complications often depends on careful reconstruction and explanation of the event and subsequent experience. The most careful preparation does not render a family or child relaxed in the face of medical problems.

The purpose of preparation is to help child and family tolerate the unavoidable anxiety while retaining a sense of trust and confidence. Only one of the more than one hundred patients in the program preferred not to be told about impending procedures because he always experienced more anticipatory anxiety than he felt he could handle. All other patients and families indicated appreciation of the careful preparation program. Preparation and support were also needed for the inevitable errors made by hospital staff, the unavoidable waiting periods, the prolonged suffering from illness, the pain of certain treatments, or, in some cases, death itself. In the dialysis-transplantation program, support is offered by a well-organized interdisciplinary team of physicians, nurses, technicians, dieticians, social workers, recreationists, and school teachers (Matthews, VanLeeuwen, and Christensen 1981; Van Leeuwen and Matthews 1975).

While research is still needed to identify the best techniques and timing of preparation programs and to demonstrate their effectiveness, already much is known that could, with benefit, be put into practice. Several good studies done in the 1950s contrast extra preparation and support given one group of patients with the standard care given a control group, in order to assess the benefits of such extra care (Jackson et al. 1952; Vaughan and Lond 1957). These studies consistently demonstrate fewer disturbances in the posthospital period for those children who received extra preparation as compared to controls who received standard care. Cassell (1965) investigated the effect of structured puppet play therapy on children between ages three and eleven undergoing cardiac catheterization. The control groups who received no special preparation showed significantly more disturbed behavior during the catheterization. Skipper and Leonard (1968) showed that children's stress can be reduced indirectly by reducing the stress of their mothers. Their experimental group of mothers received information and support from a special nurse before and after the children's tonsillectomies, while the control group received only routine management. Stress in children was measured in elevated temperatures, pulse rates, and blood pressure; postoperative vomiting; disturbed sleep following discharge; and extended periods of recovery. The children whose mothers received the information and support showed significantly less stress.

While some studies give only subjective support for preparation programs—Crocker (1980) and Siegel (1976) have rightly drawn attention to the methodological shortcomings of others—those by Melamed and Siegel (1975) and by Visintainer and Wolfer (1975) provide additional, methodologically sound evidence of the value of specific preparation programs. Most of these were done on children hospitalized for elective procedures, yet the most common hospitalization for young children is an emergency admission, which constitutes an even greater stress for children, parents, and staff than the already stressful elective admission. In spite of this fact, Roskies and associates (1975) demonstrated that in a modern pediatric hospital, the almost universal pattern was to give the child either no or misleading information about the events to be encountered.

The results of these preparation studies are remarkably consistent. However, the regular inclusion of adequate preparation programs for children is not yet a standard part of accepted hospital routine. The basis of the studies previously discussed suggest it would be fair to consider "standard care" for hospitalized children as inadequate and potentially harmful and preparation and support programs not an extra but an indispensable component of quality patient care.

SUPPORT SYSTEM

Another promising advance in the treatment of hospitalized children has been the formation of associations and foundations for almost every medical condition known today. These associations provide support in the broadest social sense, by organizing fund raising, stimulating public awareness, providing information, supporting research and service, and through political action. Although such organizations are helpful, parents are sometimes understandably reluctant to contact them, because in so doing they confront the reality of their child's diagnosis. For example, a five-year-old child with Duchenne muscular dystrophy who is still able to walk will often respond to contact with older children he has met through the Muscular Dystrophy Association by asking if he is going to end up in a wheelchair like them. Both parents and children need to be prepared for referrals to such associations and for the experiences and questions these referrals may elicit.

The list of support systems for hospitalized pediatric patients is lengthy. It includes all professional and volunteer activities in the social, religious, recreational, and educational fields. The Association for the Care of Children's Health, located in Washington, D.C., deserves special mention as a central forum for discussion of the concerns expressed in this chapter.

Finally, psychiatric consultation-liaison services to pediatric hospitals not only provide treatment for established disturbance but can offer preventive intervention as well.

Consultation-Liaison

In most pediatric hospitals child psychiatrists are available to assist in the diagnosis and management of psychiatric aspects of the problems of patients primarily cared for by pediatricians and surgeons. The traditional role of the consultant who is called to offer an expert opinion on a specific patient has expanded to include a variety of working relationships, hence the term consultation-liaison. The relationships may take many different forms, because the type of liaison depends not only on the personality style of the psychiatrist and the pediatric colleagues but also on the historical development, organization, and size of the hospital. There may be an emphasis on psychiatric service, teaching, or research as it applies to pediatric medicine. The interdisciplinary relationship may range from harmonious collaboration to uninspired coexistence (Bolian 1971; Geist 1977; Rothenberg 1968; Sarles and Friedman 1979).

In most large pediatric hospitals there are a wide spectrum of relationships: on some wards the psychiatrist may be accepted only as a traditional case consultant, while on others the psychiatrist may participate in ward rounds and be expected to promote proper psychological awareness in the management of all patients by all staff (Froese, Kamin, and Levine 1976–77; Haka-Ikse and VanLeeuwen 1976). The liaison at times takes the form of a team approach, as in the program-oriented services that exist for diabetics, fibrocystics, children with facial deformities, (Lefebvre and Munro 1978), muscular dystrophies, cancer, and so forth. The previously mentioned dialysis-transplantation program (Matthews, VanLeeuwen, and Christensen 1981; Vanleeuwen and Matthews 1975) is one example of a form of liaison where a child psychiatrist is expected to share responsibility with the nephrologist and the urologist for all the patients under their care, approaching what Caplan (1980) has termed collaboration. Of course, the actual provision of psychosocial care is carried by the larger team of physicians, social workers, nurses, teachers, and so on, as well as psychiatrists. The research in the intensive care nursery is an example of research integrated within a consultation-liaison service (Minde et al. 1980*a*, 1980*b*).

No matter how well accepted psychiatry may be, the process of referring a child for psychiatric consultation requires special consideration and is discussed in detail in chapter 30.

SUGGESTIONS FOR FURTHER READING

BAROWSKY, E. I., 1978. Young children's perceptions and reactions to hospitalization. In *Psychosocial aspects of pediatric care*, ed. E. Gellert, pp. 37–49. New York: Grune & Stratton.
Deals with children's fears and anxieties regarding hospitalization and describes how visiting, rooming-in, and methods of preparation can diminish these fears.

DANILOWICS, D. A., AND GABRIEL, H. P. 1971–72. Postoperative reactions in children: "Normal" and "abnormal" responses after cardiac surgery." *Am. J. Psychiat.* 128:185–188.
Responses of sixty-eight children undergoing cardiac surgery fell into four main groups: anxiety, anger, cooperation, and compliance. The need to evaluate a child's adjustment before and after surgery and to prepare adequately for surgery is stressed.

GELLERT, E., ed. 1978. *Psychosocial aspects of pediatric care.* New York: Grune & Stratton.
A collection of essays relating to the psychological issues in the medical treatment of children. Deals with reactions to hospitalization, surgery, and chronic and fatal illness.

HOFMANN, A. D.; BECKER, R. D.; AND GABRIEL, H. P., 1976. *The hospitalized adolescent: A guide to managing the ill and injured youth.* New York: The Free Press.
An in-depth understanding of the emotional and behavioral dimensions of adolescence and the psychodynamic effects of hospitalization on the adolescent patient. Offers practical management principles and techniques for establishing and operating adolescent health care wards, with emphasis on the need for a "team" approach.

HOWELLS, J. G., ed. 1976. *Modern perspectives in the psychiatric aspects of surgery.* New York: Brunner/Mazel.
An encyclopedic collection of articles by distinguished international contributors dealing with psychiatric aspects of all types of surgery and injuries.

KING, J., AND ZIEGLER, S., 1981. The effects of hospitalization on children's behavior: A review of the literature. *J. Assn. Care of Children's Health* 10(1): 20–28.
Provides a brief review of essential contributions to the literature, providing an adequate perspective on the various directions in the research and quality of findings.

MINDE, K. K., 1980. Bonding of parents to premature infants: Theory and practice. In *Parents-infants relationships*, ed. P. M. Taylor, pp. 291–313. New York: Grune & Stratton.
Gives a review of the current literature on the topic, providing examples from personal experiences at The Hospital for Sick Children in Toronto.

PERNILLO, M., AND SANGER, S. 1980. *Emotional care of hospitalized children: An environmental approach.* Philadelphia: J.B. Lippincott.
A general guide for any professional responsible for the care of children in hospitals or clinics. Straightforward, common-sense approach. Easy to read.

ROBINSON, C. G., AND CLARKE, H. F. 1980. *The hospital care of children: A review of contemporary issues.* New York: Oxford University Press.
A 250-page, carefully balanced work by Canadian contributors who, on the basis of psychological understanding of the child's needs, designed and implemented a range of

programs and facilities to improve hospital care and to offer alternatives for inpatient care. Helpful cost-saving aspects are included.

SIEGEL, L. J. 1976. Preparation of children for hospitalization. A selected review of the research literature. *J. Pediat. Psychol.* 1(4): 26–30.

A brief review of some of the major research studies with constructively critical comments about the quality of these studies.

THOMPSON, R. H., AND STANFORD, G., eds. 1981. *Child life in hospitals: Theory and practice.* Springfield, Ill.: Charles C Thomas.

The authors demonstrate through case studies, bibliographic resources, and personal experience the emotional needs of the hospitalized child and his or her family, while confronting the reader with the realities of administering a child life program. Particularly valuable for those who plan to implement or improve such a program.

24

Ed Pakes

The Dying Child, the Family, and the Caregivers

The professional treating the child with a potentially fatal illness must be concerned not only with the disease itself but also with the emotional reactions of child and family to the disease. Research indicates that families with a dying child constitute a high-risk group (Kaplan, Grobstein, and Smith 1976). The severe stress precipitated by a fatal illness may generate a variety of problems ranging from jealousies and unresolved grief reactions in siblings to separation, divorce, or mental illness in parents (Binger et al. 1969; Bozeman, Orbach, and Sutherland 1955; Kaplan et al. 1973).

As the acute infectious diseases come under better control, physicians and nurses must increasingly provide care for patients suffering such life-threatening and ultimately fatal illnesses as cancer, renal diseases, and certain congenital disorders.

Even the treatment of these "life-threatening illnesses" is changing. Some authors state that today cure must be considered the norm rather than the exception, with 51 percent of children with cancer remaining free of disease for more than five years (Van Eys 1977). The concept of "fighting" such a disease with unbridled determination is exemplified by the young man who ran halfway across Canada to publicize the fight and became a folk hero before his death. The possibility of a cure was close enough to make this possible (Van Eys 1977).

Doctors and nurses dealing with dying children and their families

527

experience considerable strain.* Studies have shown that physicians generally have a heightened fear of death (Feifel and Hanson 1967) and that their choice of medicine as a career may be one way of dealing with this fear (Feifel 1959, 1963). Physicians are torn between the duty to become professionally involved in the care of the dying child and family and the wish to remain emotionally detached. They may sometimes prescribe unpleasant and even unnecessary investigations and treatments even though death is inevitable, in order to protect themselves from painful feelings stirred up by their involvement and their "therapeutic" failure. While the specific reactions of child and family to the illness vary with the child's age (Easson 1968) and with factors unique to the particular family, many physicians and nurses find the process of helping child and family deal with their feelings about the illness exhausting and frustrating. Conversely, many others recognize that the possibility of doing something active and useful for the family, even if the child eventually dies, can prove helpful not only to the family but also to their own need to maintain their professional vitality.

In order to prepare to deal with such situations, some basic psychological aspects of death must be understood. Many of the issues involved in managing the chronically ill child overlap with those faced in treating dying children and their families (Anthony and Koupernik 1973; Burton 1974, 1975). As treatment improves yearly, even patients destined to die can be kept alive and in remission for increasing periods of time. The uncertainty of the future can in itself produce chronic stress for all concerned.

Factors Affecting Reaction Patterns

THE AGE OF THE CHILD

Up to the age of three, children's main concern is their fear of being separated from those they love and depend on for their security.

> Three-year-old Danny, who was dying, cried out, "I'm falling, I'm falling!" His nurse, realizing his fear of being separated, held him and replied, "I'm catching you, I'm catching you." The nurse's awareness of Danny's separation anxiety allowed her to relieve his distress in the face of death.

In middle childhood (three to seven years) children cannot conceive of the finality of death. They are, however, fearful of mutilation. They may have seen a pet run over by a car or a bird torn up by a cat. They are con-

*See Green 1976; Khan 1979; Schowalter 1970; Schowalter, Ferholt, and Mann 1973; and Weiner 1970.

cerned about the integrity of their body and frightened of anything that can destroy it. At this age children typically consider the immobility of the dead a response to external circumstances rather than a consequence of death itself. A four-year-old may say, "He cannot move because he's in the coffin," while another remarks, "Dead people close their eyes because sand gets in them." They identify death with sleep, viewing it as a response to the outside world rather than as a change in the self. Especially around the age of five and six, degrees of death are described, as by the child who said, "She could get out of the coffin if she wasn't stabbed too badly."

Since at this stage death is attributed to outside intervention and often thought of as a bogeyman (i.e., death personified) who comes to take people away, children may have a magical belief in some action that they feel can miraculously reverse the process. This is why a simple object like a Band-Aid can have such significance at this age.

> Brian, age seven, was a very bright boy with leukemia who understood that he would soon die from his disease. He experienced many procedures during his hospitalization, and prior to his death began to accuse the doctors and nurses of being murderers and killers because they stuck needles into him. To him, they were outsiders who were invading his body and causing his pain. These accusations were particularly distressing to staff, who were already feeling bad because of their inability to relieve Brian's pain and bring about a remission. When the staff could recognize and deal successfully with their own feelings of guilt, they were better able to administer his medications.

Often we do not realize that children of this age are more aware of their impending death than may seem evident (Bluebond-Langer 1978; Plank and Plank 1978). This is an age at which children frequently avoid discussing their thoughts and feelings about their illness with their parents who, they recognize, are trying to hide the truth from them.

By age eight the child can view death realistically, as a permanent biological process, for the first time. Typical of this stage would be the ten-year-old girl who likened death to the withering of flowers.

To adolescents the prospect of dying is extremely traumatic. They understand the meaning of death but often have trouble accepting the reality that they personally are about to die. Bursting with a lust for life and just on the verge of self-sufficiency, the teenager often sees death as an unfair punishment. The adolescent, more than younger children, asks, "What have I done to deserve this?" The normal age-specific emotional reaction of the newly mature to the prospect of personal death is rage. Feeling that life was just within their grasp, they see death as a ravisher and destroyer that snatches away their dreams. Both young children and mature adults can turn to others for support, but newly emancipated adolescents may have too much pride in their new-found independence to allow themselves to accept support and understanding as they approach death.

A group of medical students, well informed in clinical practice and still in touch with their own adolescence, was asked whether or not adolescents should be told they are dying. There was general agreement that they should be, since adolescence is a time when long-range plans are made and these may be unrealistic if the patient's prognosis is poor. They agreed that adolescents deserve some choice in how they will spend the remainder of their life. While physicians should avoid taking away hope that is helping an adolescent face the limited but uncertain future, too rigid a commitment to unrealistic long-term goals (e.g., preparing for college) may stand in the way of getting the most out of the time remaining.

THE LENGTH OF ILLNESS

Sudden death of a child—for example, death by accident—most frequently leads to acute grief and mourning but may result in an unresolved grief reaction, especially if the parents hold themselves responsible for the accident. The sudden infant death syndrome frequently leaves parents weighed down by guilt and wondering if they were neglectful. In such cases the parents should receive a proper explanation of the current knowledge in this field, but merely hearing the facts once may not be enough to dispel their guilt. In situations involving sudden death, it is wise to make a practice of seeing the parents at intervals following the death to assess how they are coping with their reactions to the loss. Prolonged illness, on the other hand, may eventually result in the family wishing the child dead. This too may be a source of persistent guilt, which can interfere with the completion of mourning. In either case, if the family reaction appears extreme or excessively prolonged or if relationships within the family, with members of the extended family, or with longstanding friends deteriorate drastically and show evidence of persistent strain, psychiatric referral should be considered.

THE SPECIFIC ILLNESS

Some families react to certain illnesses differently than to others. This is particularly true with genetically transmitted diseases. The parent carrying the gene feels considerable guilt, which may be accentuated by the reactions of the relatives of the nonaffected partner.

Diseases requiring extensive, continuing care, such as cases of renal failure or fibrocystic disease, generate chronic stress.

In life-long illness such as diabetes or cystic fibrosis, behavioral problems and a self-destructive failure to observe the treatment regime may represent depressive or suicide equivalents, particularly in adolescents (see chapter 14).

In an unpublished study the author, has reported on a group of leukemic children using a simple projective technique adapted from Winnicott

(1971) in which the examiner and the child, in turn, draw "squiggly" lines that the other connects to complete a drawing about which he or she then makes up a story. Each school-age leukemic child's story concerned an illness or accident, frequently including a snake that bit the child, threatening the child's life. The story continued that the "bad blood" was taken out in the hospital and "good blood" substituted. The stories of accidents and their treatment often reflected whether the child was in remission or exacerbation. Diabetic children interviewed with a similar technique emphasized aggressive eating themes in their stories, as well as frequently mentioning pin pricks and arrows, indicating the child's (at least unconscious) preoccupation with some aspects of the illness.

THE FAMILY

The psychological stress of having a dying child has a profound effect on family adaptation. In extreme cases this may cause parents to turn against each other and separate; other families, rallying to mutual support, become stronger than ever. Some families are plunged into lasting despair by the diagnosis of fatal illness. Others react to the child's diagnosis by realizing that they are not getting the most out of life and begin to live more fully than they ever have before. Some families turn to religion, friends, or the extended family for solace and support; others abruptly turn away from them in bitter alienation. Any widespread or persistent tendency toward withdrawal from previous family or social involvements may indicate that the family is having serious difficulty handling the stress resulting from the illness and is in need of supportive intervention.

Siblings

Parents often ask how best to present the facts of the child's illness to siblings. Issues such as the ages of the siblings, their level of understanding, their relationships with the sick child, and the likelihood that they may resentfully view the patient as favored because of the amount of parental time and attention focused on him or her because of the illness have to be balanced against the sick child's needs in order to arrive at the appropriate answer for a particular family. Younger children frequently believe that their hostile wishes or thoughts come true. This may cause intense guilt and remorse in response to the death of a sibling because at one time the surviving sibling was angry enough to wish the other child dead. Strong feelings of guilt or parental inability to tolerate the ventilation of hostile thoughts and feelings may result in siblings trapping their own grief inside. Should this occur, it can form the basis for later emotional disturbances.

Bereaved parents can become extremely protective of surviving children following a death in the family (Freud and Burlingham 1943). However, proper early intervention can facilitate healthy grieving and prevent future emotional illness.

> A mother who lost a five-year-old boy during heart surgery for a congenital defect requested a child psychiatrist closely involved with a self-help Bereaved Family Organization to see her eight-year-old daughter, Karen. The girl's schoolwork had deteriorated since the brother's death. She was quickly engaged in a "squiggles" drawing game. She drew and told the story of a boy who let his dog off the leash, resulting in the dog's being run over. In the story the child felt sad and responsible for the death. On a subsequent visit, Karen related a true story: she had found an injured squirrel outside. She took it to the vet only to find that it was dead. Nevertheless, she commented, "I cared and felt something inside of me that I could do something."

Karen had felt overwhelmed by responsibility for her brother's death, as was suggested in her story of the boy who let the dog off the leash only to get run over. Only by attempting to reverse the illness-death situation with the squirrel could she begin to feel in control of her world again and therefore less helpless. Following this event and its discussion with her therapist, her schoolwork began to improve and she was able to cry for short periods if reminded about her brother's absence. She was able to talk with her therapist about how helpless the brother's death made her feel and to explain how much better she felt after the incident with the squirrel.

This therapeutic experience illustrates that young children can indeed satisfactorily complete the process of mourning if given proper adult support. Intervention at the time of the death may do much to minimize for the survivors long-term psychological sequelae resulting from failure to successfully complete the work of mourning (Bowlby 1960; Cain, Fast, and Erickson 1964).

There is still some controversy, however, surrounding both the child's ability to mourn and the effects of the loss on adult emotional well-being. The issue is discussed in chapter 14 under the heading "Symptomatology of Depression in Children of Various Ages." The normal process of mourning is dealt with in chapter 4.

PREVIOUS OR OTHER CURRENT STRESSES

Because the family is preoccupied with the illness, other stresses simultaneously affecting it may receive less attention. Financial stress, marital difficulties, problems in child rearing, and neurotic difficulties of the parents that might otherwise be tolerable can become exaggerated and less accessible to resolution when compounded by a coexisting fatal illness.

THE DYING PATIENT

Patients with a potentially lethal illness often report that they are treated psychologically as if they were already dead while still very much alive. If they are depressed, they may appear uncommunicative or may make what are considered "unreasonable" demands, leading staff or family already struggling with their own feelings of inadequacy and guilt to avoid them as much as possible. Often the family, unable to deal with their feelings about the impending death, enter into a conspiracy of silence with which the dying patient consciously or unconsciously colludes.

> A young man of nineteen was dying of Ewing's sarcoma, which had metastasized throughout his body. Everyone knew he knew his prognosis except his divorced mother, who looked closer to death than he. This young man had been the "acting father" in the family since his own father had left. He felt that part of his job was to care for his mother and protect her by pretending to her that he did not know his prognosis. The rest of the family colluded with this scheme. A group discussion with the family resulted in their agreeing that mother and son should share their feelings about the impending death, as had other family members. This allowed the boy to die knowing that his mother would survive in spite of his death, and the mother, freed to mourn the loss of her son, was freed to carry on with her own life.

CULTURAL ATTITUDES

In western societies, the anger that people sometimes feel toward a dying relative is not culturally acceptable. Therefore, grieving relatives tend to turn this anger, part of the normal response to the threat of losing those we love, against each other or onto those who care for the patient. This may make it considerably harder for those providing the patient's terminal care. It should, however, not be allowed to disrupt treatment. If the source and normality of this anger are understood, staff members may be able to respond to it less personally. This will leave them free to help the family channel this frustrated energy into more constructive outlets, such as volunteer work through cancer societies.

Death as a Crisis and Opportunity for Preventive Intervention

Death in a family meets the criterion for a crisis, which, "since it cannot be easily handled by the family's commonly used problem solving mechanisms, forces the employment of novel patterns" (Glasser and Glasser 1970, p. 50). These mechanisms must be within the range of the family's capacities but may be patterns that have never been used by the family in the past (see chapter 20).

Bereaved families never forget the loss of their child, but if the opportunity presented by the crisis is constructively used, the trauma of today can eventually lead to rebuilding the family structure and relationships in a healthier manner (Hollingsworth and Pasnau 1977; Shulman 1976). At the height of their grief, however, the bereaved or soon-to-be bereaved family may feel bitter, resentful, and let down, especially by those people (relatives, friends, hospital staff) or institutions (hospital or church) whom they trusted or relied on for support in the past. Temporarily they may feel that no one who has not experienced what they are going through can possibly understand their grief. In their alienation, they withdraw from those who are trying to help them and, by repeatedly turning down others' attempts to be empathic or supportive, may further their social and emotional isolation.

Even if health care professionals find their attempts to provide support rejected, this does not mean that these families should be abandoned. Just having cared enough to remain available by trying to maintain an ongoing relationship with the family even at a time when the family cannot accept help is often remembered later as a major source of comfort and support. Physicians should look for an appropriate opportunity to refer such families to a self-help group that may hold the only credentials that the family, at that stage in its grief, may be able to recognize, namely the experience of having lost or being in the process of losing a child from the same illness. Such groups often contain one or more couples who, having had time since the death of their own child, have proceeded further in the process of mourning their loss. As they have experienced loss themselves, they are more likely to recognize the recently bereaved family's alienating behavior for what it is, an unpleasant but necessary stage in the process of mourning. They are often able to help the surviving members of the family through the difficult transition from hospital back to community, as well as to provide an ongoing contact and source of support to which the family can turn when it feels ready (Caplan and Killilea 1976; Lieberman 1979; Pakes and Fleming, in press).

GROWTH OUT OF CRISIS

A couple had requested psychiatric assistance when their daughter was diagnosed as having a rapidly growing brain tumor. In their distress at her impending death, they were distracted and preoccupied by rage at their pediatrician who had initially dismissed her symptoms as inconsequential. They threatened a lawsuit but knew that this would not change their daughter's prognosis. A joint interview with the pediatrician and parents was held, during which the physician expressed his deep regret and convinced the parents he was not at fault. This allowed them to use his services later. At the same time, the reduction in their anger resulted in her having as "good" a death as possible.

Following the death, the parents continued in counseling as a couple, although the mother suffered a severe depression that required hospitalization. They also joined a bereaved family organization whose weekly group meetings sometimes included their teenage sons. Father became a board member and trained as a group leader for newly bereaved parents. While the family members still have upsetting moments, they are functioning very well in many areas of their life. Mother, a querulous woman compared to her very giving and uncomplaining child, gradually became more like her daughter, as if she herself were keeping alive her deceased child's character.

THE CARING STAFF AND THEIR RESPONSES

All staff members react to the impending death of terminally ill patients in their own way. Since most people in the healing professions get their greatest gratification from patients who get better, the treatment of dying patients frequently becomes a source of inadequacy, frustration, and guilt rather than satisfaction (Pakes et al. 1972). The unconscious feelings might be verbalized: "I've done all I can; yet, in spite of it, this child is still dying. How can I remain involved and allow myself to care when I'm left feeling so helpless, ineffective, and guilty?"

Even though consciously aware that there are illnesses science cannot yet cure, many physicians consider themselves failures whenever a patient fails to recover in spite of their best efforts. They fail to recognize the conflict between what they know they can achieve, consciously and rationally, and what they continue to demand of themselves unconsciously. These doubts can be intensified should the physician misinterpret and take as a lack of confidence a request of the dying child's family for a second opinion or a transfer of the case to a specialist for ongoing management.

All professionals, if they are to help the child with a fatal illness, must first come to terms with their own feelings about the child's impending death and the limitations of their own therapeutic effectiveness. Many physicians deal with feelings of helplessness and passivity by intellectualization and by flights into meaningless activity. While the younger or middle-age physician may intellectualize the denial of impending death, the older physician may wonder at how fiercely and, at times, how inappropriately the young resident struggles to keep an obviously dying patient alive. Repeated unnecessary examinations and a multitude of diagnostic procedures, some of them exhausting and painful, may be performed on the dying patient in an unrecognized attempt to reduce the insoluble, emotionally unbearable problem to the level of an intellectual exercise and create for the physician the feeling that he or she is doing something worthwhile and not just standing idly and helplessly by.

A terminally ill eight-year-old was admitted to the hospital with a lump in the neck. Great lengths of time were spent trying to decide the diagnosis, but it was only casually mentioned that the father was threatening to take the patient home. He did not want his child traumatized any more. Meanwhile suggestion after suggestion was made about what lab procedures should be performed on this patient who was figuratively halfway out of the door already.

Many physicians choose to share the responsibility of treating the terminally ill child with colleagues in nursing, social work, and other allied professions. Some routinely suggest that the family might wish to have a second opinion, not that they doubt their diagnosis or plan of management but because they recognize the family's need to assure themselves that everything possible has been done. The family's request for a consultation usually stems not from dissatisfaction with the attending physician but rather from the parents' need to be certain that they have done everything possible for the child.

HEALTH CARE PRACTICES

In recent years much attention has been given to the impact on the recipients of the way in which services are provided. In pediatrics particular attention has focused on practical and simple modifications that can substantially improve the remaining life experience of the dying child. Among these are: (1) avoid hospitalization if possible; (2) substitute outpatient treatment; (3) maintain continuity of caring staff on repeat visits and admissions; (4) accept the option of the child dying at home. Recent work has illustrated that application of these principles has led to an increase in both family and patient satisfaction and in the quality of care.

Hospices may prove to be the answer to the needs of families and patients. A hospice is an institution for the terminally ill that is "committed to *caring* rather than *curing*" (National Conference on Social Welfare 1978). Characteristically, its services are directed toward reduction of pain and control of symptoms—sociological, psychological, and spiritual, as well as physical. The patient and family are regarded as the unit of care. Preparation for bereavement and support for bereaved families after the patient's death are part of the service provided by an interdisciplinary team consisting in part of volunteers. Much attention is paid, as well, to the emotional well-being of the staff. Institutional hospice care, which began in 1974 as a home care program, is designed to be a backup and a continuation in the final stages of life to home care services (Lack and Buckingham 1978). The hospice movement has grown impressively in response to a demonstrable need (DuBois 1980); as of 1978 there were 170 hospices in various stages of development in the United States (Lack and Buckingham 1978).

The National Cancer Institute is the primary source of funds for hospice development, so hospice services are directed mostly toward adult cancer patients. There are currently no services for children. DuBois (1980) suggests this is due in part to a general resistance to dealing with the plight of dying children and in part to the fact that children, having no control over their treatment, are vulnerable to the psychological need of parents and physicians for aggressive, life-preserving therapies. The presence of children at hospices is encouraged through visiting and day-care policies (DuBois 1980), and special attention is paid to the needs of the bereaved child. The National Conference on Social Welfare (1978) urges the expansion of hospice care to include a broader range of terminally ill patients, without mentioning children specifically. David Adams's annotated bibliography (1979) is a good guide to other types of care (home care, child life programs) being developed for terminally ill and chronically ill children.

Stages of Emotional Reactions to Impending Death

PATIENT AND FAMILY

Kubler-Ross (1969, 1974) has described prototypical stages of emotional reaction through which individuals progress in their adjustment to impending death. Each person and family go through these stages in their own characteristic way, though not necessarily in the stated sequence. Overlap can occur. The hospital team can do much to facilitate movement from one stage to the next and to assist the process of mourning both before and after death.

An individual can get stuck at any stage, either because of stresses whose cumulative effect exceeds the limit of tolerance or because of a preexisting vulnerability. A return visit several months to a year following the death is a useful monitoring device, providing an opportunity to give the family needed support while allowing the physician to detect unresolved grief (i.e., an arrest of the mourning process) that may become a psychiatric problem.

As defined by Kubler-Ross, there are five stages in emotional reaction to impending death: shock and denial, anger and protest, bargaining, depression, and acceptance (or adaptation). The typical first reaction, either explicitly stated or merely subjectively experienced, is that it just can't be true. This blanket denial allows patient and family to collect themselves, providing time to mobilize other less extreme defenses against the distress aroused by the diagnosis. In the anger and protest stage, the typical reactions include the repeated and bitter demand, "Why me?" or "What have I done to deserve this?" This stage begins as denial, then gradually yields to anger or protest. There is increasing use of projection, as patient and family blame their affliction and other sources of discontent, real or imagined, on others in the environment, or on God. They react as if trying to fight off whoever and whatever is around, although doing so threatens to disrupt relationships with family, friends, medical personnel, and the community at large at a time when these are most necessary to sustain functioning and avoid increasing isolation and alienation. This is the stage during which parents are frequently critical of the care their child receives. If staff members take these attacks personally and respond with hostility or rejection, they merely increase the parents' suffering.

The reaction typical of the bargaining stage is contained in the statement "I'll make a deal with you." The angry, difficult child may remember that in the past if he was good he was rewarded. In a magical way, he may attempt to bargain with the medical staff, his parents, or even God to obtain relief from his disease. He may announce or merely decide within himself that if he is a good boy for a day, his mother will take him home from hospital, he will be spared further painful treatment, or he will get better. When the bargaining does not work, the child may react with intensified anger and protest or, alternatively, with despair. The family, like the child, may revert to bargaining, responding much as the child does to their inability to alter the progress of the disease.

> Robert, a twenty-one-year-old boy with muscular dystrophy, had recently lost his younger brother to the same disease. He was obtaining great satisfaction from collaborating with a friend, an occupational therapy student, in writing a monograph describing the psychological and social effects of the disease as seen by the patient. He worked enthusiastically, anxious to communicate with people who are not chronically ill in the hope of sharpening their sensitivity to the needs of the handicapped. He began to have trouble with his breathing, which he took as a sign that his struggle against the disease was nearing the end. One night he dreamed that he had died while the monograph was not yet complete. He woke up in a panic, afraid less of dying than of the fear that his death would occur before the project that he felt was giving his life meaning was completed. The next day he told his collaborator of the dream and the anxiety it had stirred up in him. She, understanding the concept of bargaining and realizing that she had been defending herself against his coming death in the same way, replied that she was dragging out her work on the monograph as though he would not be "allowed" to die until their task was complete.

In time, inevitably, child and family can no longer avoid recognizing that the bargaining has failed, and a profound depression takes over. There are two components to this depression: (1) the struggle to accept one's losses, including all that has been missed out on either prior to or because of the illness; and (2) the attempt to prepare for possible death in the future, including an anticipatory mourning for the life that might have been.

Acceptance, the final stage of preparation for death, is reached only when the other stages have been traversed. When the illness is a fatal one, this stage is the acceptance of the inevitable.

MEDICAL TEAM

Not only the child and family but members of the medical team go through the same stages to reach the point where they are emotionally ready to accept the inevitable loss (Vachon 1982; Vachon and Pakes 1982). Like patient and family, medical staff may get stuck at any stage. Should this occur, the typical result is indicated by increasing distress and, frequently, uncharacteristic and disruptive behavior by members of the medical team. The reactions of those involved at each stage can be summarized as follows:

Members of the medical team may feel overwhelmed by the diagnosis and its implications. In their shock, they may continue to dispute the diagnosis even when the evidence is unequivocal or may seek to shield themselves from the impact of the diagnosis by prolonged laboratory investigation that no longer has either practical meaning or relevance. Dreading sharing the diagnosis with the family and fearing their ability to handle the family's upset, they may put off dealing with the parents or, alternately, may overwhelm them with more facts than they can assimilate. Much of what parents perceive as insensitivity and lack of concern on the part of physicians results, in fact, from doctors' attempts to handle their own initial shock and dismay.

Physicians frequently rebound from this initial shock and respond with resentment and even rage to the families of their dying patients. This may be directed against the family of the patient whom, with or without reason, they see as difficult, demanding, or unappreciative. Alternately, the anger may be displaced by blaming the family practitioner, surgeon or other specialist, or nurses for their supposed mishandling of the case. Rage may be vented periodically through angry explosions in the operating room or on the ward. Resentment may be displaced onto the child, who is attacked for being uncooperative or acting "like a baby," or onto the parents, who are seen as overprotective and uncooperative. At times physicians trap anger within themselves, causing draining and unproductive self-pity. They feel overworked and overloaded with more difficult cases than they can be expected to manage at one time.

Doctors and nurses, like the family, may attempt to bargain for the life of their dying patient. They may pledge to be more conscientious in the future, to read journals regularly, even (in the case of nurses) to go on night duty if only a particular child of whom they are fond can recover to go home one more time before she dies.

Physicians frequently experience short-lived frustration and discouragement that can, at times, grow into unjustified feelings of inadequacy or self-blame. At such times physicians may become unduly critical of their own work, blaming themselves because, for a while, their statistics have been worse than those reported by other centers, completely ignoring the fact that for some months previously they were better. In susceptible individuals, this self-criticism may develop into full-blown episodes of clinical depression, which may greatly interfere with functioning not only as a doctor but as a husband, wife, or parent. This is reflected in the high incidence of marriage breakdown and emotional problems in physicians' families (Vincent 1971). Alternatively, various forms of escape from the threat of emerging depression, such as compulsive overwork or abuse of alcohol or drugs, may become prominent.

Finally, most physicians reach a stage in which they recognize that they have done all they could do to prolong the life and decrease the suffering of the child and family. They may be assisted in reaching this stage by the thought that through death the child has been spared further suffering or that from what has been learned from this case physicians may be more effective in treating similar problems in the future.

Stress and the Caregivers

There is now increased recognition of staff stress and its effect on the professionals' ability to care for patients and their families. Stress on caregivers may equal or even exceed that experienced by patients and families (Vachon and Pakes 1982). When this happens, caregivers can no longer care effectively and patient/family care deteriorates as staff become demoralized and depersonalized. Supportive intervention and stress management can reduce tensions and decrease staff "burnout" (Freudenberger and Richelson 1980).

One approach to this problem is to consider separately the various factors that, acting simultaneously, can have the cumulative effect of producing incapacitating staff stress. Doing so can help staff members conceptualize the various component stresses as distinct from each other, thus rendering them less overwhelming and more amenable to change. Components to be considered include:

1. Common or universal staff reactions to the process of dying, with or without specific stresses related to a particular illness.
2. Stresses and responsibilities arising from the staff member's specific occupational role.
3. The work environment in which the professional caregiver is functioning, including such variables as staff morale and the presence and effectiveness of mechanisms for identifying and coping with the inevitable work-related tensions.
4. Psychological vulnerability of the individual staff member, including:
    (a) Psychological (i.e., intrapsychic) vulnerability.
    (b) Interpersonal stressors from relationships outside of the work milieu.

The relationship existing between these factors is represented diagrammatically in figure 24.1. This figure is a further adaptation by Vachon, Pakes, and Steinhauer of the Dohrenwends' model (Dohrenwend and Dohrenwend 1970), which translated Selye's paradigm of reactions to stress (Selye 1956) into social and psychological terms.

According to this model, the amount of stress experienced by individual staff members depends on the duration and intensity of individual stressors as well as on factors in both the individual and the work situation that either aggravate or mitigate the amount of stress experienced. These may include the personal meaning of work with dying patients to each individual team member, both cognitively and emotionally, both consciously and unconsciously (Vachon 1982). Any or all of these factors may increase or decrease each team member's vulnerability to the stressors,

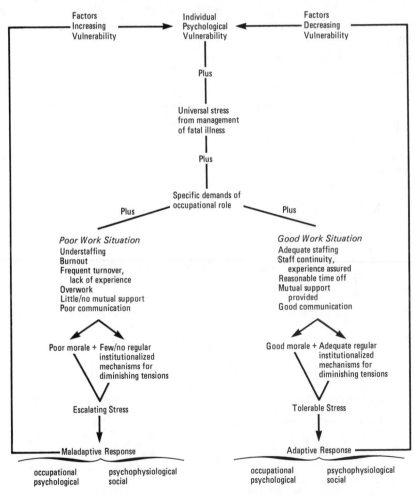

Figure 24.1 Cumulative Stress in Management of Fatal Illness

thereby predisposing him or her to either a maladaptive or an adaptive response. In an adaptive response, the net result on the individual is positive, so that the team member can tolerate the situation, continues to function well, and may even grow professionally and personally while a part of it. However, a maladaptive response will result if the cumulative effect of the various stressors exceeds the available sources of support, either psychological (i.e., internal) or social (i.e., from the work environment). In this case the individual team member's capacity for coping will be overwhelmed, his or her personal psychological vulnerability will be increased, and this will be reflected in the individual's occupational and/or personal functioning at psychological, psychophysiological, and social levels (Rabkin and Struening 1976). Hopefully, the model can be used to delineate which stresses can and which cannot be altered, thus allowing professionals to build into the system appropriate supports to facilitate coping with and adaptation to those sources of stress that cannot be avoided (Fulton 1979). It should be noted that the diagram does *not* include simultaneously occurring factors from each individual's personal life (e.g., presence or lack of financial security, marital and family relationships, presence or absence of hobbies and other interests, etc.), which may either aggravate or mitigate tensions generated in the course of work.

Fatal illness in a child is a powerful and chronic source of stress to the child, the child's family, and those providing care for the child and support for the family. Like all crisis situations, this can lead either to decompensation or to adaptation and psychological growth, depending on how the resulting cumulative stresses are managed. (See also chapter 20.)

SUGGESTIONS FOR FURTHER READING

ALBY, N., AND ALBY, J. M. 1973. The doctor and the dying child. In *The child in his family, vol. 2, The impact of disease and death,* ed. E. J. Anthony and C. Koupernik, pp. 145–157. New York: John Wiley & Sons.
    The authors concentrate on the relationships between physicians, nurses, parents and the fatally ill child, all of whom are prone to psychological stress.
BLUEBOND-LANGER, M. 1978. *The private worlds of dying children.* Princeton: Princeton University Press.
    Reports on research conducted over a nine-month period on in-hospital treatment of children with leukemia. All knew their prognosis long before death was imminent. The author discusses the five-stage process by which they acquired information about their disease, procedures, medication, and so forth, in spite of the "conspiracy of silence" that parents and doctors struggled to maintain.
BURTON, L., ed. 1974. *Care of the child facing death.* London: Routledge & Kegan Paul.
    A collection of articles on the management of terminally ill children of use to parents and all health professionals.
CAPLAN, G., AND KILLILEA, M., eds. 1976. *Support systems and mutual help multidisciplinary explorations.* New York: Grune & Stratton.

The Dying Child, the Family, and The Caregivers

As usual, Caplan is thorough, up-to-date on anything you want to know about mutual and self-help systems—at a professional level.

DOHRENWEND, B. S., AND DOHRENWEND, B. P. 1970. Class and race as status-related sources of stress. In *Social stress,* ed. S. Levine and N. A. Scotch, pp. 111–140. Chicago: Aldine.
The main use of this reference is to translate Selye's stress theories into psychosocial terms. These can usually be expanded to other stress related work situations, breaking factors into component parts to make them more manageable, that is, less stress prone.

DUFF, R. S. 1979. Guidelines for deciding care of critically ill or dying patients. *Pediatrics* 64(1):17–23.
Although medical technology is usually beneficial in the care of a sick person, it may also be intrusive, cruel, and of little value. The author proposes guidelines to aid in critically assessing its use, particularly in intensive care units.

FREUDENBERGER, H. J., AND RICHELSON, G. 1980. *Burnout: The high cost of high achievement.* Garden City, N.Y.: Doubleday & Co.
Freudenberger was one of the first to describe the burnout phenomenon—a classic study.

FULTON, R. 1979. Anticipatory grief, stress, and the surrogate griever. In *Cancer, stress and death,* ed. J. Tache, H. Selye, and S. B. Day, pp. 87–93. New York: Plenum Medical Book Co. Intertwines factors of grief, stress, surrogate grievers, cancer, and death. A useful short article.

GOGAN, J. L., et al. 1978. Treating the pediatric cancer patient: A review. *J. Pediat. Psychol.* 3(2):42–48.
Reviews the literature from 1944 to 1978 on psychosocial issues related to childhood cancer. Traces the general transition from a "protective" to an "open" approach in discussing the possibility of death with patients over four and the crucial role of family communication in facilitating the mourning process.

GOGGIN, E. L., et al. 1976. Psychological reactions of children with malignancies. *J. Am. Acad. Child Psychiat.* 15:314–325.
A study using projective techniques designed to determine how children with malignancies experience themselves and their world.

GROLLMAN, E. A., 1976. *Talking about death: A dialogue between parent and child.* Boston: Beacon Press.
A parents' guide for explaining death to children.

HOLLINGSWORTH, C. .E, AND PASNAU, R. O. 1977. The family in mourning: A guide for health professionals. pp. 63–69. In *Seminars in psychiatry,* ed. M. Greenblatt, pp. 63–69 New York: Grune & Stratton.
A consultation-liaison style approach to family mourning.

KHAN, A. U. 1979. Facing a dying child and his family. In *Psychiatric emergencies in pediatrics,* ed. A. U. Khan pp. 60–72. Chicago: Year Book Medical Publishers.
Pediatric approach to the dying child—more medically oriented.

KUBLER-ROSS, E. 1974. *Questions and answers on death and dying.* New York: Macmillan.
The classic discussion of the psychology of death and dying.

LANSKY, S. B. 1974. Childhood leukemia: The child psychiatrist as a member of the oncology team. *J. Am. Acad. Child Psychiat.* 13:499–508.
Preliminary report of an ongoing study of the leukemic child and the family. Discusses the psychological impact of prolonged anticipation of death on child and family, recommending that a child psychiatrist serve as part of the treatment team.

LIEBERMAN, M. A. 1979. Help seeking and self-help groups. In *Self-help groups for coping with crisis,* ed. M. A. Lieberman, et al., pp. 116–149. San Francisco: Jossey-Bass.
This help-oriented article "helps" to sort out the help-self-help cycle.

SAHLER, O. J. Z., ed. 1978. *The child and death.* St. Louis: C. V. Mosby.
Proceedings of a two-and-one-half-day symposium at the University of Rochester on the child and death. Deals with alternative environments, caregiver and family reactions, survivorship, and ethical and educational considerations.

VACHON, M.L.S., AND PAKES, E. H. 1981. Staff stress in the care of the critically ill and dying child. In *Childhood and death,* ed. H. Wass and C. Cours New York: Hemisphere Publishing Co.
This thorough, comprehensive chapter will be useful for any professional working in the field of death and dying. The introduction can be universally applied. The elaboration of the Selye, Dohrenwend, Vachon, Pakes stress model can be reapplied to the reader's own setting, and the reader's specific area of interest can be easily identified.

VERNICK, J. 1973. Meaningful communication with the fatally ill child. In *The child in his family,* vol. 2, *The impact of disease and death,* ed. E. J. Anthony and C. Koupernik, pp. 105–119. New York: John Wiley & Sons.
The author reports on how fatally ill children learn about their disease, medication, life expectancy, and so forth. Vivid examples show their varied responses to the threat of death, such as fear, anger, puzzlement, and even humor. A clear demonstration of how a sensitive therapist deals with dying directly and authentically.

25 *Simon Kreindler and Harvey Armstrong*

The Abused Child and the Family

Physical Abuse

The "battered child syndrome," first described in 1962 (Kempe et al. 1962), refers to a constellation of signs and symptoms seen in children who have suffered nonaccidental injury, nutritional deprivation, or physical or emotional neglect as a result of acts of commission or omission on the part of their parents or guardians.

Acts of physical or emotional abuse and/or neglect generally indicate more pervasive family pathology, particularly in the parent-child relationship but commonly also in the spousal relationship. In many cases the children's physical injuries are less noxious than the pathological home environment in which they occur. Consequently, any assessment or attempted treatment of an abused child must take this family perspective into account (Gelles 1973; Newberger 1973).

INCIDENCE

In spite of increased public and professional awareness of the problem and the recent introduction of mandatory reporting legislation in many jurisdictions, the incidence of child abuse still cannot be accurately assessed. Although the number of cases identified has increased dramatically in recent years, best estimates place the incidence at ten cases per thousand live births (Minde et al. 1975). Several extensive studies suggest that the actual incidence of abuse substantially exceeds officially re-

545

ported figures (Gelles 1979; Helfer and Kempe 1974; Robertshaw 1981; Smith 1975). Boys and girls are equally likely to be abused, although prior to age twelve boys outnumber girls in every age group, whereas girls significantly outnumber boys among teenagers (Gil 1973). Contrary to what is commonly believed, child abuse is not confined to very young children, although the most serious injuries and fatalities occur in the under-three age group (Gil 1973).

Child abuse occurs within all ethnic groups and socioeconomic levels of society. The large number of cases reported among ethnic minorities probably reflects discriminatory reporting attitudes (Newberger and Daniel 1976), as well as the higher incidence among these families of socioeconomic deprivation or familial dysfunction, both of which are strongly associated with child abuse (Gil 1973).

DIAGNOSIS

The research of Klaus and Kennell (1976) has demonstrated the important long-term effect of parent contact with the newborn child in the first few days of life and of parent-infant bonding. Premature babies or newborns with serious complications requiring prolonged hospitalization are particularly vulnerable to subsequent abuse and/or neglect because of the medically necessitated interruption in the parent-infant bonding process (Lynch and Roberts 1976; Minde et al. 1975; see also chapter 8). Failure of bonding of the parent to the baby is assumed to increase the risk of subsequent child neglect and, in some cases, abuse.

Recent research indicates that the detection of high-risk parents—that is, those likely to have difficulty with parenting, caring for, and nurturing their children—can be significantly improved by observing parent-infant interaction during the immediate postnatal period (Klaus and Kennell 1976). Significant here are observations of lack of maternal bonding as reflected in the mother not wanting to hold, feed, or name her baby. The absence of cuddling, rocking, eye contact, or talking to the baby are equally important. Other behaviors of concern include negative comments about the baby being ugly, mean, or bad, or rough handling of the baby with minimal interaction or warmth (Schmitt 1980).

Physical abuse, emotional neglect, nutritional deprivation, and sexual exploitation of children are all part of a larger spectrum of deviant parenting behavior that has multiple etiological roots. It is not uncommon to find more than one of these coexisting within the same family, and while at times just one child is mistreated, it is equally common to find one or more siblings who have also been abused and/or neglected.

The following findings are, by themselves, only signals to be alert to. The more of them are present in a given case, the more child abuse/neglect should be suspected (adapted from Kempe and Helfer 1972).

When the parent:

1. Presents a history that does not adequately explain the child's injury, which changes significantly from time to time or is otherwise contradictory.
2. Is hostile, evasive, and uncooperative in providing information.
3. Has delayed unduly bringing the child for medical examination or hospital care.
4. Seems detached and inappropriately unconcerned by the seriousness of the child's injury.
5. Seems primarily concerned with establishing his or her innocence of wrongdoing at a time when this is not even being questioned.
6. Refuses hospitalization of the child or further diagnostic studies.
7. Inappropriately leaves the child in the hospital, either during the emergency examination or immediately following admission.
8. Takes the child to different hospitals for injuries sustained on different occasions.
9. Takes the child to the hospital on numerous occasions for seemingly insignificant illnesses.
10. Does not visit the child in the hospital or visits only infrequently.
11. Does not relate well to the child during visits; does not hold, feed, change, touch, or play with the child.
12. Lacks the usual concern regarding the child's progress.
13. By the handling of the child evokes criticism from the hospital staff.
14. Is often difficult to locate by telephone and frequently moves the family to new locations.
15. Gives a history that indicates he or she has suffered serious emotional deprivation or physical abuse.
16. Has an unstable marital relationship.
17. Has few friends and no reliable sources of outside help to turn to when under stress.

When the child (adapted from Kempe and Helfer 1972):

1. Has an unexplained injury.
2. Shows overall evidence of poor care.
3. Shows evidence of dehydration and/or malnutrition without a demonstrable organic cause.
4. Rapidly gains weight in the hospital when given adequate nutrition.
5. Demonstrates developmental delays, particularly in the area of gross motor activity and speech and language development.
6. Has been given inappropriate food, drink, or drugs.
7. Appears unusually fearful or passive and withdrawn on initial medical examination.
8. Looks to others (hospital staff) for cues as to how to behave.
9. Does not look to parents for reassurance and may show little distress about being separated from them.
10. Seeks the attention of adults indiscriminately.
11. Responds with appeasing behavior; smiles at inappropriate times at anyone who approaches.
12. Is apprehensive when other children cry.
13. Seems hyperalert to the environment.
14. Shows injuries that are not mentioned in the history provided by the parents.
15. Shows evidence of previous injury and repeated recent injury.
16. Shows evidence of multiple and/or old fractures.
17. Shows a pseudomature ability to respond to parental expectations.

18. Is viewed as "different" or "bad" by parents, regardless of the reality.
19. Refuses to offer any explanation as to how the injury occurred (in the younger child), gives a contradictory history, or parrots the parental explanation of the injury.
20. Denies the existence of parental conflict or family problems when these are obviously present.
21. Denies previous abuse, even when this may have been well documented.

PSYCHODYNAMIC FACTORS

Parents who abuse their children may demonstrate almost any type of psychopathology (Helfer and Kempe 1968). Except for a small number who are clearly sociopathic or psychotic, the majority do not fall into any one diagnostic category. They do have many features in common. Parents who abuse children frequently show a pattern of behavior that can exist either separately or in combination with other psychological disorders (Lee 1976). Characteristic findings include the following.

Abusive parents have major deficits in their own self-esteem. Instead of being responsive to the needs of their children, they look to their children to gratify their needs and not frustrate them. When this (role reversal) occurs they feel more cared for and, therefore, more worthwhile. If ever the children fail to meet their excessive demands, or behave in a way that is annoying or frustrating, the parents' past feelings of inadequacy, worthlessness, and frustration are stirred up and may result in violent outbursts of uncontrolled rage (Vesterdal 1978).

Parents with these characteristics usually have a high potential for being abusive. Battering rarely occurs, however, without the simultaneous interaction of at least two other variables. The first of these is a characteristic of the child who is abused. Abused children are somehow special—for example, because of prematurity, a difficult temperament, a specific physical defect, or because the parents view them as psychologically different from other normal children (Solnit 1978; Vesterdal 1978).

Finally, there is often a crisis. This may be a major event such as abandonment by the spouse or partner, death of a parent, an unwanted pregnancy or loss of a job, or a seemingly more minor disappointment such as a hairstyle that did not come out just right or an imagined rejection when one parent feels that the other prefers one of the children to him or her.

Many abusive parents have a history of being raised in much the same way that they are raising their own children. Many of them never received the kind of parenting necessary to develop a sense of self-worth or a capacity to trust others (Vesterdal 1978). This deprivation, which results in their intense feeling of never having been cared for in those crucial early years, can and often does occur in spite of considerable maternal attention and material abundance.

The practical and the mechanical aspects of mothering—the feeding, holding, clothing, and cleaning of the infant—and the more subtle emotional ingredients of tenderness, responsiveness, and emotional interaction with the child must be distinguished. Failure in the more mechanical aspects of mothering seems to result in the neglected child or the infant with "failure to thrive." On the other hand, physical abuse is associated with a failure in the development of the empathic relationship between parent and child (Helfer and Kempe 1974; see discussion of reactive attachment disorder, chapter 8.)

TREATMENT

Once the diagnosis of physical abuse has been made, or when it is only possible to have a high degree of circumstantial evidence, a multifaceted treatment approach must be instituted. The abused child may require medical and/or surgical treatment for which hospitalization may be necessary. If hospitalization is not necessary, it must be decided whether the child can safely be returned home or whether a temporary alternative placement is indicated. At the same time, the child's development and psychological status should be assessed to decide whether any form of psychological intervention seems necessary. If the child has been hospitalized, a pediatrician may have already discussed with the parents the physical findings and any further investigations that are planned. Concurrent with the immediate pediatric and environmental management of the child, the parents (or parent) must be approached in a sympathetic, nonpunitive way. There is a great temptation to react to suspected or known abuse either by identifying with the child and responding with anger toward the parent or by identifying with the parent and denying the possibility that he or she could have abused the child. Neither approach is helpful. Physicians, nurses, or workers attempting to help abusing parents must remain empathic even in the face of their sometimes considerable anger and must, at the same time, be prepared to discuss the situation fully and directly. They must convey to the parents their real desire to understand the kinds of psychological, familial, social, and economic stresses with which they have, albeit unsuccessfully, been attempting to cope (Gelles 1973).

The immediate management of the parents usually involves the intervention of a caseworker from a social agency that has the legal authority to protect and, if necessary, provide alternate care for children neglected or abused in their own families. In addition to providing a supportive or therapeutic relationship for the abused child and the abusing parents, these agencies (children's aid societies or child welfare associations) can help to arrange for a number of environmental supports such as homemakers, day-care or nursery placement for the abused child and/or siblings, assistance with finding and/or paying for a babysitter, help in finding employment, assistance in arranging educational upgrading, and so forth. Later, referral to self-help groups such as Parents Anonymous should be considered. In some cases referral of one or both parents for marital counseling or individual psychotherapy may be indicated. In many jurisdictions mandatory reporting of suspected abuse is required.

In the vast majority of cases, a lengthy involvement by the child welfare worker is needed to bring about any change in abusing parents. The doctor may directly treat the parent or child, may be called on to act as a consultant to the worker responsible for the case, or, at other times, may make recommendations regarding the management of the abused child and/or the siblings. All physicians, nurses, and workers should be aware that many children raised in an abusive environment may demonstrate such marked developmental delays of one sort or another that they may be diagnosed retarded. If the source of the delay is recognized early enough, this sort of functional retardation can be reversed by placing the child in a loving foster home, therapeutic nursery, or preschool program, which can provide the previously lacking stimulation and/or remediation. The longer the condition goes unrecognized, the harder it is to reverse the problem. Even when the functional retardation has been diagnosed early, it may take several months before improvement is seen. For instance, it has been noted that over a three- to six-month period, a previously abused child with what appears to be below-normal intellectual potential will start to demonstrate increased attention span, imitativeness, and interest in problem solving; a more positive response to praise and more creative play; and a greater interest in the people and things around him or her (Martin 1976). Once these new behaviors start to appear, the child may show accelerated development. However, it may be six more months before demonstrated changes are reflected in test scores.

A major task in helping abused children's subsequent development is related to the superficial quality of their relationships with others. On the surface, these children often seem fairly normal. When observed over longer periods, however, it becomes clear that they relate only superficially to peers and have great difficulty forming relationships of genuine trust with someone special. Instead of reacting spontaneously, these children often rely on cues from others to determine their responses at a particular time. Only if they learn to take the risks involved in behaving naturally and spontaneously can they develop a healthy self-esteem and, as adults, a capacity for intimacy.

Once an adequate plan of management has been instituted, it may be necessary to reconsider the child's placement. In general, it is not safe to return the abused child home until there is strong evidence that the parents are obtaining enough satisfaction and pleasure in their adult lives that they no longer need to turn to the child to satisfy their emotional needs. The parents' capacities to help each other and to accept professional help in times of crisis are good indicators of the safety of the home. If the parents continue to have a distorted perception of the child and unrealistic expectations, return home is contraindicated. Parental pressure on the child welfare agency or court to return the child because of fears of public or family disapproval probably indicate that little has changed as far as the safety of the child is concerned.

The following guidelines (apapted from Kemp and Helfer 1972) can be used to assess the safety of the home when return of the child is being contemplated. Again, the more of these present, the stronger the likelihood that the child can be replaced safely. The home is more likely to be safe if:

1. The parents have demonstrated their willingness and ability to accept help in time of need or crisis.
2. The parents are developing some outside-the-home interests.
3. The parents are developing an improved self-image.
4. Help is available to the parents on an on-call basis twenty-four hours a day.
5. The spouse is able to recognize when his or her partner needs help and is willing to do something about it.
6. Obvious, previous crises such as housing, food, job, illnesses, and so forth, have been resolved.
7. Obstacles to getting help are minimal (for example, a telephone is available).
8. The parents no longer perceive the child as bad or different.
9. The parents' expectations of the child are more realistic.
10. The child is pleasing to the parents and is seen as an individual with needs of his or her own.
11. The parents are willing to accept help to meet any special needs (medical, social, psychological) of the child.
12. The parents have been conscientious in keeping follow-up appointments for the child and themselves (Kempe and Helfer 1972).

Finally, it must be remembered that the child under three is statistically at a much higher risk of being reinjured than the child over three.

After the child has been returned home, however, it is essential that treatment continue.

> When all has gone well, the parents have improved and the child returned home, there is often a tendency for parents or worker or both to consider that everything is now all right and treatment should be discontinued. This should never be done. The continuation of treatment is crucially important at this time. Not only is there a need to consolidate gains which have already been made, but it is necessary to follow through and see that the inevitable shifts in emotion and changes in living patterns caused by the return of the child can be managed without regression to previous unhealthy patterns. The purpose of treatment was not just to get the child back, but to improve the total living pattern of the family and significantly change the parent-child interactions. (Kempe and Helfer 1972, p. 20)

PROGNOSIS

The prognosis in cases of child abuse depends on many variables. Probably more than 50 percent of abused children have been abused prior to the incident that brought them to medical attention. In fact, it has been suggested that physical abuse of children is more often than not an indication of a prevailing pattern of caregiver-child interaction in a given home than an isolated incident (Helfer and Kempe 1974). It is also estimated that there is a 25 to 50 percent risk of permanent injury or death when an abused child is returned home without intervention (Schmitt and Kempe 1975). Where intervention occurs, the prognosis for the child depends not only on the accessibility of the parents to rehabilitation but also on the type and severity of the injury. Obviously the effects of severe head trauma, longstanding physical neglect, and emotional deprivation will be much more severe than those of a broken leg or bruised buttocks.

Abusive parents, unfortunately, are generally "poor patients" in the traditional sense. Those who actively resist all therapeutic involvement have the worst prognosis. These parents generally compose the least stable families, with frequently changing adult partnerships, abuse of drugs and alcohol, unemployment, and frequent moves from one community to another. The prognosis becomes increasingly guarded as the number of these adverse variables increases (Kreindler 1976) and is probably poorest where the situation is compounded by a parent who is either sociopathic or frankly psychotic. For parents who can tolerate a therapeutic involvement and can learn to call for help in time of crisis, the prognosis is much better, particularly if they develop a more realistic view and can accept the child as an individual with capabilities and needs of his or her own. If the parents can, in addition, develop a sense of themselves as more worthwhile, the prognosis is the most optimistic.

PREVENTION

Prevention measures to be undertaken to combat child abuse include the following:

1. Cultural and legal sanctions against the use of violence or physical force in child rearing or education.
2. The elimination of poverty, and the assurance of an equal opportunity to enjoy life for all members of society. This measure would involve adequate income, health care, social services, housing, educational, cultural, and recreational facilities for all members of the community without discrimination.
3. Comprehensive family-planning programs, including available abortions in order to reduce the number of unwanted and rejected children, who are the major victims of child abuse.
4. Family life education and counseling programs for adolescents and young adults preparing for marriage and parenthood.
5. The monitoring of parental (maternal) behavior in hospital obstetrical wards, both antenatally and in the early postnatal period, for indications of rejecting behavior or high risk for bonding failure associated with subsequent abuse and/or neglect (Gray et al. 1976).
6. High-quality, locally available social and medical child welfare and protection services, which can decrease the environmental and internal stress on family life.

7. Improved cooperation and communication between family physicians, hospitals (particularly emergency services and family practice units), children's aid societies or child welfare associations, police, courts, and community agencies.

Sexual Abuse

Sexual abuse of children raises even stronger reactions in those encountering it than does physical abuse. There are good reasons for this. Child sexual abuse is accorded one of the strongest taboos in most societies (Freud 1946; Lindzey 1967; Malinowski 1953; White 1948). The very idea of adults having sexual feelings toward children, though exploited in advertising and promoted by kiddie-porn groups, is usually denied with repugnance by most people in most societies. These powerfully internalized taboos generate considerable anxiety when sexual abuse is encountered in the real world. The resulting condemnation and legal sanctions against sexual abuse of children are so punitive that this is often one of the least exposed and understood forms of sexual behavior.*

DEFINITION AND CLASSIFICATION

Sexual abuse of children encompasses a wide range of behaviors in the child and in the responsible adults. A useful classification divides sexual abuse into three categories: sexual abuse, sexual misuse, and incest.

In *sexual abuse,* an older person forces sexual activity on a minor in any context. *Sexual misuse* involves the exposure of a child to sexual stimulation inappropriate for the child's age, level of psychosexual development, and role in the family. *Incest* is defined as the occurrence of sexual intercourse between two persons whose marriage, if they were adults, would be prohibited by law. Each category includes many possible behaviors, and all three can occur in a single situation, as when a child is physically or psychologically forced to submit to incest following that child's involvement in some form(s) of sexual misuse.

INCIDENCE

Forcible or sadistic sexual assault on children by strangers is the rarest but perhaps best-known form of child sexual abuse. The details of the crime and the hunt for the abuser are often sensationalized by the media, and this evokes emotional responses and attitudes that color how other

*See Groth 1978; Kinsey, Pomeroy, and Martin 1948; Kinsey et al. 1953; Landis 1956; and Mohr, Turner, and Jerry 1964.

forms of sexual involvement with children are viewed. Most often, in 50 to 80 percent of cases, the abuser is someone known to the family—often a relative, neighbor, family member—or to the child, as a group leader or teacher (DeFrancis 1971; Ellerstein and Canavan 1980; Groth 1978; Scherzer and Padma 1980). Most frequently, the abuser is an older sibling or a parental figure, with abuse occurring more frequently in foster, step-, and adoptive families (Kubo 1959).

Estimates of the frequency of sexual abuse have increased over the years. It is not known whether this reflects true increase in frequency or higher visibility and reporting. Most of those working in the field suspect it represents the latter, since many adult patients in the past have reported childhood sexual experiences that were dismissed as fantasy without any serious investigation or attempt at confirmation (Freud 1962; Nasjleti 1980; Raphling, Carpenter, and Davis 1967; Rush 1980).

More recently, surveys of such high-risk groups as prostitutes and female drug abusers have given histories of childhood sexual abuse in up to 48 percent of cases (Lukianowicz 1972; Malmquist, Kiresuk, and Spano 1966), while as many as 30 percent of large surveys of college students (Landis 1956) recalled sexual abuse in its broadest context at some point during childhood or adolescence (Howard 1957; Malmquist, Kiresuk, and Spano 1966). In most studies the frequency of reported abuse was ten times higher in girls than boys (DeFrancis 1971; Ellerstein and Canavan 1980). A lower percentage of the boys recalled that legal or therapeutic action was taken by a responsible adult at the time of abuse. Young children reported the abuse to adults less frequently than did adolescents.

Children of either sex and any age may be abused, though pubescent or early-adolescent girls are more frequently involved (Berry 1975; Browning and Boatman 1977; Ellerstein and Canavan 1980). The child victim may have no active role in the abuse, although children who lack nurturing, support, and closeness with adults either inside or outside the home may play a role either passively or actively in encouraging or prolonging the contact (Halleck 1962; Henderson 1972; Maisch 1972).

Despite previous belief, sexual abuse is not limited to lower socioeconomic classes (Giaretto 1976; Giaretto, Giaretto, and Sgroi 1978; Weinberg 1955). Recent estimates in communities with specially designed programs to deal with sexual abuse report it occurring in one in ten to one in one hundred middle-class families (Giaretto 1981). Other reports from Ontario indicate that 35 percent of all reported abuse cases are sexual in nature (Ontario Child Abuse Register 1981).

Reasons for inaccurate and underreporting include the shame and guilt of the participants or the reluctance of parents, child, and professionals to face the anxiety related to what society considers scandalous behavior. These, combined with a low index of suspicion and the threat of legal sanctions, contribute to the obscuring and hiding of sexual abuse (Rush 1980).

Criminal prosecution can result in a jail or penitentiary term, either of which may involve the physical assault or killing of the abuser by other inmates. Following incarceration, the family is temporarily or even permanently left without a breadwinner and may disintegrate under the resultant strain. Thus the family as a whole is victimized, and the sexually abused child may be made a scapegoat who is blamed for all the family's misfortunes.

FAMILY STRUCTURE AND DYNAMICS

There is little evidence that a single sexual assault of a child by a stranger is related to family pathology, but children who develop prolonged sexual relationships with adults outside their own families do so as a result of feeling unsupported, alienated, and deprived within their families (Gebhard et al. 1965; Geiser 1979; Guthiel and Avery 1977). Children's need for nurture, dependency, and support makes those who are deprived more vulnerable to the nurturing and the blandishments offered in exchange for sexual favors by the person who is simultaneously abusing them (Peters 1976; Stechler 1980; Tilelli, Turek, and Jaffe 1980).

Alcoholism, drugs, brain damage, mental retardation, and severe character pathology may play a role in triggering assaults on children by adults unfamiliar to them (Gebhard et al. 1965; Groth 1978). Feelings of sexual inadequacy and a sexual preference for children often characterize those who use a position of authority and trust to seduce children and to maintain the relationship until it is exposed or until the child has reached puberty. The sexual gratification and release obtained is extremely reinforcing, so that pedophilia often becomes the favored mode of sexual release (Mohr, Turner, and Jerry 1964). Sexual abuse involving strangers is less common, however, and there are significant differences between it and sexual abuse occurring within the child's family, as incestuous fathers and brothers are not pedophilic (Fox 1962; Fox 1980; Mohr, Turner, and Jerry 1964; Santiago 1973).

Father-son, mother-son incest is seldom reported in the literature, and those few reports usually involve psychotic mothers and absent or very uninvolved fathers. Much more is known about father-daughter incest. (Dixon et al. 1978).

Many studies have demonstrated that incest is a family affair rather than just the expression of one family member's psychopathology (Giaretto 1976; Kaufman, Peck, and Taquiri 1954; Maisch 1972; Peters 1976). Among the features typical of the incestuous family are the following: a history of incest in previous generations, (Meiselman 1979; Raphling, Carpenter, and Davis 1967; Weinberg 1955); a mother who was rejected by her own mother and who has identified with her own mother's rejecting attitudes by rejecting her daughter. Thus the mother acts out her rage at her own mother by displacing this onto her daughter, whom she then deprives and rejects. At the same time the mother rejects her sexual role as wife and demands instead to be mothered by her daughter, thus disrupting intergenerational boundaries within the family (Berry 1975; Guthiel and Avery 1977; Henderson 1972).

The fathers in incestuous families are often authoritarian but immature and may have psychopathic qualities that allow them to rationalize their own behavior and accept deviant sexual norms. They are usually fearful of adequate females, and for this reason establish a relationship with a wife whose feelings of inadequacy allow them to continue in a dominant role, thus avoiding the threat of their own unrecognized but powerful need to be dependent (Cavallin 1966; Gebhard et al. 1965; Meiselman 1979). Their sexual relationships with their wives, while at first adequate, deteriorate over time as both husband's and wife's sexual involvement with each other declines. The husband's sexual interest is at some point displaced from the wife onto one of the children, often the oldest daughter, although the carnal nature of his involvement with her often develops gradually and may at first be denied or rationalized away. Eventually, however, the frankly sexual nature of the enmeshment can no longer be denied and the child, already deprived by her mother, forced into a woman's sexual role for which she is in no way prepared but trapped within the family by her age, her lack of confidence, and the gap contributed by the family's isolation from others, turns to the father for gratification of her dependency needs. Through his reinforcement she soon finds that her feminine behavior and sexual cooperation allow her effective leverage to have her father meet her needs. This encourages her to rely more and more on her special position to obtain favored status and concessions. Over time, as the relationship becomes more intimate, the wish to totally displace the ungratifying mother is facilitated by the father's sexual interest in the daughter and reinforced by her own need for validation, nuturance, support, and emotional warmth. Once the overtly sexual nature of the relationship is established, the daughter experiences shame and guilt. She hides the relationship from others for fear of losing the gratification and emotional support that it provides, mindful of the consequences for both herself and her father if it is revealed. The mother is often a witness to many subtle clues as to the incestuous nature of the father-daughter relationship but, like others who can also see them, she refuses to believe them or take them seriously. This may be because she does not see the situation as serious due to her own deviant sexual upbringing or because of her fear that exposing and dealing with the issue will destroy the family (Bagley 1969; Guthiel and Avery 1977; Howard 1957; Weiner 1962).

Other children in the family are often aware of the ongoing situation. If they are girls, they are often being groomed to take their turn at serving in a sexual role (Meiselman 1979). They often collude by covering up the ongoing incestuous relationship or may be simultaneously involved. Boys are often bribed to keep the secret and may themselves take part in incestuous behavior with their sisters (Raphling, Carpenter, and Davis 1967).

The Abused Child and the Family

The passage of thousands of children through the offices of skilled professionals without detection of reported sexual abuse indicates the difficulty in diagnosis. In intrafamilial sexual abuse, child and parents conspire with each other to protect the family secret (Kaufman, Peck, and Taguiri 1954). When sexual abuse occurs from outside the family, fear of the trauma of repeated questioning or of the humiliation involved in a court appearance often deters parents from taking actions that are likely to cause stress and publicity for themselves and the child.

Presenting symptoms are variable. Occasionally the child may speak frankly about the nature of the sexual abuse to a parent or other trusted adult, only to feel betrayed when this attempt to break out of the situation is negated by the lack of an appropriate response. Other presenting signs and symptoms can be classified into medical, emotional, behavioral, and educational symptoms in the child. There are also some suggestive familial presentations.

Medical symptoms, which should be regarded as likely evidence of sexual abuse until proven otherwise, include: evidence of trauma to any part of the child's body (Ontario Child Abuse Register 1981); trauma to the genitals or anus (Braut and Tisza 1977); infections of the vagina, rectum, or urethra (Brant and Tisza 1977); pregnancy in a young adolescent (Cormier, Kennedy, and Sangowicz 1962); and presence of any venereal infection (Brant and Tisza 1977).

Sexual abuse should be considered among the possible causes for one or more of the following signs and symptoms appearing at school (note, however, that these in no way constitute proof that abuse is occurring): academic failure (Cowie, Cowie, and Slater 1968; Kubo 1959; Felice 1978); school refusal and frequent absences (Browning and Boatman 1977); poor peer relations (Bagley 1969); seductive or fearful behavior with male teachers (Cormier, Kennedy, and Sangowicz 1962); refusal to undress for physical education classes or showers; refusal to stand in front of the class for oral presentations; and removal from extracurricular activities.

Emotional presentations that again may suggest inquiring about possible sexual abuse especially when combined with some of the medical, behavioral, or familial presentations described include: psychosomatic symptoms (Meiselman 1979; Molnar and Cameron 1975); shyness, anxiety, depression, suicide (Felice 1978; Kaufman, Peck, and Taquiri 1954); extreme pseudomaturity (Browning and Boatman 1977; Lustig et al. 1966); hysterical seizures (Goodwin, Simms, and Bergman 1979); amnestic states; genital anesthesia; frequent bathing and handwashing; absence of peer relationships (Browning and Boatman 1977; Meiselman 1979); fantasies of pregnancy; and frank psychotic behavior (Peters 1976).

Behavioral problems that may be associated include: running away from home (Browning and Boatman 1977; Halleck 1962; Maisch 1972); delinquency of any kind (Cowie, Cowie, and Slater 1968; Meiselman 1979); promiscuity (Sloane and Karpinski 1942; Malmquist, Kiresuk, and Spano 1966); and the involved child having excess amounts of money.

The following family constellations are frequent in families in which sexual abuse is occurring: psychopathy, alcoholism, and drug abuse in parents (Cavallin 1966; Lukianowicz 1972; Meiselman 1979); a divesting of maternal responsibility onto the child (Browning and Boatman 1977; Kaufman, Peck, and Taguiri 1954); extreme closeness, overprotection, and indulgence of the child by the father (Browning and Boatman 1977; Cormier, Kennedy and Sangowicz 1962); jealousy and the cutting off of peer contacts and dating by the father (Bender and Blau 1937; Lukianowicz 1972); and serious disorganizing mental illness in the mother (Browning and Boatman 1977).

The more of the preceding signs are present, the more carefully the possibility of recurrent sexual abuse should be considered. Often, however, even when many of these signs are present, the anxiety and inhibitions of the human service professional prevent the direct consideration of possible sexual abuse. As a result, sensitive interviewing of the child about sexual activity with adults is avoided. The question "Have you ever had any sexual activity with a member of your own family or with another adult?" is perhaps the easiest and most direct way of breaking through the anxieties of both the professional and the child in order to invite an open discussion of the topic.

MANAGEMENT

When the child or adolescent gives a history of sexual abuse, the professional should remain calm and nonjudgmental. So great is the child's and family's anxiety and guilt that any reinforcement of it will be detrimental to future management. After getting a detailed and complete history of the child's involvement, the professional should meet with the parents to discuss the situation. In many jurisdictions there is a legal requirement that child welfare authorities be notified in all cases of suspected sexual abuse, as they play an important role in the continued management of such cases. Child welfare authorities are also often the only agency able to provide the necessary extended supervision, the legal advice, the out-of-home child protection, and the continued follow-up of the case over a long period of time. They may also supply preventive services for the other children in the family.

Management of sexual abuse requires considerable time, effort, resources, and skill. At first, family members may deny the child's accusations and refuse to deal with the issue. At this point it is necessary to inform the family that child welfare authorities will have to be notified. After their notification, a temporary decision as to whether the child and/or the abusing parent should remain home or be placed elsewhere must be made. Some determination must be made of whether returning the child home is likely to expose him or her to further pressure to retract what was said or to a risk of further abuse. The option of placement away from home should be discussed with the child at the time of diagnosis.

The child's wishes in this regard should be given respect, along with other relevant factors such as the willingness of the parents to acknowledge and deal with the problem, the parental psychopathology, the family structure, and the nature of the abuse. Any accusations by the child should be taken seriously and not prejudged. Many such accusations are true, although in rare cases the charge may result from a child's fantasy or lying in an attempt to punish the family. The investigating professional must be open to both possibilities and decide on appropriate management following an adequate investigation, not on the basis of personal discomfort or a refusal to consider seriously either major alternative. The next step is to evaluate the parental pathology and the family's strengths and weaknesses with as much care, sympathy, and humanity as possible. At times a more sensible and just interim action is the removal of the abusing adult from the home.

If the father or other offender is severely inadequate or psychopathic, he may deny the child's accusations and refuse to participate in any proposed intervention. This results either from guilt, shame, or from the realistic fear that admitting what has occurred may open the way to legal charges if information gathered in the assessment or therapy is used as evidence against him in a court of law. Should the offender refuse to participate in any exploratory or therapeutic involvement, it may be necessary for the child welfare agency to bring the issue before the court. Sometimes cooperation of the police, the prosecuting attorney, and the court can be sought to make participation in assessment and treatment a condition of probation or a suspended sentence. Should the abuser be a member of the child's family, the professional would need to determine whether and under what circumstances it would be in the child's best interests for the family to continue to live together as before. If this is contraindicated, he or she would then have to determine whether the child or the abusing adult should be the one to live apart from the rest of the family (DeFrancis 1971; Scherzer and Padma 1980; Stechler 1980; Tilelli, Turek, and Jaffe 1980).

If the abuser has a long history of pedophilic offenses and is someone unrelated to the family, the professional must consider which of the possible interventions to recommend. Occasionally prolonged penal separation from society with long-term treatment may seem the only reasonable alternative, and even this can fail.

MEDICAL INTERVENTION

A thorough history and physical examination of the child should be conducted with the consent of either parents or child welfare agents. If there has been recent sexual abuse, examination of the body for evidence of physical abuse is essential. Taking of clothing, fingernail scrapings, loose pubic hair, vaginal swabs for sperm and sperm mobility, examination for phosphatase and ABO blood typing, and cultures for veneral disease should be obtained from any area involved in the sexual act (Herjanic and Wilbois 1978; Rosenfeld 1979; Tilelli, Turek, and Jaffe 1980). Sgroi (1978) describes in detail the procedure to be followed during such an examination.

Thorough recording and note taking is essential, as the examining physician may be called to give evidence in court (Giaretto 1976; Giaretto, Giaretto, and Sgroi 1978; Sgroi 1978; Stechler 1980).

TREATMENT

The cardinal rule in treatment is to be as nonthreatening as possible, to both child and family. Otherwise the intervention may be more damaging than the experience itself, particularly if the child ends up in care, the father in prison, and the family on welfare (Giareto, Giareto, and Sgroi 1978; Meiselman 1979).

To gain the cooperation of child and family in investigating the situation, the professional must begin with a thorough history and evaluation of various family members and of the marital relationship. Children must have a chance to talk about what has occurred and to deal with any guilt and sense of personal responsibility that they may feel. They need the opportunity to explore and try to improve the relationship with the mother, who is often ambivalent if not hostile, and to develop adequate peer relationships and plans for the future.

The mother must have an opportunity to face and deal with her feelings about her child having had a sexual relationship with another adult, often her own husband. She must also deal with her sense of failure as a person, a mother, and a wife. Mothers often feel rage about having been displaced by one of their own children and guilt for having colluded to allow the situation to continue as long as it did (Giaretto 1976; Topper 1979). Denial of sexual abuse rather than any active role in it is the cause of her failure to act.

The father needs an opportunity to express his feelings about the situation. Intense guilt and shame may be evident immediately or may be a major factor contributing to ongoing defensiveness. The father should be helped to acknowledge his own responsibility for what has happened and, if possible, to transmit his acceptance of responsibility to the child involved. Other children in the family should be informed about what has been going on in the family at a level that they can understand and cope with emotionally. They should be helped to express what life has been like for them in the family, including their reactions to the turmoil precipitated by the situation having being discovered and investigated; their frequent fears or experience with sexual abuse; their guilt for knowingly, through their silence, having colluded with the ongoing abuse of a sibling; their shame about what has occurred; or their fears for the future of any individual family member or the family as a whole. They should be encouraged to express and work through ambivalent feelings (pity and guilt) along with resentment and rivalry with the maternally rejected but paternally indulged child (Berry 1975; Giaretto 1976; Giaretto, Giaretto, and Sgroi 1978).

Techniques for achieving these ends vary. Some experienced therapists prefer meeting with the family as a group in order to identify and improve aspects of family functioning, without seeing individual family members separately (Groth 1979). Others recommend seeing each major participant in individual psychotherapy, supplementing this with family and marital therapy as indicated (Anderson and Shafer 1979). Finally, group therapeutic approaches have been developed for sexually abusive fathers as well as for the mothers, fathers, and children involved (Lubell and Soong 1982; Tsai and Wagner 1978). These may be less available in smaller communities or where the incidence and/or detection rate are less.

PREVENTION

Prevention must involve the provision of support systems for children in dysfunctional families; reducing the catastrophic consequences for both the sexually abused child and the family in criminal courts; the creation of therapeutic support systems for families one or more of whose members have been sexually abused; and increased cooperation between medical, child welfare, legal, and enforcement agencies so that sexual abuse is dealt with more constructively (Giaretto 1976; Meiselman 1979; Scherzer and Padma 1980).

Early education and instruction about how children should respond if exposed to inappropriate sexual behavior should be encouraged in families through parent education programs and should be taught in the schools (Geiser 1979).

All professionals who work in primary contact with children should receive training in the prevention of and dealing with, at least on a "first-aid" basis, real or suspected child sexual abuse (Geiser 1979; Scherzer and Padma 1980).

OUTCOME

The results of sexual abuse of females depend on many factors. Brief sexual encounters between prepubertal brothers and sisters are least, if at all, damaging and require the least intervention (Cowie, Cowie, and Slater 1968; Fox 1962; Santiago 1973). If the abuse is violent and sadistic, the impact on the child may be extreme, causing depression, shame and guilt, social withdrawal, multiple fears, and constriction of life. Brief sexual contact between a caring adult and a very deprived child may have little negative impact and may even have some positive effect on the child's life (Landis 1956; Meiselman 1979; Peters 1976). Prolonged incestuous contact within the family, however, even if it is partially caring in nature, is accompanied by a warping and distortion of the child's developmental experiences. It creates distorted attitudes and feelings about heterosexual relationships; it often compounds maternal deprivation (Kaufman, Peck, and Taguiri 1954) and results in conduct disorders, depression, shame and guilt, anxiety, and a more difficult family life for the victim and her children in the next generation. In some cases the shame, guilt, rage, and sense of betrayal that remain as a family secret even years after the cessation of actual sexual molestation can, if not resolved, be more damaging in the long run than the abuse itself (Nasjleti 1980; Rush 1980; Sloane and Karpinski 1942).

So far, controlled follow-up studies have been done only for girls who have been victims of incest (Felice 1978; Meiselman 1979; Molnar and Cameron 1975; Nasjleti 1980). They show that most girls involved in incestuous relationships develop sexual and conduct disorders, though a direct causal link cannot be demonstrated. A few have neurotic symptoms, while a very small minority do not see the experience as having been damaging. Many of these victims had not experienced any familial intervention, so that in their cases it was not the intervention itself that produced the difficulties. Their problems were more likely the result of the abnormal family structure and the distorted developmental experiences that both caused and resulted from the ongoing sexual abuse. Controlled follow-up studies of children exposed to other types of abuse are much needed.

SUGGESTIONS FOR FURTHER READING

ANDERSON, L. M., AND SHAFER, G. 1979. The character-disordered family: A community treatment model for family sexual abuse. *Am. J. Orthopsychiat.* 49:436–445.

A collaborative approach to treatment that views the sexually abusive family as analogous to the "character-disordered" individual. This model assumes that effective intervention requires authoritative control and coordination of all professional activity.

BURGESS, A. W., et al. 1978. *Sexual assault of children and adolescents.* Toronto: Lexington Books.
A handbook to guide workers involved with the offenders or victims of sexual assault. The major themes are the individual's stress and trauma, community program planning, and interagency cooperation.

EEKELAAR, J. M., AND KATZ, S. N., eds. 1978. *Family violence: An international and interdisciplinary study.* Toronto: Butterworth Publishers.
Proceedings of an international conference covering the broad spectrum of family violence with a heavy emphasis on child abuse. The response of the social and legal systems in different countries is highlighted.

ELLERSTEIN, N. S., ed. 1981. *Child abuse and neglect: A medical reference.* New York: John Wiley & Sons.
A very comprehensive, well-illustrated book containing detailed information on medical issues that confront clinicians dealing with abused and neglected children.

GARBARINO, A., AND STOCKING, S. H. 1981. *Protecting children from abuse and neglect: Developing and maintaining effective support systems for families.* San Francisco: Jossey-Bass.
Child abuse is a problem not only of individuals but also of environments. This book is the first coordinated, interdisciplinary study of the ecology of child abuse and neglect—a discussion revealing new, cost-effective strategies that promise significant improvements in the prevention and treatment of this serious social problem.

GELLES, R. J. 1979. Violence against children in the United States. In *Critical perspectives on child abuse,* ed. R. Bourne, and E. H. Newberger, pp. 53–67. Lexington, Mass: Lexington Books.
A report on the incidence, modes, and patterns of parent-to-child abuse in the United States, dealing both with reported abuse and with the wide range of aggressive acts between spanking and grievous assault, an area hitherto largely unresearched.

HELFER, R. E., AND KEMPE, C. H. 1973. *The battered child.* Chicago: University of Chicago Press.
This study sets forth the essential medical, social, and legal framework through which the problem of child abuse must be faced.

KEMPE, C. H., ed. 1977. *The Int. J. Child Ab. & Neg.* New York: Pergamon Press Ltd. (Published quarterly since 1977.)
Contains reprints of most of the papers presented at the annual International Congress on Child Abuse and Neglect. Probably the best source of up-to-date data (epidemiology, clinical intervention, legal issues, etc.) on the subject.

KEMPE, R. S., AND KEMPE, C. H. 1978. *Child abuse.* Cambridge, Mass: Harvard University Press.
These pioneer investigators report the results of their innovative work with parents and children. They discuss the varieties of abuse, the complex social and familial conditions for abuse, and short- and long-term treatment. Of great interest is their reported success in identifying high-risk parents before abuses occur.

KROTH, J. A. 1979. Family therapy impact on intrafamilial child sexual abuse. *Child abuse and neglect* 3(1):297–302.
A family therapy treatment program evaluated using a cross-sectional longitudinal design. The generally positive outcomes related to psychosomatic symptomatology, emotional disturbance, and social isolation in the victims and to aberrant behavior and marital relationships among the parents are discussed.

LUBELL, D., AND SOONG, W.-T. 1982. Group therapy with sexually abused adolescents. *Can. J. Psychiat.* 27(4):311–315.
The authors' therapy group for young adolescent girls focused on improving self-image and developing social skills. The girls' group experiences, as well as the major themes and organizational issues in running a group of this type, are discussed.

MEISELMAN, K. C., 1979. *Incest.* San Francisco: Jossey-Bass.
A discussion of adult and adolescent adjustment difficulties of childhood incest victims. The author integrates studies of the last fifty years with her own new research on psychotherapy patients reporting incestuous experiences. Guidelines and recommendations for the evaluation and treatment of incest cases are included.

TSAI, M., AND WAGNER, N. N. 1978. Therapy groups for women sexually molested as children. *Arch. Sexual Behavior* 7:417–527.

Therapy groups were established for the alleviation of sexual guilt and shame and for the clarification of emotional and behavioral consequences of molestation. Clinical findings and the nature of the curative effect of group therapy are discussed.

WEITZEL, W.; POWELL, B.; AND PENICK, E. 1978. Clinical management of father-daughter incest. *Am. J. Dis. Child.* 132:127–130.

The characteristics of the daughter are discussed—her position in the family, her experience of guilt or shame, and her reasons for reporting the incest to an outsider.

26 Quentin Rae-Grant and George Awad

The Effects of Marital Breakdown

Separation and Divorce

In a century characterized by major political, social, and economic changes, none is more striking or widespread than those involving the concept of marriage. These changes have had a major impact not only on the adults who dissolve a marriage but also on the increasing number of children who are inevitably affected by separation, divorce, and, frequently, remarriage procedures. The divorce rate has been climbing steadily in most Western countries, but despite the many lamentations, exhortations, and dissertations on the topic, there has been little scientific study of the causes and the impact of the sociological, epidemiological, and psychiatric factors related to this major revision of the social structure.

HISTORICAL PERSPECTIVE

It is difficult to study separations in an epidemiological way since the term *separation* is used in so many different ways, and there is no uniform mode of standardized recording of data specifically about marital separations. Marriage, divorce, and remarriage rates are recorded, however, and those for women provide the best data and serve as reliable markers to review trends. The divorce rate has been rising steadily throughout this century, peaking immediately following World War II when alliances made under wartime conditions were dissolved as their civilian inappropriateness became obvious. Since then, however, and particularly since the middle 1960s, the divorce rate has risen steadily while the first-marriage rate has dropped. This has led to a situation in California where there are as many divorces in a year as there are first marriages. Until recently most of those who divorced tended to remarry, although the older people are at the time of divorce, the less likely this is. The remarriage rate has begun to drop, and the concept of serial, state-sanctioned monogamy no longer represents the social norm.

LIKELIHOOD OF DIVORCE

Although divorce rates have increased throughout the population, divorce seems disproportionately high in those who marry before the age of twenty, those of lower educational status, those who are socioeconomically disadvantaged, and members of minority groups (U.S. Bureau of the Census 1972). The most significant change is in the increased number of children affected by divorce. In 1975 there was an average of 1.08 children per divorce decree in the United States (National Center for Health Statistics 1977), from a high in 1964 of 1.36. Nevertheless the absolute number of children affected by divorce has increased, as the decline in family size has been outweighed by the increased frequency of divorce.

According to Canadian statistics, the ratio of divorce to marriage in 1974 was one to four, while in 1979 it was approximately one to three. In 1977, 1,123,000 Canadian children experienced parental divorce (Statistics Canada 1979).

REASONS FOR DIVORCE

Reasons for divorce can be conceptualized under the headings of attractions, barriers, and alternatives.

Attractions

Prior to the twentieth century, divorce was an expensive, prolonged process. It was, therefore, a formal mechanism for marriage dissolution available only to the wealthy. This changed early in the twentieth century

TABLE 26.1

U.S. Statistics

	First-Marriage Rate (per 1,000 single women) 14–44 years	Divorce Rate (per 1,000 married women) 14–44 years	Remarriage (per 1,000 widowed and divorced women) 14–54 years
1921–23	99	10	98
1936–38	98	13	83
1945–47	145	24	163
1954–56	120	15	129
1966–68	107	20	166
1975–77	85	37	134

Adapted from P.C. Glick and A.J. Norton, *Population Bulletin*, 325, 1977. U.S. Census Bureau.

so that currently, within middle-income levels, the higher the husband's income the less the likelihood of divorce (Levinger 1979). However, the higher the income of the wife the more commonly divorce occurs, since women with independent means are less likely to stay in an unsatisfactory marriage.

Although a smaller proportion of the population is remaining married, marriage still conveys social status to those involved and provides a degree of comfort for friends and colleagues who remain married. In general, high occupational status decreases the proneness to divorce, although particular occupations seem to be particularly vulnerable, perhaps because of the hours worked and, therefore, the competition between the job and family life (Cutright 1971; Vincent 1961). Where the partners have similar social and economic backgrounds, are of the same religion, and have only a slight difference in age, the chances of the alliance lasting are correspondingly increased (Bumpass and Sweet 1972; Kerckhoff 1974). Different religious affiliations, even if one of them is strongly opposed to divorce, increase the likelihood of marital breakdown (Bumpass and Sweet 1972).

Sexual satisfaction is generally associated with marital satisfaction (Wallin and Clark 1958), but its absence has not been clearly linked to marital instability. In fact, divorcing couples not infrequently report an improvement in their sexual relationship, at least temporarily, after the finalization of the divorce. Joint property, particularly major investments such as home ownership, may be a deterrent to divorce or at least a reason to pause for reconsideration.

Barriers

Reinforcing the advantages of continuing the partnership are the economic and symbolic barriers to its dissolution. Divorce is expensive. Maintaining two residences and providing for children following separation are major economic concerns. The process of divorce itself, even when "amicably" arrived at, is often enough to discourage or reverse precipitate decisions.

Psychological penalties must be considered as well. Increasingly well known is the sense of loneliness, the difficulty and insecurity involved in finding alternative, appropriate partners, and the emotionally wrenching cost to children of separation and divorce. Religion, as well, often holds together unsatisfying marriages, with the strength of the tie reflecting the attitude of the religion toward divorce (Wallin and Clark 1958). But religious opposition is only one of the social forces opposing marital dissolution. Kinfolk, family, and community, particularly small tight-knit or rural communities, still frown on and exert pressures against those who choose divorce as an alternative.

Alternatives

In many ways, alternatives are increasing, particularly as women enter the work force in larger numbers at pay that is equal and nondiscriminatory. Many wives, therefore, are now in a position to live on their own rather than having to feel totally trapped because of years of not having worked or of having unmarketable or rusty employment skills. Even so, for most, separation and divorce involves substantial financial hardship. Many, particularly if they have children, join the "working poor" or eventually have to rely on welfare. However, reentry into the job market increases their range of social contacts and chances of remarriage.

Many women in traditional marriages yearn for freedom, independence, and self-actualization and see marriage and continued domination by the demands of the spouse as the major obstacle to achieving these. The independence they achieve through separation, however, may prove to be either real or illusory. In those cases where it is primarily the spouse's domination that has restricted their independence, separation may indeed present many new and long overdue opportunities for success and fulfillment. However, for those who project onto their spouses the responsibility for their personal dissatisfaction with themselves, separation may initiate a lonely and depressing period marked by disapproval from friends and family and the need to assume responsibilities for which they are unprepared. At the same time, in the absence of the spouse, they may be forced to recognize for the first time their personal unreadiness for independence. Like all crises, the one precipitated by separation may have either a positive or negative outcome.

The process of marital dissolution has become less laborious and traumatic as legal changes have gradually been brought into line with social custom. The concept of no-fault divorce avoids the elaborate maneuvers or fabrications in which one party was made to assume the "guilt" even when everyone was aware that marriage breakdown is a shared responsibility. The debilitating concept of life-long alimony is gradually being replaced by that of providing interim support to allow a period of rehabilitation and restoration of skills, particularly where one spouse has given up a working career to raise the couple's children. In addition, the time required for separation prior to divorce action on the grounds of mutual incompatability is gradually being reduced. Divorces have even been granted to couples remaining in the same home but maintaining clearly separate geographic boundaries within it. More recently family law reforms have emphasized the couple's joint responsibility for the care of the children and have begun to assign their custody to that partner considered best equipped to raise them. The concern of the courts and the state in this process is not only for the welfare of the children but also, though covertly, to ensure that they do not become a public expense.

PROCESS OF DECISION TO DIVORCE

There are few married couples who have not, in moments of strife, threatened separation or divorce as the ultimate step in conflict resolution. Such conversations may frighten children who hear them out of proportion to any real threat to the marriage. In many marriages, however, the bleak prospect of a continuing relationship becomes rapidly apparent to at least one partner as the glow that brought them together dissolves and the reality of what each partner really is like becomes evident.

Certain circumstances seem to make separation more likely as a way of resolving marital disputes. A history of divorce in the previous generation is associated with a higher chance of divorce in the present one (Pope and Meuller 1979), as is relative economic freedom of both partners. Families of origin often support separation, particularly if they never really approved of the match in the first place. An angry, hostile atmosphere at home can lead to one or both partners spending more and more time away from home, often using work either as the reason or as the excuse for this withdrawal. This also increases the opportunity for developing alternative sexual relationships. The actual incident that precipitates the separation may be less the cause than the final straw, or excuse, on which a move that has become increasingly inevitable is finally justified.

Trial separations and trial reunions that frequently precede the final breakup may give the contesting partners a chance to assess the consequences of separation but are often steps toward the still unrecognized but inevitable outcome of a permanent dissolution. The period of separation is in many ways a period in limbo. The adults are not legally free to develop new relationships. If they do so, there is often an element of surreptitiousness built into them. They remain attached, at least by legal fiction. The lack of a final decision may accentuate the issues and contentions between the couple, causing conflicts around the division of income, the ownership of property, and visiting rights and access to the children.

Most lawyers representing clients in a contested action for divorce believe strongly in the value of the adversarial process, feeling that only in this way can justice be achieved. This contributes to an unfortunate potential for escalation, particularly if the contestants seek legal involvement before resolving these basic issues. This fact is beginning to be recognized by many lawyers practicing family law, who try to direct their clients to mediators trained to help them arrive at reasonable decisions regarding custody, access, property division, and visiting rights.

The divorce itself is not more than a legal statement. The assumption that this ends the marital bond is frequently untrue (Weiss 1979). The emotional bond may remain, even though love may have long since disappeared. Where the relationship has been a stormy one, the battles can continue long after the legal process has supposedly resolved them (Weiss

1979). In these battles the children often become the shuttlecocks between the parents, as they may provide the only avenue through which the parents can continue to compete with and get back at each other. Both parents usually have ample opportunity to feel legitimately aggrieved and to handle their residual anger and distress through conscious or unrecognized (i.e., acting-out) sabotage of access and visiting agreements. Custodial parents are often unhappy and frustrated at having to be the sole disciplinarian and to assume responsibility for all parenting routines, while the visiting parent is free to use a time-limited contact to take the children on interesting and exciting trips. The visiting parent often spends much time missing the children and feels particularly aggrieved and manipulated when visits are repeatedly cancelled for real or fabricated reasons. Nor are children necessarily entirely the innocent victims of such intrigues. Children can be resentful and are often determined to reunite the separated parents. They can be both ingenious and, at times, highly successful at arousing guilt, which they can utilize to punish the parents or to pressure them toward a reconciliation that neither parent wants. Their efforts to break up new relationships can also be extremely effective.

IMPLICATIONS FOR MENTAL HEALTH

Broken families, including increasing numbers of separated and divorced parents, are nonspecifically but highly correlated with many of the major mental illnesses of children and adolescents (Garfinkel and Golombek 1974) and with delinquency (Offord et al. 1979).

Adults who are divorced or separated are disproportionately overrepresented in psychiatric records. Marriage and living together appear to have considerable influence in protecting those involved from psychiatric illness, although the possibility that a single common underlying factor predisposes both to marital breakdown and mental instability, or that the marriage breakdown is predisposed to by personal instability, cannot be ruled out. In epidemiological terms, nevertheless, the differences are striking, with mental illness rates for the separated and divorced frequently in the range of twenty times as high as those for the married (Grad and Sainsbury 1966; Srole et al. 1962). The association of marital status with suicide and homicide is also striking. (National Center for Heath Statistics 1970). Those who are divorced are also prone to physical illness, particularly those in which social factors are at least one known contributing factor, such as alcoholism, diabetes, and some neoplasms (National Center for Health Statistics 1970a).

The emotional impact of separation on adults is just beginning to be studied systematically. The emphasis is on the marital bond that persists long after the separation and divorce, either as lingering affection or as continuing hostility and disparagement. Attachment is different from love and can endure long after love and even liking have faded. The reactions of the adults involved in separation and divorce, then, are frequently responses to the loss of a major attachment figure and may include feelings of fear, panic, depression, rage, restlessness, hyperalertness, and a host of contradictory and opposing feelings still associated with the lost figure (Bumpass and Sweet 1972; Parkes 1972). Somatic complaints, such as difficulty sleeping or loss of appetite, may be symptoms of an underlying though significant depression. The mental state following separation or, in more muted form, after divorce is characterized by ambivalence: a sense of loss combined with anger at the lost object; a relief, yet one often combined with regret. While there may be periods of euphoria at being free from an impossible or destructive relationship, these usually yield in time to signs of depression and distress colored by loneliness, panic, and concern about the future; poor self-esteem in the present; and feelings of failure in the past. This depression can severely restrict functioning capacity and responsiveness and is often accompanied by the repetitive ventilation of anger, either appropriately or inappropriately, toward the ex-spouse. Indeed, the continuing battles over children, finances, and property seem at times to be instigated to keep alive at least some kind of relationship between the two spouses.

This disruption in functioning will continue until the separated partners have undone the emotional bond that still unites them and are ready to move on to other interests and relationships. For this to occur, the work of mourning the loss of the attachment figure from whom separation has occurred must be completed. Time is usually the best healer. How long any individual will need to complete the emotional detachment from the ex-spouse to be free to form new interests and relationships will vary with a number of factors, including the intensity of the bond to be undone, the circumstances of the undoing, the psychological resources of the individual, the extent of that individual's capacity to tolerate loss, and the amount of support from others available to assist the individual through the transitional state. Until this process of disengagement is complete, the individual is not psychologically ready to form new alliances, except on the rebound.

Rebound relationships are notoriously unstable, as the new partner is not seen or selected for his- or herself but rather is used to fill the void left by the loss of the ex-partner to whom the rebounding individual remains strongly attached. Such relationships rarely, if ever, work. In time, the realization comes that the new relationship is not what is wanted, at which point the substitute, like a prop in a play that is over, has no further value and is discarded. Disengagement usually has to precede the formation of new relationships, unless these are entered on with a clear understanding that they are formed for immediate replacement and mutual satisfaction but without any implication of long-term commitment or a more formal and lasting relationship.

Very few divorces can be accomplished without major traumatic effects on all individuals concerned. However, this must be balanced against the fact that in time, most of those involved do recover and may even function at a better level than previously. The restoration takes time: time to adjust to a new economic level; time to enter or reenter the employment market; time to develop a new set of friends, as most of the couple's friends will remain friendly with one or other of the separating pair but rarely with both; time to restore self-confidence by successfully accepting new challenges and finding new directions; time to resolve feelings of loss, depreciation, and failure.

Some divorced persons—or children of families that have undergone a divorce—may require counseling or psychiatric care to assist the work of mourning or in order to avoid developing a full-blown clinical depression.

THE EFFECTS OF DIVORCE ON CHILDREN AND ADOLESCENTS

Until recently, our knowledge about the effect of divorce on children depended on case studies. It is only in the last ten to fifteen years that serious research on large samples has been available. Currently our knowledge comes from two sources: child psychiatric populations and nonclinical groups of youngsters whose parents are divorcing.

Studies from Child Psychiatric Clinics

The epidemiological studies of McDermott (1970), Kalter (1977), Kalter and Renbar (1981), and Schoettle and Cantwell (1980) compare two groups of clinic children, one with divorced parents and the other with parents who have remained married.

McDermott studied children referred to a children's psychiatric hospital from 1961 to 1964. There were 116 children whose parents were divorced and 1,349 whose families were legally intact. There were more first-born, only, and black children but fewer Catholics in the divorced group. This group's presenting problems were of shorter duration and their complaints were more sharply defined, with identifiable maladjustment specifically at home and in school. There were clusters of symptoms associated with delinquency as well as depression. Many children blamed themselves for the marital break, and many seemed to take on the characteristics of the absent parent, the father in all cases. This was interpreted as an attempt to deal with the father's loss through identification.

Kalter's study of 387 children generally confirmed McDermott's study, demonstrating that children of divorce had a higher rate of antisocial and delinquent problems, specifically drug taking and sexual behavior (Kalter 1977). In addition, the proportion of children of divorce in the clinic group was higher than in the general population. However, Kalter found that more specific features emerged when the data were analyzed by sex and age (under seven, seven to eleven, and twelve up). Thus girls with a stepfather were referred at a much higher rate; girls who had been through their parents' divorce when between seven and eleven had a higher incidence of subjective psychological symptoms; girls over twelve showed problems in the sexual and drug areas. Boys over twelve who had been through a divorce had more frequent conflict with the law. The only finding common to all groups of divorced children was the higher incidence of aggression toward parents.

Schoettle and Cantwell (1980) compared 1,043 children of divorce with 1,172 children from intact families. The divorced children more frequently came from low-income, nonreligious families and were most often the only or firstborn child. Children of divorce also had more frequent behavior and socialization problems.

Studies of Nonclinical Samples

There are two major ongoing studies of nonclinical samples, that of Wallerstein and Kelly in California and those by Heatherington in Virginia. These children were studied because they were children of divorce, not because of any problems that necessitated psychiatric intervention.

Wallerstein and Kelly (1980) studied 131 children (63 boys and 68 girls) ranging in age from one to twenty-two years. The children were from sixty families who came for a six-week free divorce counseling service advertised as child-centered, preventive, planning oriented, and voluntary. The main findings indicate the different responses at different ages. Preschool and kindergarden children (three to five years old) regressed. They showed fear that they might be left alone; returned to using their security blanket again; lost their newly acquired toilet training; were bewildered and had macabre fantasies to explain the separations. Guilty and blaming themselves for the separation, they showed either increased aggressive behavior or the opposite, a total inhibition of aggression. All showed a diffuse need for physical contacts, nurturance, and protection (affect hunger).

The young school-age children (six to eight years old) were notable for their sadness. They were afraid of being abandoned and felt deprived of food or toys. Yearning for the departed parent (mostly father), they were angry at the custodial mother, while inhibiting their aggression at the father. They were involved in a loyalty conflict, but very few felt responsible for the separation.

The older school-age children (nine to twelve years old) perceived their family disruptions with soberness, clarity, and distance. They were resourceful in their efforts not to be overwhelmed by their feelings and attempted to submerge their anxiety through activity and play. This group was most clearly distinguished by its anger, which was well organized and clearly directed. They had a shaken sense of their own identity, showed somatic symptoms, and aligned themselves with one or other parent.

For adolescents (thirteen to eighteen years old), the divorce produced major changes in the parent-child relationship and increased the adolescent's worry about sex and marriage. These adolescents experienced a profound sense of loss, anger, and loyalty conflicts. Some showed greater maturity and a more realistic view of money. Some attempted to distance themselves from the family crisis and their parents through a degree of detachment that verged on aloofness. A number failed to cope and were delayed in their psychosocial adolescent development. The comparison thus far made in these studies looks at different reactions at different developmental stages. The numbers do not yet allow a finer analysis of the differences between boys and girls.

The second major study of nonclinical groups is a series of studies by Heatherington and her colleagues (1979*a,b*) of thirty-six nursery school boys and thirty-six nursery school girls and their divorced parents (twelve to fourteen). Custody was with the mother, and there was a control group of the same number of children and parents from intact families. A battery of tests, questionnaires, and observations was done at two months, one year, and two years following divorce.

At one year, children from divorced families were functioning less well than children from high-discord nuclear families, who, in turn, showed more problems than low-discord nuclear families. In addition, boys of divorced families still showed aggressive, oppositional, dependent, impulsive behavior. Research concluded that the impact of divorce seems more pervasive and long lasting for boys than for girls. In addition to these general findings regarding behavior, there were differences on specific measures. Thus while there was no difference in the children's IQ at two months and at one year, children of divorce had a lower performance IQ at two years. While girls showed no difference in their sex-role preference at two years, divorced boys at two years scored lower than previously on male preference and higher on female preference scales. In the first year following divorce, disruptions were found in both play and social relations for both boys and girls. While the effects had disappeared in girls at two years, they were more intense and enduring for boys. The play patterns of divorced children were less socially and cognitively mature. The children showed limitations and rigidity in their fantasy play. One year after the parental divorce, both boys and girls showed high rates of dependent, help-seeking, and acting-out, noncompliant behavior. In general, boys from divorced families, even when they improved, were viewed and responded to more negatively by peers and teachers than were children from nondivorced families or girls from divorced families.

SUMMARY

It is not unusual, therefore, for children to show a variety of signs of emotional distress or behavioral disorder in response to parental separation or divorce (Heatherington, Cox, and Cox 1979*a,b;* Wallerstein and Kelly 1980). Often, over time, the children adjust to the situation and their symptoms recede. Should these symptoms be so extensive as to cause serious disruption in the child's ongoing functioning and development, or should there be no evidence that the child is beginning to adjust to the altered situation within a reasonable time, a psychiatric assessment with or without some periodic or ongoing therapeutic involvement of child and/or family is indicated. If in doubt, it is safer to err in the direction of seeking assessment rather than allowing an undue delay (Heatherington, Cox, and Cox 1979*a,b*).

Custody and Access

The custody of and access to children after separation are the focus of some of the most bitter disputes between ex-spouses. Fortunately, many divorcing parents are able to make major and sensitive decisions regarding custody and/or access with minimal acrimony and dispute. Some couples can reach such decisions by themselves, while others can use counseling or clinical services constructively to do so. Unfortunately, there is a group of parents whose disputes about custody and access linger on, at times for years, despite legal and clinical interventions. The effect of such disputes on both children and parents is often destructive (Watson 1969).

DEFINITIONS

The person(s) with *custody* has the power over and responsibility for a child's upbringing. Three areas are most often disputed: care and control, residence, and the freedom to move out of the court's jurisdiction.

Care and control refers to the parental power to influence the child, either through daily interactions or through making major decisions on matters such as schooling, religious upbringing, and socializing activities. During marriage, both parents share custody. However, following a divorce, one parent might be awarded full custody or the custody might be limited in certain areas, such as the ability to move with the child out of the jurisdiction of the court that granted custody without the other parent's permission.

Access refers to the time that the noncustodial parent has with the child. The types of access vary tremendously. Some divorced couples are able to terminate their marital relationship but continue their parenting relationships without major difficulty. Thus, between themselves and the child, they can work out a flexible visiting schedule that takes everyone's needs into account. When this cannot be achieved, access can become an area of conflict and dispute requiring external adjudication. For a minority, the continuing conflict is so serious, and the resulting situation so detrimental, that access for one parent may have to be terminated.

The way society and courts have viewed parental rights to custody has changed throughout history (Derdeyn 1976*a,b*). Greek and Roman law gave the father absolute control over his children whom he could desert, sell, or even kill with impunity. This absolute right was carried on unchanged into English law until the fourteenth century, when the father's absolute power was reduced, although his right to custody was not. The concept of custody involving both rights and responsibilities began to evolve in the eighteenth century. In 1839 the doctrine of parens patriae gave British courts the power to decide custody of infants under seven and to assume jurisdiction over the welfare of children. Some fathers, such as the poet Percy Shelley, lost custody of their children. The right of the mother gradually increased, until the Guardianship of Infants Act of 1925 proclaimed the equality of the father and mother with respect to custody. Even though the law gave both parents equal rights, for most of the twentieth century the presumption has been that mothers make better parents of young children.

FACTORS CONSIDERED IN DETERMINING CUSTODY*

In determining custody, the "best interest of the child" was the guideline used until recently. The following were the main four criteria considered as defining the child's best interest:

1. A young child should be placed in the custody of the mother.
2. A girl should be placed in her mother's custody, while a boy should be in that of his father if he no longer requires his mother's constant care.
3. If the child is old enough to form an intelligent judgement, his or her choice of custodian should be given consideration.
4. The noncustodial parent should have the right of visitation. The right of visitation should be refused only where its exercise would cause serious harm to the child.

With the major social and economic changes of the past decade, there are no longer any definite criteria regarding the inherent advantage of one parent over another. Instead, it is hoped that custody decisions take into account the child's needs, particularly the need for continuity in key relationships. Goldstein, Freud, and Solnit (1973) have suggested the term "least detrimental alternative" as a better guideline for custody determination, on the grounds that this would keep the focus on currently available alternatives. This would demand a realistic comparison of potential dispositions rather than encourage wishful and often unrealistic fantasy about what might conceivably at some point in the future be in the child's best interest.

Several criteria in both the clinical and the legal literature and statutes

*See Benedek 1972; Derdeyn 1975; and McDermott et al. 1978.

have evolved over the past few years. They share an intention to safeguard the child's need for continuity of care (Saxe 1975).

There has been a *recognition of the emotional tie between parent and child.* Goldstein, Freud, and Solnit (1973) suggest that psychological and not biological parenting should be the criterion used in deciding custody. While this concept is very helpful, theoretically useful, and of major practical importance in child welfare cases (e.g., deciding on custody between foster parents and biological parents), its applicability after divorce is often limited since both parents are usually psychological parents. It is, therefore, desirable to continue contact with both parents, unless specific and major contraindications exist. Instead what needs to be decided if possible is with which parent the child's ties are stronger.

The capacity of the parent to provide for the emotional and physical well-being of the child has to be taken into account. Knowledge of this capacity is derived from a general psychosocial profile of each parent, involving a thorough assessment of past as well as current psychological, social, and parental functioning. The assessment of parenting capacity is quite different from a psychiatric assessment of the parents: the latter is a cross-sectional assessment of the parents' current mental status, while the former contains a combination of a longitudinal assessment of the parents' continuing function as parents with a cross-sectional assessment of the person as a parent and as a member of the family system (Awad 1978; Steinhauer 1981).

The preference of the child must be considered. While the child's preference must be determined, its strength and the reasons for this preference also must be assessed. The child may choose one parent because of a stronger attachment or because that parent is lenient and imposes no limits or bribes the child with money. Generally speaking, the older the child, the more weight should be given that child's preference.

The need for continuity—of intrafamilial relationships and, to a lesser extent, with the environment (neighborhood, school, etc.)—must be recognized. The less disruptive an arrangement, the better.

These criteria cannot be considered mechanically or given numerical value. Many situations are extremely complicated, as these factors can be contradictory. For example, the attachment of the child could be toward a less competent parent or to a parent who, if given custody, would disrupt the child's continuity with other important relationships and with the environment. In general, custody should be determined on a global evaluation of these factors.

Other factors currently considered include preference toward either parent, parental mental illness, and parental "morality."

Regarding *preference toward either parent,* in today's society neither parent is inherently preferred as the custodial parent. As explained previously, the preference of mothers as custodial parents is a recent phenomena. However, it is a preference that made sense in the context in which it was applicable, namely one in which fathers worked while mothers stayed at home and raised children. Today that context has changed, so there is no inherent reason why mothers should always have custody or necessarily have better "parenting" capacities.

Mental illness of the parent should be investigated during a custody dispute. However, a parent with a mental illness is not axiomatically at a disadvantage. The relationship between mental illness and the capacity to parent is a complex one. There is no relationship between diagnosis and the capacity to parent. For example, a schizophrenic might be a more capable a parent than one with the diagnosis of psychoneurosis, which is generally considered a "milder" illness. More helpful than the psychiatric label is a detailed investigation of the psychosocial functioning of each parent and how that affects the child.

Considerations of the *"morality" of the parent* is an area fraught with personal judgment. To some people any life style different from their own is immoral. In addition, until recently a double standard was legally sanctioned to the disadvantage of women. Unless the life style or behavior of a parent affects that individual's parenting capacity, the life style should not be considered a factor in custody. For example, the fact that a women has an affair or decided to leave her husband and live with another man is unrelated to her parenting ability. On the other hand, any behavior that influences the parenting capacity of a parent, such as erratic, impulsive, and inadequate arrangements for the children's care, should be considered.

ACCESS

No single access plan is ideal. A useful plan should take into account the parents involved, their ability to negotiate with each other, their places of residence, their employment demands, the child's age and wishes, as well as the child's psychological, educational, and leisure-time needs (Awad and Parry 1980). In addition, any of these factors can change over time, so the plan should be flexible.

It is important, wherever possible, to encourage parents and children to negotiate and reach mutually agreeable plans on their own. If they can do so, their plan should be accepted even if it is unorthodox or unusual. At times parents seek professional help to arrange an access plan, either because they want to discuss plans with an expert or because they are referred to resolve a dispute. If they are reasonable enough to use clinical help to resolve conflict and improve their communication, the following general principles can be discussed with them.

1. An access plan should allow for uninterrupted and frequent access for the visiting parent.
2. For the preschool child, frequent brief visits are preferable to day-long or overnight visits.
3. For the school-age and older child, allowing the child increased control of the frequency and duration of visits is desirable.

4. Issues related to the child's daily routines, health care, education, leisure-time activities, and religion should be agreed on jointly by the separated parents, then supported both in the custodial home and during access visits.

Some parents, however, remain in serious conflict about access and are unable to negotiate or resolve their disagreement. In some such situations, a clinician can help by suggesting a clear plan that is either court-ordered or accepted by both lawyers (Saxe 1975). Such a plan should be very precise, spelling out all the details that cannot be changed without agreement. Five general principles should guide decision making in these disputed access situations.

First, the child belongs in one home, the home of the custodial parent. This is where the child spends most time, keeps most belongings, and from which most activities originate. Custody arrangements should clearly support the child's feeling that he or she lives with the custodial parent and visits the noncustodial parent.

Second, the custodial parent carries the primary responsibility for bringing up the child. The daily routines, education, religion, health care, and leisure-time activities are the prerogative of the custodial parent. Should the custodial parent remain open to considering the views, feelings, and suggestions of the noncustodial parent in major decisions, this will usually be to the child's advantage, but the final say is that of the custodial parent. Support of these plans during access visits is expected of the noncustodial parent.

Third, the age of the child should be a primary factor in planning length, location, and frequency of visits. As noted earlier, the needs of the preschool child differ from those of the older child or adolescent. If access is to be productive for the child and satisfying to the parent, the arrangements need to be suitable for age.

Fourth, changes in visiting arrangements should be expected and planned for in response to changes in the child's activities or illness of the child or either parent. Visiting time should disrupt the child's normal routine as little as possible. In other words, the visiting parent should fit in with the child's schedule and not vice versa. Arrangements for unexpected changes in visiting plans should be preset, requiring minimal negotiation by the parents.

Finally, visiting parents should avoid making visits into "special" occasions. It is better for parent and child to join in normal activities. To maintain visits as "special" places a strain on the noncustodial parent and limits the opportunity for the development of a natural parent-child relationship.

JOINT CUSTODY

One of the most recent and probably one of the most controversial ideas regarding child custody has been the concept of joint custody. Part

579

of the controversy may be the difficulty in defining what joint custody means. A recent handbook (Joint Custody 1979) published by proponents defines it as "the legally enforceable right of both parents to continue to act as parents and to share in making decisions affecting their child after divorce." Few people would disagree with the general concepts expressed in this definition, but what does "sharing" mean? Does it give both parents "equal rights"? If so, how is "equal" defined? Another area of concern is the enforcibility of this order when one parent, usually the custodial parent, does not want the agreement. It is difficult to imagine an arrangement that requires a lot of cooperation and reasonable working together between two equal parents to succeed when one of them is opposed to it. Finally, and perhaps the most controversial point, is the way some people interpret equal sharing to mean equally sharing everything, including time spent with the child. Thus there are arrangements whereby the child moves between parents' homes in order to spend equal time with each parent. Such a child might change residence every three or four days or every week. The objection to such an arrangement is that it serves primarily the parents' needs rather than those of the child. Children feel lost moving back and forth between two homes and often end up feeling that they do not belong to either. Despite these objections, it is becoming clear that for some parents a joint custody arrangement can be successful. Two recent studies have tried to delineate the factors that contribute to the success of joint custody arrangements, where the child spends equal time with both parents (Arbanal 1979; Steinman 1981). The factors needed for the success of such an arrangement included parental commitment to the arrangement, parental mutual support and valuing of each other, and flexibility and agreement on the implicit rules of the arrangement. Both studies found that the children were not torn by intense loyalty conflicts and that the moving between homes was the most troublesome aspect of the arrangement. Thus the successful joint custody arrangement involves parents with shared values, attitudes, and behavior.

Stepfamilies

The problems faced by a newly married couple in meshing their lives, adjusting to each other, and negotiating a compatible way of living together have been summarized in chapter 3. This adjustment is by no means an easy task. The circumstances become very much more complicated and convoluted, however, in families where one adult is not a birth parent of the children. Acclimatization requires time and inevitably presents difficulties and conflicts that must be overcome, but understanding from the beginning that this is a difficult process increases the likelihood of a successful outcome.

The term stepparent has, in our culture and its mythology, a very negative connotation. Our literature and folklore are peppered with images of the stern and punitive stepfather and the rejecting "wicked witch" stepmother. These communal fantasies recognize the difficulties but compound them by reinforcing the negative sterotype. There are no birthday or greeting cards to stepparents (Visher and Visher 1979). Most school forms that parents are required to fill in make no provisions for information on, and do not recognize the status of, the nonbiological parent. Alternative terms, such as the reconstituted family, remarried family, or blended family are euphemisms intended to decrease the aspersions implied by the term stepfamily. As used here, "stepfamily" will apply to any union, formal or informal, in which two adults live together in an at least semipermanent state that includes offspring belonging biologically to at least one other individual.

The number of people involved in stepfamilies has been increasing, although the formal process of remarriage, as figures given previously reflect, may have dropped. While accurate estimates are difficult, figures suggest that between 13 and 15 percent of unions are stepfamilies, involving a very substantial number of children (Population Reference Bureau 1977; Roosevelt and Lofas 1976). As divorce has risen in incidence and frequency, so has the frequency of stepfamilies, thus increasing the number of children who have multiple parent figures (Goldstein, Freud, and Solnit 1973).

Unlike the intact nuclear family, which both adults enter on equal terms and at the same time, one stepparent is always a newcomer to the stepfamily that disrupted the original family. The newcomer is often treated as an alien, an intruder, a possible competitor, as a threat to the established homeostasis that has resulted from the death or, much more frequently nowadays, from the separation and divorce. The family, indeed, may have been strengthened, supported, and brought closer together by sharing the adversity of separation together (Rosenbaum and Rosenbaum 1978). The introduction then of someone new into the family presents further complications. Like any foreign body, the newcomer can be dealt with by (1) encapsulation, (2) isolation, (3) extrusion, and (4) incorporation.

ENCAPSULATION

The stepparent may have a clearly defined and circumscribed role within the new family, but other parts of the usual parental role are often ambivalently offered or covertly withheld. For example, while a stepfather may be explicitly told that he is now the father of the family, any of his attempts to act like a father or to utilize a father's authority may be resented and undermined. Stepparents are part of the reconstituted family system; however, their right to full and equal status in family decision making is frequently overtly or covertly inhibited. This is particularly likely to become an issue around the management and discipline of children (Visher and Visher 1979). The stepparent is assigned a role yet at the same time denied the scope or authority to discharge that role. Some children quickly accept the invitation to play on these mixed messages and rapidly become skilled at playing one parent off the other (Bohannan and Erickson 1978). Their actions at least temporarily isolate the newcomer, who is made to feel unwanted, inferior, and a second-class family member. Unless these role conflicts are worked out, the stepparent will, of necessity, be excluded from full membership in the reconstituted family. Any suggestion, however appropriate, to alter or modify well established family customs may be regarded as trying to "take over" rather than as fitting into the existing family system (Stern 1978). Some couples manage to achieve a working balance in their relationship, but if one partner continues to exclude the other from full and autonomous participation in child rearing, the new marriage itself will be undercut. Should this occur, the family will function as a double system with all the confusion, ambiguity, inconsistency, and tension that this entails for the children (Visher and Visher 1979).

ISOLATION

Stepparents may find themselves being blamed and scapegoated when things go wrong within the family. Brushed aside as unfamiliar with the family's overt or covert rules, they are in a no-win situation, regarded as distant, ineffective, or undermining if they remain uninvolved or intrusive and interfering if they try to participate fully in family affairs. This isolation is further emphasized if they are unfavorably compared to their predecessor, the absent biological parent. These factors lead to an inhibition of spontaneity, and the resulting alienation and distancing become increasingly intolerable even for those children who initially vigorously opposed the entry of this new adult into their family life.

EXTRUSION

Stepparents are sometimes seen as competitors for the biological parent's total attention. The competition between a mother and her adolescent daughter, by no means unusual, is generally moderated by the mother's enjoyment of her daughter's budding adulthood. But where a stepmother and daughter are close in age, the competition for the father's attention may be greatly exaggerated. The teenage daughter may have been the woman of the house until displaced by a rival with a greater claim on her father. Thus her role, as she sees it, is usurped by the newcomer. Similarly, the older boy who may have been cast in the role of the man in the family will frequently resent the intrusion of a stepfather who displaces him from his position of number-one male and who determines, in many ways, the direction of family activities and emphasis. When this occurs, children may actively band together and deliberately form an alliance against the stepparent. The greater their effectiveness, the more destructive such an alliance can be. Just as children may feel responsible for (1) the separation, (2) the divorce, and (3) attempts to bring their natural parents back together again so, particularly in middle childhood, they may feel responsible for keeping out intruders in order to preserve at least their fantasy that the original family may get together again. At least for most children, the new union marks the final point at which this struggle to preserve what no longer exists is eventually relinquished (Simon 1964).

The end point of these active extrusions or passive encapsulations is that the stepparent becomes isolated and, even if the relationship with the new marital partner was initially good, often withdraws more and more into his or her own occupation, activities, or group of friends or gives greater emphasis to the children of a former marriage. The eventual outcome of this is often what everyone has feared, although many of their actions seem to invite it—namely another separation and the inevitable experience of further loss that accompanies it (Visher and Visher 1979).

Both parents face a similar set of conflicts. They can be so wary of the results of disagreement and dispute that they avoid any confrontation whatsoever. To do this the birth parent may take on the role of a middleman between the new spouse and the birth children. The birth parent's intent may be to protect the children from the new parent, because he or she feels guilty and responsible if conflict arises. Conversely, the birth parent may protect the stepparent from the children, fearful that any conflict could presage another marital breakdown. Such families do not solve problems well. Instead they tend to scapegoat the children, particularly a child who already has some constitutional or psychological vulnerability. That child is then used as a lightning rod on whom all family conflict is focused until the family presents to a professional or a clinic for help with the "identified patient."

INCORPORATION

Hopefully, by a process of trial and error combined with both parents' insistence on the stepparent's role as a full member of the family and through clarification by both parents acting together of roles and expectations for all, in time the newcomer's right and contribution to the family unit as another parent who can be expected to respond to realistic expectations with realistic involvement is comfortably accepted. Many children, particularly when they have friends in a similar situation, seem able, after a period of wariness or direct opposition, to accept the presence of the stepparent in the family, probably even as "mother" or "father." Some stepparents, if given a chance to do so, can provide more satisfaction and responsiveness than the children ever received from the absent parent, who is often idealized in fantasy (Rosenbaum and Rosenbaum 1978).

Children living with a stepparent of whom they become fond often have the problem that the more they like the stepparent, the more they feel disloyal to their own absent parent. This feeling is reinforced when the natural parent reacts with hostility and negativism toward the ex-spouse's new partner. For the child this ambivalence is not easy to tolerate or resolve. It is exaggerated when the absent parent remarries and introduces a new set of stepsiblings who have to be included in activities and consideration.

In contrast with the original nuclear family, stepfamilies have much more diffuse and poorly defined boundaries between themselves and the outside world. At least one of the members belongs to another family elsewhere. The boundaries of the stepfamily must stretch periodically to include members of one or, not infrequently, two other families who do not live with them but do contain children or siblings of at least some members of the reconstituted group. Thus a child or parent may have some but different status in several different family groupings, in one of which the person lives while being just a visitor in others. Whereas the nuclear family had a sense of "us" versus "them," the stepfamily has an "us," "them," "half us," "half them" feeling about many of the blood relatives who live elsewhere within other family groupings (Messinger, Walker and Freeman 1978; Rosenbaum and Rosenbaum 1978).

Stepparents often try hard to win the affection of their new children and may go out of their way to gain rapid acceptance. However, it is preferable to allow the children to approach at their own pace, as they disengage sufficiently from the absent parent to begin relating comfortably to the stepparent. Aggressive attempts to reach out in a desperate effort to win the love and esteem of those children who, from the beginning, are prejudiced against the new parent usually fail. Other children, equally bruised and battered by separation and divorce, may indeed welcome new stepparents, particularly if they can provide more satisfaction than came from the original parent. Older children and adolescents especially can often realize that the more successful the marital relationship, the better the outlook for the total family (Visher and Visher 1979).

These complications often come to a head around visiting privileges and the strain of sharing the children between two no-longer-married partners. Where children from two previous marriages are involved, the complexity of visiting arrangements and weekend and holiday activities becomes extremely complicated and like a chess game, in that the various "pieces" must be maneuvered by different sets of ground rules and expectations. In addition, visiting the absent parent can prove stressful when the children are expected to bear stories of the success or lack of it in the new union, or are discouraged from—or made to feel guilty about—

forming new attachments to stepparents. For stepparents, loving new children may raise feelings of disloyalty to their own children who, by this time, may have been programmed to resent and respond negatively to them. Whereas in nuclear families bonds of love are encouraged and promoted, in stepfamilies increasingly close and enriching relationships inevitably arouse questions of loyalty and guilt.

One issue that pervades all reconstituted families is that of loss (Simon 1964). Many of their members have experienced loss, sadness, and depression. The memory of this may lead to fear and an avoidance of forming new relationships lest they too break down, causing a repetition of the pain previously encountered. This sense of loss is reactivated by children's visits to natural parents, by comments, by birthdays and holidays when there is competition as to where the child will be or which parents will put on the more spectacular display of caring. A parent may continue to feel attached to a former spouse. Particularly if the spouse has died, he or she may be idealized, approaching in death a perfection never achieved in life, one with which the present spouse could never successfully compete (Simon 1964). Alternately, the survivor may hold back from a total involvement because of lingering thoughts of what a further loss or failure might entail. Thus many members of the reconstituted family are haunted by memories of previous loss and hyperalert to the possibility of future loss and further distress (Visher and Visher 1979).

The complexity of the situation lies in the fact that many more individuals, at times in competition with each other for the child's loyalty and affection, are involved in the reconstituted family than in the original nuclear family. Demands for attention are correspondingly greater, as are the continuing obligations to the previous family, including major financial ones. Thus the divorced and remarried partner may be required to support the former spouse and children while unable to provide adequately for the current spouse and offspring. This common source of resentment can become a major bone of contention. Visher and Visher (1979) suggest that this conflict of loving, combined with a feeling that giving to one group leaves less for the other, is probably the primary issue in stepfamily discomfort.

The absent family members may contribute to this discomfort by deliberately or inadvertently fostering comparisons. The absent parent's rivalry with the custodial parent may be exaggerated by the latter's remarriage. The new stepparent develops a relationship with the children, is encouraged to compete to be a better parent than the absent parent, and inadvertently inflames the continuing conflict between the birth parents. Children can become skilled at manipulating, at least to their material advantage, the competing suitors for their affection and loyalty. The absent father, for example, becomes super-Dad who tries each visit to impress the children with what he is doing, how he can provide for them, the interests in his life. Because his visits are brief, he can indulge them without the necessity of disciplining them. The custodial parent is forced to make demands and provide controls. These differences can be interpreted by the children as a measure of who loves them most. Loss and anticipated loss, a lack of clear boundaries, different sets of alliances, and the tug and pull of these on members of the family are compounded and cemented by the guilt feelings engendered by the various different kind of likings that grow up. The guilt can be dealt with by withdrawal, by clear favoring of natural children through giving priority to their activities and their needs, by complaining of the demands made by the new family, or by overcompensating and offering more than is needed or expected. This emphasizes the need for building clear communicative pathways by which either relative neglect or overindulgence can be identified and fairly and evenly balanced, so that obtainable goals are set and achieved without reneging on existing and competing obligations (Visher and Visher 1979).

Two further considerations seem more prominent in the stepfamily than in the natural family situation. Children may be very much aware of the new sexual relationship, which may be more obvious than that of their natural parents. This is particularly true when the children go through the courtship, trial marriage, and then marriage period aware of the intense involvement between the adults. Where the parents are comfortable in their own sexuality and their mutual enjoyment, this can form a solidifying bond that eventually becomes supportive for the children, provided it is not so overemphasized as to be inappropriately stimulating or challenging. It can help children accept their own sexuality and deal with the other issue inherent in the stepfamily situation, that of living with other children with whom they have not grown up and with whom the more usual incest taboos do not operate (Visher and Visher 1979). While this listing might appear to suggest that the stepfamily must face and overcome a virtually insurmountable set of challenges, most reconstituted families do achieve a way of living together that satisfies most of the needs of their participants. Despite the initial confusion and even anguish, in time the reconstituted family has a good chance to develop the comfort and security that can allow it to become "the" family (Duberman 1975).

As society becomes increasingly comfortable with these arrangements, there is increased social acceptance of the new groupings, formal and informal. The difficult role facing any adult moving into such an already established family is easier and more socially supported than in the past.

In summary, the problems that stepfamilies face in working out a modus vivendi are much more complicated than the process by which the nuclear family goes about creating the same bonds. The continual comparison, competition, and contrast between absent parents and their stepparent replacements increase the possibility of continuing conflict. However, just as intact nuclear families are often capable of making the changes necessitated by the addition of a new family member (see chapter 3), so in stepfamilies some of the same processes can prevail. Reasonable expectations, particularly on the part of the adults, and allowing children to approach at their own rate usually leads to the stepparent being comfortably included in what can, in time, become a truly blended family.

SUGGESTIONS FOR FURTHER READING

ABARBANEL, A. 1979. Shared parenting after separation and divorce: A study of joint custody. *Am. J. Orthopsychiat.* 4(2):320–329.

One of the few articles in the field to take a positive stand on joint custody. Arbanal reports on successful joint custody arrangements and draws conclusions on what makes a successful arrangement.

BERELEK, E. P., AND BERELEK, R. S. 1972. New child custody laws: Making them do what they say. *Am. J. Orthopsychiat.* 42(5):825–834.

An in-depth look at the new child custody laws in Michigan that set a precedent by looking after the best interests of the child rather than the convenience of the parents. Implications for behavioral scientists are discussed, as well as a general outline of the cooperation needed for effective functioning of the laws.

GOLDSTEIN, J.; FREUD, A.; AND SOLNIT, A. J. 1973. *Beyond the best interest of the child.* New York: The Free Press.

An authoritative and definitive statement on criteria for decision making with regard to children's interests in custody and access situations based on the extensive experience of highly respected authors. Deals with the issues from both a legal and a psychological-psychoanalytic viewpoint. A standard reference in this field.

HEATHERINGTON, E. M.; COX, M.; AND COX, R. 1979. Family interaction and the social, emotional and cognitive development of children following divorce. In *The family: Setting priorities,* ed. V. Vaughn and T. Brazelton, pp. 71–87. New York: Science and Medicine.

Reports the results of intensive psychological testing and investigation of the impact of separation and divorce and represents a different approach from Wallerstein and Kelly's to the collection of information on the short- and long-term impact of these social events.

LEVINGER, G., AND MOLES, O. C. 1979. *Divorce and separation.* New York: Basic Books.

An extremely useful book that incorporates the opinions of many experts—including Weiss; Norton and Glick; Levinger; and Pope and Mueller—into a comprehensive handbook for anyone dealing with divorce or separation. Views are presented from psychological, psychiatric, and legal standpoints. Highly recommended.

VISHER, E. B., AND VISHER, J. S. 1979. *Step-families: A guide to working with step-parents and step-children.* New York: Brunner/Mazel.

Drawn from personal and clinical experience, this work covers the often difficult process of reconstituting a family from the viewpoint of each person involved. Also included are chapters directed toward working with the individuals concerned and general guidelines for people involved in the stepfamily situation.

WALLERSTEIN, J. S., AND KELLY, J. B. 1980. *Surviving the breakup: How children and parents cope with divorce.* New York: Basic Books.

Summarizes the experiences and careful investigation of the impact of parental separation and divorce on children at different ages. Provides the ongoing results of one of the few definitive studies currently underway using primarily a clinical interview and follow-up approach.

WEISS, R. S. 1979. The emotional impact of marital separation. In *Divorce and separation,* ed. G. Levinger and O. C. Moles, pp. 201–210. New York: Basic Books.

An excellent review of the psychosocial and emotional concomitants and implications for family members involved in divorce and separation.

PART V

Principles of Intervention

27

Naomi Rae-Grant

Prevention

The Case for Prevention

The gap between the demand and supply of mental health services for children and adolescents seems to be increasing despite the decreased number of children in the population. Various estimates suggest that only about 10 percent of children needing service receive it. Questions as to which forms of treatment provided by personnel with what kinds of disciplinary background are most effective for which kinds of children are still hotly debated. A consensus is developing, however, at least that assessments on which interventions are based should be conducted according to some classification commonly used in child mental health circles. The term child mental health is used advisedly, since only a small fraction of all child mental health services is specifically psychiatric. Over the past decade several studies have emphasized the limited effectiveness of treatment of children and adolescents with conduct and personality disorders, who in spite of it often continue as adults not only to be disturbed but frequently to be the parents of the next generation of problem children (Shamsie 1981; Warren 1978). Factors correlated with these child and adolescent conditions most difficult to treat are beginning to be identified (Offord, Allan, and Abrams 1978; Robins 1966; Rutter et al. 1975). A recent study of over 600 particularly "hard to serve" children and adolescents emphasizes the frequency with which they had experienced poor parenting, multiple placements, and poor educational achievement (Report on the Hard-to-Serve Child in Ontario 1981).

The idea that physical and emotional well-being are closely interrelated is by no means a recent one. Two thousand years ago, Juvenal coined the phrase *mens sana in corpore sano.* Until comparatively recently, the number of medical treatments available to cure disease was so limited that the psychosocial aspects of medical care—the "art" of medicine, consisting largely of comfort and wise counsel—was most of what average family physicians had at their disposal to support patients through illnesses and to help them come to terms with their disabilities. During the past fifty years, however, the increasing emphasis on specialization, subspecialization, and the "technicalization" of medicine has largely obscured the understanding of the interaction between mind and body in western medicine. Recently, however, the situation has improved as the concepts of stress, stress effects, and the results of adverse life styles on physical and mental health have been recognized and reported in the popular as well as in the professional press. For over twenty years it has been recommended that at least part of available health resources should be devoted to primary prevention (Caplan 1976; Hobbs 1975). It is clear that the incidence of high-risk pregnancies and birth problems can be reduced; that sociocultural mental retardation is largely preventable; and that children's competence to deal with their environment can, to some extent, be enhanced. Yet despite some definite and encouraging activity and in spite of a host of papers, commissions, task forces, and mounting interest, the actual implementation of programs and training of mental health personnel in primary prevention has been woefully inadequate.

Barriers to Prevention

There have been a number of reasons for the delay in developing preventive programs. For one thing, there is the dilemma of definition. In any discussion of prevention, someone will inevitably say, "But you must know what you want to prevent before you can begin to prevent it!" The concept of specific protection is appropriate when considering the eradication of smallpox, rubella, or polio, but in the mental health field, specific techniques for averting mental illness, personality disturbance, and their sequelae are much less obvious.

Until recently there was little public demand for preventive activities. Children and adolescents, although a significant proportion of the population, do not vote and so far have not established an effective lobby for improving the quality of their lives.

The balance between the rights of children and the rights of parents is just beginning to be addressed seriously. In the past children have been regarded as the property of their parents, and no special knowledge or skill has been considered necessary for adequate parenting. Rather parenting is thought to be something that all can do instinctively, and any attempt to direct or criticize styles of parenting, regardless of the destructive effects of those patterns on children, is still interpreted as a violation of parental rights.

In the mental health field, a variety of genetic, organic, psychological, and environmental factors act together in varying combinations to produce often quite dissimilar mental, emotional, and behavioral disturbances. As a result of this "systemic complexity" (Broskowski and Baker 1974), "specific interventions are difficult to design or often become trivial or inconsequential over time" (Bower 1977).

In retrospect it is surprising, for example, that the brief exposure of four-year-olds to Head Start Programs as they were originally set up could have been expected to enhance children's learning skills sufficiently after just a few short weeks to allow children to cope in spite of the continuing exigencies of inadequate and underfunded school systems and unchanged disadvantage and discrimination in home and neighborhood.

Thus, to be effective, primary prevention programs must take into account the total social system in which the population lives. Although a number of early efforts at prevention were not very effective, some recent studies do exist that convincingly demonstrate that preventive interventions can be effective and, over time, demonstrate considerable cost benefit.

In the past it was sometimes difficult to determine clearly defined groups of "at risk" children who had an increased probability of developing psychological handicaps and who could, therefore, serve as a target population for preventive interventions. The term was used originally to describe those infants who, because of antenatal, perinatal, and postnatal factors, were considered at high risk for the development of later sensory, motor, or mental handicaps. But while the concept helped identify important variables contributing to later infant mortality or morbidity, it was not helpful in predicting the future for any particular child. In several prospective studies correlations between single perinatal or postnatal events and later handicaps have been found to be surprisingly low (Buck et al. 1969; Niswander et al. 1966; Parmalee and Haber 1973). It is now clear that there is an ongoing transactional effect between infants and their families that may, if the family is sufficiently supportive, outweigh the effect of the child's potential vulnerability.

While research has already provided enough facts to allow us to improve the quality of life and reduce the level of cumulative risk to the child population, it seems to take an inordinate time for such information to reach those who work directly with children, to produce the desired changes in medical, social work, nursing, or teaching practice. This is particularly so when research findings are derived from different specialties by researchers of different disciplines and are published in different journals. The information explosion has made it more difficult to sift facts from fantasies, to translate technical jargon into plain English, and to disseminate information to those actually working with children on a day-to-day basis.

Although many child welfare and children's mental health agencies have begun to carry out and evaluate primary prevention programs, traditional funding patterns have not supported such efforts, nor until very recently have government or agency boards encouraged a shift in emphasis toward preventive programming. In the medical field, funding patterns are one of the biggest barriers to preventive involvements. For example, the fee-for-service funding by which most Canadian child psychiatrists are rewarded for direct service to individuals and families discourages rather than supports the more economical use of child psychiatrists as agency consultants using their skills and knowledge to provide backup to other professionals working on the front line with children, the so-called "multiplier effect" (Eisenberg 1961).

The complexity of our society and the emphasis on "treatment" in the social and health services have been major factors in the relative lack of research and of emphasis on finding effective forms of prevention. The causes of psychopathology have been much better studied than have those factors that protect some children coming from similar adverse circumstances, allowing them to escape relatively psychologically unscathed.

Definitions

The term primary prevention includes any activity that reduces the incidence of disorder, dysfunction, or disability that would otherwise interfere with social, emotional, or intellectual functioning in children. Bloom (1968) subdivided prevention into two distinct processes which are commonly carried out by two different groups of people. These are specific protection and health promotion.

Specific protection is what is generally thought of as prevention. It includes activities that protect individuals from the effects of an adverse environment. Examples include the immunization of all women of child-bearing age in order to reduce the incidence of rubella (German measles), a major cause of birth defects in the first three months of pregnancy; the provision of adequate nutrition and health care during pregnancy to reduce the incidence of premature and low–birth-weight infants vulnerable to a whole range of reproductive casualties; the provision of adequate obstetric care to known high-risk mothers and high-quality neonatal care to their babies immediately upon delivery, to reduce the incidence of birth damage.

In the widest sense of the term health, promotion helps individuals cope with their environment, thus increasing their potential for optimal intellectual, emotional, social, and physical growth. Examples of health promotion include the provision of infant development programs and readily available, enriched day care to encourage optimal development for children of retarded and other high-risk mothers; teaching social competence to preschool children; teaching pregnant mothers to anticipate, understand, and respond appropriately to the physical, emotional, and differing temperamental needs of their infants; and improving school facilities and teacher training to produce school environments more responsive to children's educational, emotional, and social needs.

Specific protective activities are usually provided by health care professionals, whereas activities promoting health, generally less well conceptualized and developed in our culture, are more "educational" in nature. They may be supplied by professionals or volunteers with a wide variety of skills.

In summary, then, prevention includes any activity undertaken before individuals are defined as "cases" or "clients." It then selects a target group seen as being at high risk and tries to reduce that group's vulnerability to stress or to enhance its capacity to cope with an adverse or stressful environment. The characteristics of primary prevention are summarized in table 27.1, and prevention is contrasted with treatment in table 27.2.

TABLE 27.1

Characteristics of Primary Prevention

Reduces the incidence of new cases of disorders, disabilities, and dysfunctions in a population.
Targets groups rather than individuals.
Reduces stress in the environment.
Raises individual or group immunity to stress.
Aims at the development of optimal potential.
Promotes individual or group competence in its broadest sense (Toffler's "copability").
Improves the quality of life in targeted populations.
Raises the general health of the childhood population.

TABLE 27.2

Differences Between Prevention and Treatment

Treatment	Prevention
Focuses on individual	Focuses on group or population
Referred patients or clients	Unreferred persons or groups
Identified "problem"	At risk
Aim is remedial	Aim is protective
Restores status quo	Enhances competence

Basic Concepts in Prevention

It is now quite evident that adverse conditions in the growing child's environment do not necessarily produce adverse outcomes. Instead, outcomes depend on a number of factors, which may be summarized as follows.

1. The number of stresses in the environment that exert a cumulative effect. (Rutter 1979).
2. The vulnerability of the child.
3. Protective factors in the child (i.e., resilience).
4. Protective factors in the environment.

Sameroff and Chandler (1975) have described this interaction between factors in the child and the family as a transactional model of development. (See figures 27.1 and 27.2). Modifying a formula suggested by Albee (1979), it could be said that the

$$\text{incidence} = \frac{\text{organic factors} + \text{stress}}{\text{competence} + \text{coping skills} + \text{available supports}}.$$

Rutter (1979) demonstrated that certain children are more negatively affected by adverse conditions than others. In other words, there is an interaction between the vulnerability of the child and the degree of risk in the environment. Children may be vulnerable because of their constitutional or genetic endowment, temperament, sex, physical or mental defect, prenatal or perinatal insults, or environmental circumstances. Sameroff and Chan-

FIGURE 27.1

Transactional Models of Development

Caregiver's mode of functioning

Specific characteristics of the individual child

FIGURE 27.2

Abuse-prone Parents	+	Vulnerable Child (Source of more than usual stress)	+	→	Child Abuse
Aggressive		Premature	Additional stress		
Impulsive		Difficult temperament			
Immature		Handicapped			
Self-centered		Sick			
Critical of self/others					
Unreasonable expectations					
History of abuse					
As a child					

dler (1975) postulated a continuum of care-taking casualty; at one end were environments supportive enough to strengthen even the most vulnerable of children, while at the other end were environments too disordered to meet the needs of even the most resilient child. The majority of family environments lay somewhere in between, providing parenting "good enough" to allow the average child to grow and develop reasonably well. For example, premature infants do well in stimulating, nurturing home environments, whereas such children reared in less supportive conditions have much lower levels of intelligence and school performance (Robinson 1972). Hertzig (1979) suggests that the cohesive, well-functioning family intuitively provides extra stimulation for the high-risk, premature infant during the first year of life, thus assisting that child to compensate for quite severe difficulties at birth. This is illustrated in figure 27.3.

Rutter (1974) has demonstrated that not all adverse variables have the same potency; some are merely additive—the effect of two stresses is cumulative (i.e., one plus one equals two); some are transactional—if one is present, the likelihood of another being present is increased (e. g., the presence of socioeconomic disadvantage increases likelihood of premature birth). Finally, some are potentiating—for example, psychosocial disadvantage plus more than one hospitalization before age six results in a markedly increased incidence of later emotional disturbance (i.e., one plus one equals more than two).

The notion of reducing environmental stress while simultaneously increasing children's competence to cope with stress suggests a two-pronged strategy; first the professional assesses the potential stress in a particular environment and attempts to reduce that level by careful planning; second, he or she attempts to enhance the child's capacity to cope with that environment. For example, the effects of hospitalization in young children can be decreased by reducing separation from the parents. This can be done by providing accommodation and encouraging parents to stay with the child and by minimizing the length of stay (see chapter 24). At the same time, children's ability to cope with hospitalization can be increased by explaining to them what to expect before beginning all investigative and treatment procedures and by providing enough opportunities to discharge tension about what is in store through play sessions with someone experienced (e.g., child-life worker). Part of increasing the child's ability to cope

FIGURE 27.3

Continuum of Care-taking Casualty

Adaptive Environment (Meets need of most distressed infant)	⟷	Range of Average Environments ("Good enough" parenting)	↔	Disordered Environment (Does not meet needs of least distressed infant)	⟷	Distress (Emotional, Financial, Social, Economic)

From A.J. Sameroff and M.J. Chandler, 1975.

with the stress involves obtaining adequate information, having the opportunity to discuss fantasies and clear up misconceptions, being able to prepare for unknown and frightening situations by practising new behavior in the presence of a supportive person and, finally, by having the chance to reevaluate the experience afterward. These, incidentally, are among the same basic factors isolated by Marmor (1975) in looking at the factors common to eight different types of psychotherapy.

Points of Possible Intervention in the Life Cycle

Kessler and Albee (1977) have suggested that anything that improves the quality of children's lives can be considered within the realm of primary prevention. If the number of adverse factors could be reduced and children's competence simultaneously increased, it is possible that the level of cumulative stress could be decreased enough to cause a significant drop in the incidence of emotional and conduct disorders in the childhood population. It is possible to intervene at any point in the life cycle, and the relative merits of various interventions at any given point can be argued, as can the question of which of the possible interventions can be most beneficial to the largest percentage of the population. The focus can be primarily on the individual at different stages of development; on the family at the various normal stages in its evolution; on the family, but only at times of crises (e.g., when parents separate, when a family member dies, when parents become unemployed, or when moving into a new culture). Alternatively, the focus could be on the environment in which the family lives (community, subculture); on those institutions (e.g., day nurseries, schools) and agencies that have an impact on the developing child; or at the level of the broad social scene. Intervention at any of these levels may ameliorate the environment and/or subsequently facilitate more competent functioning. (See table 27.3.)

FOCUS ON THE DEVELOPING CHILD AND FAMILY

The parental, child, and environmental factors that place children "at risk" in their physical and emotional development are beginning to be understood. Although it cannot yet be predicted exactly which child should be the target for early intervention, groups of children likely to be at risk can be identified. At the same time, some of the protective factors that promote psychological well-being even in remarkably adverse environments have been identified (Rutter 1979). Kornberg and Caplan (1980) have recently reviewed risk factors and possible preventive interventions at vari-

TABLE 27.3

Intervention at Different Levels

Focus on Intervention	Level	Nature of Intervention
Individual child and/or Family	Case level	Intrapsychic Intrafamilial Interpersonal
Group (type) of children or families	Class level	Family/subcultural
Local environment (e.g., institutions agencies, neighborhoods)	Community level	Socio/Cultural
Wider environment areas	Central level	Sociopolitical

ous stages in development. In this chapter only interventions recommended for implementation during pregnancy and the preschool years will be discussed.

Preconception

Ryan (1972) has stressed the relationship between a mother's health status prior to pregnancy and the subsequent health of her children. He pointed out that the fact that many women of child-bearing age are in poor physical condition is inevitably reflected in an increased incidence of prenatal and perinatal problems. He suggested a concerted effort to improve the health and to establish habits of adequate nutrition and exercise in high school teenagers, thus setting a pattern for adult life. Routine immunization would eliminate mental retardation caused by the most common infectious diseases during pregnancy. The measles eradication program in Massachusetts has demonstrated the effectiveness of an all-out campaign to improve the immunization status of a childhood population. Over the six years after the launching of the drive (i.e., 1965–1971), the number of reported measles cases dropped by 98 percent (Fotheringham and Morrison 1976).

Prenatal Period

It is well documented that the incidence of premature births and birth complications in at-risk populations can be reduced by nutritional advice, dietary supplements, and good prenatal care of all (Ryan 1972). Nations providing outreach health programs have been able to reach as much as 98 percent of the population (Fox 1978). The dangers of smoking, alcohol, drugs, and radiation during pregnancy, now well established (Fotheringham and Morrison 1976), should be made known to prospective parents.

Early identification of complications of pregnancy such as multiple pregnancy, toxemia, placenta previa, combined with arrangements for specialized care of such high-risk pregnancies can reduce the incidence of birth problems and resultant damage and disability in children (Wynn and Wynn 1976). This can be achieved through a good primary care service available to all pregnant mothers, along with the ensured provision of regional specialized perinatal units.

The psychosocial aspects of prospective parenthood are equally important. The stress of severe continuing personal tensions, especially marital discord during pregnancy, has been identified as closely associated with ill health, neurological dysfunction, developmental lag, and behavioral disturbances in childhood (Stott 1973). Sameroff and Zax (1977) have found that psychiatrically distrubed women have more problems in pregnancy and delivery and are more likely to have babies with difficult temperaments than mothers whose index of pathology is low. Regional health units that provide childbirth education classes for prospective parents could also be used to teach them about normal child development and basic aspects of child care. More outreach prenatal services that emphasize the psychosocial as well as the physical aspects of antenatal care are urgently needed.

Perinatal Period

The possibility of reducing the incidence of premature births by early identification and adequate care of high-risk pregnancies and the effectiveness of specialized regional facilities in reducing neonatal morbidity and mortality in high-risk births have already been demonstrated (Swyer 1970). Recently attempts have been made to facilitate bonding between parents and child and attachment between child and parents in the perinatal period. Klaus and Kennell (1976) have stressed contact between mother and newborn infant in the early minutes of life. Minde and associates (1980), studying the interactions of mothers and their premature infants, were able to identify mothers who were at risk of providing inadequate stimulation for their infants at home. A group of mothers led by a nurse and the mother of an older "preemie" helped mothers express their frustration and disappointment around the premature birth and prepared them to care adequately for their infants following discharge from the hospital. Broussard and Hartner (1970) demonstrated how mothers' early perceptions of their newborn child as average or below average were reflected in the child's functioning as a preschooler, and that it is possible to improve maternal functioning by perinatal intervention. Ideally, adequate staff support and rooming-in of mothers with infants, which should be routinely available in any obstetric unit, can help inexperienced or anxious mothers understand their infant's biological rhythms and needs, thus improving their competence and confidence, teaching them the basics of child care, and getting breast feeding established.

Infancy—Preschool Years

Physically and emotionally healthy parents who themselves have had adequate parenting are most likely to produce well-functioning, competent children. Ideally parents should be emotionally mature enough to meet the physical and emotional demands of infants and toddlers and should have available to them an adequate support network of friends and relatives. Unfortunately, in modern urban society with its high geographic mobility and increasing incidence of family breakdown, many parents lack such supports. The identification of high-risk families, the provision of babysitting services, crisis relief, and opportunities for companionship with others might significantly reduce the inevitable stress of their isolation.

The routine health and developmental assessment programs carried out in France, Sweden, and Finland are estimated to have saved millions of dollars in health care. The Sixth French Plan, carried out between 1971 and 1976, was designed to reduce handicapping conditions in childhood (Wynn and Wynn 1976). It saved the French government an estimated seven billion francs—a cost/benefit ratio of seven or eight. This study concluded that regular contact between parents and the service, along with special training of the health care personnel, were essential for a child health service to have any economic benefit. Such regular contact was achieved by introducing a system of child allowances paid to parents contingent on medical examinations. Other conclusions were that any child health service should teach parents when to ask for help and have guidelines as to which systematic examinations were cost effective (Wynn and Wynn 1978). An important finding was that 90 percent of the remedial handicaps identified at the nine-month and two-year assessments had not been recognized by the parents. To be effective, any such developmental service must involve specialized training for the medical and nursing personnel.

The importance of a safe, stimulating learning environment that encourages language and cognitive development has been well recognized (White 1978). The most competent three-year-olds are those whose mothers frequently talk to them while, at the same time, providing a safe environment that allows exploratory behavior and rewards with their approval the mastery of each new developmental skill. Data now available about successful learning environments from home observers of normal mothers (White et al. 1977), from successful interventions with retarded mothers (Heber 1978), and from studies of stimulating environments in good day-care centers (Kagan, Kearsley, and Zelazo 1978) should make it possible to reduce the ravages of sociocultural deprivation by a combination of prospective parent education and judicious early intervention with mothers and children identified as high risk. Two recent findings are important in preparing prospective parents and others who work with children and families to understand the ongoing transactions between children and the environment. The first, the identification of enduring temperamental traits by Thomas and Chess (1977), allows parents to be taught to identify and respond more appropriately to their child's basic temperament. The second is the recognition of the transactional model of interaction between child and environment and the ways that each influences the responses and development of the other in an ongoing way.

Support for Families in Crisis

Our culture prepares people poorly for much of the social and emotional side of life. The inevitable changes, responsibilities, joy, or loneliness caused by changes in physiological, social, or vocational status are seldom, if ever, discussed. Preparation for such major changes as adolescence, marriage, separation, divorce, serious illness, retirement, and death is either haphazard or, often, nonexistent. Yet such major changes call for major shifts in both individuals' and families' habitual methods of coping and defending, shifts that disrupt the steady state and typically arouse considerable discomfort and anxiety (see chapter 3). Nevertheless, present status continues to be regarded as if it were permanent rather than a transition on the way to something else. Toffler (1970) suggests it would be more helpful to view people not as what they are but to anticipate what they are becoming, in order to prepare them to cope better with the inevitable crises of life and the changes in technology and society.

Providing services that prepare people to cope with transitional states should effectively reduce reactions to stress, either physical or emotional. There is a growing literature on the effects of crisis on individuals, some of it describing ways of helping adults through crisis transition and deficit states (Romeder 1981) (see chapter 20). Examples include seminars for the separated; discussion groups about divorce; self-help groups for single parents, bereaved parents (e.g., Compassionate Friends), and the widow-to-widow program in the United States. Comparatively little is known, however, about how transitional states affect children, and even less has been done to provide support systems to help children and their families through such states. For example, parents who have lost a spouse are usually so overwhelmed with their own grief that they are often not able to comfort their children and help them complete the work of mourning (see chapter 4). Thus children who have lost a parent, either through death or family breakdown, would probably benefit from the chance to discuss their common situation and feelings with a small group of others in various stages of adjusting to a similar loss.

Some parents have set up their own associations for mutual support in coping with the stress of living with a handicapped child. Such associations, often organized by groups of parents whose children have a common disease or disability, have achieved a great deal in working with professionals and governments toward improving services and facilities for affected children and families. At the same time participating parents share information about how to manage and what to expect and prepare for in the future, about resources and forms of assistance available to help children like theirs. Activity in such an organization helps many parents overcome the overwhelming feelings of passivity and hopelessness that can otherwise sap their vitality. Working together with other parents with a similar problem helps many feel less singled out, alone, and bitter. Such associations may organize facilities and groups for afflicted children or for their nonafflicted siblings, who often feel neglected and out of place because of the family's preoccupation with the disabled child and the inevitable associated problems. These activities may assist the children much as those of the parent association support and prepare the parents.

Other groups of families in transitional states are vulnerable to being overwhelmed by too much stress at a given time. An example would be the families of recent immigrants. In coming to a new land, most immigrants must first face the loss of family, friends, financial security, social status, and membership in a community in which they felt they belonged and with whose customs they were familiar. The period following immigration is one of crisis for almost all immigrant families. Contributing to this crisis are the need to arrive at new and culturally appropriate role definitions, to reconcile the social and religious traditions of the old world with those of the new, to modify patterns of behavioral control to ones acceptable within the new society. As with all periods of transition, the stress generated by the demand for such rapid change is considerable. New immigrant families often lack the friends and extended family networks to support them through the transition. Particularly painful and divisive is the gap between adolescents committed to assimilation and their parents clinging to old world traditions. As this gap widens, it often provides the battleground on which the adolescent's struggle toward individuation is fought. Some such adolescents seek support within a group of alienated, antisocial youth formed along ethnic or subcultural lines. Immigrant families then are families at risk. What can be done to minimize disruption and to extend their ability to cope?

In many communities, there are immigrants' associations composed of members of each national group who, having been in the host country longer, are therefore further on in the process of acculturation. Such associations may need to reach out repeatedly to new immigrant families that, if left to their own devices, may withdraw into self-imposed isolation just when a bridge to the new community is most needed. If informed by immigration services of the arrival of a new family in its area, the association could welcome it and provide, possibly in a group with other recent immigrants, important information about the community, available social services, housing and employment opportunities, schools and health facilities, religious institutions, and ethnic organizations the family might be encouraged to join. The children's transition might be eased by setting up a "buddy system" to team up new arrivals with others from the same ethnic background already well established in the new community. Different immigrants have different problems, which are probably best understood by members of the same ethnic community who have been through them. The experiences of Italian, Greek, and Portuguese immigrants, where tensions between assimilated teenagers and traditionally oriented parents are common, differ substantially from those of the West Indian immigrant child left behind on the islands to be brought up by a grandmother in a closely knit neighborhood community, who suddenly is sent for by parents who, now financially established, want to reunite their family. Such children, separated from the grandmother and other familiar adults who have become an extended family, and often still reacting to the original separation from parents with feelings of alienation, frustration, and resentment of the parents' expectations for gratitude and obedience, may reply with even more difficult, disturbing, and antisocial behavior (DaCosta 1975).

Immigrant families may often have difficulty accepting service from the usual mental health facilities. Wherever possible, workers, religious leaders, and volunteers from the same ethnic background, with backup of professional mental health consultants who have been through or who are at least sensitive to the problems typical of the particular immigration, may be best equipped to assist the family through the transitional periods. At the same time the opportunity can be used to help them anticipate and therefore prepare for the future, thus strengthening their ability to cope. (Silverman 1978).

Caplan (1976) suggests that social planning do everything possible to support extended families. The term family is used in the sense of people who live in the same household or related persons frequently in touch with each other and bound together by affection. Community organizations, recreation associations, and churches should also modify their facilities and activities to cater to entire families rather than to individual age groups. Caplan gives examples of original ways of helping families, such as the use of retired people to provide liaison between professionals and families or training families to provide help as a group not only to their own members but also to other families.

Children and Social Environments

Children and Schools

How children adjust to the outside world and its institutions (e.g., schools) depends on a number of variables, including how well their families have provided them with the language, social, and emotional preparation needed to master the more formal "curriculum" of the school. Are the security and trust derived from family relationships enough to allow the child to trust and relate to other adults in less familiar environments? The greater the disparity between the intellectual and social skills taught at home and those expected by the school, the more likely a child is to have difficulty adjusting to school. This difficulty may be compounded by the school's reaction to the child. Some schools, especially those that are more curriculum-centered than child-centered, are much less sensitive to the varying needs, abilities, and skills of incoming students. The child who has developed confidence in a supportive family is more likely to approach school enthusiastically, expecting it to be helpful and the teachers to show goodwill. In contrast, the child who has learned that relationships with adults usually bring rejection and disappointment is liable to transfer that suspiciousness into the school. Rutter (1979) has shown that schools can enhance or detract not only from cognitive development and educational achievement but also from social and behavioral development. He and his colleagues demonstrated that certain schools, even in the most disadvantaged areas, promoted not only superior educational achievement but also a reduction in antisocial behavior, truancy, and dropout rates in their students. The variables that seemed to contribute to these significant differences included the cumulative effect of emphasis on an academic atmosphere, student responsibility, and immediate positive rewards for effort. These combined to develop a school ethos that improved not only educational achievement but also behavioral functioning (Rutter et al. 1979).

Children and Hospitals

Ways of minimizing the potentially damaging effects of repeated long-term hospitalization on children have been discussed in detail in chapter 24. The major principles involve avoiding hospitalization whenever possible, preparing children adequately for hospitalization, ensuring that each period in the hospital be as brief as is medically possible, providing the community support services to allow this, and training families to assume as much as possible of the total care of chronically ill children with the assistance of visiting nurses, homemakers, and so forth when required (Shore and Goldston 1978; see also chapter 24).

Continued research is needed into the relative effects of different ways of preparing children both for hospitalization and for therapeutic procedures. Efforts to minimize the potential trauma of these experiences and to enhance children's competence to cope with them should become a regular component of standard pediatric management, not a frill to which lip service is paid. To achieve this, doctors, nurses, and hospital administrators should be trained in the techniques and importance of psychosocial aspects of pediatric care.

Children and the Child Welfare System

The effects on children coming into the care of the child welfare system and ways of preventing or minimizing long-term detrimental effects have been discussed in some detail in chapter 4. Basic principles involve strengthening family life to avoid whenever possible taking children into care; protecting the child's need for continuity of relationships to major attachment figures; assisting children to complete as fully as possible the work of mourning; preparing child and foster parents adequately for placements; and using visits and follow-up support to minimize unnecessary breakdowns and replacements (Steinhauer 1977).

A knowledge and application of the special care required in adoptions of older children (i.e., those beyond six months of age) needs to be more generally appreciated by both social workers and adoptive parents. Additional research is needed to clarify the indications for adoption of such children as opposed to subsidized adoption or planned permanent foster care (foster care with tenure). In the meantime, adoptive parents and adoptee may need time, information, and the assurance of continuing support if they are to develop lasting relationships (see also chapter 4).

THE WIDER ENVIRONMENT

Large metropolitan areas have recently experienced a breakdown of community networks and affiliation—the "sociocultural disintegration" described by Leighton (1971). Where this occurs, it is associated with an increased incidence of psychiatric disability, alienation, and violence in the population, irrespective of socioeconomic background. The incidence of depression, particularly in mothers of young children, also increases, thus compounding the risk of resultant emotional if not physical neglect of those children, many of whom subsequently show behavioral and personality disturbances. The risk of impaired mental health under such circumstances has been identified by Mead (1977) and Coelho and Stein (1977); the effects of family breakdown and the loss of a sense of community in causing a failure to bond to society and resultant predisposition to continuing alienation, depression, vandalism, and violence by Rakoff (1980) and Steinhauer (1980); the effects of cumulative stress on children by Rutter and associates (1974*b*); and the effects on physical health of family disruption by Lynch (1977). It has been suggested that changing social conventions can have similar effects. Wolff (1978) found an increased incidence of cardiac problems among adults coincident with the breakdown of the close extended family, religious, and community networks that had long existed in the town of Roseto, Pennsylvania. To avoid an even greater incidence of stress-related psychological, psychosomatic, and somatic illness in our adult population and of learning problems and behavior disorders in our children, some kind of supportive community network must be reestablished so that individuals can feel respected and supported as children and needed, competent, and responsible as adults.

Any discussion of the wider social environment must include consideration of the availability of ample opportunities to obtain employment compatible with personal expectations. The importance of this is demonstrated by the improved social functioning and reduction in the incidence of psychiatric disorders in a community in which new industry provided jobs for the first time in years (Leighton 1971). In his recent comprehensive review of the literature on the management of antisocial youth, Shamsie (1981) has stressed the degree to which long-term employment seems to protect against antisocial behavior. Although the technological revolution threatens to reduce drastically the work force needed, there is as yet little evidence of planning for alternative activities that will supply the sense of achievement and the financial security needed to provide status and self-esteem. Despite much rhetoric to the contrary, the work ethic is not dead. People in western society still tend to be typed by, to anchor their identity to, and to obtain a major part of their self-esteem from the job they do and the status that they have achieved.

Types of Prevention Programs

Bloom (1968) emphasized that there are three main types of prevention programs: high risk, cohort, and community-wide ones.

High-risk programs target individuals or groups known to be at risk for developing a condition. Examples include genetic screening, the use of amniocentesis in mothers in the high-risk age groups, and programs for pregnant teenagers. During the perinatal period, examples include the identification before discharge from the hospital of high-risk mothers who are observed having difficulty bonding to their newborn babies. A reduced incidence of sociocultural retardation could be achieved by involving both identified high-risk mothers and infants in focused interventions started within the first few months of life and combined with a program of enriched day care.

Cohort programs involve interventions with groups at particular stages of their development, for example, at birth, at school entry, or on entering high school. Examples include assessments of immunization status and screening for vision and hearing impairment at school entry and the use of periodic health and developmental assessments in preschoolers, as is done in France.

Community-wide programs are addressed to everyone living in a particular community or area. The use of newspapers, television, radio, and printed publications are obvious but as yet unevaluated methods of reaching people, although the Ministry of Community and Social Services in Ontario is currently attempting to determine the value of commercial-type television spots about child rearing. The Ministry is also utilizing popular children's products (e.g., disposable diapers) to bring pamphlets about various aspects of child rearing to parents' attention. For several years every family of a first-born child in Louisiana was sent brochures containing information on child development at regular intervals until the child entered the first grade. The same series of brochures has been widely used in other states and in parts of Canada. The province of Alberta is just beginning an attempt to evaluate the effectiveness of these pamphlets in changing child-rearing practices.

Implications for Training

We do not know yet which types or combinations of interventions are most likely to pay off. We may find that helping neighbors become involved with each other so that their neighborhood becomes a community will allow adults, children, and adolescents to use their creative and helping capacities and skills to support each other. Dispelling loneliness and facilitating the development of relationships may, for example, prove to be the most effective of preventive interventions while requiring the least in terms of cost.

The implications of primary prevention, when the kinds and types of expertise needed are considered, are enormous. As we learn more about the effects of such environmental influences as pollution, noise, and overcrowding, the need to consider the "human factor" in developing housing, institutions, and city planning becomes more apparent. The effects on people of changing legislation will require more forethought on the part of politicians. Concern for health and prenatal and perinatal development will involve nutritionists, public health personnel, physicians, obstetricians, and pediatricians. People trained in infant stimulation, early childhood education, and parent training will be needed to facilitate child development in the early years. The humanizing of institutions may require changing attitudes and practices rather than an infusion of funds, but the implications for professional training and the need to inculcate respect for other professional disciplines is apparent. Psychiatry, psychology, and social work can contribute less through direct service than by providing, in a consultative capacity, knowledge about people, about their development and their needs, and about life crises and methods of prevention and response. People who have themselves successfully negotiated life crises such as bereavement, separation, divorce, unemployment, and retirement may be those best qualified to help others deal more effectively with similar crises, but they will still need professional backup to avoid subjective distortion and unnecessary burnout. Inevitably, observers, monitors, and evaluators will also be needed to provide baseline and follow-up data, if the relative effectiveness of various preventive programs is to be determined systematically.

Implications of Primary Prevention for Child Psychiatry

The focus on primary prevention requires a significant shift in attitude from one concerned with treating psychopathology to one directed toward competence promotion; from an individual to a group orientation; from accepting referrals for assessment from other agencies to working with other agencies in joint planning to develop appropriate preventive programs. Child psychiatrists should be in a position to make these shifts because they have been prepared to be concerned not only with the individual child but with that child's family, school, and community, knowing that the child who has difficulty in learning will often develop a secondary emotional or behavioral disorder that will, in turn, place major stress on the family. The child psychiatrist should be aware that the learning environment provided during the crucial early years of a child's development will vary with the family's capacity for successful nurturing, depending on the emotional status of the parents; the success of the relationship between them; the levels of stress in the family; the presence, involvement, or absence of the father; and the presence or absence of other significant adults in the child's environment. The child psychiatrist is in a natural position to bridge some of the difficult interface areas between children and families at risk and those with whom they come in contact, for example, between hospital and family, between family and school, between home and agency, between agency and institution. Child psychiatrists can play an important role in consultation with, in liaison to, and in the education of other physicians and agencies. Finally, they can help identify areas requiring research needed to expand our knowledge about those protective factors that allow many children to develop surprisingly well in spite of grossly unsatisfactory environments as well as those correlated with the development of emotional and behavioral disorders.

SUGGESTIONS FOR FURTHER READING

KESSLER, M., AND ALBEE, G. W. 1977. An overview of the literature of primary prevention. In *Primary prevention of psychopathology: The Issues,* vol. 1, ed. G. W. Albee and J. M. Joffe, pp. 351–399. Hanover, N.H.: University Press of New England.
Recommended for general reading. This chapter presents an excellent synopsis of the major issues in the prevention field from the micro- to the macrolevel; it covers the range of possible strategies, suggests possible intervenors, and discusses the notion that anything that improves the quality of life for children is in the area of prevention.

MARMOR, J. 1975. The nature of the psychotherapeutic process revisited. *Can. Psychiat. Assn. J.* 20(8): 557–565.

Recommended for health care professionals. The author describes several features of the psychotherapeutic process that are common to a wide spectrum of therapeutic modalities, from psychoanalytic to behavioral.

RUTTER, M. 1974. Epidemiological strategies and psychiatric concepts in research on the vulnerable child. In *The child in his family,* vol. 3, *Children at Psychiatric risk,* ed. E. J. Anthony and C. Koupernik, pp. 167–179. New York: John Wiley & Sons.

Recommended for health care professionals. Emphasizes the importance of a data base from which to plan programs. Discusses the interaction of concepts such as risk, stress, vulnerability, and invulnerability.

SAMEROFF, A. J., AND CHANDLER, M. J. 1975. Reproductive risk and the continuum of caretaking casuality. In *Review of child development research,* vol. 4, ed. F. D. Horowitz, et al., pp. 187–244. Chicago: University of Chicago.

Recommended for all health care professionals. Suggests that there is an interaction between factors in the child and those in the family environment and that families may provide a range of environments, from ones that are so good that they can meet the needs of the most vulnerable infant to those that are so inadequate that they cannot meet the needs of the healthiest, most competent baby.

SHORE, M. F., AND GOLDSTON, S. E. 1978. Mental health aspects of pediatric care—Historical review and current status. In *Psychological management of pediatric problems,* vol. 2, ed. P. R. Magrab, pp. 15–53. Baltimore: University Park Press.

Recommended for general reading. Describes the ways in which hospitalization can be reduced and the hospital environment can be ameliorated to reduce stress for the child patient. Includes recommendations about such factors as length of stay, preparation for procedures, and involving parents and child in decision making and care and discharge planning.

28

David N. Mushin

General Principles of Treatment in Child Psychiatry

Introduction

The previous chapters have described children and their development, their relationships within the family and in the broader social context, and the nature of their psychological disorders. While children have much in common with people of all ages, certain features unique to childhood and adolescence need to be considered in planning treatment.

First, it must be recognized that, by and large, children do not seek—and often do not want—treatment for their psychological problems. Generally parents initiate treatment, sometimes in response to the child's asking for help but more often because of their or other adults' concern or discomfort with the child's symptoms and behavior. Adolescents may seek help on their own, but usually the referral defines the child's problems as seen through adult eyes. The clinician should always try to distinguish what the child sees as treatment needs from those of the referring adults. Treatment planning requires intervention at appropriate levels, according to need.

Jane, age four, was referred because of defiant behavior toward her parents. Her mother especially was concerned that Jane would grow up to be unsocialized. On evaluation, Jane was a lively and inquisitive girl who frequently feared punishment and disapproval. Her mother, an inhibited and prudish woman, was threatened by Jane's openness and down-to-earth manner. Elsewhere, for example in kindergarten, Jane was seen as well liked and normal. Rather than changing Jane's behavior, treatment sought to help the mother relax her need to control Jane, which stemmed from her own exaggerated defenses against sexual and aggressive impulses, the extreme repression of which was causing marital conflict. Concurrently Jane's therapist sought to decrease her fear of punishment for any show of initiative.

Second, and as the example demonstrates, clinicians must remember how dependent children are on their environment and especially on their families. Children are not yet ready to function autonomously. As more is learned about family dynamics, it becomes increasingly clear that no one develops independent of family and social influences. Adults, and to some extent older adolescents, can often learn in treatment to deal differently with internal (psychological) problems and to improve their handling of family and social pressures. But in spite of their relative independence, family and social pressures still significantly affect their response to therapy. These social influences are greatly intensified in children, particularly young ones. Ongoing family pressures are a continuing source of stress that can aggravate or perpetuate children's psychological problems. Because of their dependence on their parents, children have less room than adults to withdraw by opting out of the family. The family, without even realizing it, may be determined to keep the focus on the child's problems to divert attention from other even more serious family difficulties. Thus the continuing influence of ongoing family pathology and resistance to change in the child identified as the patient may either support or undermine the treatment. Work with the family and, perhaps, other social systems may be essential to help individual children. If treatment substantially changes any family member, this will put pressure on the existing family equilibrium, unless the family system is adaptable enough to incorporate the change by making compensatory adjustments when necessary.

Third, it must be understood that developmental changes in children are more rapid, more dramatic, and perhaps more fundamental than those that occur later in life. These developmental changes and their impact on child and family are discussed in chapters 1, 2, 3, 9, and 12. From a treatment perspective, a child's developmental status is significant in a number of ways.

The significance of a child's behavior will depend on the child's stage of development. As discussed in chapter 9, normal children periodically show signs of stress related to conflicts intensified by developmental pressures characteristic of a particular stage. The significance of a symptom, for example, depends on whether it is occurring in a two-year-old or a ten-year-old. Temper tantrums are expected in two-year-olds, but the ten-year-old who has repeated tantrums probably has a diagnosable developmental, neurotic, or incipient personality disorder. This fact has major implications for management. When dealing with normal developmental stress, clinicians may just need to reassure or educate the parents, while extensive individual or possibly family therapy would be indicated for one of the more serious conditions.

> Five-year-old Nadia's parents complained of her aggressiveness toward her younger sister. They said she lied, particularly when she had done something wrong, frequently resisted going to bed, and was slow at learning to read. Evaluation revealed that Nadia's development was appropriate for her age. Her parents, though well educated, had little knowledge of developmental norms. Following the assessment, they were reassured about Nadia and given some appropriate reading material. After their anxiety about Nadia had settled somewhat, they could better acknowledge and deal with those marital problems that were the source of much of the anxiety that had been displaced to Nadia.

Emotional and behavioral problems in turn affect children's ongoing development. Because of depression, an eight-year-old may do poorly in school and invite rejection from peers. The resulting learning problems and isolation from peers will further undermine developmental progress. In planning treatment, removing the presenting symptoms may be less important than removing factors blocking ongoing development.

A child's developmental level will also affect the choice of treatment. A three-year-old with very little capacity for conceptualization and abstract expression can best express and resolve troublesome thoughts and feelings through play (i.e., play therapy), whereas most ten-year-olds are better able to discuss issues more directly. Thus the child's developmental level becomes important in choosing the most appropriate way for therapist and child to communicate with each other. As therapy progresses, however, the child may temporarily regress. For many children, this is essential for their treatment. For example, a pseudomature twelve-year-old who initially shunned the playroom might develop, during treatment, an interest in play and in other childish activities that he or she would use to express conflicts and concerns.

Finally, clinicians must recognize that since children's emotional, behavioral, and cognitive problems arise from an interplay of biological, psychological, and social factors (Thomas 1981), all these parameters must be considered before a plan of management is decided on.

> Joseph, at age six, was referred because of hyperactivity. Diagnosed as having minimal brain dysfunction, he had been treated with methylphenidate. Although his behavior had improved, he remained overactive, did poorly at school, could not make or keep friends, and did not pay attention in class. Assessment revealed that in addition to the organic reasons for his overactivity, there were other important factors to consider. Joseph badly lacked self-esteem and was convinced that anything he tried was doomed to failure. He was constantly angry that others didn't appreciate his difficulties but feared asking for help for fear of exposing his deficiencies. This left him a ready target for blame in his family, while in the classroom he was frequently berated for his poor

performance and disruptive behavior. Joseph's parents were ashamed of his difficulties and resented what they felt as the school's blaming them for Joseph's problems. Psychological testing revealed specific learning disabilities that were interfering with academic achievement.

Joseph's treatment involved simultaneous intervention at a number of levels. His medication was continued, but he also began to be seen in individual psychotherapy to improve his self-confidence, his ways of dealing with his many conflicted relationships, and control of his aggressiveness when frustrated. Concurrently Joseph's parents met regularly with a social worker, to understand Joseph and his problems better and to resolve some of the guilt, frustration, and shame his behavior had caused the family. A consultation was arranged with Joseph's school to help the boy, his parents, the teachers, and his therapist work better toward their common goal. Remedial education programs were designed to help Joseph compensate for his learning disability. Both Joseph and his parents were encouraged to set more realistic overall expectations.

These, then, are general factors to consider in planning management for a particular child. The management discussed in this chapter deals largely with secondary and tertiary intervention, as primary intervention is discussed in chapter 27. Although a team of professionals working in a child psychiatric setting was directly involved in Joseph's case, many of a child psychiatrist's interventions do not require direct involvement. Frequently child psychiatrists provide advice and consultation to help parents, physicians, teachers, social workers, and others cope more effectively with children who are either reacting to difficult situations (e.g., marital breakdown) or to periods of heightened developmental stress. With appropriate backing and advice, a family may be able to help a child cope with the loss of a parent (Adam et al. 1982), a pediatrician can handle successfully many conflicts arising from chronic illness or anxiety-provoking diagnostic procedures, and teachers can more effectively manage disruptive classroom behavior.

Direct Forms of Treatment

BIOLOGICAL THERAPIES

Biological therapies in child psychiatry include medication, electroconvulsive therapy, and psychosurgery. The latter two therapies are rarely used with children, as there is little evidence of their effectiveness. Recent advances in knowledge have allowed medication to be used more selectively and effectively, almost always in combination with other forms of intervention. Medication can be particularly helpful in dealing with problems of behavior (e.g., hyperactivity, poor control of aggression; bizarre psychotic behavior). Its use in child psychiatry is discussed in chapter 29.

PSYCHOLOGICAL THERAPIES

Psychological therapies attempt to effect change through the relationship between the therapist and an individual patient, a family, or a group. All therapeutic relationships have a number of common attributes.

One attribute is that a need for help is seen by the patient and/or family. Sometimes the family or the school, not the child or adolescent, perceives the need for help. In such cases, unless the therapist takes time and is able initially to clarify this need with the child, it will be hard to obtain the cooperation and commitment needed for successful treatment.

> Robert, age sixteen, was sent for therapy by his parents because of underachievement at school, rebellious behavior at home, and excessive drinking. Robert insisted that he had no problems but said that neither his parents nor his teachers understood him. He rationalized his drinking as the current social norm for his age group. In the family there was serious marital difficulty and problems between parents and children. Robert repeatedly tried to find out what his parents had said about him to the therapist and what they thought of him. When this was explored, it became clear that he felt unaccepted by others and, in particular, by his parents. Since he remained extremely dependent on them, their approval was crucial to his self-acceptance, and he had internalized their disapproving view of him. His initial bravado changed to a more subdued attitude as he began to express his depression. At this stage he could see that he required help for his difficulties just as his parents did for theirs.

Another attribute of therapeutic relationships is that as they work together, patient and therapist form a particular relationship, sometimes termed a therapeutic alliance. This begins when the patient acknowledges a need for help and looks to the expertise, knowledge, and commitment of the therapist to meet this need. Initial ventilation of problems to an accepting, nonjudgmental adult who tries to understand matters from the child's point of view provides relief from anxiety, increasing the hope that the therapy may succeed. Over time—and it may take a great deal of time—the patient develops an increasing trust and gradually allows the therapy to become increasingly important. Confidence that the therapist has the situation under control, that unacceptable impulses will not get out of hand and that, wherever possible, the therapist will respect the child's wish to keep their discussions confidential further enhance the relationship. To establish the therapist's reliability, children frequently need to test the relationship. For example, Robert, the sixteen-year-old just discussed, mentioned various incidents of drug taking early in therapy, then checked to see if this information was relayed to the parents. It was only after he had convinced himself of the therapist's trustworthiness that he could relax his guard and begin using the therapeutic alliance productively.

A third attribute is that the therapy occurs in a particular setting that can be counted on to provide the materials and structures that the patient needs. The therapist is regularly available at predictable times; play material is provided; and consistent behavioral guidelines are established and maintained. This provides a consistency and security that allow the child to experience the treatment as a "corrective emotional experience."

> Susan was an extremely disturbed six-year-old with poor impulse control and disorganized behavior in a family where the parents were rigid, demanding, and punctilious. There were extreme demands for conformity, cleanliness, and politeness, which Susan was unable to meet. Early in her therapy Susan was guarded and avoided messy materials such as paint, sand, or water. As she gradually gained confidence that the therapist could accept her even if she sometimes made a mess, she began to experiment with these activities but soon had trouble controlling her urge to mess everything in sight. The therapist made it clear that it was fine to have fun as long as her mess was contained within the sandbox, sink, and paint areas. Susan repeatedly returned to such play with pleasure. At about the same time, her parents began to report to their therapist that her behavior at home had become more organized, with fewer uncontrollable outbursts of aggression. It was as if Susan had utilized the material, limits, and acceptance available in her therapy to learn first to tolerate and then to handle successfully her exaggerated fear of losing control of her messiness, which, to her, was associated with almost certain rejection.

The final attribute of all therapeutic relationships is that during the course of therapy, the therapist uses certain strategies to help the patient resolve emotional, cognitive, or behavioral problems. The strategies utilized depend partly on the therapist's theoretical perspective, partly on how the therapist perceives and formulates the patient's needs, and on the therapist's knowledge of which of the available treatments are most likely to succeed. Much of the psychiatric literature describes various intervention strategies and the guidelines for their use. Various examples can be given. In behavior therapy certain target behaviors are identified and strategies evolved to eliminate them. In conjoint family therapy problems within the family system are identified and methods evolved to change family structure and functioning to allow the family to resolve these. Attention may be deliberately focused away from the identified patient and onto the family as a whole. Negative behaviors may be presented with more understanding, in order to change the atmosphere from one of blaming to one geared toward mutual understanding and problem solving. With very resistant families, the therapist may effect change by maneuvering the family into situations where it is extremely difficult not to change (Palazolli et al. 1978). In psychodynamic psychotherapy the therapist encourages a therapeutic alliance and then uses it to understand the thoughts, feelings, defense mechanisms, and conflicts, many beyond conscious awareness, that affect the patient's behavior. The child's responses are clarified and interpretations made to increase the awareness of unconscious feelings and motives that are so often important in perpetuating consciously repudiated behavior. Along with this there is the constant expectation that what patients recognize they can learn to take control over and change. Thus insight can be used to increase understanding but is constantly combined with the expectation that the patient will use the increased understanding to find more successful ways of dealing with problems. These general comments apply to all psychological treatments, but various forms of psychotherapy differ from one another in their theoretical basis and in the techniques they use to bring about change. There are two main groups of psychotherapies: therapies aimed at modifying behavior without directly attempting to identify or resolve conflicts contributing to that behavior, and those aimed at dealing with conflicts and modifying defense patterns to allow for more adaptive (i.e., successful) behavior.

Therapies Aimed at Modifying Behavior Without Directly Attempting to Resolve the Conflicts Leading to That Behavior

Behavior therapy, which falls under this heading, assumes that all behavior, including symptoms, represents a response to stimuli that can be clearly identified and then altered. Unlike dynamically oriented psychotherapists, behavior therapists do not see the need to view behavioral symptoms as an outward expression of inner conflicts. They are less interested in learning about past conflicts and the origins of pathological behavior than in identifying, measuring, and modifying specific "target behaviors" that they will attempt to change.

The behavior therapist takes as a basic model the fact that a stimulus provokes a response. Take, for example, the classic experiment in which Watson had a young child play with a white rat in the laboratory (Watson and Rayner 1920). Watson then repeatedly handed the rat to the child while simultaneously making a loud noise. This invariably frightened the child (i.e., the noise, an unconditioned stimulus, always produced a fear response). As the child learned to associate the appearance of the rat with the occurrence of the noise, the fear became associated not just with the noise but also with the rat. By this stage, the presence of the rat even without the noise was enough to frighten the child, who had learned (i.e., had been conditioned) to fear the rat. The rat's presence was now a conditioned stimulus evoking a learned fear response. Another way to condition the child to fear the rat would have been to punish the child each time the rat was presented (negative reinforcement). Similarly, if the child's mother had screamed and jumped on a chair every time the rat was presented, the child might model him- or herself on mother and develop a fear of white rats. That fear might extend to include other white furry animals (stimulus generalization). If the rat was then presented repeatedly in the absence of any fearful stimuli, the child might in time lose the fear through the process of extinction. If it was presented along with a pleasant stimulus, or if playing with the rat was accompanied by a reward, the child might lose the fear through counterconditioning. The child's mother might also help overcome the fear by playing calmly with the rat in the child's presence, thus providing a model, this time for a nonfearful response.

These concepts are basic to learning theory and its systematic application in behavior therapy. Good descriptions of its use as a treatment technique are provided by Werry and Wollersheim (1967), Brown (1972) and Yule (1977). An important part of behavior therapy is clear problem definition. Certain "target" symptoms—behaviors or feelings that are most distressing to the patient, the parents, or others—are identified. These might be isolated symptoms—for example, temper tantrums or a fear of dogs—or they might form part of a more generalized pathological process—for example, stealing as a symptom of long-standing feelings of emotional deprivation or disruptive classroom behavior that masks a learning disability. The problem is analyzed to define stimuli that elicit the behavior and responses that either sustain or alter it. Thus temper tantrums may occur when a child is ignored by the mother and may be intensified when she becomes frustrated and throws up her hands in despair or yells and spanks the child. On the other hand, they may diminish when she firmly has the child remain in his or her room until the child is ready to deal reasonably with what is upsetting.

The factors in the relationship between therapists and patients described earlier also apply to behavior therapists. Someone—either the child, the family, or another important person in the child's life—feels a need for help. A cooperative relationship is set up between child and therapist. Initially therapist and family (hopefully including the child) agree on the target behaviors to be changed and work together to define factors that evoke and maintain them. The therapist, using his or her knowledge of the family and of learning theory, proposes ways to eliminate the target behaviors. These might include: (1) identifying and eliminating stimuli that perpetuate the target behavior; (2) avoiding responses that positively reinforce the target behavior; (3) prescribing a regime that fails to reinforce or punishes unwanted behavior (thus encouraging its extinction), while positively reinforcing (rewarding) more desired forms of behavior (an approach called operant conditioning).

> Melody, aged twelve, resisted chores around her group home and was antagonistic and quarrelsome with everyone. If the staff attempted to hold her to her responsibilities or to explore why she was so oppositional, she responded with endless arguments, accusations, and blaming of others, followed by storming out of the home. Melody had recently resumed shoplifting, and the staff were unable to persuade her to behave in a less antisocial manner. Things had reached the point where she was about to be discharged from the group home. Neither she nor the staff wanted this. The staff were feeling helpless, resentful, and out of control. Melody was frightened, angry, and, at that point, incapable of modifying her behavior. Since the usual treatment strategies of the group home were not helping, it was decided to institute a behavior modification program.

Accordingly, Melody was told by the staff that unless she controlled her behavior, her placement would break down. Melody agreed. The staff suggested a behavior modification program, which Melody accepted. Together they drew up a list of target behaviors to be eliminated (e.g., messy room, disobedience, fighting, swearing, stealing). For each occurrence of these behaviors, Melody would spend a set amount of time sitting alone in her bedroom (i.e., time out). Failure to serve her time, arguing, or leaving the group home when there was time to be served would automatically lead to additional time out. All unacceptable behaviors and the time allotted to each were charted and posted on the kitchen wall. On a second chart was a list of points that Melody could earn for approved behaviors, such as cleaning up her room, washing the dishes, doing one hour's homework, earning a satisfactory school report, and so on. These could be used to earn privileges otherwise unavailable. The "rate of exchange" had been negotiated in advance; Melody must earn 5 points to go downtown on her own, 2 points to wear makeup, and so on. Each week Melody and the staff would meet to adjust penalties, rewards, and the ways in which Melody could spend points to keep the program both fair and therapeutically effective.

This example illustrates how Melody and the staff members clearly identified target behaviors they wished to extinguish. They combined both negative reinforcement of unacceptable behavior (time spent in the bedroom) and positive reinforcement of desirable behavior (points to be exchanged for privileges). As a disruptive or socially unacceptable behavior was relinquished, the environment—staff, peers, teachers—spontaneously reinforced the change. Generalization occurred; for example, Melody was negatively reinforced only for agreessive or antisocial behavior occurring within the group home, but she began to behave more acceptably outside the home as well. Her relationships with children in the neighbourhood and at school also improved.

Another form of behavior therapy involves extinguishing unwanted behavior or feelings via desensitization. This has proved useful in treating phobias and certain somatic conditions. First the child is trained to relax him- or herself deeply. This feeling of relaxation is then used to alter the relationship between a feared stimulus and response. A hierarchy of situations affecting the fear stimulus is drawn up, ranging from the least to the most frightening. These are gradually and sequentially presented to the child during periods of relaxation, starting with the least threatening. The child may use the technique of relaxation to overcome fear or discomfort occurring outside the therapy session.

Michael, age nine, became phobic about riding in elevators. He was initially taught to relax and instructed to paractice this at home. This in itself gave him some control over his fears. He was then encouraged to imagine riding in elevators while in a relaxed state but was told to relax whenever he was becoming anxious. The therapy then moved to sitting outside elevators when relaxed, looking inside a stationary elevator, standing inside a stationary elevator, riding an elevator with the therapist, riding an elevator with his mother, and finally his working an elevator by himself. Michael's refusal to ride in elevators had

619

been a particular source of conflict with his mother, and with the removal of his phobia their relationship improved.

While behavior therapy may be performed in a clinic setting, it is frequently extended by training parents to continue the program at home. Parents are taught to identify and manipulate the contingencies that perpetuate (i.e., reinforce) target behaviors occurring in the home. Changing the parents' attitude and behavior may provide positive models for the child. In some cases, intermittent reinforcement of the desired behavior will be necessary to prevent extinction of the change.

> Three-year-old Helen refused to eat despite her mother's constant encouragement and concern about her low weight. It was so important to the mother that her children eat large amounts of food that mealtime became a battle between mother and daughter. In addition, Helen received much attention from her parents by refusing to eat, but the frustrated parents spent little time with her except when she was misbehaving. The parents were instructed to feed Helen only as much as she wanted and to let her take as long as she wished to eat. Concurrently the parents were told to spend set periods each day playing with Helen, giving her attention at these times. Soon after Helen began getting the attention she needed in neutral or pleasant situations instead of through struggles over food, she gradually began asking for more food at mealtimes and the battles with the parents greatly decreased.

Behavior therapy is helpful in modifying unwanted symptoms and behavior in a variety of conditions including neurotic disorders (e.g., phobias), psychophysiological disorders (e.g., enuresis and asthma), conduct disorders, and psychoses (e.g., autistic children). Before instituting a behavioral regime, the therapist should evaluate child and family thoroughly to establish which target behaviors to modify and which contingencies (i.e., factors within the family that are positively and negatively reinforcing them) to utilize. Melody's antisocial behavior was treated successfully using behavioral techniques. However, had her behavior been a symptom of severe depression, it would not have been enough just to eliminate the surface behaviors; some way of helping Melody deal more successfully with the underlying depression would have had to be found.

Therapies Aimed at Dealing with Conflicts and Modifying Defense Patterns to Allow More Adaptive Behavior.

Chapters 9 and 12 deal with the determinants of childhood psychopathology as seen primarily from a psychodynamic, developmental, and family systems point of view. The constitutional makeup of the child, the vicissitudes of development, and the child's interaction with the family and the outside world determine how each child mediates between biological drives and external demands and, later, those of the developing conscience. The process of mediation is aided by the example (role modeling) and the caring qualities of parents, and by various defense mechanisms (see chapter 12). The therapies discussed in this section are based on the assumption that symptoms of both behavioral and/or emotional disturbance result from underlying psychopathology derived from developmental and neurotic conflicts (see chapter 12). Thus these treatments deal with the child's internal psychological structure and not just with external stimuli, even though the latter contribute to and may also perpetuate symptomatic behavior.

> Roger, age five, was referred because he lit fires secretly and in potentially dangerous places, for example, under the house. As a result, his mother needed to keep close watch over him. There was a direct connection between the fire-setting and the rewards that came from the increased attention and concern of his mother, who otherwise remained preoccupied with her own problems, paying little attention to her children. Further investigation revealed that Roger was confused and frightened about his parents' recent marital separation. He felt abandoned by both parents, and nurturing parent figures played little part in his play. He did, however, express strong angry and destructive feelings by repeatedly destroying parent figures by accidents or fires in his play. In drawing his family, Roger portrayed himself hiding in the fireplace among the flames, which he said couldn't hurt him. His parents acknowledged their difficulty coping with the dependency needs and the aggressive behavior of their children.

Roger's fire-setting seemed to have a number of determinants.

1. It allowed him to express the rage he felt but could not direct at his parents.
2. It served as a counterphobic defense, that is, it helped him ward off feelings of powerlessness and helplessness by doing things that, in his fantasies, helped him feel invulnerable and indestructable.
3. It enabled Roger to feel in control of the dangerous situation at home. The fires that might destroy the family were of his making, while the disruption of the parents' marriage was beyond his control. This helped him deny his feelings of anxiety and helplessness concerning the family breakup.
4. As often occurs with young children, Roger felt partially responsible for breaking up his parents' marriage. Setting fires and being punished for them allowed him some relief from guilt, by shifting the focus from the more threatening situation of the marital breakdown to the more tangible one of his fire-setting.
5. The fires were considered Roger's attempt to communicate to his mother his perception of the dangerousness of the family situation and of his own aggressiveness and hostility.
6. The setting of fires had obviously provided increased attention from his parents, who had previously tended to ignore his needs.

The therapist recognized early in the therapy as Roger began to express his fantasies, at times verbally and at times in symbolic form in play, that he was not consciously aware of the determinants of his fire-setting. Therapy was designed to deal with these unconscious processes so as to help Roger cope better with his life and to decrease interference with his ongoing psychological development. In instituting therapy, a key role was played by the attributes of the therapeutic relationship common to psychological therapies.

Such psychodynamically oriented psychotherapies vary according to the depth of the unconscious processes they seek to unravel, the patient's capacity to benefit from understanding conflicts (i.e., insight), the therapist's theoretical orientation, the family's level of functioning, and certain practical considerations such as the family's willingness and ability to attend treatment sessions regularly.

As previously mentioned, children are inevitably involved in family relationships. To help a child, other family members, at least the parents, must somehow be involved in the therapeutic process. It would be counterproductive to teach Roger to recognize and express directly feelings of abandonment and rage if the parents, unable to accept those feelings, became more punitive and rejecting. Unresolved personal conflicts that each parent brings into a marriage or ongoing marital conflicts may cause major distortions in the parents' ability to perceive accurately and respond effectively to children's needs. Disturbed children are frequently disturbing, and parental anxiety and distress often interfere despite even the parents' conscientious attempts to understand and meet their children's needs. Thus it is essential that when children are seen in individual psychotherapy, parents are concurrently involved in appropriate counseling or therapy. Depending on the nature of the problem, the parents may need help in any or all of the following ways.

1. They may need help to recognize and understand a child's conflicts, needs, and developmental requirements and to tolerate the direct expression of previously repressed feelings and needs.
2. Marital conflicts may need to be mediated or resolved in order for the child to be helped.
3. The parents may need to examine and, when necessary, modify their expectations and attitudes toward their child. These may in part be distorted by the child's stirring up in them intense feelings and conflicts left unresolved from their experiences in their families of origin.

As a child, Mrs. S had been repeatedly rejected and degraded by her own mother. Any criticism by her six-year-old daughter Edna provoked intense rage and physical abuse of Edna. Mrs. S complained that Edna was selfish and did not do enough for her. Edna's normal behavior was reawakening in her mother intense feelings of deprivation and rage, originally experienced at the hands of her own mother but now distorting her perceptions of and relationship to her daughter.

4. One or both parents may require personal psychotherapy to resolve psychological difficulties that, as well as affecting both that parent's life and marriage, are having major and destructive effects on that individual's ability to parent.
5. Many children and adolescents find early in their therapy that having repressed feelings stirred up is an unpleasant and painful experience. They often try to avoid this discomfort and escape from therapy by trying to convince the parents that the therapist they have selected is "no good" or that they "never say a word, so it's a complete waste of time and money sending me there." Parents

often fail to realize that many such children, while ambivalent about their therapy, are nevertheless using it well. Unless the parents understand this as the child's way of trying to sabotage the therapy, they may fall into the trap and either terminate it or transfer the child to another therapist. Instead they should be encouraged to recognize this for what it is—a not unusual resistance to facing and dealing with painful personal conflicts in therapy—and should point out to the child that their family is obviously having difficulties and that it is up to each of them, the child included, to see to it that the sources of conflict and tension are discussed openly and frankly in their treatment.

The child whom the family identifies as the patient may be seen in individual psychotherapy, collaborative therapy, conjoint family therapy, or group therapy.

Individual Psychotherapy. Individual psychotherapy involves direct interaction between a therapist and a child, directed toward resolution or improved handling of the child's intrapsychic problems. The therapist first tries to form a therapeutic alliance with the child. The use of this alliance then varies, depending on whether primarily intensive (i.e., exploratory) or primarily supportive psychotherapy is intended.

In *intensive psychotherapy,* the therapist emphasizes helping the child recognize and understand the nature of conflicts and the ways that the anxiety and defenses they generate distort perceptions and interfere with functioning. Roger, for example, would be helped to understand his problems dealing with his aggression and his feelings of guilt concerning his parents' failed marriage. He would also be helped toward an understanding of his own defenses, for example, that he needed to deny the dangerous nature of fires and that it was safe in therapy to express some of his rage and to allow himself to be vulnerable in the presence of the therapist even thought she could, had she not understood Roger's weaknesses, attack or reject him as had others in the past. There would be appropriate objects and toys available for Roger to facilitate play activities and, depending on his age and level of maturity, he and his therapist would communicate with each other either verbally or through the metaphor of play. An intense relationship between Roger and his therapist would develop. This might require that Roger be seen two to three times per week, with the therapist choosing to remain relatively nondirective to allow Roger to develop and project (or transfer) his own fantasies onto the therapist, minimally contaminated by the reality of what the therapist was really like. The therapist would continue to accept Roger in spite of immature and infantile behavior but would limit those behaviors when appropriate and would help him explore the determinants of those behaviors to find other, less destructive ways of expressing feelings and resolving the related conflicts. Under such circumstances, invariably there would be times in which Roger viewed the relationship with the therapist in distorted ways. Roger, in fact, became furious at his therapist at the end of every session, indicating through his play that the therapist did not care for him. Actually she cared about him a great deal, but by avoiding expressing this directly, she encouraged Roger to project (or transfer) onto her his feelings of not being cared for, which echoed earlier experiences with other important figures. Roger's feelings of rejection by the therapist were an echoing of feelings of rejection the boy originally experienced from his mother. His feeling that his mother did not care about him was unconsciously transferred onto the therapist. Therapists can use feelings of rejection and abandonment currently being experienced within the therapeutic alliance to help a child become aware of how much his or her perceptions of current relationships are contaminated and distorted by feelings left over from the past. A child may be more able to look objectively at the relationship with the therapist than at the more conflict-laden one with the parents. Strategies of intensive psychotherapy include clarifying for children the nature of their actions and responses and interpreting issues apparent to the therapist, though not consciously understood by the patients.

Play therapy is not a separate and distinct form of treatment, but rather individual or group therapy in which both patient and therapist utilize play rather than talking to communicate with each other. In most therapy with children, communication between child and therapist is sometimes verbal and sometimes nonverbal, through play. In general, the younger the child, the more likely play is to be the major medium of communication. The essential process of play therapy, however, is the same as that of individual or group therapy. The cases of Roger and Susan give examples of how a child and a therapist can use play to communicate with each other.

Intensive psychotherapy requires a patient able to continue to function reasonably in the face of a process that temporarily stirs up periods of regressive (i.e., less mature) feelings and behavior, while bringing up to the surface impulses that have long been repressed. Both child and family must be able to cope with the anxiety-provoking material that is elicited. When conducted on an outpatient basis, intensive psychotherapy also requires that the child learn to differentiate her reactions to the therapist from those to the parent; that is, the patient must have some capacity to understand, tolerate, recognize, and learn from distortions occurring in her perceptions of the therapist. Such therapy is time consuming and involving. It is reserved for children with entrenched neurotic and personality disorders and occasionally for older psychotic children who are able to establish appropriate therapeutic relationships.

Supportive psychotherapy attempts less to uncover conflict and develop insight than to use the therapeutic alliance to direct the child away from conflict toward more appropriate patterns of behavior. Therapy is used to drain off anxiety and to help the child learn to deal with day-to-day problems in a realistic and effective manner. In supportive psychotherapy, the therapist is more likely to answer questions directly and to indicate personal opinions. Fantasy material is deemphasized by the focus on the child's handling of day-to-day problems. Supportive rather than intensive psychotherapy is indicated for the child in danger of being overwhelmed by the turmoil of daily living; for the child whose intellectual limitations stand in the way of working out the questions posed in intensive psychotherapy; or for families and children who are not psychologically minded and who, therefore, are unprepared to explore conflict situations in depth. Supportive therapy is also indicated where a child's symptoms seem to result from a developmental crisis (see chapter 20) in the life of child or family, following the resolution of which normal developmental patterns and interactions will be reestablished. After a period of supportive psychotherapy, some patients are better able to cope with their feelings and to tolerate their internalized conflicts. At that stage, the therapist might decide either that no further treatment is indicated or shift to a more exploratory type of therapy.

> James, age eight, quickly became paranoid in therapy sessions, imagining that spies were hiding in the wall, that there were secret cupboards, and that he would be taken from sessions and placed in jail. After repeated reassurance regarding the confidential nature of his sessions, and sensing the therapist's acceptance of him, his play began to feature sequences where people would be drowned or killed in accidents. This play was poorly structured and had many sadistic elements. At first his therapist tried to help James structure his play and look for solutions to the problems that the play figures were encountering, for example, ways to prevent them from drowning. After a series of such interventions, the play became more organized, and James began to talk about his feeling of being an unworthy person who might easily be rejected by his parents, his therapist, and anyone else to whom he felt close. As he subsequently showed more ability to tolerate discussion of internal conflicts, the therapist's role became less one of providing structure and more one of encouraging James to bring forward his conflicts.

Intensive and supportive psychotherapy as defined represent two ends of a spectrum. Most psychotherapy with children contains both exploratory and supportive elements. In addition, some children are seen in planned short-term psychotherapy in which a prior decision is made to treat a child for a predetermined number of sessions—usually six to ten. The therapist actively and directly engages the child (and/or family) in treatment and then, in a structured way, focuses the therapy to help the child and family identify and learn more effective ways to deal with a selected and limited number of key conflict areas.

Collaborative Therapy. As previously mentioned, when children are seen individually, it is important also to involve the parents in the therapeutic process. Especially in more supportive types of therapy, the same therapist frequently sees both child and parents. In more intensive psychotherapy, it is important that the relationship between child and therapist develop without being contaminated by the therapist learning about the child from what the parents say. Rather the therapist must allow the child to bring things into the therapy at his own rate, and the child should know that the therapist is his ally, not the parents'. In such situations a second therapist or counselor, often a social worker, works with the parents. Both therapists then collaborate together between therapeutic contacts. Feedback to the child's therapist may warn of impending crises in the family or help the therapist conceptualize more clearly the interpersonal component of the child's behavior, the reason and motives behind parental attitudes and behavior, and so forth. Feedback to the parents' therapist may provide some warning that the child is undergoing particular conflicts in therapy that may for a while cause difficult behavior in the home.

It is not infrequent that parents decide to terminate their child's psychotherapy prematurely if they are made anxious by changes in the child's behavior for which they have not been prepared. Parents concerned about a withdrawn, shy child who has difficulty with normal self-assertion and getting along with others may have difficulty as their child begins to express more directly feelings, concerns, anger, and so on. Many families need to retain one child as the "sick" member of the family (see discussion of scapegoating, chapter 3). Removal of the scapegoated child's symptoms often aggravates the parents' difficulties, intensifying their anxiety and precipitating a premature withdrawal and termination. Collaboration between child's and parents' therapists helps each maintain an overall perspective of the treatment process, minimizing parental anxiety and the risk of such disruptions.

Conjoint Family Therapy. In conjoint family therapy, one or more therapists treat the family as a unit rather than concentrating on the psychopathology of an individual family member whom the family has identified as the patient. Thus while the individual psychotherapist deals primarily with the internalized psychopathology of individuals, the family therapist treats the family system to which these individuals identified as patients belong. This is not an either/or situation, as both intrapsychic and interpersonal pathology can usually be found in the families of children who have emotional or behavioral problems. It is rather a question of viewing the same situation from two different vantage points and therefore intervening at two different points of entry.

Family therapists intervene primarily at the interpersonal level, assuming that if the family can identify and resolve its interpersonal and structural difficulties, its members will be freed to function more successfully, both individually and collectively, without further help. Family therapists deal indirectly with the psychopathology of individuals. While many concede that one determinant of disturbed interpersonal functioning is the behavior resulting from intrapsychic conflict, their prime concern is with manifest behavior, the relationships between family members, and the pathological structure of the family system. Family therapy implies that if pathological family structure and interaction can be modified, the psychopathology of individual family members will in turn be relieved, even without having been confronted primarily and directly. To do this the therapist must first make family members aware of the gaps and distortions in their communications. Family therapists can accomplish this in the following ways.

1. By their personal response to each family member, by establishing rapport, empathy, and communication between themselves and the family, and by serving as a model of someone who listens as well as talks.
2. By providing an atmosphere in which issues can be examined and discussed rather than argued. By listening to everyone, family therapists help family members hear one another. By supporting silent members to speak up, they encourage ventilation of negative feelings and serve as both a safety valve and a mediator. They promote the clear, direct expression of both positive and negative feelings but avoid scapegoating. They help convert concealed conflicts into open expressions of feeling that, when denied an outlet, serve as foci of mounting tension that is periodically discharged in an indirect, unclear, explosive, and destructive manner.
3. By helping family members identify the basic issues around which they have been struggling in a confused, frustrating, and nonproductive manner. Family therapists do this by locating and counteracting the various barriers, sources of confusion, and defensive maneuvers that perpetuate the family's confusion. This allows them to help the family identify the real problems, and to relate day-to-day issues to recurrent patterns and chronic sources of vulnerability. In so doing, they use confrontation and interpretation to undermine resistances and to reduce circular conflict, guilt, and fear.
4. By serving as an educator and a reality tester. In this way they focus family members' attention on how they communicate with one another. They make family members aware of covert levels of their own communication, thus encouraging them to communicate more fully, more directly, and more clearly with one another. If the family can do so, it will have a safety valve to use to identify precisely areas of conflict and to work together to find appropriate and generally acceptable solutions.
5. By bringing out into the open power struggles within the family. Family therapists do this by making families aware of the covert and frequently pathological ways in which they manipulate or dominate each other. This often helps members recognize (a) why others react to "innocent" requests or remarks as they do; (b) why minor incidents are continually being inflated into major ones; (c) how much disagreements are settled on the basis of who is boss rather than what is appropriate.
6. By demonstrating to family members how and why so little clear communication occurs. Family therapists clarify, for example, the degree to which members talk but do not listen (i.e., two monologues rather than one dialogue); the degree to which they battle over irrelevancies, upsetting each other but never identifying or resolving the basic issues; the degree to which disagreements, rather than being resolved, are merely sidestepped by a false consensus in which one member appears to give in to keep the peace, only to sabotage the false agreement later.

Some families respond readily to a therapist's attempts to clarify the nature of their difficulties and can, with relatively little resistance, use what they have learned to find newer and more effective ways of communicating and problem solving. In other families, the homeostatic principle (see chapter 3) may evoke considerable resistance to any proposed change.

These are families who may demand more time and involvement than many primary physicians or counselors have available. They might be considered for a referral for psychiatric consultation and psychotherapy.

An example of the therapeutic utilization of the observed family interaction follows.

> A family consisting of the parents and two teenage children was seen in family therapy. The identified patient was fifteen-year-old John, who was underachieving at school and defiant of his parents. In a particular session John, who resented the treatment, sat quietly scowling, refusing to respond to other family members or the therapist. Both parents complained that this deliberate noninvolvement was typical of his behavior at home.
>
> Near the end of the session, John complained about how destructively his parents and brother behaved at times. His father then became extremely angry, stating that this was how John always wasted family time by avoiding the main subject, namely his school problems. The therapist pointed out that the father became angriest just as John did what he (the father) had expected of him, namely join in and communicate his opinions and feelings to the family. They then discussed how unacceptable it was for John to point out conflicts or difficulties in family members other than himself. Thus John was placed in a double bind: they were angry at him if he avoided speaking up, but when he did so, they would get angry unless he said what they wanted to hear.

This important family dynamic might have been harder to detect and demonstrate if family members were not seen together.

Treating the family as a unit almost always intensifies ongoing family interaction by focusing on pathological areas of functioning. This tendency, which contributes so much to the effectiveness of family therapy when properly selected and applied, can be destructive and may even contribute to family breakdown if used inappropriately or ineffectively.

Contraindications to treatment of the family as a unit include:

1. Evidence of a malignant and irreversible trend toward breakup of the family, except where "separation counseling" is indicated.
2. Unwillingness or inability of the family as a unit or of key family members (especially the parents) to tolerate open discussion of contentious issues in a manner that allows all members and the therapist the right to question, to disagree, and to express how they feel.
3. An inability to obtain the involvement of all family members whose presence the therapist considers essential to the success of treatment.
4. The therapist's inability to avoid being drawn into transactional games according to the family's rules, thus causing a loss of objectivity and perspective as the therapist becomes part of the pathological family system rather than a separate and objective observer.
5. Should the family situation or the behavior or adjustment of any individual member continue to deteriorate in spite of ongoing family treatment, psychiatric consultation is indicated.
6. Should severe scapegoating persist or intensify as the examiner tries to explore other sources of family tension, a temporary shift to a collaborative approach should be considered.

Group Therapy. Group therapy is of particular value in treating children with problems in peer relationships. The format varies with age and the needs of the children in the group. Whereas younger children may play together in the presence of the therapist (activity group therapy), adolescents are more likely to discuss their difficulties more directly. Therapeutic groups are usually balanced to include some children who are overcontrolled and others who are frequently overwhelmed by explosive outbursts of intense feeling. The more inhibited members may benefit from the stimulation obtained from their more volatile peers, while at the same time serving as a damper on the impulsiveness of members whose controls are precarious. Group members help each other both by serving as models for each other and by confronting others with unacceptable behavior and directing them toward new ways of managing. The exposure to other group members stimulates and supports emotional expression, and the bonds formed between the children in a group may be important in enhancing self-esteem and in helping them develop the confidence and social skills they need to risk themselves in less protected social situations.

Therapeutic Nursery Schools. Another alternative specifically designed to address the treatment needs of the emotionally disturbed preschool child is the therapeutic nursery school. Programs vary from setting to setting, and even within the same setting. Therapists and teachers take on many roles, interacting with the children individually and in groups, offering support, providing structure and limits, and encouraging affective expression through play and verbalization (Enzer 1979). For most preschool children, peer-group interaction contributes to the overall therapeutic effort. Interactions with nonfamily members reveal different aspects of a child's functioning, daily conflict shifts, and means of coping with them (Furman 1979).

Many programs involve parents, particularly mothers, and some provide group or individual therapy for the parents (Enzer 1979). Therapeutic nursery schools are often recommended so that the parents can be actively involved in helping their child. The schools provide some respite from the strain of living with a severely disturbed child without necessitating removal of that child from the family. This is extremely beneficial for the parent-child interaction. Teachers and therapists serve as role models, helping parents develop greater sensitivity to their child's needs. Parents may also find comfort in the realization that their child poses a problem even for the "professional" (Enzer 1979).

Many serious problems in a preschooler can be treated in a therapeutic nursery school. Pervasive disorders, problems in separation from the mother or persisting responses to earlier separations, conduct disorders that are most apparent outside the family, and disorders in children whose parents, due to prominent blind spots, are unable to recognize and deal appropriately with the child's behavior, are disorders for which therapeutic nursery schools may prove particularly helpful (Furman 1979).

Summary of Psychotherapies

The various forms of psychotherapy are not mutually exclusive. The choice of therapy for a particular child is a complicated issue, involving many factors. For any child or family the therapy of choice may change depending on that family's need at a given time. The decision to employ one or more of the psychotherapeutic techniques described herein does not necessarily preclude the selective use of social intervention, educational techniques, medication, or behavior modification, under appropriate circumstances.

SOCIAL INTERVENTION

As children are more dependent on the environment than adults, they may be more vulnerable to pathogenic surroundings and less able to deal successfully with the resulting stresses without outside help. Substandard housing and poverty may play an important role in family disintegration. Some families benefit greatly if directed toward community resources that can provide support and improve their living conditions. Help is needed, particularly in times of crisis and transition. Immigrant families who move into communities where even the language is strange find that the life style, which their teenagers rush to embrace, clashes with their own old world and religious traditions (see chapter 27). Social and ethnic agencies may help such parents make contact with a similar ethnic group within the new community with which they can identify, a group that may be able to interpret the customs and mores of the larger community and provide them with the security they need to avoid alienating their adolescents permanently. Schools and teachers can do much either to alleviate or to aggravate learning or behavioral problems. Even if organic or psychological components of such a problem exist, a modified approach or special placement by the school may be necessary to salvage a child's potential for learning and adjusting.

Finally, some children are rejected, neglected, or abused emotionally and even physically by their parents. Such situations may urgently demand some form of community intervention, though the exact form of this may vary from counseling the family or providing a specially trained homemaker to, in the last resort, taking the child into care as a ward of a children's aid society or child welfare association (see chapter 4).

RESIDENTIAL TREATMENT OF CHILDREN

Wherever possible, children should not be removed from their own families in order to receive treatment. Sometimes, however, it is necessary to remove a child, at least temporarily. Some parents are so depriving and abusive—usually they too were similarly deprived and abused as children—that their children need placement for their own protection. Sometimes children are so upsetting to the family and community because of severe conduct disorders or symptoms of psychosis that, despite attempts to support and guide the family, they provoke severe family and even community disorganization, rejection, and attack. Other cases may have proved refractory even to an adequate trial of outpatient therapy. In any of these situations, it may be appropriate to admit the child to a treatment setting more suited to his or her physical, emotional, and therapeutic needs. This step should not be taken lightly, as the very act of removing a child from the family may prove more damaging than the situation from which relief is sought.

A variety of resources provide alternative living situations; these range from foster homes and group homes, which provide some degree of supervision, guidance, and support, to the more structured, staff-operated group homes and treatment centers.

The term residential treatment center includes a wide range of environments, each with its own standards for admission. The same clinical picture might guarantee a child's admission to one treatment center yet exclude her from another, depending on general factors such as age and sex and on specific factors such as "treatability" and "fit," both of which are highly subjective. "Treatability" refers to what is seen as the child's potential for responding to treatment, while "fit" defines the child's compatibility with other patients and suitability for the particular therapeutic milieu (Noshpitz 1975).

Treatment centers can provide more external controls over the child's total living environment. Many have cottage or group home arrangements with eight to ten children of the same age in each unit. Trained child-care workers assigned to each group serve both as surrogate parents and as therapists who help the child cope with emotional and behavioral difficulties as they occur in the course of daily living. This form of treatment is known as *milieu therapy*. It may be supplemented by medication, direct psychotherapy of the child, or therapeutic involvement of the entire family. This treatment is usually provided by an interdisciplinary team consisting of a psychiatrist, psychologist, social worker, and child-care workers. The team evaluates the child's status and progress at various times, reformulates treatment goals and the roles of the various team members, and works out techniques of intervention for best achieving goals. In the residential treatment center, round-the-clock interventions are used to identify and attempt to resolve the child's conflicts as they occur or to modify behavior through the application of learning theory. Residential settings can sometimes assist the autistic child toward socialization, more appropriate behavior, and the development of speech. For the severely retarded child, a protective environment with constant nursing care may be required.

Children are often placed in residential treatment more because of external factors not directly related to their psychopathology than from a predictable response to universally acceptable diagnostic criteria (Sackin and Meyer 1976). Political, economic, and community pressures often have more influence than clinical considerations. The expense of residential treatment is prohibitive for many families, and when such treatment is subsidized, the claim on public funds can lead to confusion or conflict between courts and treatment facilities (Steinhauer 1978). In numerous jurisdictions strong and often predominantly economic pressures toward deinstitutionalization have led to the closing of training schools and massive reductions in available treatment beds. Predictably, this has resulted in many seriously disturbed and antisocial youngsters being accommodated, often inadequately, in foster and group homes that are already overextended and often poorly equipped to deal with them (see chapter 4). When such placements break down in crisis, it becomes increasingly difficult to find a setting or agency able and prepared to accept responsibility for the child. All too often such youngsters continue to deteriorate while being shunted here and there in a mental health system unable to accommodate them (Holden 1976). At the other extreme, many children are admitted to residential institutions because appropriate facilities were not available for them (Pappenfort and Kilpatrick 1969). Despite warnings against inappropriate referrals for residential care simply because no other service is convenient or available, psychiatrists often feel forced to admit children because of a lack of appropriate alternative resources.

Probably the major point of general agreement is that residential treatment is indicated when the child's psychopathology warrants removal from the usual familial and social environments (Rinsley 1974) to protect the family from the child, to protect the child from the environment, to protect the child from his or her own destructiveness, or others from the child's misbehavior (Noshpitz 1975), because the family can no longer endure the distress caused by the child's behavior, (Sackin and Meyer 1976) or because medical management is one aspect of the treatment needed. Residential treatment is not indicated when separation from the family would prove more catastrophic than the child continuing to live with the symptoms (Noshpitz 1975).

In summary, as long as family and community feel that they can cope with even a seriously disturbed child's behavior, such a child can be maintained in the community. Most referrals for admission occur when those immediately responsible for the child feel helpless, angry, frightened, and no longer able to cope. Most admissions occur when the admitting officer is convinced of an existing or impending crisis that nothing short of removal from the home and placement in a stable but actively therapeutic environment will alleviate. Thus, in the final analysis, the decision for admission may be determined more by the environment's inability to cope than by the child's psychopathology.

Most seriously disturbed children can be treated best without separating them from their families. If residential treatment is required, the very act of removing the disturbed child from the family may produce a sense of relief that a thorn has been removed from the family flesh. Ideally clinicians will use this period of relief to help the family work to create a more stable situation to which the child will eventually return. It is not uncommon for the family to see the child's placement as proof that the child alone is the problem. This may cause family members to resist attempts to involve them in ongoing counseling or therapy, as they close ranks to permanently exclude the "bad" or "sick" child. Thus removal of a child from the family may create a crisis in that child's relationship with the family. Therefore, every effort should be made to keep family and child involved with each other and with the therapeutic program.

SUGGESTIONS FOR FURTHER READING

ADAMS, P. L. 1974. *A primer of child psychotherapy.* Boston: Little, Brown & Co.
    A brief and extremely clear description of the process of assessment and treatment. Intended for the beginner but a good review for the experienced practitioner as well.
ALDRICH, C. K. 1975. Psychotherapy for the primary care physician. In *American handbook of psychiatry,* 2nd ed., vol. 5, ed. D. X. Freedman and J. E. Dyrud, pp. 739–756. New York: Basic Books.
    After discussing the role of the primary care physician, provides an excellent review of major issues involved in the process of diagnosis and psychotherapy. Clinical examples and bibliography.
ANTHONY, E. J. 1974. Psychotherapy of adolescents. In *American handbook of psychiatry,* 2nd ed., vol. 2, ed. G. Kaplan, pp. 234–250. New York: Basic Books.
    A clear, readable discussion of the preconditions for psychotherapy and the problems and techniques of individual psychotherapy with adolescents.
BARTEN, H. H., AND BARTEN, S. S. 1973. *Children and their parents in brief therapy.* New York: Behavioral Publications.
    The papers included illustrate a range of short-term approaches to psychotherapy with children and their families.
BIJOU, S. W., AND REDD, W. H. 1975. Behavior therapy for children. In *American handbook of psychiatry,* 2nd ed., vol. 5, ed. D. X. Freedman and J. E. Dyrud, pp. 319–344. New York: Basic Books.
    Presents a number of theoretical models and discusses a variety of therapeutic procedures. Extensive bibliography.
BLOS, P., AND FINCH, S. M. 1975. Psychotherapy with children and adolescents. In *American handbook of psychiatry,* 2nd ed., vol. 5, ed. D. X. Freedman and J. E. Dyrud, pp. 133–162. New York: Basic Books.
    A clear, well-organized description providing theoretical framework and discussing many issues and technical problems involved in psychotherapy with children and adolescents. An excellent introduction to the area with an extensive bibliography.
BROWN, D. G. 1972. Behavior modification with children. *Mental Hygiene* 56(1):22–30.
    A clear statement of behavior modification in the treatment of children.
DARE, C. 1977. Dynamic treatment. In *Child psychiatry: Modern approaches,* ed. M. Rutter and L. Hersov, pp. 949–966. Philadelphia: Lippincott.
    A good overview of the major issues involved in dynamically oriented psychotherapy, written by a prominent British psychoanalyst.
DEWALD, P. A. 1969. *Psychotherapy: A dynamic approach.* New York: Basic Books.
    A good basic textbook on psychotherapy and its underlying dynamic considerations.

FREUD, A. 1975. *The psychoanalytic treatment of children.* New York: International Universities Press.
An authoritative description of psychoanalytic treatment of children from one of the pioneers in the field.

GLENN, J., AND SCHARFMAN, M. 1978. *Child analysis and therapy.* New York: Jason Aronson.
A recent and highly technical book that approaches the analysis of children from the perspectives of both child development and psychoanalytic theory. The applications of psychoanalytic principles to other related areas (e.g., prevention, psychotherapy, tutoring for cognitive deficits, nursery school) are explored. Recommended for the experienced therapist or serious student of child analysis or psychotherapy.

HAWORTH, M. R., ed. 1964. *Child psychotherapy.* New York: Basic Books.
A well-edited collection of authoritative articles examining the theory and practice of psychotherapy with children, including extensive discussion of play.

HIRZ, R. H. 1980. The preschool child: Approaches in psychiatric diagnosis and treatment. *Psychiat. Clin. N. Am.* 3(3):547–561.
Discusses developmental stages in the preschool period and characteristics that are particularly important to diagnosis and treatment strategies with preschool children and their families.

HOLMES, D. J. 1964. *The adolescent in psychotherapy.* Boston: Little, Brown & Co.
While not a recent book, this is still one of the best discussions on the particular factors concerned in the psychotherapy of adolescents.

KAHN, D. C., AND BOYER, D. N. 1980. Inpatient Hospital Treatment of Adolescents. *Psychiat. Clin. N. Am.* 3(3):513–545.
A review of the literature on adolescent inpatient treatment over the past ten years and the results of the authors' survey of aspects of adolescent treatment at facilities across the United States.

NOSHPITZ, J. D. 1975. Residential treatment of emotionally disturbed children. In *American handbook of psychiatry,* 2nd ed., vol. 5, ed. D. X. Freedman and J. E. Dyrud, pp. 634–651. New York: Basic Books.
A good introduction to issues of administrative structure, selection, and fit of parents; good discussion of milieu therapy and life space interviewing; some discussion of role of psychotherapy, problems in role clarity, collaboration, and accountability; issues around school and discharge.

ROSENTHAL, A. J., AND LEVINE, S. V. 1971–72. Brief psychotherapy with children: Process of therapy. *Am. J. Psychiat.* 128:141–146.
Examines techniques and content of brief psychotherapy with children.

SANDLER, J.; KENNEDY, H.; AND TYSON, R. L. 1980. *The technique of child psychoanalysis: Discussions with Anna Freud.* Cambridge, Mass.: Harvard University Press.
A systematic introduction to child psychoanalysis and its contributions to the development, psychopathology, and psychotherapy of children. Describes and illustrates the structure of all stages in the treatment process, emphasizing particularly the relationship and interaction between patient and therapist.

WEINER, I. B. 1970. *Psychological disturbance in adolescents.* New York: John Wiley & Sons.
Chapter 9 is a concise presentation of specific aspects of psychotherapy with adolescents.
————. 1975. *Principles of psychotherapy.* New York: John Wiley & Sons.
A recommended discussion of the basic principles of psychotherapy.

WOLMAN, B. B., ed. 1972. *Manual of child psychopathology.* New York: McGraw-Hill.
Good chapters on various modalities of treatment of children.

YULE, W. 1977. Behavioural approaches. In *Child psychiatry: Modern approaches,* ed. M. Rutter and L. Hersov, pp. 923–948. Philadelphia: Lippincott.
Describes the basic problem-solving approaches and discusses the rapidly expanding principles and techniques of behavior modification as applied to children's disorders. Particular attention is paid to the advances of many parents and teachers in the use of these techniques and to advances in application to areas that have proved resistant to more traditional therapies.

29

Robert Carr

The Role of Medication in the Treatment of the Disturbed Child

Introduction

What is the current status of pediatric psychopharmacology more than four decades after Charles Bradley's seminal article on the use of d,l-amphetamine (Benzedrine) in behaviorally disordered children (Bradley 1937)? In brief, psychopharmacologic agents are at times shamefully abused and at others equally shamefully disavowed and withheld. Abuse does occur (Maynard 1970; Sprague 1977), though not nearly to the extent suggested by the 1970 *Washington Post* report that between 20 to 25 percent of children in the Omaha, Nebraska, school district were receiving stimulants for hyperactivity. Abuse occurs most often when drugs are used not as one ingredient in a well-formulated treatment plan but rather as a specific and sufficient treatment in and of themselves. Thus drugs are more likely to be abused when other services—psychological, educational, or social—are not available, and when there is undue emphasis on cost in the cost/benefit formula. Abuse is greatest, then, in areas poorly served such as remote areas, inner cities, and large, poorly staffed institutions. In addition, some professionals place very heavy emphasis on biological considerations and downplay the usefulness of support and psychological therapies. For those with this bias, drugs are the obvious answer.

On the other hand, those who consistently avoid psychopharmacologic agents often do so out of fear and ignorance. Recent advances in psychiatric practice, based on a clearer understanding of etiology and a broader concept of formulation, have led to a long overdue rediscovery of biological issues. This has underlined what Freud himself believed, namely that as knowledge advanced, the biological underpinnings of psychological disturbance would gradually become clearer.

Yet even though the biological components of psychological processes are better understood, they still describe the process by which psychological disturbance develops only at a different—not necessarily at a better—level. However, this understanding does make possible useful interventions at that level. Clinicians can no longer afford to act as if biology and psychology were totally unrelated, by pursuing an "either-or" approach and using either medication or psychotherapy alone when, in fact, their young patients' needs may best be served by a judicious combination of the two (Harrison 1978).

Advances in the psychopharmacology of adult patients have generally preceded advances in pediatric psychopharmacology. The work of Philip May (1976, 1981), for instance, clearly demonstrated the superiority and higher cost/benefit ratio of antipsychotic medications over psychotherapy in relieving the distressing hallucinations and delusions of adult schizophrenia. However, the demonstration of this fact should not lead to an unqualified enthusiasm for antipsychotic drugs to the point where they are considered not just a specific but a sufficient treatment for schizophrenia. Such enthusiasm may contribute to a devaluation of tried and tested interventions, specifically psychotherapies and milieu therapy, which have never been as quickly or even as demonstrably effective. It is only now, after several decades of increasing sophistication in the use of antipsychotics, that an awareness of their limitations as well as their dangers (e.g., tardive dyskinesia and the depersonalization of treatment associated with the exclusive use of medication) are emerging (Seeman 1981).

Pediatric psychopharmacology has an interesting parallel in the treatment of what is now termed attention deficit disorder with hyperactivity. Although the capacity of stimulants to increase the ability to focus attention and to modulate excessive motor activity and impulsivity has been proven, the immediate improvement in these symptoms has not been reflected in equally dramatic improvements in long-term prognosis. As the unbridled enthusiasm of the past two decades has begun to abate, these agents are just now beginning to find a more balanced place in our armamentarium (Weiss 1981). As Winnicott (1965) has stated, it is primarily through ongoing relationships, whether parental or therapeutic, that the most devastating handicaps—those in interpersonal relationships—may be corrected. Medications, through their modulating effects, can help relationships work. Through their effects on level of arousal, intensity of drive, anxiety, and emotional control; through their support of the child's conscience and psychological defense mechanisms; and through their enhancement of the child's capacity for attention, memory, and reflection, the appropriate use of medication can increase the child's frustration tolerance and impulse control, thus favoring more adaptive, socially acceptable, and therefore gratifying relationships with others.

Many issues—such as that of diagnostic uncertainty; of the symptomatic nature of drug treatment; of the combined use of several different therapeutic modalities which raise the question of which is doing what; of the nature of the perception of the child's handicap; of the ecology of drug use; and of the principle of *primum non nocere* ("above all, avoid causing harm")—continue to make the clinical practice of psychopharmacology complex and challenging.*

History of Pediatric Psychopharmacology

In the early 1930s children with hyperkinetic impulse disorders showed improved behavior when administered thyroid extract (Lourie 1977). Bradley (1937) was the first to report on the beneficial effects of d,1-amphetamine (Benzedrine) on the mood and behavior of a heterogeneous group of behaviorally disordered children. Modification of behavior by amphetamine was confirmed by Bender and Nichtern (1956), who also noted that dextroamphetamine (Dexedrine) was equally effective at half the dose of amphetamine.

Diphenylhydantoin was introduced for epilepsy in 1938 and subsequently was evaluated for possible benefit in behavior-disordered children. Although individual reports suggested improvement, there are no well-controlled, established indications for its use in nonepileptic disorders (Stores 1978).

Methylphenidate (Ritalin) was introduced in 1954, and Knobel and Lytton (1959) reported its usefulness in hyperkinetic children. The 1950s also saw the introduction of the antipsychotics and antidepressants, which have since been applied in a variety of conditions running the gamut of diagnostic categories. For example, haloperidol was reported as useful in Gilles de la Tourette's syndrome (Seignot 1961).

With the advent of antidepressants, there was revived interest in de-

---

*See Gittelman-Klein, Spitzer, and Cantwell 1978; Minde 1980; Sandberg, Weiselberg, and Shaffer 1980; Schachar, Rutter, and Smith 1981; and Shepherd 1980.

pression in children and the development of increasingly sophisticated drug trial methods. Alleged drug misuse use led to caution and much greater selectivity (Sprague 1977; Sterling 1979). However, on close examination the extent of use was considerably lower than reported—1.73 percent of school-age children (Krager and Safer 1974) versus the 20 percent 1970 figure. There remains still cause for concern about reported high percentages (60–65 percent) of institutionalized children receiving psychotropic medication (Sprague 1976).

Neuroanatomy and Neurophysiology

Nervous tissues effect the rapid conduction of signals through complex electrophysiological and biochemical changes that lead to the release of neurotransmitters across synapses. These in turn affect the discharge potential of the postsynaptic neuron. Neurotransmitters exert one of two effects on the postsynaptic cell: they may lead to excitation (by depolarizing the cell membrane) or to inhibition (by hyperpolarizing the membrane). The final state of the membrane reflects the balance of up to several thousand synaptic inputs acting on a single neuron.

Whatever affects neurotransmitter metabolism, cell membrane permeability, or the number and sensitivity of receptors can affect the function of the neurons involved. While a great number of neurotransmitters have been demonstrated (Cohen and Young 1977; Iversen 1980) in the brain (e.g., norepinephrine, dopamine, serotonin, histamine, gamma-aminobutyric acid, endorphins, etc.), probably only 1 to 5 percent of brain neurotransmitters are known (Kolata 1979). Therefore, most investigators consider current theories of how drugs work a gross oversimplification.

In most of the psychiatric syndromes, drugs probably achieve results mostly by altering the energizing (reticular activating) and feeling (limbic) systems (Briant 1978).

Although it has been postulated that excesses or deficiencies in these systems are associated with individual disease states, it has not been proven that this excess or deficiency is the fundamental defect. An excess or deficiency of transmitter could be a result rather than the cause of the psychiatric syndrome, just as placebos may affect the levels of endorphins in the brain consequent to their evoking higher cortical input to the limbic system. Also, because drugs have many different effects, clinical improvement with a medication does not unequivocally prove one specific theory of metabolic dysfunction. However, since it is in the reticular activating and limbic systems that norepinephrine (NA), dopamine (DA), and serotonin (5-HT) are most heavily concentrated, these few transmitters have been intensely studied in psychiatric disorders. A schematic neuroanatomic localization of the neural tracts for norepinephrine, dopamine-, and serotonin-containing neurons is presented in figure 29.1 with more detailed description of the pathways in table 29.1.

Specific psychiatric and neurologic syndromes are currently associated with some of these pathways. Thus in Parkinson's disease the nigrostriatal pathway seems to show selective degeneration. The monoamine theory of affective disorders suggests that a decrease in the functional activity of the noradrenaline or serotonin neurons results in symptoms of depression, while an increased activity in this system appears in mania. The dopamine hypothesis of schizophrenia holds that an increased activity in the mesolimbic neurons is the biological basis for schizophrenia. The attention deficit disorder may represent a functional underactivity in the noradrenergic (reticular activating system) or dopaminergic (mesolimbic; mesocortical) systems. A schematic representation of the postulated excess and deficiency states in these disorders is presented in table 29.2.

The drugs used to treat these conditions act either by blocking or enhancing the action of these neurotransmitters in the synapse or at their receptors (see table 29.3).

The site and mode of action of these drugs also helps to predict which "treatment-emergent" side effects may occur. Thus dopamine-blocking agents (antipsychotics) used to treat the excess states of schizophrenia or Gilles de la Tourette's syndrome can result in dopamine-deficiencylike states such as Parkinsonism due to their action on the nigrostriatal tract. Catecholaminergic enhancers such as amphetamines and tricyclic antidepressants used to treat attention deficit disorder and depression can result in catecholaminergic excess states such as amphetamine psychosis (action on mesolimbic system), tics (action on nigrostriatal tract), and mania (action on ascending noradrenergic tract).

However, neurotransmitter physiology cannot yet provide a general theory of normal or deviant development. Snyder has given the analogy of an electrical circuit: "The fact that a dangerous short circuit can be abolished by tripping a circuit breaker does not mean that the short is in the breaker—it may be anywhere in the circuit." (Kolata 1979).

Psychotropic drugs are used predominantly, if not exclusively, symptomatically rather than matched to any one specific diagnostic category, with the possible exception of attention deficit disorder (Gittelman-Klein, Spitzer, and Cantwell 1978). The DSM-III diagnostic categories do not lead immediately to selection of the appropriate drug by category. Drug selection is based on the specific signs and symptoms that the professional seeks to modulate. Thus success in using drugs depends more on carefully defining the target signs and symptoms to be modulated than on diagnosis. If the most common pitfalls and sources of failure in the use of psychopharmalogic drugs were to be identified, they would be the unsystematic use of drugs and the inadequate monitoring of responses.

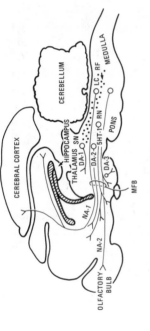

FIGURE 29.1

Neuronal Localization in the Brain

Type	Path	Function
Noradrenaline		
NA-1 (Dorsal Bundle)	Locus Coeruleus- - - MFB- - -Cerebral Cortex; Hippocampus	Arousal
NA-2 (Ventral Bundle)	Brain stem- - - - -MFB- - -Hypothalamus; Limbic System	Affective
		Modulation
NA-3 (ARAS)	Reticular Formation- - - Diffusely- - -Forebrain	Arousal
Dopamine		
DA-1 (Nigrostriatal)	Substantia Nigra- - - - -Caudate; Putamen	Motor
DA-2 (Mesolimbic)	Midbrain- - - - -Nucleus Accumbens; Olfactory tubercle	Limbic
DA-3 (Tuberoinfundibular)	Arcuate Nucleus (Hypothalamus)- - -Median Eminence	Neuroendocrine
Serotonin		
5HT-1	Raphe Nuclei- - - - - -Hypothalamus; Amygdala; Cerebral cortex	Regulate sleep-wakefulness

LC = Locus Coeruleus   MFB = Median Forebrain Bundle   SN = Substantia Nigra
RN = Ralphe Nuclei   RF = Reticular Formation (NA-3)   ARAS = Ascending Reticular Activating System.

TABLE 29.1

Major Neuronal Pathways of Dopamine, Norepinephrine, and Serotonin

Neurotransmitter	Tract	Path	Function (Hypothesized)
Dopamine (DA)	1. Nigrostriatal (Motor) DA-1	Substantia nigra to corpus striatum and amygdala	Extrapyramidal modulation of motor responses
	2. Mesolimbic (Emotional) DA-2	Dorsal to interpeduncular nucleus (tegmentum midbrain) to nucleus accumbens and olfactory tubercle (also cingulate and frontal cortex)	Behavioral arousal, motivation, emotional control
	3. Tuberoinfundibular (Endocrine) DA-3	Arcuate nucleus to median eminence (hypothalamus)	Control of releasing hormones to the pituitary
Norepinephrine (NA)	1. Ascending reticular formation NA-3		
	a. Caudal (inhibitory)	a. Caudal-lateral reticular formation of medulla (inhibitory)—diffusely to cortex	Screen out irrelevant stimuli and focus attention
	b. Rostral (facilitatory)	b. Rostral-reticular formation of medulla and pons (facilitatory)—diffusely to cortex	
	2. Dorsal Bundle NA-1	a. Locus coeruleus to cerebral cortex, cerebellar cortex, and limbic system	Wakefulness
	3. Ventral Bundle (reward pathway) NA-2	b. Ventral bundle—to hypothalamus and limbic system	Reward system; affective modulation
Serotonin (5-HT)	Raphe system	Midline nucleii of pons and medulla to:	
	a. Caudal group	a. Spinal cord	Regulate sleep-wakefulness
	b. Rostral group	b. Hypothalamus, limbic areas, neocortex	

The systematic use of drugs involves:

1. Identification of target signs and symptoms.
2. Choice of a single agent with the least potential for serious toxicity.
3. Starting with a low dose, which is gradually raised until the desired therapeutic effect is achieved or until side effects or toxicity preclude a further increase (i.e., to tolerance).
4. If unsuccessful, moving to the next least toxic drug and repeating the procedure.

Adequate monitoring of response involves the use of target symptom goal attainment scales (e.g., Conners' ten-point Parent Teacher Questionnaire), which can be used by parent, teacher, and clinician, thus allowing for three independent and transsituational assessments of response (Conners 1973).

The relationship between a target phenomenon and the selection of agents is summarized in Figure 29.2.

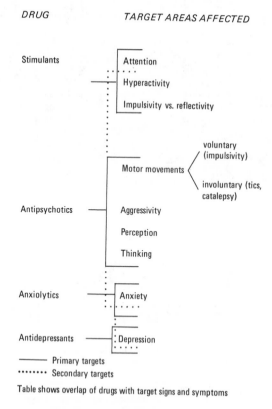

DRUG	TARGET AREAS AFFECTED

——— Primary targets
······· Secondary targets

Table shows overlap of drugs with target signs and symptoms

Figure 29.2

Drug Categories

The systematic use of drugs in children can only be undertaken after an adequate initial diagnostic assessment. This should result in a category diagnosis. However, since the drugs will be aimed at specific target symptoms, these must be identified before beginning treatment. Identification by history from the parents and by office observation should be cross-checked for reliability by obtaining information from the school. If the symptoms are detectable from two of these three sources, a drug trial may be warranted. Wherever possible, it is wise to establish a treatment baseline of two to four weeks before beginning medication. Some authors suggest beginning with a placebo since 18 to 45 percent will respond positively due solely to this effect (Barkley 1977a). The lowest initial dose of the drug, which may be half the minimum recommended dose, should be tried first. Dosage is increased systematically; short-acting drugs (e.g., the stimulants) may be increased every one to two days, while longer acting drugs (e.g., the phenothiazines) should be increased only every four to five days. Clinical effects should be monitored; this can be done using such instruments as the Abbreviated Symptom Checklist (Conners 1973). Side effects should also be noted and vigilence kept for the most serious toxic effects of the drug.

Major drug categories used in children are the stimulants, antipsychotics, and antidepressants.

STIMULANTS

Dextroamphetamine and methylphenidate are the stimulants used with children, principally and perhaps specifically for those with attention deficit disorder.

Amphetamine
(asymmetric carbon with d- and l- forms)

Methylphenidate
(piperidine derivative of amphetamine)

Amphetamine has d- and l- forms, but only the d- form is a central stimulant (Seeman, Sellers, and Roschlau 1980). The racemic (d, l) mixture (i.e., amphetamine sulfate) has only half as much effect as an equivalent weight of the d- form dextroamphetamine sulfate (Dexedrine). Within the nervous system, dextroamphetamine causes release of and blocks the reup-

TABLE 29.2

Postulated Excess and Deficiency States in Clinical Disorders

Deficiency States	Excess States
Attention Deficit Disorder	**Schizophrenia** (90 percent limbic; 10 percent basal-motor)
System: Norepinephrine (? and dopamine) (recticular activating plus mesocortical)	*System:* Dopamine (mesolimbic plus mesocortical)
Abnormality: Amount of transmitter release is decreased.	*Abnormality:* Amount of transmitter is normal but there is an increased number of receptors.
Effect: Information processing is underfocused.	*Effect:* Information processing is overfocused.
Treatment: Stimulants enhance release and block reuptake.	*Treatment:* Antipsychotics block dopamine receptors.
Parkinsonism	**Tardive Dyskinesia**
System: Dopamine (nigrostriatal)	*System:* Dopamine (nigrostriatal)
Abnormality: Selective degeneration of nigrostriatal neurons.	*Abnormality:* Increased number of receptors plus dying dopaminergic cells lead to denervation hypersensitivity.
Effect: Loss of inhibitory modulation of extrapyramidal functions (leads to akinesia plus rigidity).	*Effect:* Hypermotility.
Treatment: Dopamine enhancers (e.g., levodopa; amantadine) or anticholinergic (e.g., benztropine) restore dopamine/acetylcholine balance.	*Treatment:* No good agent; drug holidays.

Deficiency States	*Excess States*

Depression

System: Norepinephrine and/or Serotonin (? Dopamine; ?Acetylcholine)

Abnormality: Reduced NA or 5-HT release, plus increased number of postsynaptic receptors.

Effect: Dysregulation of affect through limbic system.

Treatment: Four groups of antidepressants
1. tertiary amines—↑5-HT (e.g., imipramine and amitriptyline).
↑2. secondary amines—NA (e.g., desipramine and nortriptyline).
3. Mianserin—antagonist of NA at presynaptic; inhibitory receptors.
4. Monoamine oxidase inhibitors.

Gilles de la Tourette's Disease (90 percent basal-motor; 10 percent limbic)

System: Dopamine (nigrostriatal)

Abnormality: Excess dopamine.

Effect: Hypermotility.

Treatment: Dopamine receptor blockers; NA agonist (e.g., clonidine) that stimulates presynaptic inhibitory receptors

Mania

System: Norepinephrine and/or serotonin (?dopamine; ?acetylcholine)

Abnormality: ?Opposite that of depression, that is, NA excess plus increased number of postsynaptic receptors.

Effect: Disregulation of affect through limbic system.

Treatment: Lithium blocks vesicle–membrane fusion and subsequent release of dopamine.

take of catecholamines (NA and DA). The enhanced noradrenergic activity, probably affecting the reticular activating system or presynaptic inhibition of the dopaminergic system, may account for its general arousing and attentional focusing effects (Barkley 1977*b*; Satterfield, Cantwell, and Satterfield 1974; Shelty and Chase 1976). Enhanced dopaminergic activity, probably in the nigrostriatal and mesolimbic systems, may account for some aspects of motor activity (stereotypies, tics) and paranoid hallucinosis seen with higher doses (Lucas and Weiss 1971). However, some of the psychotic effects may be the result of increased release of serotonin at high dosages (Gilman, Goodman, and Gilman 1980).

Methylphenidate, the piperidine derivative of amphetamine, has more prominent effects on mental than on motor activities or appetite (Gilman, Goodman, and Gilman 1980). After oral administration, the effects of

TABLE 29.3

Hypothesized Actions and Side Effects of Major Drug Groups Used with Children

Drug	Hypothesized Action	Result of Excessive Administration
Antipsychotics	Block the functioning of dopaminergic systems by binding competitively to receptors for dopamine.	Excess administration can block excessively, producing symptoms of dopamine deficiency (e.g., Parkinsonism).
Stimulants	Enhance the release *and* block the reuptake of norepinephrine and dopamine. Arousal effect (noradrenergic excitation) in reticular activating system, which is thought to be underaroused in attentional disorders.	Excess levels can invoke involuntary motor movements by effect on nigrostriatal (dopamine) system *and* hallucinations by effect on mesolimbic system.
Antidepressants	Inhibit reuptake of norepinephrine and serotonin. Reversal of postulated deficiency of these biogenic amines in depression (i.e., catecholamine hypothesis of depression) *also* Enhance arousal in attention disorders and in enuresis where they are presumed to effect the depth of sleep.	Swing to mania.

dextroamphetamine sulfate and methylphenidate appear in one-half to one hour, reach their peak concentrations in plasma in about two hours, and have a half-life in plasma of one to two hours. Thus the therapeutic effect is quite short, lasting about four hours. The equivalent dose ratio between methylphenidate and dextroamphetamine sulfate is about two to one.

The clinical target signs and symptoms for which these stimulants are most useful are short attention span, poor concentration, impulsivity, and hyperactivity. Methylphenidate has now been approved for use in children under the age of six, and Millichap (1973) has concluded that it is generally superior to dextroamphetamine sulfate in terms of overall effectiveness and fewer side effects.

The recommended dosage of methylphenidate is between 0.24 and 2.0 milligrams per kilogram per day to a maximum of 60 milligrams per day. The difference between the high and low dose appears significant, and may be related to the major locus of action (e.g., presynaptic inhibition versus postsynaptic enhancement) at varying dosages (Sprague and Sleator 1977). Enhancement of learning appears to peak at a dose of 0.3 milligrams per kilogram per dose. As the dose is increased, the effect on learning is decreased, although social behavior seems most improved at a dose of 1.0 milligrams per kilogram per dose. Thus different target behaviors respond best at different doses. However, due to variability in pharmacokinetics in individual patients, basing doses on milligrams per kilogram makes the drawing of these conclusions questionable without blood level determinations. If this differential effect on learning versus behavior is confirmed, it carries major implications, since children are more often treated for undesirable social behaviors that are improved at dosages of stimulants which may adversely effect attention and learning.

Although methylphenidate has a short half-life, it should be started as a single morning dose. Often a noon dose is not necessary. This single initial morning dose also allows some comparison of morning and afternoon performance and behavior. The initial dose for one week is low (e.g., 5 mg methylphenidate before breakfast daily). It is then increased weekly, first by 5 milligrams before lunch, then 10 milligrams at breakfast and 5 milligrams at noon, and then increasing serially until a total of 60 milligrams total per day is reached. While parents frequently report a rebound hyperactivity after school, they are generally prepared to accept this if school behavior improves. An afternoon dose may be given at four o'clock if the after school period becomes intolerable to parents, but then increased benefits must be balanced against the risk of sleep-onset difficulties.

The most commonly reported side effects of methylphenidate are anorexia (especially at doses over 20 mg/day), sleep-onset insomnia, and emotional lability (tearfulness and withdrawal) (Kugel et al. 1975). Less often stomachache and headache are reported. Tachycardia and increased blood pressure may occur and should be watched for. Tics and psychotic behaviors have occasionally been reported.

Pemoline (Cylert) is an oxazolidine that is structurally dissimilar to methylphenidate but has similar effects on the nervous system. Still under investigation, it is not yet available for general use but offers more sustained effects since its half-life is about twelve hours. The onset of clinical effectiveness may be delayed by three or four weeks. However, it does offer significant advantages through a single daily dose, more even therapeutic effect, and minimal side effects on the cardiovascular system.

The height and weight suppression scare in response to methylphenidate initially reported by Safer and, more recently, by Greenhill remains unresolved Greenhill et al. 1981; Safer, 1972). Although the bulk of the evidence to date suggests that it is not of great clinical significance, the height and weight of children receiving methylphenidate should be monitored.

A summary of target symptoms, dosages, and precautions in using stimulants is given in table 29.4.

ANTIPSYCHOTICS

The antipsychotics are used in children with attention deficit disorder, Gilles de la Tourette syndrome, severe anxiety states and conduct disorders, as well as in childhood psychoses.* Some would argue that the use of these agents in any conditions other than adolescent or adult-onset schizophrenia represents a "shotgun" pharmacology approach (Seeman 1981). When used in children the target signs and symptoms include psychomotor agitation (including hyperkinesis), unmodulated anxiety, stereotypies, impulsive aggressivity, and disorganized thinking.

The phenothiazines and butyrophenones have been used primarily, although the thioxanthines have also been studied.

Although there are many different phenothiazines and butyrophenones, they differ little except in side effects, that is, all are dopamine blockers. Essentially all these drugs selectively block dopamine receptors by adopting a configuration identical to that of dopamine; they all overlap with the dopamine molecule and compete at its receptors. (See figure 29.3.)

The main actions and side effects of these drugs are determined by the blockade of the main dopaminergic pathways. Thus they have motor (nigrostriatal), emotional (limbic), and endocrine (tuberoinfundibular) effects. In Gilles de la Tourette's disease the postulated overactivity of the

---

*See Campbell et al. 1978; Cohen et al. 1979; Gittelman-Klein et al. 1976; Werry and Aman 1975; White 1977; and Winsberg and Ypes 1978.

TABLE 29.4
Drug Category—Stimulants

Target Signs and Symptoms	Specific Drugs	Dosage Range	Precautions (For All Members of Group)	Side Effects (For All Members of Group)
1. Poor attention span 2. Poor concentration 3. Hyperactivity 4. Impulsivity 5. Emotional lability	1. Methylphenidate 2. Dextroamphetamine 3. Pemoline	5–60 mg/day 2.5–40 mg/day 37.5–112.5 mg/day	1. Monitor growth (height/weight) 2. Rebound effect on withdrawal	1. Anorexia and weight loss 2. Insomnia 3. Decreased growth rate: both height, weight decreased 4. Irritability and restlessness 5. Abdominal pain and headaches 6. Sadness, crying, and withdrawal 7. Increased blood pressure, tachycardia 8. Rare complications: thrombocytopaenia toxic psychosis tics

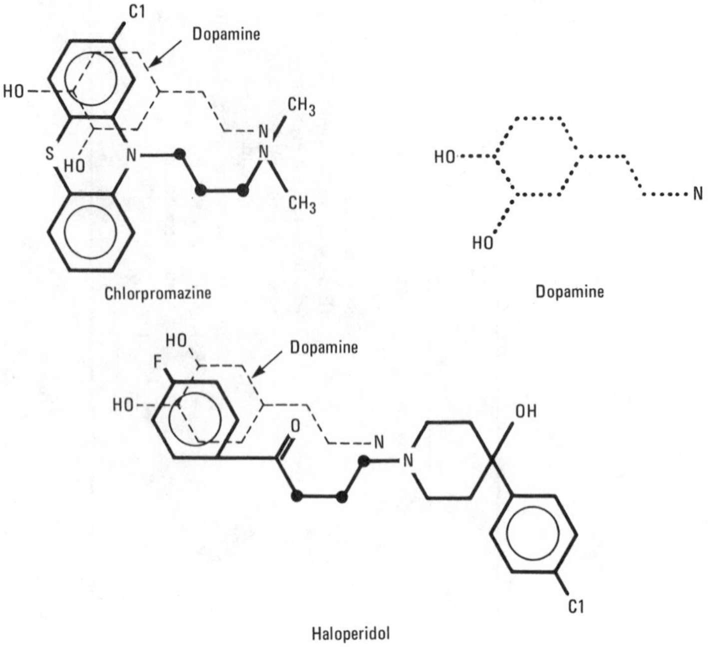

Figure 29.3

nigrostriatal system is blocked, and in schizophrenia and mania the over-activity in the mesolimbic and mesocortical areas is blocked. Parkinsonism is a predictable side effect, as it represents a "hypodopaminergic" state that can be induced by excess dopamine blockade in the nigrostriatal pathway.

The relative potencies of oral doses of the various phenothiazines are primarily related to their different solubilities in fat (including cell membranes). Table 29.5 shows the relative potency of antipsychotics compared to a 100 milligram oral dose of chlorpromazine.

Psychomotor slowing and affective indifference are the two main side effects of the antipsychotics. Thus external stimuli do not effect the normal degree of arousal; emotional responses mediated through the limbic system are less pronounced. Toxic effects of these medications include:

1. Extrapyramidal—due to dopamine blockage; children are particularly sensitive.
   a. Parkinsonism—akinesia, rigidity, tremor.
   b. Acute dystonic reactions—torticollis, oculogyric crisis.
   c. Akathisia (restlessness)—may be confused with worsening psychotic or hyperactive symptoms.
   d. Tardive dyskinesia (Gualtieri et al. 1980).
   e. Withdrawal dyskinesia—lasts only a few weeks.

These are most marked in agents with predominant dopamine-blocking action (e.g., haloperidol and trifluoperazine) without counterbalancing anticho-

The Role of Medication in the Treatment of the Disturbed Child

TABLE 29.5

Prescribing Information Regarding Antipsychotic Drugs

| Name of Drug | Relative Potency | | Starting Dose in Children |
	Comparable Dose	Relative Strength	
Chlorpromazine	100 mg	1X	10–25 mg b.i.d.*
Thioridazine	100 mg	1X	10–25 mg b.i.d.
Perphenazine	10 mg	10X	
Trifluoperazine	5 mg	20X	1 mg b.i.d.
Fluphenazine	1.8 mg	50X	
Haloperidol	2.5 mg	40X	0.5 mg b.i.d.

*If used for attention deficit disorder, doses of chlorpromazine in excess of 75 mg/day (or equivalent with other antipsychotics) may result in mental dulling and decreased cognitive performance. However, doses of up to 200 mg chlorpromazine or equivalent can be helpful in containing the frequently associated hyperactive and impulsive behavior. Thus varying the dose will determine which of the two target systems will be addressed.

linergic effects (e.g., thioridazine and chlorpromazine). These effects can be modified by restoring the cholinergic-dopaminergic balance using anticholinergic agents (e.g., benztropine).

2. Drowsiness and postural hypotension—related to alpha adrenergic blockade and so worse with the aliphatic (e.g., chlorpromazine) and piperidine (e.g., thioridazine) phenothiazines.
3. Blood dyscrasias (e.g., neutropenia and agranulocytosis) are rare, and usually occur between the fourth and tenth week of treatment; a biweekly and then monthly complete blood count is recommended with prolonged use.
4. Jaundice—occurs rarely (i.e., 1 in 1,000 patients). The jaundice is of the obstructive type and is thought to be a hypersensitivity reaction, since it is not dose-related.
5. Photosensitivity and dermatitis—occur occasionally (about 4 percent of patients).
6. Weight gain is common, probably due to an effect on hypothalamus.
7. Seizures at high dosage; probably only in latent epileptics.

The mental dulling—especially seen with the alpha adrenergic blockers (e.g., chlorpromazine and thioridazine)—presents a problem in treatment because of the interference with cognitive performance. Werry and Aman (1975) studied the differential effects on behavior and cognitive performance on high (0.05 mg/kgm/day) and low (0.025 mg/kgm/day) doses of haloperidol. Both doses were effective in reducing behavioral symptoms, but the higher dose led to diminished cognitive performance.

Starting doses for these drugs are approximately 10 to 25 milligrams twice a day for chlorpromazine and thioridazine; 1 milligram twice a day for trifluoperazine; and 0.5 milligrams twice a day for haloperidol. After a few days the doses can be combined into a single nighttime dose. There are no absolute upper limits to these drugs, if tolerated, but the ususal maximum range is up to about 500 milligrams of chlorpromazine or its equivalent below the age of twelve.

Table 29.6 summarizes the targets, types, and precautions when administering antipsychotics.

ANTIDEPRESSANTS

At this time the only antidepressant drugs used with children are the tricyclics. The monoamine oxidase inhibitors are not acceptable for use in children under age sixteen, although Frommer (1967) did report their use in childhood depression. The clinical syndromes for which the tricyclics have been investigated and used include: enuresis (Rapoport et al. 1980); attention deficit disorder (Werry, Aman, and Diamond 1980); depression (Puig-Antich et al. 1979); separation-anxiety disorder (school phobia) (Gittelman-Klein and Klein 1973); and autism (Campbell et al. 1971).

To date, none of these syndromes has shown a sufficiently clear or superior response to antidepressants to warrant their routine use.

The basic structure of the tricyclic antidepressants is similar to the phenothiazines; however, the sulfur atom is replaced by an ethylene ($-CH_2-CH_2-$) bridge.

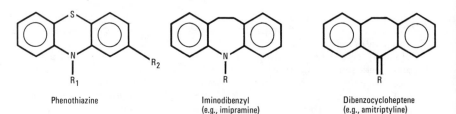

| Phenothiazine | Iminodibenzyl (e.g., imipramine) | Dibenzocycloheptene (e.g., amitriptyline) |

Figure 29.4 Molecular Structure Demonstrating Ethylene Bridge of Tricyclic Antidepressants

The antidepressant effect has been considered related to the antidepressants' inhibition of the reuptake on noradrenergic and serotonergic pathways by reversing the relative deficiencies of these transmitters. However, more recent studies have shown that they also cause changes in the number and sensitivity of monoamine receptors (B-receptor subsensitivity) or affect monoamine transmission by decreasing presynaptic inhibition (Crews and Smith 1978; Sulser 1979). Thus although mood disorders are thought to reflect problems in the balance and stability of neural regulation, the site and mode of action remains controversial. Other neurochemical mechanisms including dopamine, acetylcholine, hormones, and brain peptides have also been implicated (Risch, Kalin, and Murphy 1981). The effects of antidepressants on monoaminergic systems have also been postulated to explain their usefulness in attention deficit disorder (catacholaminergic), enuresis (reticular activating system), and autism (serotonergic). Their side effects represent an extension of their pharmacologic activity. These side effects include:

TABLE 29.6
Drug Category—Antipsychotics *

Target Signs and Symptoms	Drugs Utilized	Characteristics of Subgroups	Dosages	Side Effects
1. Psychomotor agitation (including hyperkinesis)	1. Phenothiazines	*High Dosage* Greater anticholinergic activity. More sedating. Extrapyramidal side effects less often.	See Table 29.8	1. Extrapyramidal effects: Parkinsonian rigidity and tremor Acute dystonias Akathisia Oculogyric crises (?)Tardive dyskinesia
2. Unmodulated (?intolerable) anxiety	a. Aliphatic subgroup, (e.g. chlorpromazine)			2. Hepatotoxicity: (rare) cholestatic jaundice (hypersensitivity)
	b. Piperidene subgroup (e.g., thioridazine)			
3. Stereotyped behaviors	c. Piperazine subgroup (e.g., trifluoperazine, perphenazine, fluphenazine)	*Low Dosage* Less anticholinergic activity. Less sedation. Extra pyramidal side effects more common.		3. Effects on blood and vascular system: agranulocytosis (rare) hypotension
4. Impulsive aggressivity				4. Skin disorders: photosensitivity (4%) eczema
5. Disorganized thinking	2. Butyrophenones (e.g., haloperidol)			5. Anticholinergic: dry mouth constipation blurred vision
				6. Appetite increased (100 %)

*The antipsychotics are used in children most often in nonpsychotic disorders. They are used in: attention deficit disorder, Gilles de la Tourette syndrome, severe anxiety states, conduct disorders, and childhood psychosis.

1. Anticholinergic—blurred vision, dry mouth, urinary retention, constipation.
2. Cardiovascular—hypotension, tachycardia, heart block, and arrythmias.
3. Neurological—drowsiness, seizures, swings from depression to mania.
4. Allergic reactions (rare)—cholestatic jaundice, rashes, agranulocytosis.

An overdose of tricyclic antidepressants can be lethal, and their increasing use by both children and adults represents an escalating risk for accidental or intentional self-poisoning. Although their use in attention deficit disorder, prepubertal depression, and school phobia has been reported, their routine use for these conditions cannot as yet be recommended (Gittelman-Klein and Klein 1973; Puig-Antich et al. 1979; Werry, Aman, and Diamond 1980), except in particularly refractory cases.

The effectiveness of antidepressants in enuresis has been well demonstrated but is often shortlived, and the problem often recurs on stopping the drug. For this reason, imipramine is recommended only to defuse the situation when the enuresis is causing concern and severe negative interaction in the family, and to initiate a more healthy and positive family-child interaction.

The empirical dose range is between 1.5 and 3.5 milligrams per kilogram per day. Doses in excess of 3.5 milligrams per kilogram per day may cause severe cardiovascular effects (Saraf et al. 1978).

Table 29.7 summarizes the targets, types, and precautions when administering antidepressants.

LITHIUM

Lithium salts (lithium carbonate) are used for manic depressive disease in adults. The lithium ion (Li^+) is thought to interfere with the actions of the sodium ion (Na^+) associated with the excitability of nerve cells. Most likely it prevents release of dopamine by blocking vesicles in the dopaminergic nerve terminals from fusing and discharging. Theoretically, it should be useful in blocking schizophrenic psychosis, Gilles de la Tourette's disease, and tardive dyskinesia as well. It has been reported useful in uncontrollable aggression in adults and children, in hyperkinetic reaction, and in childhood schizophrenia.[*] However, at this time its use in children should be confined to recurrent manic depressive disease in adolescence (Campbell, Schulman, and Rapoport 1978; Steinberg 1980; Youngerman and Canino 1978).

ANTIANXIETY DRUGS AND SEDATIVES

Included in the category of antianxiety drugs and sedatives are nonbarbiturate sedatives (e.g., chloryl hydrate), antihistaminics (e.g., diphenhy-

[*]See Campbell 1973; DeLong 1978; Greenhill et al. 1981; Platt, Campbell, and Cohen 1981; and Sheard et al. 1976.

TABLE 29.7

Drug Category—Antidepressants

Target Signs and Symptoms*	Drugs Utilized	Dosage Range	Side Effects
1. Enuresis	1. Tricyclic antidepressants only	1.5–4.5 mg/kg/day	1. Anticholinergic: dry mouth constipation blurred vision
2. Poor attention span; poor concentration	Monoaminoxidase inhibitors not acceptable for use under age 16, though some disagree (Frommer 1967)	Total dose should not exceed 100 mg/day	2. Cardiovascular: prolonged QRS complex increased conduction time increased blood pressure decreased cardiac output possible arrhythmias and arrest (especially if dose exceeds 3.5 mg/kg/day)
3. Depression			
4. Separation anxiety			3. Seizures

*Syndromes for which antidepressants have been investigated in children include enuresis, attention deficit disorder, depression, and separation-anxiety disorder.

dramine and hydroxyzine), and benzodiazepines (e.g. chlordiazepoxide, diazepam). The use of the antihistaminics and benzodiazepines in anxiety disorders of childhood has been reviewed and their effectiveness has clearly not been substantiated (Gittelman-Klein 1978). Chloryl hydrate at doses of 50 milligrams per kilogram (maximum 1,000 mg) is a useful hypnotic. Diazepam is useful in pavor nocturnus. (See chapter 9.)

SUMMARY

Table 29.8 attempts to summarize the drugs, target symptoms, dosage, and adverse reactions of the most commonly prescribed drugs, excluding the anxiolytic and sedatives.

Diagnostic Categories (DSM-III)

MENTAL RETARDATION

There is no drug that specifically treats the deficit in mental retardation, except perhaps where a specific etiologic defect such as hypothyroidism, pyridoxine deficiency, or dependency states, or lead poisoning is identified. However, the retarded child may experience any coincident condition for which psychopharmacologic intervention is effective. Thus attentional, conduct, anxiety, and tic disorders accompanying the mental defect can be treated psychopharmacologically just as though they were the primary diagnosis.

ATTENTION DEFICIT DISORDER

The stimulants are the drugs of choice for attention deficit disorder (ADD). Approximately 75 percent of children show an acute response with decreased hyperactivity, increased concentration and attention, and decreased impulsivity (Barkley 1977a). ADD appears to be lifelong—that is, while the hyperactivity may decrease following adolescence, the same is not true of the attention deficit (MacKay, Beck, and Taylor 1973; Wood et al. 1976). The greatest handicap is basically an inability to stop, look, and listen. Long-term follow-up studies of children with this disorder are disappointing in their demonstration that drug treatment has a significant lasting impact on major social, academic, or psychological adjustment. As an adjunctive treatment, stimulants do optimize the chance that the child may be taught, befriended, and generally tolerated by those whose influence will encourage developmental progress. Controversial issues remain with regard to dosage (0.3 mg/kgm/day vs. 2.0 mg/kgm/day); safety (effects on growth); and long-term benefit.

Alternative drugs that cannot at present be recommended for routine use include the tricyclic antidepressants (imipramine and amitriptyline). Antipsychotics (chlorpromazine, thiroidazine, haloperidol) have been carefully investigated but should be reserved for those cases that respond poorly to stimulants or in whom side effects of the stimulants preclude attainment of an optimal dose. Attention must be paid to their possible mental dulling effect and decreased cognitive performance (Werry and Aman 1975).

CONDUCT DISORDER

The diagnostic category of conduct disorder remains troublesome because of its overlap with attention deficit disorder (Sandberg, Weiselberg, and Shaffer 1980). If a clear diagnosis of ADD can be made, treatment of that disorder with stimulants is indicated. However, more frequently in children with a conduct disorder, the impulsive-aggressiveness is the target symptom most in need of medication. For this symptom both the antipsychotics and, more recently, lithium have been used, although at present lithium cannot be recommended for routine use in conduct disorders (Platt, Campbell, and Cohen 1981).

ANXIETY DISORDERS

The use of anxiolytics in overanxious and separation anxiety disorders has not been systematically studied (Gittelman-Klein 1978). The tricyclic antidepressants have been reported useful in cases of school phobia in which an underlying separation anxiety exists. However, this recommendation is based on a single study and should not be considered routinely (Rapoport, Mikkelson, and Werry 1978).

Although their effectiveness has not clearly been demonstrated, the anxiolytics empirically may be useful when used briefly (two to four weeks) to assist in getting school-phobic children back to school.

STEREOTYPED MOVEMENT DISORDERS

Gilles de la Tourette's disorder shows some response to the dopamine blockers (e.g., haloperidol) in about 75 percent of cases (Cohen et al. 1979).

ENURESIS

Enuresis shows a rapid initial response to tricyclics (e.g., imipramine) but often reappears after cessation of the drug. For this reason, condition-

TABLE 29.8

Summary of Major Prescribed Drugs

Target Symptoms	Half-life ($t_{1/2}$) (hours)	Drug	Dosage m/day	Adverse Reactions.	Comments
I. Stimulants					
1. Short attention span 2. Impulsivity 3. Hyperactivity	2–7	1. Methylphenidate	Range: 5–60 mg Median: 20 (10 mg bid)	*Common*: Anorexia, insomnia, tearfulness, irritability, stomach and headaches.	Specific mg/kgm doses are not useful due to wide variability of individual kinetics.
	5	2. Dextroamphetamine	Range: 2.5–40 mg Median: 10 mg (5 mg bid)	*Rare*: Growth retardation, toxic psychosis, Gilles de la Tourette's syndrome.	Growth retardation appears secondary to decreased caloric intake.
	12	3. Pemoline	Range: 37.5–112.5 mg Median: 75 mg in A.M.		Pemoline not available for use in Canada

Target Symptoms	Half-life (t ½) (hours)	Drug	Dosage m/day	Adverse Reactions	Comments
II. Antipsychotics					
1. Psychomotor agitation 2. Mood Lability 3. Agressive/Destructiveness 4. Stereotypies and motor verbal tics 5. Thought disorder 6. Hallucinations	10–20	1. Phenothiazines Aliphatic (e.g., chloropromazine) Piperdine (e.g., thioridazine) Piperazine (e.g., trifluoperazine) 2. Butyrophenones (e.g., haloperidol)	 Range: 25–500 mg Range: 25–200 mg Range: 0.25–20 mg Range: 0.5–20 mg	Common: Drowsiness, increased appetite, anticholinergic (esp. thioridazine) Extrapyramidal signs: parkinsonism; akathisia; acute dystonias; Cardiovascular: postural hypotension; cardiac conduction abnormalities Rare: Photosensitivity (4%) (esp. chlorpromazine), allergic skin rashes, agranulocutosis, cholestatic jaundice.	High dose/low potency drugs produce more sedation and cardiovascular effects. Low dose/high potency drugs produce more extrapyramidal effects. Tardive dyskenisia may not develop in persons under 20 years of age although withdrawal dyskinesias are seen transiently (2 weeks).
III. Antidepressants Tricyclics Enuresis ?Separation-anxiety ?Prepubertal depression Attention deficit disorder	10–17		Range: 25–75 mg 25–150 mg 25–150 mg	Common: Anticholinergic tremors, increased blood pressure, EKG changes, decreased seizure threshold. Rare: Hypotension	Conditioning techniques are preferable to tricyclics for enuresis. Doses greater than 3.5 mg/kgm/day should have EKG monitoring.

ing techniques are considered preferable (Esman 1977; Rapoport et al. 1980).

PERVASIVE DEVELOPMENTAL DISORDERS

The neurochemistry and neurophysiology of autism and childhood-onset pervasive developmental disorders remain much less well understood than adult psychotic disorders, to which they may or may not be related (Ritvo 1977). Thus drug treatment is symptomatic rather than specific. The antipsychotics ameliorate hyperactivity, mood lability, and excitability, but the social and language impairments are not reversed (Campbell et al. 1978).

SPECIFIC DEVELOPMENTAL DISORDERS

Children with specific developmental reading disorders and other "specific learning disorders" do not show a long-term academic improvement in response to stimulants (Gittelman 1980). In spite of this, the use of stimulants in these disorders is widespread. However, it should be discouraged.

AFFECTIVE DISORDERS

Typical manic and, more frequently, depressive disorders have been reported in prepubertal children (Loranger and Levine 1978). Much research into this area is currently underway. At present, however, the elective use of antimanic and antidepressive agents cannot be advised as the treatment of choice.

SUMMARY

Table 29.9 reviews the major syndromes for which drugs have been prescribed and adds qualifying remarks.

Conclusions

Recent advances in neurophysiology and neurochemistry have just begun to allow a review of some of the normal and disordered biological functions of the brain that underlie behavior. Understanding the normal mechanisms suggests ways in which biological interventions might modulate these functions when they become disordered. Conversely, effective biological treatments give clues about structure and function.

TABLE 29.9

Some Common Psychiatric Syndromes and Drugs Used in Their Treatment

Syndrome	Drugs Utilized	Remarks
Attention Deficit Disorder	1. Stimulants methylphenidate dextroamphetamine 2. Antipsychotics	Respond positively to both stimulants and antipsychotics.
Specific Learning Disabilities	Stimulants commonly used	Specific learning disabilities do *not* respond to stimulants.
Conduct Disorders	Stimulants commonly used	Conduct disorders are *not* responsive to stimulants unless there is a clearly associated attention deficit disorder.
Childhood Psychosis	Antipsychotics	Hyperactivity, mood lability, and excitability are often improved, but social and language impairments are not reversed.
Anxiety Disorders	1. Anxiolytics 2. Tricyclic antidepressants	Anxiety disorders have not been systematically studied for response to anxiolytics but *separation-anxiety* has been reported to respond to tricyclic antidepressants.
Enuresis	Tricyclic antidepressants	Often respond quickly but symptom may appear after cessation of drug so that conditioning techniques are considered preferable.
Depressive Disorders	Tricyclic antidepressants	These are just starting to be systematically studied in prepubertal children, with some suggestion that the tricyclics may be effective.

Although the use of psychopharmacologic agents to treat childhood disorders is now in its fifth decade, their administration remains highly empirical and directed toward groups of target symptoms that grossly impair adaptation, not toward specific disease or diagnostic entities.

Recent major advances in our knowledge of the psychopharmacology of childhood disorders and the increased research being done suggests that the frontiers of our knowledge will continue to expand rather rapidly. Several generations of child psychiatrists, including most of those who trained prior to the late 1970s, were never exposed to this knowledge, and few were routinely expected to consider psychopharmacologic agents as a potentially important adjunct to treatment. As a result, those unfamiliar and uncomfortable with these recent advances often resist integrating psychopharmacological interventions into their overall approach to patients. While psychopharmacologic agents are rarely, if ever, a specific and sufficient treatment in and of themselves, current knowledge has reached the point where their potential contribution should always be considered in formulating a treatment plan.

SUGGESTIONS FOR FURTHER READING

AMAN, M., AND SINGH, N. 1980. The usefulness of thioridazine for treating childhood disorders—fact or folklore? *Am. J. Men. Def.* 84:331–338.
A critical look at the disparity between clinical experience and established scientific fact in the use of this commonly employed antipsychotic; suitable for most readers.

BARKLEY, R. 1977. Hyperkinesis, autonomic nervous system activity and stimulant drug effects. *J. Child Psychol. & Psychiat.* 18:347–357.
A comprehensive review of the use of stimulants in hyperkinesis; clearly organized and covering major areas of interest and concern; suitable for most readers.

BLAU, S. 1978. A guide to the use of psychotropic medication in children and adolescents. *J. Clin. Psychiat.* 39:766–772.
Very compact and useful guide from a research and clinical group of investigators; a very good clinical presentation.

COHEN, D., AND YOUNG, G. 1978. Neurochemistry and child psychiatry. *J. Am. Acad. Child Psychiat.* 16:353–411.
Update of neuroanatomy and neurotransmitter physiology as it may explain some of the abnormality in childhood psychopathology; most suitable for those with some background in neurosciences.

GREENHILL, L., et al. 1981. Growth hormone, prolactin, and growth responses in hyperkinetic males treated with D-amphetamine. *J. Am. Acad. Child Psychiat.* 20:84–103.
Cautions about the growth retarding effect of stimulants are reawakened.

GUALTIERI, C. et al. 1980. Tardive dyskinesia and other movement disorders in children treated with psychotropic drugs. *J. Am. Acad. Child Psychiat.* 19:491–520.
Looks at the risk for supersensitive movement disorder secondary to antipsychotic drug use in children; level of concern remains high.

MINDE, K. 1980. Some thoughts on the social ecology of present-day psychopharmacology. *Can. J. Psychiat.* 25:201–212.

The Role of Medication in the Treatment of the Disturbed Child

Explores many of the complexities and complications in the use of psychotropic drugs in children.

PUIG-ANTICH, J. 1980. Affective disorders in childhood: A review and perspective. *Psychiat. Clin. N. Am.* 3:403–424.

Review of current area of intense investigation by one of its foremost researchers; helps summarize burgeoning new area.

WERRY, J. 1982. An overview of pediatric psychopharmacology. *J. Am. Acad. Child Psychiat.* 21:3–9.

Excellent up-to-date review of the field.

WERRY, J., ed. 1978. *Pediatric psychopharmacology: The use of behavior modifying drugs in children.* New York: Brunner/Mazel.

The best textbook in the field today.

WHITE, J. H. 1980. Psychopharmacology in childhood: Current status and future perspectives. *Psychiat. Clin. N. Am.* 3(3):443–453.

Psychopharmacological treatment in childhood psychiatric disorders is always directed toward amelioration of target symptoms rather than cure. Its aim is to return the child as rapidly as possible to a functioning state, thus preventing academic and social failure.

30

Quentin Rae-Grant

The Primary Care and Referral of Children with Emotional and Behavioral Disorders

Parents and others responsible for children with emotional or behavioral difficulties have available to them a number of channels, formal and informal, through which they may seek help for their children or themselves. Generally they turn first to other family members or to close friends seeking either confirmation of their worries or reassurance that there is nothing basically wrong and no cause for concern. When convinced that some help is needed, they may then turn to a trusted clergyman, family practitioner, or pediatrician. Because these individuals already know the family and have an ongoing rapport with them, they are in many ways more able to quickly establish a working relationship that can be used to help solve the problems. However, because of the social aspect of the relationship the family has with the person to whom they turn for help, they may withhold certain very personal and emotionally charged but important information out of a sense of reticence or embarrassment. Thus the personal relationship, while facilitating the early contacts, may impede the investigation and examination of more intimate areas.

664

Pathways of Help

The majority of behavioral problems and emotional disorders are, and will continue to be, dealt with by resources other than mental health facilities. Depending on the nature of the symptoms, where they present problems for other people, and the judgment that the children require help, they may enter the service system by many different channels. Children often first show problems and difficulties on school entry. These same difficulties may not be present at home or may be within the parents' tolerance. Teachers also have, from experience, a broader concept than individual parents of what constitutes the need for help and the range of normality and abnormality. In the early school years social problems and later academic difficulties may lead the teachers to indicate to the parents the need for investigation and possibly intervention. The initial stages of evaluation and intervention utilize the knowledge of the teacher, the principal, or school-associated services, such as guidance counselor, school psychologist, or psychiatrist. If the child's antisocial behavior is troublesome to the community, the problem may first be brought to the attention of the police and the juvenile court system. While many cases are dealt with appropriately by reprimand and admonition or by a court appearance with a warning or conditions of probation, if the problems continue and the degree of behavioral disturbance is such that removal from home is a court-considered alternative, a mental health evaluation is often requested to advise the court on appropriate action (see chapter 13).

Should physical symptoms be the manner of presentation, it is likely that the family practitioner, pediatrician, public health nurse, or medical outpatient department may be the first to be consulted. Many physical symptoms have no underlying organic cause but are an expression of emotional disturbance in the child or in the family. Abdominal pain is a frequent initial complaint, for example, in cases of school phobia (see chapter 12). The physical symptoms of anorexia nervosa almost invariably are the first manifestations of the underlying psychological and family issues (see chapter 19).

A substantial proportion of general and pediatric practice involves problems that are emotional or developmental in origin or occur in conjunction with or as a consequence of a physical illness of a family member. With the advances in modern pediatrics, the number of children who survive previously fatal conditions is increasing; thus in pediatric practice the issues are not only treatment of the physical condition but also of the family's reaction to it and its impact on the child and other family members and their relationships (see chapter 21).

If abandonment, neglect, or physical or sexual abuse occur or are suspected, a child welfare organization is likely to be the initial resource involved, with in more severe cases simultaneous medical investigation and treatment. Indeed, in most jurisdictions, anyone suspecting child abuse or sexual abuse is required by law to report this suspicion to the authorities. This requirement overrides the question of confidentiality, and penalties for nonreporting are provided although rarely implemented (see chapter 25).

With the increasing number of children attending day-care centers and nursery schools, the staff there may be the first to identify at this early age that the child is in need of help and to suggest appropriate action to the parents. Adolescents are often brought by parents because of the difficulties and oppositional behavior that create problems for the parents. Older adolescents may seek help on their own from facilities clearly designated for them, particularly drop-in centers that have a variety of formal and informal services tailored to the needs of this age group (see chapter 5).

Thus a variety of professionals working in a variety of settings may be selected, at times on a random basis, to provide primary, or frontline, care. Since the number of children in need of help is at least ten times the number that can be served by the available mental health resources, the continuing importance of primary care and the need for primary resources to have available adequate mental health and psychiatric services for backup and consultation when required is obvious. It has to be recognized that, with the multiple alternative pathways to help, the choice of a particular pathway may inadvertently determine the nature of treatment provided. Each of the systems of care has preferred methods and tends to utilize these for most of the cases served. Thus two children with the same symptoms and the same underlying problems may receive quite different interventions depending on the source from which their families seek help. The cross-overs between the service systems are becoming increasingly flexible, and smooth transmission implies the knowledge of how to refer and how to lay the ground for alternative intervention when this is clearly indicated. This chapter will address the questions of general principles of intervention at the primary care level, when to refer and what to expect on referral.

Evaluation of the Problem

Symptoms of emotional disorder are really only signals of underlying distress. They indicate an imbalance between internal and external forces to which, at times, they may provide a partial solution. Most symptoms occur in a transient form in normal children during the course of development,

666

particularly at times of internal change (e.g., adolescence) or external change (e.g., leaving home to go to school or in response to illness or death of a family member; see chapter 9). In fact, if the "symptoms" in a normal population are compared with those in a clinic caseload, the difference lies not in the presence or absence of symptoms but in the number, degree, intensity, and duration of the symptoms in those identified as needing help.

The first question to decide then is whether symptoms are normal and age-appropriate and, therefore, likely to disappear in time. Second, the kind of response that these symptoms are evoking from the environment must be clarified, as even a "normal" symptom that elicits an overreaction of concern or hostility may become a fixed and more enduring pattern. Thus the longer the duration and the greater the inability of the environment to cope with the child's symptoms, the stronger the indication for intervention. Should it be that more than the normal developmental difficulties are at the root of the issue, the more immediate the identification of the underlying problem, the more likely intervention will be successful, and the more quickly it will prove effective.

Appropriate intervention is based on a comprehensive history and examination of the child and the crucial systems affecting him or her, particularly the family and the school. Accepting the symptoms at face value may ignore the underlying problem. Indeed, it may also ignore the part of the system most requiring help. Children's behavior often is used as the admission ticket for help when the issue may actually lie in the parental relationship, such as a bad marriage or threatened separation or indeed a major emotional disorder in one of the parents, which is a less socially accepted reason for seeking help. Parental alcoholism and depression are prime examples.

The objectives of the evaluation are to develop a working understanding of how each family member functions as an individual, a knowledge of how members relate to and influence one another, and some idea of their potential strengths as well as their areas of difficulty. Clinicians may begin by tracing developmentally the appearance of the behavior, who first identified it as a matter of concern, the various opinions expressed about it, what has been tried to ameliorate the behavior, and the degree of success. Simultaneously, the primary caregiver can explore the interest of the family and of the child in working toward change, given the time and energy that this requires. The family that does not recognize the behavior as a problem and comes only because someone else has identified it as one, or those who do not see that they have had any part in its origin and feel that they can do nothing to effect change, are unlikely to understand the need for their involvement or to be motivated to take part in any remedial program to the extent necessary for its success. At the other end of the scale is the family that assumes some responsibility for the production of the difficulties, is willing to work, and motivated to change.

Primary Care Interventions

Although people come expressing a desire for help, they may also bring an underlying fear of criticism and a sense of failure, since they themselves have not been able to solve the problem. Seeking help confirms this sense of inadequacy and so may be combined with a covert hope that perhaps the counselor too will fail, since insofar as he or she is helpful, this success can be taken as proof of the client's inadequacy.

Any request for help represents an opportunity for intervention. The greater the anxiety level of the family—that is, the closer the family appears to be approaching a state of crisis—the more receptive the family may be to a relatively brief intervention (see chapter 20). Generally, the avenues available for intervention include review, environmental manipulation, reassurance, and counseling.

REVIEW

Frequently the taking of a fairly complete individual and family history may in itself have important therapeutic effects. In the process of stock taking and with the help of the interviewer, the central issues and the areas in which change is required may become very clear. Therefore, the appropriate therapeutic modalities to be employed may become obvious.

ENVIRONMENTAL MANIPULATION

Environmental manipulation still has a respected place, provided the professional can clearly demonstrate the relationship between the component in the environment to be altered and the behavior attributable to it, as in removing the dependent and clinging child from the parents' bedroom. Change for the sake of change is rarely effective, and may be contraindicated if it obscures or complicates the problem, as in a change of school or school refusal (see chapter 12). Usually environmental manipulation is effective only when all parties agree to its potential value, for example when patents and school concur on the child repeating a school grade.

REASSURANCE

Many parents seek reassurance because of concern for their child's future and doubts about their own competence. If, following adequate exploration of the child's behavior, general adjustment, and the overall family situation the worker is sure that reassurance is justified, supplying it may do much to decrease parental anxiety and to provide a more relaxed and healthy environment in which the child can grow. The three-month-old colicky child with an anxious and uncertain parent shows dramatic improvement when the mother is effectively reassured (see chapter 9). However, premature or false reassurance is *never* justified, as it may invalidly dismiss behavior that merits more extensive intervention. Although counselors often use reassurance for their own convenience or to save time, false reassurance rarely helps in the long run. (For further elaboration and examples, see discussion of reassurance in chapter 20.)

COUNSELING*

Counseling is a two-way process of helping individuals and families define problems in relationships, recognize what they are doing to one another, elicit alternatives, and develop new skills for coping. Counselors cannot impose their ideas, as they will be rejected unless they coincide with those of the parents. Counselors do not have all the answers, nor should they allow themselves to be placed in the position of having to provide the solutions. Counseling is a joint endeavour—counselors guide but cannot mandate; they may suggest, they may have to repeat, and they must always be prepared to revise the direction of their advice. Counselors commit themselves to work with people as they struggle, effectively or not so effectively, with their problems. From the beginning, the counselors' position contains a number of potential pitfalls.

The process of counseling is not a popularity contest. It is based on a sense of trusting and a willingness to explore and change with the help of a relationship that guarantees respect to the individuals seeking counseling. They have often done their very best to handle the situation and should not be blamed or scapegoated for what they have been unable to do without help. At times, however, it becomes necessary for counselors to point out clearly and directly issues that are being avoided and that, when brought up in discussion, may provoke very negative feelings, antagonism, and even temporary open hostility, including pointed criticisms of the alleged incompetence or error of the counselors. It is important, however, to distinguish between the raising of an issue when it seems crucial to the progress of treatment and the deliberate provocation employed by some muscular therapists in which honesty is not a vehicle but a weapon. Counseling is a therapeutic alliance. It goes through phases. Counselors may be placed on a pedestal of knowledge and acumen on one occasion. On another they may be roundly lambasted for not being helpful or for raising unpleasant topics. Both reactions are distortions of the reality. Indeed the examination of how and why the counselor is being placed in these positions plays an important part in understanding the dynamics of the situation. Counselors are perceived and dealt with in ways that recapit-

---

*The term counselor will be used generically to describe anyone providing the services defined herein. There is obvious overlap with certain forms of psychotherapy, casework, and much that goes on within the doctor-patient relationship.

ulate and reflect other key relationships from the present or the past. The process of help involves recognizing these distortions as projections and examining their origins.

> The first day that Dr. S walked onto the ward he noticed that Michael, age fourteen, was carefully watching him and constantly keeping him at a distance. Later he learned that Michael, who had been through fourteen foster homes, was mistrustful and hostile to all adults. Dr. S worked intensively with Michael for over a year. He had forgotten the circumstances of their initial meeting until one day Michael, who had become rather friendly, commented that when Dr. S had first walked onto the ward, "I just took one look at you and your face was so mean, I just knew you were a son of a bitch." When Dr. S asked how he looked now, Michael laughed and replied, "You look okay. I didn't even know you then. I just figured you'd be mean, because you were a grown-up." Clearly, Michael was projecting onto Dr. S feelings derived from past relationships with adults. From that time on, much of Michael's therapy consisted of demonstrating ways in which his distorted perceptions and hostile behavior in response to them interfered with his relationships and provoked others to punish and reject him.

Only when counselors have been able to remain neutral and objective, neither flattered by the plaudits nor devastated by the antagonism, can they make the projective nature of these feelings clear as they occur. Counseling implies maintaining a position of neutrality, particularly in situations involving conflict between two sides that see the same issue from very different vantage points. Each side competes for the counselor as an ally, inviting him or her to confirm that its opinions are correct. Once counselors lose their objectivity, they lose their credibility and usefulness and become co-opted into the ongoing struggle. It is particularly dangerous to reach conclusions and act on them having heard only one side of an issue. In cases involving child custody, for example, the picture given of one parent by the other may be factually correct but emotionally distorted (see chapter 26). The same is true where adolescents and parents are in conflict. To become the ally of one side, and therefore the antagonist of the other, is an invitation frequently extended and rarely justified. Counselors should recognize that the child's or adolescent's description of the parents is only his or her perception of them rather than an accurate presentation of the parents as they are.

Counselors need not work in isolation, nor indeed should the clients. There are many helping agencies available for families—the school, social agencies, recreation services—and simultaneous involvement of the family and child with these agencies may facilitate what counselors can do individually. Effective collaboration with these agencies assists in sharing the burden, particularly in dealing with multiproblem families.

A more recent development in sources of aid are the self-help groups in which families who have children with various illnesses, physical or emotional, meet together to support each other. Families can benefit from sharing with others in a similar predicament their anxiety, frustration, and problems. The feeling of not being alone in the situation is an additional reassurance. Many families with disturbed children are socially isolated, and involvement in community social groups, particularly with activities for parents as well as for the children, expands their support system. This support system used to be provided by the extended family or small communities. In large cities, those most in need often have difficulty in providing and finding alternatives and need help and encouragement to seek out the many sources of support available.

Counselors also can benefit from support, particularly with difficult cases. This can come from ongoing sharing with colleagues facing similar problems, or by meeting regularly with a mental health consultant for guidance.

Senn and Solnit (1968) have listed a number of common errors in case management. Many of these relate to issues of time—for example, the interview that is late in starting or has to be cut short because of other commitments. This leads to a feeling that the interview is hurried. The informants are not given time or a sense of comfort in dealing with more personal issues and respond to the pressure that they sense on the counselor. The counselor may be tempted to speed up the process, to accept the obvious as the essential and to look for *the* cause rather than recognize that most situations occur from multiple factors, including temperamental, personality, interpersonal, cultural and family values. The temptation to dismiss problems as a stage of development can be particularly misleading. In cases of what used to be called adolescent turmoil, on follow-up it was clear that many of the cases required substantial help. The turmoil may be not simply normal adolescent opposition to authority and personal discomfort but the first indication of more serious pathology, such as depression or early stages of psychosis (see chapter 15).

Other pitfalls that Senn and Solnit point out are the counselors' loss of objectivity previously mentioned and their failure to understand and accept the limits of their capacity to intervene. This factor may also inhibit or delay referral to other resources when necessary and cause failure to prepare for the referral. Direct advice is sometimes valuable when it is based on a careful review of the situation. Theoretical discussions have little place in the treatment process, but all families are entitled to ask what is involved, what alternatives are available, the competence of the counselor to conduct what is proposed, and, particularly in the area of the use of medication, side effects that may occur and of which they should be aware. The public is now well informed, although sometimes erroneously, about the hazards of medication. These hazards are often grossly exaggerated. For example, recent work has shown the use of anxiolytics to be justified in reducing anxiety level enough to allow other therapy to proceed. The pendulum is again swinging to the moderate use of these drugs and away from withholding them on theoretical grounds (see chapter 29). Patients' questions, however, are legitimate. The asking and answering of them honestly is an essential part of intervention (Rosenbaum 1982).

Referral

Referral may be indicated for a number of reasons. During the course of evaluation, major diagnostic questions may arise that counselors feel are beyond their competence to answer, or the skills they have available may not be those required by the case. The reason for referral, however, may come later in ongoing counseling, when a certain stage seems to have been reached and further progress stalemated. Then referral for consultation or continuing treatment by someone else is indicated.

When a person has been counseling a case over a period of time, it may be difficult to consider referral and natural to view it as a reflection on his or her own work. Yet good counselors are those who have learned to understand and accept the limits of what they personally can do. Not all people are able to deal with all issues with the same equanimity and effectiveness. To recognize that one works better with certain conditions and not as well with others is an indication of maturity and skill as a counselor. Referral can be both helpful and necessary, but it can also be used in a punitive way. The counselor's discomfort about the need or request for referral may lead to its being done in an abrupt, curt, and mechanical fashion that decreases the likelihood of its being followed through. If presented with annoyance, the referral is likely to be interpreted as punishment for failure to improve despite the best help that the counselor could provide. Implicit in the process of successful referral is the preparation of people for disengagement from current attachments and helping them get ready to pick up with others who bring different skills. Since often the referral is made as much for the counselor's purpose as for the client's, it is important to give attention to how the issue is raised and to what it means for those to whom it is suggested. Clients should have an opportunity to work through their concerns and should terminate feeling free to return when and if this seems appropriate.

REASON FOR REFERRAL

The patient, client, or family should be referred to more specific mental health and psychiatric resources in the following situations:

1. When the endeavors of the counselor or practitioner do not seem to be helping, or where a plateau at which no further improvement is occurring seems to have been reached.

2. When a major diagnostic question arises on which the counselor wishes either a more specialized opinion or further investigation—for example, differentiation of severe neurosis from psychosis, brain damage, or retardation.
3. When the counselor is faced with certain crisis situations that the family cannot control or tolerate even with his or her help, such as serious suicide attempts or threats or massive and continuing aggressive or antisocial behavior. Nonresponsive cases of anorexia nervosa and other psychosomatic disorders are also best referred to settings where the physical and emotional components can receive attention simultaneously (see chapter 19).
4. When the counselor's own sense of discomfort about what is being dealt with or what he or she is doing begins to mount, the counselor is wise to seek further advice on case management. Too often these feelings are partially recognized by the practitioner but ignored so that action is delayed. In general, it is better to err on the side of referral than to delay until a crisis forces one's hand.
5. When the initial evaluation indicates that the degree and number of problems will require more time than the primary caregiver is willing or able to offer.

Referrals can only be recommended; they cannot be forced on the family or the patient. Without the clients' willing cooperation, the referral is not likely to be helpful. Their cooperation will have to be solicited, and child and family may need to discuss the referral over a period of time before they are able to accept it for what it is, namely a move in their own interests, suggested and supported by the counselor. This support may have to continue after the other facility is involved, as the process of transfer is not an easy one, and often the original counselor occupies a position of trust, which the new therapist has yet to win. The degree to which a referral may prove helpful is often determined by this process of preparation and the time given to resolving the doubts, answering the questions, and providing the incentive.

Children who are referred should be told whom they will be seeing and the reasons for the referral. The more clearly they understand why they are being referred, the more likely they are to benefit from the referral. Often parents are anxious about seeking help from a psychiatrist and may communicate this anxiety to the child. There is often realistic concern about how the peer group will react if the psychiatric meetings become known. Adolescents in particular may feel apprehensive about having to see a psychiatrist, and frequently the resolution of this initial anxiety is the essential first phase of therapeutic work.

Sometimes it is helpful for children and adolescents to develop and rehearse a cover story to tell their peers. While their friends do not need to know the details of the child's treatment, unless they are given some information they become curious; this curiosity may lead to further teasing and scapegoating. The child returning to school after an absence needs to have a reasonable explanation to give to friends. In helping the child to develop one, the counselor may help to avoid secondary social consequences and stigma (see chapter 12).

The practitioner also has a part to play in smoothing the way for people at a referral source. He or she should provide the mental health or psychiatric facility with the reasons for the referral, something of the background of the family and the problem, what has gone on already, and, in particular, whether or not the practitioner wishes to remain involved in the situation (that is, is this a request for consultation?) or expects the psychiatrist or mental health center to pick up the treatment. A message via nurse or secretary often leaves many of these questions unanswered, leading to later misunderstanding. Most mental health facilities prefer direct contact either by telephone or letter. The most successful referrals generally occur when the two people or agencies involved know each other, have worked together on cases previously, and have developed a sense of trust in each other's competence.

Many mental health facilities, following such a discussion, will ask that a member of the family phone to set up the initial appointment. This request is partly to involve the family in making the contact right from the beginning and partly out of the knowledge that the family that lacks motivation to follow through on a suggested referral is not yet sufficiently prepared to benefit from it.

In referring a case to either an individual consultant or a multidisciplinary setting, the referring practitioner or counselor has some legitimate expectations of the agency, including the agency's formulation of the case and treatment recommendations. The counselor also can expect to be kept up to date with case progress, as not infrequently parents will check back with the original trusted individual. More frequently these days, the referring individual is invited to participate in conferences that analyze the findings or review progress, particularly toward the time of case closing and referral back to the initial counselor for further follow-up.

Mental Health Professional Roles

In the heyday of the child guidance clinics, the roles of the psychiatrist, psychologist, and social worker had an artificial distinction and clarity. The *psychiatrist* was the physician on the team. He or she physically examined and psychiatrically assessed the child. The psychiatrist also provided the medical component of treatment including psychotherapy and medication, if indicated. The *psychologist,* though also at times serving as a child therapist, primarily contributed during the assessment, defining the child's intellectual functioning through intelligence tests and assessing emotional development and delineating areas of conflict through projective tests. The *social worker* was responsible mainly for taking a history from the parents, for obtaining information on social functioning, and for providing casework (counseling) for the parents. Together these three constituted a *thera-peutic team,* working with each other on a collaborative basis as one person treated the child and another the parents. The psychiatrist, as team leader, assumed responsibility for the team's developing and maintaining an integrated approach to treatment.

The picture has changed considerably as the various professionals involved redefine their aspirations and areas of expertise. Psychologists have moved from a heavy reliance on projective testing to more specific testing in the cognitive areas, particularly useful in delineating difficulties in learning. They have also developed to a greater extent than most psychiatrists and social workers the techniques of behavior modification. With the increasing range and effectiveness of psychopharmacological agents and an increased emphasis on the art of consultation, many psychiatrists are less involved in ongoing psychotherapy, which they frequently delegate to other members of the enlarged treatment team. In most hospital-associated facilities, the contributions of *occupational therapists,* both diagnostically and therapeutically, have been recognized. A major role is often assigned to *speech pathologists,* and *nurses* with specific training in the mental health area are frequently involved in providing group and milieu therapy. In this their function may overlap with that of the *child-care worker* (milieu therapist), who has community college training in preparation for on-the-spot care of children, particularly in residential treatment. The child-care worker often has taken further training in group or family therapy. Thus roles have become blurred. Each discipline brings its own contributions and complements the areas of expertise of the others. No single discipline has all the answers or all the resources. While there remain cases requiring long-term intervention, the pressure of mounting service demands and changing philosophies and techniques of treatment have led to a shift from the traditional fascination with psychopathology and intrapsychic clarification to an increasing emphasis on functioning and coping capacities and short-term and crisis approaches to treatment. Within the same setting, a similar service may be provided—and provided with a varying degree of skill and sophistication—by a number of professionals from a variety of disciplines.

New roles are gradually evolving, with that of the child psychiatrist increasingly emphasizing the integration of physical, psychological, and psychiatric findings to develop an overall biopsychosocial synthesis of the case. In medical considerations the psychiatrist is by law required to assume the final responsibility of the case and be accountable for this.

In addition, the expanding field of psychopharmacology requires the psychiatrist's medical background and knowledge to prescribe efficiently and to know the appropriate monitoring procedures and blood levels that are the benchmark for thoughtful use of medication. As chapter 29 indicates, effectiveness is much improved and side effects are avoided by having blood levels tested regularly rather than relying on dosage as related to weight, which has been the mechanism thus far. The gaps that existed or were created between child and adult psychiatry and pediatrics are rapidly being bridged, and for children and adolescents with more serious disorders, this integrated approach that also uses several developing disciplines such as biochemistry and clinical psychopharmacology provides more comprehensive treatment and greater safety.

Mental health facilities have operated in isolation for too long. This isolation was partly of their own choosing and partly because of the social discomfort about mental illness. However, when this distancing extended even to other mental health facilities, it created a series of unrelated centers of competence rather than a continuum of care through which children and families could move according to their needs at particular times. The emphasis also was often on treating intensively small numbers of patients rather than applying basic principles of parsimony in intervention (Rae-Grant and Hollister 1972). Intervention ideally should be the least intrusive, the least expensive, the least intensive, and the shortest in duration required to produce the needed restoration of competence to function and to grow productively. As children's and families' needs change with time, so the appropriate source to provide this continuing help and appropriate service also changes. The challenge facing all jurisdictions is the integration of a continuum of service.

SUGGESTIONS FOR FURTHER READING

BALINT, M. 1957. *The doctor, his patient, and the illness.* New York: International Universities Press.
Describes and gives details on what has become one of the major models of collaboration between mental health professionals and primary caregivers. It focuses, most specifically, on doctor-patient relationships, but the principles are applicable to the development of an ongoing support system and further education in clinical practice and handling of emotional and psychological issues. A classic in the field.

BERMAN, S. 1974. The relationship of the private practitioner of child psychiatry to prevention. *J. Am. Acad. Child Psychiat.* 13:593–603.
Discusses the contribution of the child psychiatrist in private practice to child mental health services and the importance of coordinating his or her participation with programs to institutions, mental health legislation, and mental health training.

HODGE, J. R. 1975. *Practical psychiatry for the primary physician.* Chicago: Nelson-Hall.
Useful for the medical practitioner who needs an understanding of basic psychiatry.

RICHMOND, J. B., AND SCHERL, D. J. 1975. Research in the delivery of health services. In *American handbook of psychiatry,* 2nd ed. rev., vol. 6, ed. D. A. Hamburg and H. K. H. Brodie, pp. 731–755. New York: Basic Books.
Highly technical review of major issues related to research into the delivery of health services, covering such areas as research design, evaluative indices, and studies and consumer participation.

RIEGER, N. I., AND DEVRIES, A. G. 1974. The child mental health specialist: A new profession. *Am. J. Orthopsychiat.* 44:150–158.
Describes a training program for child mental health specialists that is recommended as

essential for nationwide implementation if adequate preventive and treatment services are ever to be produced.

ROSENBAUM, J. F. 1982. Current concepts in psychiatry: The drug treatment of anxiety. *N. E. J. Med.* 306(7):401–404.

One in a series of four articles that summarizes succienctly the current state of knowledge about the administration of psychopharmacological agents for the treatment of psychosis, depression, anxiety, and other psychiatric conditions.

SENN, M., AND SOLNIT, A. J. 1968. *Problems in child behavior and development.* Philadelphia: Lea and Febiger.

A most practical and useful text for pediatricians and practitioners that presents diagnosis and intervention within a developmental framework. Highly recommended.

Discusses the contribution that the practicing child psychiatrist can make to a child welfare association or children's aid society through ongoing consultation.

STEISEL, I. M., AND ADAMSON, W. C. 1974. The use and training of allied mental health workers in child guidance clinics. *J. Am. Acad. Child Psychiat.* 13:524–535.

Discusses the importance and various roles of allied mental health workers in enhancing the delivery of care to children in child guidance clinics.

TIZARD, J. 1974. The upbringing of other people's children: Implications of research and for research. *J. Child Psychol. & Psychiat.* 15:161–73.

Discusses the association between the behavior of children in residence and the formal organizational structure and child-care practices of institutional settings, exploring both theoretical and practical issues related to child development.

LIST OF ABBREVIATED

JOURNAL TITLES

Acad. Therap.   Academic Therapy
Acad. Therap. Quart.   Academic Therapy Quarterly
Act. Psychiat. Scand.   Acta Psychiatrica Scandinavia
Adol.   Adolescence
Adv. Teratol.   Advances in Teratology
Am. Anthrop.   American Anthropologist
Am. Fam. Physician   American Family Physician
Am. J. Clin. Nut.   American Journal of Clinical Nutrition
Am. J. Dis. Child.   American Journal of Diseases of Children
Am. J. Ment. Def.   American Journal of Mental Deficiency
Am. J. Nur.   American Journal of Nursing
Am. J. Ob. Gyn.   American Journal of Obstetrics and Gynecology
Am. J. Orthopsychiat.   American Journal of Orthopsychiatry
Am. J. Psychother.   American Journal of Psychotherapy
Am. J. Psychiat.   American Journal of Psychiatry
Am. J. Pub. H.   American Journal of Public Health
Am. Psychol.   American Psychologist
Am. Sociol. Rev.   American Sociological Review
Ann. Med. Psychol.   Annales Medico—Psychologiques
Ann. Adol. Psychiat.   Annals of Adolescent Psychiatry
Ann. Clin. Res.   Annals of Clinical Research
Ann. Int. Med.   Annals of Internal Medicine
Ann. Neurol.   Annals of Neurology
Ann. N.Y. Acad. Sci.   Annals of the New York Academy of Science
Arch. Dis. Child.   Archives of the Diseases of Children
Arch. Gen. Psychiat.   Archives of General Psychiatry
Arch. Neurol. Psychiat.   Archives of Neurological Psychiatry
Arth. & Rheum.   Arthritis and Rheumatism
Aust. & N.Z. J. Psychiat.   Australia and New Zealand Journal of Psychiatry
Austr. J. Ment. Retard.   Australian Journal of Mental Retardation

Behav. Disord.   Behavioural Disorders
Behav. Neuropsychiat.   Behavioral Neuropsychiatry
Behav. Sci.   Behavioral Science

List of Abbreviated Journal Titles

Behav. Therap. Behavior Therapy
Biochem. Pharm. Biochemical Pharmacology
Biol. Psychiat. Biological Psychiatry
Brit. J. Ed. Psychol. British Journal of Educational Psychology
Brit. J. Hosp. Med. British Journal of Hospital Medicine
Brit. J. Med. Psychol. British Journal of Medical Psychology
Brit. J. Med. British Journal of Medicine
Brit. J. Ob. Gyn. British Journal of Obstetrics and Gynecology
Brit. J. Psychiat. British Journal of Psychiatry
Brit. J. Sociol. British Journal of Sociology

Can. Ment. Health Canada's Mental Health

Can. Fam. Physic. Canadian Family Physician
Can. J. Psychiat. Canadian Journal of Psychiatry
Can. Psychiat. Assn. J. Canadian Psychiatric Association Journal
Child Dev. Child Development
Child Psychiat. & Hum. Dev. Child Psychiatry and Human Development
Child Wel. Child Welfare
Clin. Ob. Gyn. Clinical Obstetrics and Gynecology
Clin. Ped. Clinical Pediatrics
Cur. Therap. Res. Current Therapeutic Research

Dev. Med. & Child Neurol. Developmental Medicine and Child Neurology
Dis. Ner. Syst. Diseases of the Nervous System

Electroencephal. & Clin. Neurophysiol. Electroencephalography and Clinical Neurophysiology
Except. Child. Exceptional Children

Fam. Therap. Family Therapy
Fam. Therap. Coll. Family Therapy Collections
Fam. Plan. Persp. Family Planning Perspectives
Fam. Process Family Process

H. & Soc. Work Health and Social Work
Hosp. Prac. Hospital Practice

Inf. Ment. Health Infant Mental Health
Int. J. Child Ab. & Neg. International Journal of Child Abuse and Neglect
Int. J. Eat. Disord. International Journal of Eating Disorders
Int. J. Ment. Health International Journal of Mental Health
Int. J. Psychiat. Med. International Journal of Psychiatry in Medicine
Int. J. Psychoanal. International Journal of Psychoanalysis
Int. J. Soc. Psychiat. International Journal of Social Psychiatry
Int. Rev. Psychoanal. International Review of Psychoanalysis
Int. U. P. International Universities Press
Iss. Ment. Health Nurs. Issues in Mental Health Nursing

J. Abnorm. Child Psychol. Journal of Abnormal Child Psychology
J. Abnorm. Soc. Psychol. Journal of Abnormal Social Psychology
J. Amer. Acad. Child Psychiat. Journal of the American Academy of Child Psychiatry
J. Am. Med. Wom. Assn. Journal of American Medical Women's Association
J. App. Behav. Anal. Journal of Applied Behavior Analysis
J. Aut. & Childhood Schiz. Journal of Autism and Childhood Schizophrenia
J. Behav. Therap. & Exper. Psychiat. Journal of Behaviour Therapy and Experimental
Psychiatry
J. Child Psychol. Psychiat. & All. Discip. Journal of Child Psychology Psychiatry and
Allied Disciplines

J. Child Psychol. & Psychiat.   Journal of Child Psychology and Psychiatry
J. Child Wel. Leag. Am.   Journal of Child Welfare League of America
J. Chron. Dis.   Journal of Chronic Diseases
J. Clin. Psychol.   Journal of Clinical Psychology
J. Comp. & Physiol. Psychiat.   Journal of Comparative and Physiological Psychiatry
J. Cons. & Clin. Psychol.   Journal of Consulting and Clinical Psychology
J. Cons. Psychol.   Journal of Consulting Psychology
J. Epidem. & Comm. H.   Journal of Epidemiology and Community Health
J. Exper. Child Psychol.   Journal of Experimental Child Psychology
J. Exper. Ed.   Journal of Experimental Education
J. Fam. Prac.   Journal of Family Practice
J. Gen. Psychol.   Journal of Genetic Psychology
J. Learn. Disab.   Journal of Learning Disabilities
J. Marr. & Fam. Therap.   Journal of Marital and Family Therapy
J. Marr. & Fam. Counsel.   Journal of Marriage and Family Counselling
J. Marr. & Fam. Liv.   Journal of Marriage and Family Living
J. Marr. & Fam.   Journal of Marriage and the Family
J. Med. Gen.   Journal of Medical Genetics
J. Nerv. & Ment. Dis.   Journal of Nervous and Mental Disease
J. Neur. Trans.   Journal of Neural Transmission
J. Ob. Gyn. & Neonat. Nurs.   Journal of Obstetric, Gynecological and Neonatal Nursing
J. Pediat. Psychol.   Journal of Pediatric Psychology
J. Pediat.   Journal of Pediatrics
J. Pers. & Soc. Psychol.   Journal of Personality and Social Psychology
J. Prev.   Journal of Prevention
J. Psychiat. & Law   Journal of Psychiatry and Law
J. Psychosom. Res.   Journal of Psychosomatic Research
J. Rheum.   Journal of Rheumatology
J. Sch. Health   Journal of School Health
J. Soc. Iss.   Journal of Social Issues
J. Soc. Ser. Res.   Journal of Social Service Research
J. Spec. Ed.   Journal of Special Education
J. Am. Acad. Psychoanal.   Journal of the American Academy of Psychoanalysis
J. Am. Acad. Child Psychi.   Journal of the American Academy of Child Psychiatry
J. Am. Optomet. Assn.   Journal of the American Optometric Association
J. Am. Psychoanal. Assn.   Journal of the American Psychoanalytic Association
J. App. Behav. Anal.   Journal of Applied Behavioral Analysis
J. McLean Hosp.   Journal of the McLean Hospital
J. Ont. Assn. Child. Aid Soc.   Journal of the Ontario Association of Children's Aid Societies
J. Youth & Adol.   Journal of Youth and Adolescence
J. Am. Med. Assn.   Journal of the American Medical Association

Lang. & Speech   Language and Speech

Mat.-Child Nurs. J.   Maternal–Child Nursing Journal
Mayo Clin. Proc.   Mayo Clinic Proceedings
Med. J. Austr.   Medical Journal of Australia
Millbank Mem. Fund. Quart.   Millbank Memorial Fund Quarterly
Mod. Med.   Modern Medicine
Mono. Soc. Res. Child Devel.   Monograph of the Society for Research in Child Development
Mt. Sinai J. Med.   Mount Sinai Journal of Medicine

Nat. Found. Ed. Res.   National Foundation for Educational Research
N. E. J. Med.   New England Journal of Medicine
N. Y. State J. Med.   New York State Journal of Medicine
Nova Scot. Med. Bull.   Nova Scotia Medical Bulletin

List of Abbreviated Journal Titles

Ont. Med. Rev.   Ontario Medical Review

Pediatr.   Pediatrics
Pediatr. Ann.   Pediatric Annals
Pediatr. Clin. N. Am.   Pediatric Clinics of North America
Percep. & Mot. Skills   Perceptual and Motor Skills
Proc. Roy. Soc. Med.   Proceedings of the Royal Society of Medicine
Psychiat. Clin. N. Am.   Psychiatric Clinics of North America
Psychiat. Neurol.   Psychiatric Neurology
Psychiat. Quart.   Psychiatric Quarterly
Psychiat. Quart. Supp.   Psychiatric Quarterly Supplement
Psychiat. & Neurol. J. Spec. Med.   Psychiatry and Neurology Journal of Specialist Medicine
Psychoanal. Stud. Child   Psychoanalytic Study of the Child, The
Psychol. Bull.   Psychological Bulletin
Psychol. Med.   Psychological Medicine
Psychol. School   Psychology in the Schools
Psychopharmacol. Bull.   Psychopharmacological Bulletin
Psychophysiol.   Psychophysiology
Psychosom. Med.   Psychosomatic Medicine
Psychotherap. & Psychosom.   Psychotherapy and Psychosomatics
Psychiat. Res. Rep.   Psychiatric Research Report

Rehab. Coun. Bull.   Rehabilitation Counselling Bulletin
Rehab. Lit.   Rehabilitation Literature
Rehab. Med.   Rehabilitation Medicine
Rev. Fran. Psychanal.   Revue Française de Psychanalyse

Scand. J. Rheumatol.   Scandanavian Journal of Rheumatology
Sem. Hematol.   Seminars in Hematology
Sem. Psychiat.   Seminars in Psychiatry
Soc. Psychol. Quart.   Social Psychology Quarterly
Soc. Sc. & Med.   Social Science and Medicine
Soc. Work   Social Work
Soc. Rev.   Sociological Review
Suicide & Life Threat. Behav.   Suicide and Life Threatening Behavior
Trans. Am. Neurol. Assn.   Transactions of the American Neurological Association
Trends Pharmacol. Sc.   Trends in Pharmacological Sciences

REFERENCES

ABRAMS, J.C., and KASLOW, F. W. 1976. Learning disability and family dynamics: A mutual interaction. *J. Clin. Child Psychol.*, 5(1): 35–40.

ACHENBACH, T.M. 1980. What is child psychiatric epidemiology the epidemiology of? In ed. F. Earls, *Studies of children*. pp. 96–116, New York: Prodist.

———, and EDELBROCK, C.S. 1978. The classification of child psychopathology: A review and analysis of empirical efforts. *Psychol. Bull.* 85(6): 1275–1301.

ACKERMAN, N.W. 1958. *The psychodynamics of family life*. New York: Basic Books, pp. 15–25.

———. 1961. Prejudicial scapegoating and neutralizing forces in the family group with special reference to the role of family healer. *Int. J. Soc. Psychiat. Spec. Ed.*, 2: 90–96.

ADAM, K.S., LOHRENZ, J.G., HARPER, D., and STREINER, D. 1982. Early parental loss and suicidal ideation in university students. *Can. J. Psychiat.* 27(4) June: 275–81.

ADAMS, C.E. 1980. Psychotherapy with a blind patient. *Am. J. Psychother.* 34(3): 426–33.

ADAMS, D.W. 1979. *The psychosocial care of the child and his family in childhood cancer: An annotated bibliography*. Hamilton, Ont.: McMaster University Medical Centre.

ADAMS, J.E., and LINDEMANN, E. 1974. Coping with long-term disability. In *Copying and adaptation* ed. G.V. Coelho, D.A. Hamburg, and J.E. Adams, 127–38. New York: Basic Books.

ADAMS, P.L. 1979. Psychoneuroses. In *Basic handbook of child psychiatry*, Vol 2. ed. J. Noshpitz, pp. 194–235. New York: Basic Books.

ADAMSON, W.C., and ADAMSON, K.K. (eds.) 1979. *A handbook for specific learning disabilities*. Toronto: Gardner Press.

ADELMAN, H.S. 1978. Diagnostic classification of learning problems: Some data. *Am. J. Orthopsychiat.* 48(4): 717–26.

ADELSON, J. 1980. *Handbook of adolescent psychology*. New York: Wiley-Interscience.

ADER, R. 1980. Psychoimmunology. *Psychosom. Med.,* 42(3) (May): 307–17.

———, and FRIEDMAN, S.B. 1965. Differential early experiences and susceptibility to transplanted tumor in the rat. *J. Comp. Physiol. Psychiat.* 59: 361–64.

AGER, S. 1972. Luding out. Letter to Editor, *N.E.J.Med.,* 287: 51.

AGUILERA, D., and MESSICK, J. 1974. *Crisis intervention: Theory and methodology*. St. Louis: C.V. Mosby.

AICHHORN, A. 1925/1971. *Wayward youth*. New York: Viking Press.

AINSWORTH, M.D.S., BLEHAR, M.C., WATERS, E., and WALL, S. 1978. *Patterns of attachment: A psychological study of the strange situation*. Hillsdale, N.J.: Lawrence Erlbaum.

AINSWORTH, M.D.S., and WITTIG, B.A. 1969. Attachment and exploratory behaviour of one year olds in a strange situation. In *Determinants of infant Behaviour*, Vol. 4. ed. B.M. Foss. London: Methuen.

AISENBERG, R.B., WOLFF, P.H., ROSENTHAL, A., and NADAS, A.S. 1973. Psychological impact of cardiac catheterization. *Pediat.,* 51: 1051–59.

References

ALBEE, G.W. 1979. Primary prevention. *Can. Ment. H.* 27(2): 5–9.

ALBY, N., and ALBY, J.M. 1973. The doctor and dying child. In *The child in his family.* Vol. 2, *The impact of disease and death.* ed. E.J. Anthony and C. Koupernik, New York: Wiley. 145–57.

ALDERTON, H.R. 1977. Psychoses in childhood and adolescence. In *Psychological problems of the child and his family.* ed. P.D. Steinhauer and Q. Rae-Grant, pp. 165–91. Toronto: Macmillan.

ALDRICH, C.K. 1975. Office psychotherapy for the primary care physician. In *American handbook of psychiatry,* ed. S. Arieti and G. Caplan. Vol. 5. 2nd ed., pp. 739–756. New York: Basic Books.

ALDRIDGE, M.J., and CAUTLEY, P.W. 1975. The importance of worker availability in the functioning of new foster homes. *J. Child Wel. Leag. Am.* 54 (January): 444–53.

ALEXANDER, F. 1962. The development of psychosomatic medicine. *Psychosom. Med.* 24(1): 13–24.

ALEXANDER, J.F. 1973. Defensive and supportive communication in normal and deviant families. *J. Cons. & Clin. Psychol.* 40: 223–31.

———, and PARSONS, B.V. 1974. Short-term behavioral intervention with delinquent families: Impact on family process and recidivism. In *Annual review of behavior therapy: Theory and practice.* Vol. 2. ed. C.M. Grancks and G.T. Wilson, pp. 472–85. New York: Brunner/Mazel.

ALLEN, F.H. 1942. *Psychotherapy with children.* New York: W.W. Norton.

AMAN, M.G., and WERRY, J.S. 1975. Methylphenidate in children: Effects upon cardiorespiratory function on exertion. *Int. J. Ment. H.* 4:119–31.

AMERICAN ACADEMY OF PEDIATRICS: Committee on Adoptions. 1971. Identity development in adopted children. *Pediat.* 47(5) (May): 948–49.

———: Committee on Fetus and Newborn. 1975. Report of the ad hoc task force on circumcision. *Pediat.* 56 (October): 610–11.

———: Committee on Hospital Care. 1978. *Hospital care of children and youth.* Evanston, Ill.: American Academy of Pediatrics.

AMERICAN FAMILY PHYSICIAN JOURNAL. 1979. M.D.'s can help children with learning disabilities. *Am. Fam. Physician* 19(1): 223–24.

AMERICAN PSYCHIATRIC ASSOCIATION. 1968. *Diagnostic and statistical manual of mental disorders (DSM-II).* Washington, D.C.: American Psychiatric Association.

———. 1980. *Diagnostic and statistical manual of mental disorders (DSM-III).* Washington, D.C.: American Psychiatric Association.

———. 1980. Identity related disorder. In *Diagnostic and statistical manual of mental disorders* (DSM-III). Washington, D.C.: American Psychiatric Association.

———. 1980. Anorexia nervosa. In *Diagnostic and statistical manual of mental disorders* (DSM-III). Washington, D.C.: American Psychiatric Association, pp. 67–69.

———: Committee on Public Information. 1975. *A psychiatric glossary.* 4th ed. New York: American Psychiatric Association.

ANASTASIOW, N. 1981. Early childhood education for the handicapped in the 1980's: Recommendations. *Except. Child* 47(4) (January): 227–82.

ANDERS, T.F. 1978. Home recorded sleep in 2 and 9 month-old infants. *J. Am. Acad. Child Psychiat.* 17:421–32.

———. 1982. A longitudinal study of night time sleep–wake patterns in infants from birth to one year. In *Frontiers in infant psychiatry,* ed. J.D. Call and E. Galenson New York: Basic Books.

———, and WEINSTEIN, P. 1972. Sleep and its disorders in infants and children: A review. *Pediat.* 50:312–24.

ANDERSON, C. 1956. Early brain injury and behavior. *J. Am. Med. Wom. Assn.,* 11:113–19.

ANDERSON, E.W., KENNA, G.C., and HAMILTON, M.W. 1960. A study of extramarital conception in adolescence. *Psychiat. Neurol.* 139:313–62.

ANDRULONIS, P.A., GLUECK, B.C., STROEBEL, C.F., VOGEL, N.G., SHAPIRO, A.L., and ALDRIDGE, D.M. 1981. Organic brain dysfunction and the borderline syndrome. *Psychiat. Clin. N. Am.* 4(1) (April): 47–66.

ANGLIM, E.E. The politics of permanency planning for children. Paper presented at the Annual Meeting of American Orthopsychiatric Association, Toronto, Canada, April, 1980.

ANTHONY, E.J. 1957. An experimental approach to the psychopathology of childhood: Encopresis. *Brit. J. Med. Psychol.* 30:146–75.

———. 1958. An experimental approach to the psychopathology of childhood: Autism. *Brit. J. Med. Psychol.* 31:211–25.

683

———. 1964. Communicating therapeutically with the child. *J. Am. Acad. Child Psychiat.* 3:106–25.

———. A clinical evaluation of children with psychotic parents. *Am. J. Psychiat.* 126 (August):177–84.

———. 1974*a*. *The child and his family.* New York: Wiley.

———. 1974*b*. Psychotherapy of adolescence. In *American handbook of psychiatry,* Vol. 2. ed. G. Caplan. 2d ed. pp. 234–49. New York: Basic Books.

———, and KOUPERNIK, C. (eds.). 1973. *The child in his family* Vol. 2. *The impact of disease and death* New York: Wiley.

ANTHONY, J., and SCOTT, P. 1960. Manic depressive psychosis in childhood. *J. Child. Psychol. Psychiat.* 1:53–72.

APLEY, J. 1976. Recurrent abdominal pain in children: A physician's views. In *Topics in paediatric gastroenterology,* ed. J. A. Dodge, pp. 181–87. Kent, Ohio: Pitman.

ARAJARVI, T., PENTTI, R., and AUKEE, M. 1961. Ulcerative colitis in children. I. and II: A clinical, psychological and social follow up study. *Ann. Clin. Res.* 7:1 (part 1); 7:259 (part 2).

ARBANAL, A. 1979. Shared parenting after separation and divorce: A study of joint custody. *Am. J. Orthopsychiat.* 49(2): 320–29.

ASSOCIATION FOR THE CARE OF CHILDREN'S HEALTH 1981. *The family in child health care.* Selected papers from the 14th International Conference of the ACCH. ed. P. Azarnoff and C. Hardgrove. New York: Wiley.

ATKIN, M. 1974. The "doomed family"—Observations on the lives of parents and children facing repeated child mortality. In *Care of the child facing death,* ed. L. Burton, pp. 60–73. London: Routledge & Kegan Paul.

AWAD, G., and PARRY, R. 1980. Access following marital separation. *Can. J. Psychiat.* 25(5):357–65.

AYLLON, T., LAYMAN, D., and KANDEL, H.J. 1975. A behavioral–educational alternative to drug control of hyperactive children. *J. App. Behav. Anal.* 8:137–46.

BACHARA, G.H., and ZABA, J.N. 1978. Learning disabilities and juvenile delinquency. *J. Learn. Disab.* 11(4): 242–46.

BAER, D.M. 1970. An age-irrelevant concept of development. *Merrill-Palmer Quart. Behav. & Dev.* 16: 238–45.

BAGLEY, C. 1969. Incest behaviour and incest taboo. *Soc. Probs.* 16: 505–19.

BAHNSON, C.B. 1969. Psychophysiological complementarity in malignancies: Past work and future vistas. *Ann. N.Y. Acad. Sci.* 164: 319.

BAKWIN, H., and BAKWIN, R.M. 1966. *Clinical management of behavior disorders in children.* 3d ed. Philadelphia: W.B. Saunders.

———. 1972. *Behavior disorders of children.* Philadelphia: W.B. Saunders.

BALDWIN, B.A. 1978. A paradigm for the classification of emotional crises: Implications for crisis intervention. *Amer. J. Orthopsychiat.* 48(3): 538–51.

BALDWIN, W., and CAIN, V. 1980. The children of teenage parents. *Fam. Plan. Persp.* 12(1) (January/February): 34–43.

BALIKOV, H., and FEINSTEIN, C.B. 1979. The blind child. In *Basic handbook of child psychiatry.* Vol. 1. ed. J. D. Call, pp. 413–20. New York: Basic Books.

BALSER, B.H. 1957. *Psychotherapy of the adolescent.* New York: International Universities Press.

BARBARA, D.A. 1954. *Stuttering: A psychodynamic approach to its understanding and treatment.* New York: Julian Press.

BARGLOW, P., BORNSTEIN, M., EXUM, D.B., WRIGHT, M.K., and VISOTSKY, H.M. 1968. Some psychiatric aspects of illegitimate pregnancy in early adolescence. *Am. J. Orthopsychiat.* 38: 672–87.

BARKER, P. 1975. Haloperidol. *J. Child Psychol. Psychiat.* 16: 169–72.

———. 1980. *Basic child psychiatry.* 3d ed. London: Granada.

BARKLEY, R.A. 1977*a*. Hyperkinesis, autonomic nervous system activity and stimulant drug effects. *J. Child Psychol. Psychiat.* 18: 347–57.

———. 1977*b*. A review of stimulant drug research with hyperactive children. *J. Child Psychol. Psychiat.* 18: 137–65.

———. 1978. Recent developments in research on hyperactive children. *J. Pediat. Psychol.* 3(4): 158–63.

References

————. 1979. Dose effects of Ritalin on the mother–child interactions of hyperactive children. Unpublished manuscript. Medical College of Milwaukee, Wisconsin.

————, and CUNNINGHAM, C.E. 1979. The effects of Methylphenidate on the mother–child interactions of hyperactive children. *Arch. Gen. Psychiat.* 36: 201–208.

BARNES, A.B., COHEN, E., STOECKLE, J.D., et al. 1971. Therapeutic abortion: Medical and social sequels. *Ann. Inter. Med.* 75 (December): 881–86.

BAROWSKY, E.I. 1978. Young children's perceptions and reactions to hospitalization. In *Psychosocial aspects of pediatric care,* ed. E. Gellert, pp. 37–49. New York: Grune & Stratton.

BARRACLOUGH, B.M. 1974. Are there safer hypnotics than barbiturates? *Lancet,* 1: 57–58.

BARROWS, T.S., et al. 1977. *Procedures document for psychoeducational diagnostic services for learning disabled youths.* Prepared under Grants 76 NI-99-0133 and 76-99-002 from the National Institute of Juvenile Justice and Delinquent Prevention, Law Enforcement Assistance Administration, U.S. Department of Justice. Princeton, N.J.: Educational Testing Service.

BARTEN, H.H. and BARTEN, S.S. (eds.). 1973. *Children and their parents in brief therapy.* New York: Behavioral Publications.

BARTROP, R.W., LAZARUS, L., LUCKHURST, E., KILDH, L.G., and PENNY, R. 1977. Depressed lymphocyte function after bereavement. *Lancet,* 1: 834–36.

BATESON, C., JACKSON, D.D., HALEY, J., and WEAKLAND, D.J. 1956. Toward a theory of schizophrenia. *Behav. Sci.* 1: 251–64.

BAUER, D.H. 1976. An exploratory study of developmental changes in children's fears. *J. Child Psychol. Psychiat.* 17: 69–74.

BAUER, R.H. 1979. Memory, acquisition, and category clustering in learning disabled children. *J. Exper. Child Psychol.* 27(3): 363–83.

BAXLEY, G.B., and LeBLANC, J.M. 1976. The hyperactive child: Characteristics, treatment, and evaluation of research design. In *Advances in child development and behavior,* Vol. 2 ed. H.W. Reese. New York: Academic Press.

BAYLEY, N. 1969. *The Bayley scales of infant development.* New York: Psychological Corp.

————. 1970. Development of mental abilities. In *Carmichael's manual of child psychology,* vol. 1. 3d ed. ed. P.H. Mussen, pp. 1163–1209. New York: Wiley.

BEAR, D.M. 1979. Interictal behaviour in temporal lobe epilepsy: Possible anatomic and physiologic bases. In *Epilepsy: Neurotransmitter behaviour.* Canadian League Against Epilepsy.

BECK, A.T., SETHI, B.B., and TUTHILL, R.W. 1963. Childhood bereavement and adult depression. *Arch. Gen. Psychiat.* 9(3): 295–302.

BECKER, W.C. 1971. *Parents are teachers.* Champagne, Ill.: Research Press.

BEGAB, M.J. 1966. The mentally retarded and the family. In *Prevention and treatment of mental retardation,* ed. I. Philips, pp. 71–84. New York: Basic Books.

BEIER, D. 1964. Behavioral disturbances in the mentally retarded. In *Mental retardation: A review of research,* ed. H.A. Stevens and R. Heber. Chicago: Univ. of Chicago Press.

BEISER, H.R. 1955. Therapeutic play techniques. Symposium 1954—Play equipment for diagnosis and therapy. *Am. J. Orthopsychiat.* 25: 761–70.

BELSKY, J., and STEINBERG, L.D. 1979. The effects of day care: A critical review. *Child Dev.* 49: 929–49.

————. 1979. What does research teach us about day care: A follow-up report. *Child. Today* July–August: 21–26.

BEMPORAD, J.R., PFEIFER, C.M., GIBBS, L., CORTNER, R.H., and BLOOM, W. 1971. Characteristics of encopretic patients and their families. *J. Am. Acad. Child Psychiat.* 10: 272–92.

BENDA, C.E. 1952. *Developmental disorders of mentation and cerebral palsies.* New York: Grune & Stratton.

BENDER, L. 1942. Childhood schizophrenia. *Nerv. Child.* 1:138–40.

————. 1947. Childhood schizophrenia. *Am. J. Orthopsychiat.* 17: 40–56.

————. 1953. Childhood schizophrenia. *Psychiat. Quart.* 27: 663–81.

————. 1970. The life course of schizophrenic children. *Biol. Psychiat.* 2: 165–72.

————. 1980. Attitudes toward disabled people. *Dev. Med. Child Neurol.* 22 (August): 427–28.

————, and BLAU, A. 1937. The reactions of children to sexual relations with adults. *Am. J. Orthopsychiat.* 7:500–18.

BENDER, L., and FARETRA, G. 1972. The relationship between childhood schizophrenia and adult schizophrenia. In *Genetic factors in schizophrenia,* ed. A.R. Kaplan, pp. 28–64. Springfield, Ill.: Chas. C Thomas.

References

BENDER, L., FREEDMAN, A.M., GRUGETT, A.E., and HELME, W. 1952. Schizophrenia in childhood: A confirmation of the diagnosis. *Trans. Am. Neur. Assn.* 77: 67–73.

BENDER, L., and GRUGETT, A.E. Jr. 1956. A study of certain epidemiological factors in a group of children with childhood schizophrenia. *Am. J. Orthopsychiat.* 26: 131–45.

BENDER, L., and HELME, W.H. 1953. A quantitative test of theory and diagnostic indicators of childhood schizophrenia. *Arch. Neurol. & Psychiat.* 70: 413–27.

BENDER, L., and NICHTERN, S. 1956. Chemotherapy in child psychiatry. *N.Y. State J. of Med.* 56: 2791–96.

BENEDEK, E.P. 1972. Child custody laws: Their psychiatric implications. *Am. J. Psychiat.* 129(3): 326–28.

———, and BENEDEK, R.S. 1972. New child custody laws: Making them do what they say. *Am. J. Orthopsychiat.* 42(5): 825–34.

BENTOVIM, A. 1970. The clinical approach to feeding disorders of childhood. *J. Psychosom. Res.* 14: 267–76.

BERG, G., and KELLY, R., 1979. The measured self-esteem of children from broken, rejected, and accepted families. *J. Divorce.* 2(4): 363.

BERGER, M.M. (ed.) 1978. *Beyond the double bind.* New York: Brunner/Mazel.

BERGMAN, P., and ESCALONA, S.K. 1949. Unusual sensitivities in very young children. *Psychoanal. Stud. Child.* 3(4): 333–52.

BERGMANN, T., and FREUD, A. 1966. *Children in hospital.* New York: International Universities Press.

BERGSTRAND, C.G., and OTTO, U. Suicide attempts in adolescence and childhood. *Acta Paediat.*, 51: 17–26.

BERMAN, A. 1974a. Delinquents are disabled. In *Youth in trouble,* ed. B. Kratoville, pp. 39–43. Proceedings of a Symposium, Dallas–Fort Worth Regional Airport, May, 1974. San Raphael, Calif.: Academic Therapy Pubs.

———. Delinquents are disabled: An innovative approach to the prevention and treatment of juvenile delinquency. Final Report of the Neuropsychology Diagnostic Laboratory at the Rhode Island Training Schools, December, 1974b.

———. Speech before the symposium on the Relationship of Delinquency to Learning Disabilities Among Youth. Little Rock, Ark., December, 1974c.

BERMAN, E.M., and LIEF, H.I. 1975. Marital therapy from a psychiatric perspective: An overview. *Am. J. Psychiat.* 132(6) (June): 583–92.

BERMAN, G. 1982. Personal communication.

BERNAL, J. 1973. Night waking in infants during the first 14 months. *Dev. Med. Child Neurol.* 15: 760–69.

BERNAL, M.E., and MILLER, W.H. 1970. Electrodermal and cardiac responses of schizophrenic children to sensory stimuli. *Psychophysiol.* 7:155–68.

BERNSTEIN, B. 1962. Social class, linguistic codes, and grammatical elements. *Lang. & Speech.* 5: 221–40.

BERNSTEIN, N.R. 1976. *Emotional care of the facially burned and disfigured.* Boston: Little, Brown.

———. 1979. The child with severe burns. In *Basic handbook of child psychiatry,* ed. J.D. Call. Vol. 1. *Normal development.* pp. 465–74. New York: Basic Books.

BERRY, S.W. 1975. Some clinical variations on a classical theme. *J. Am. Acad. Psychoanal.* 3: 151–61.

BERSCHEID, E., and WALSTER, E. 1972. Beauty and the beast. *Psychol. Today,* 5(10): 42–46, 74.

BETTER HEALTH FOR OUR CHILDREN: A NATIONAL STRATEGY. 1981. The report of the select panel for the promotion of child health. Washington, D.C.: The U.S. Department of Health and Human Services.

BIJOU, S.W., and REDD, W.H. 1975. Behavior therapy for children. In *American handbook of psychiatry,* vol. 5. 2d ed. eds. D.X. Freedman and J.E. Dyrud, pp. 319–44. New York: Basic Books.

BINGER, C.M. 1973. Childhood leukemia: Emotional impact on siblings. In *The child in his family.* Vol. 2. *The impact of disease and death.* eds. E.J. Anthony and C. Koupernik, pp. 195–209. New York: Wiley.

———, ALBIN, A.R., FEUERSTEIN, R.C., et al. 1969. Childhood leukemia: Emotional impact on patient and family. *N. E. J.Med.,* 280(8): 414–18.

BIRCH, H.G., and WALKER, H.A. 1966. Perceptual and perceptual-motor dissociation: Studies in schizophrenic and brain-damaged psychotic children. *Arch. Gen. Psychiat.* 14: 113–18.

686

References

Birch, Hon. Margaret. 1979. *The family as a focus for social policy.* Toronto: Ontario Government Book Store.

Blakely, W.P. 1969. An exploratory study of emotional responses related to reading. Unpublished paper, Drake University, Des Moines, Iowa.

Blau, A. 1936. Mental changes following head trauma in children. *Arch. Neurol. Psychiat.* 35: 723–69.

Blehar, M. 1974. Anxious attachment and defensive reactions associated with day care. *Child Dev.* 45 (September): 683–92.

Bloodstein, O.A. 1969. *A handbook on stuttering.* Chicago: National Easter Seal Society for Crippled Children and Adults.

Bloom, B.L. 1968. The evaluation of primary prevention programs. In *Comprehensive mental health.* ed. L.M. Roberts, N.S. Greenfield, and M.H. Miller, p. 117. Madison, Wis.: Univ. of Wisconsin Press.

Blos, P. 1963. *On adolescence.* New York: The Free Press of Glencoe.

———, and Finch, S.M. 1975. Psychotherapy with children and adolescents. In *American handbook of psychiatry.* Vol. 5, 2d ed., ed. D.X. Freedman and J.E. Dyrud, pp. 133–62. New York: Basic Books.

Bluebond-Langer, M. 1978. *The private worlds of dying children.* Princeton: Princeton Univ. Press.

Blum, R.G., and Associates 1969. *Society and drugs, Drugs I: Social and cultural observations.* San Francisco: Jossey-Bass.

Blumer, D. 1977. Treatment of patients with seizure disorders referred because of psychiatric complications. *J. McLean Hosp.* (June): 53–73.

———. 1979. Psychiatric aspects of temporal lobe epilepsy: A review. In *Epilepsy: Neurotransmitter behaviour.* Canadian League Against Epilepsy

Bohannan, P., and Erickson, R. 1978. Stepping in. *Psychol. Today.* 11 (January): 53–59.

Bohman, M. 1970. *Adopted children and their families.* Stockholm: Propius.

Bolian, G.C. 1971. Psychiatric consultation within a community of sick children: Lessons from a children's hospital. *J. Am. Acad. Child Psychiat.* 10: 293–307.

Bolton, F.G., Jr., Laner, R.H., and Kane, S.P. 1980. Child maltreatment risk among adolescent mothers: A study of reported cases. *Am. J. Orthopsychiat.* 50(3) (July): 489–504.

Boone, J.E. 1975. Overview of developmental disabilities. In *Early Intervention,* Monograph No. 6, Canadian Psychiatric Research Institute. London, Ont.: Canadian Psychiatric Research Institute.

Bosaeus, E., and Sellden, U. 1979. Psychiatric assessment of healthy children with various E.E.G. patterns. *Acta Psychiat. Scand.* 59: 180–210.

Boszormenyi-Nagy, I. 1965. A theory of relationships: Experience and transaction. In *Intensive family therapy,* ed. I. Boszormenyi-Nagy and J.L. Framo. New York: Harper & Row.

———, and Spark, G.M. 1973. *Invisible loyalties.* Cambridge, Mass.: Harvard University Press.

Boszormenyi-Nagy, I., and Ulrich, D.N. 1981. Contextual family therapy. In *Handbook of family therapy,* ed. A.S. Gurman & D.P. Kniskern. New York: Brunner/Mazel, pp. 159–86.

Boutourline Young, J. 1971. The physiology of adolescence (including puberty and growth). In *Modern perspectives in adolescent psychiatry,* ed. J.G. Howells, pp. 3–27. Edinburgh: Oliver & Boyd.

Bowen, M. 1960. Family concept of schizophrenia. In *Etiology of schizophrenia,* ed. D.D. Jackson. New York: Basic Books.

———. 1978. *Family therapy in clinical practice.* New York: Jason Aronson.

Bower, E.M. 1977. Mythologies, realities, possibilities, in primary prevention. In *Primary prevention of psychopathology,* Vol. 1, *The Issues.* ed. G.W. Albee and J.M. Joffe, pp. 24–41. Hanover, N.H.: Univ. Press of New England.

Bowlby, J. 1952. *Maternal care and mental health.* 2d ed. Switzerland: World Health Organization. Monograph No. 2.

———. 1960. Grief and mourning in infancy and early childhood. *Psychoanal. Stud. Child.* 15: 9–52.

———. 1961. Process of mourning. *Int. J. Psychoanal.* 42: 317–40.

———. 1963. Pathological mourning and childhood mourning. *J. Am. Psychoanal. Assn.,* 11:500–41.

———. 1969. *Attachment and loss.* Vol. 1, *Attachment.* New York: Basic Books.

———. 1973. *Attachment and loss.* Vol. 2, *Separation: anxiety and anger.* New York: Basic Books.

———. 1980. *Attachment and loss.* Vol. 3, *Loss: sadness and depression.* New York: Basic Books.

Bozeman, F.M., Orbach, C.E., and Sutherland, A.M. 1955. Psychological impact of cancer and

687

its treatment: III. The adaptation of mothers to the threatened loss of their children through leukemia, Part I. *Cancer,* 8:1–33.

BRADLEY, C. 1937. The behavior of children receiving benzedrine. *Am. J. Psychiat.* 94: 577–85.

———. 1941. *Schizophrenia in childhood.* New York: Macmillan.

———. 1957. Characteristics and management of children with behavior problems associated with organic brain damage. *Pediat. Clin. N. Am.* 4:1049–60.

BRADLEY, S., and SLOMAN, L. 1975. Elective mutism in immigrant families. *J. Am. Acad. Child Psychiat.* 14: 510–14.

BRANDON, S. 1970. Crisis theory and possibilities of therapeutic intervention. *Brit. J. Psychiat.* 117: 627–33.

BRANSTETTER, E. 1969. The young child's response to hospitalization: Separation anxiety or lack of mothering care? *Am. J. Pub. H.* 59(1): 92–97.

BRANT, R.S.T., and TISZA, V.B. 1977. The sexually misused child. *Am. J. Orthopsychiat.* 47(1): 80–90.

BRAZELTON, T.B. 1961. Psychophysiologic reactions in the neonate: I. The value of observation of the neonate. *J. Pediatr.* 58: 508–12.

———, KOSLOWSKI, B. and MAIN, M. 1974. The origins of reciprocity: The early mother–infant interaction. In *The effect of the infant on its caregiver,* ed. M. Lewis and L.A. Rosenbaum, pp. 49–76. New York: Wiley.

BRESLAU, N., WEITZMAN, M., and MESSENGER, K. 1981. Psychologic functioning of siblings of disabled children. *Pediatr.,* 67(3) (March): 334–53.

BRIANT, R. 1978. An introduction to clinical pharmacology. In *Pediatric psychopharmacology: The use of behavior modifying drugs in children,* ed. J. Werry. New York: Brunner/Mazel.

BRILL, R. 1977. *Implications of the conceptual level matching model for treatment of delinquents.* Paper presented at the First Conference of the International Differential Treatment Association, Rensselaerville, New York.

BRODER, E.A. 1975. Assessment, the foundation of family therapy. *Can. Fam. Phys.* 21: 53–55.

BRODY, E. 1974. Aging and the family personality: A developmental view. *Fam. Process* 13: 23–37.

BRONFENBRENNER, U. 1974. A report on longitudinal evaluations of preschool programs. Vol. 2, Is early intervention effective? Washington, D.C.: U.S. Department of Health, Education and Welfare. Office of Human Development, Office of Child Development, Children's Bureau.

BROSKOWSKI, A., and BAKER, F. 1974. Professional, organizational and social barriers to primary prevention. *Am. J. Orthopsychiat.* 44(5): 707–19.

BROUGHTON, R.J. 1968. Sleep disorders: Disorders of arousal? *Science* 159 (March): 1070–78.

BROUSSARD, E.R., and HARTNER, M.S.S. 1970. Maternal perception of the neonate as related to development. *Child Psychiat. & Human Dev.* 1: 16–25.

BROWN, B.S., and COURTLESS, T.F. 1971. The mentally retarded offender. Washington, D.C.: U.S. Department of Health, Education and Welfare, publication No. (HSM) 72–9039.

BROWN, D.G. 1972. Behavior modification with children. *Ment. Hyg.,* 56(1): 22–30.

BROWN, J.K. 1977. Migraine and migraine equivalents in children. *Dev. Med. Child. Neurol.* 19: 683–92.

BROWN, J.L. 1960. Prognosis from presenting symptoms of preschool children with atypical development. *Am. J. Orthopsychiat.* 30: 382–90.

———. 1963. Follow-up of children with atypical development (infantile psychosis) *Amer. J. Orthopsychiat.* 33: 855–61.

———. 1969. Adolescent development of children with infantile psychosis. *Sem. Psychiat.* 1: 79–89.

BROWNING, D.H., and BOATMAN, B. 1977. Incest: Children at risk. *Am. J. Psychiat.* 134: 69–72.

BRUCH, H. 1973. *Eating disorders.* New York: Basic Books.

———. 1974. Perils of behavior modification in treatment of anorexia nervosa. *J. Am. Med. Assn.* 230: 1419–22.

———. 1977. Psychotherapy in eating disorders. *Can. J. Psychiat.* 22 (April): 102–108.

BRUUN, R.D., SHAPIRO, A.K., SHAPIRO, E., SWEET, R., WAYNE, H., and SOLOMON, G.E. 1976. A follow-up of 78 patients with Gilles de la Tourette syndrome. *Am. J. Psychiat.* 133: 944–47.

BRYAN, T., and BRYAN, J.H. 1977. The social–emotional side of learning disabilities. *Behav. Disord.,* 2(3) (May): 141–45.

References

BRYAN, T.H. 1978. Social relationships and verbal interactions of learning disabled children. *J. Learn. Disab.* 11(2) (February): 107–15.

BRYCE, M.E., and EHLERT, R.C. 1971. 144 foster children. *Child Welf.,* 50(9): 499–503.

BUCHLER, P. 1978. Children from incomplete families: A preliminary empirical study of the literature. *Schweitzerische Zeitschrift fur Soziologie.* 4(2): 33.

BUCK, C., GREGG, R., STAVRAKY, K., SUBRAHMANIAM, K., and BROWN, J. 1969. The effect of single prenatal and natal complications upon the development of children of mature birthweight. *Pediat.* 43 (June): 942–55.

BUMPASS, L., and SWEET, J. 1972. Differentials in marital stability: 1970. *Am. Sociolog. Rev.* 37 (December): 754–66.

BUNNEY, W.E., Jr. 1977. The switch process in manic–depressive psychosis. *Ann. Inter. Med.* 87: 319–55.

BURKE, E.C., and STICKLER, G.B. 1980. Enuresis: Is it being overtreated? *Mayo Clin. Proc.* 55: 118–20.

BUROS, O.K. (ed.) 1972. *The seventh mental measurements yearbook.* Vol. 1. Highland Park, N.J.: Gryphon Press.

BURT, C. 1958. The inheritance of mental ability. *Am. Psychol.* 13: 1–15.

BURTON, L. (ed.) 1974a. *Care of the child facing death.* London: Routledge & Kegan Paul.

———. 1974b. The family coping with a heavy treatment regime. In *Care of the child facing death.* ed. L. Burton, pp. 74–84. London: Routledge & Kegan Paul.

———. 1975a. *The family life of sick children.* London: Routledge & Kegan Paul.

———. 1975b. The loss of a child. In *The family life of sick children.* London: Routledge & Kegan Paul.

BUXBAUM, E. 1959. Psychosexual development: The oral, anal and phallic phases. In *Readings in psychoanalytic psychology,* ed. M. Levitt, pp. 43–56. New York: Appleton.

BUXTON, M. 1976. Applying the guidelines of "beyond the best interests of the child." *Child Psychiat. Hum. Dev.* 7(2): 94–102.

BYRNE, G. 1981. Personal communication.

CADORET, R.J. 1978. Psychopathology in adopted-away offspring of biologic parents with antisocial behavior. *Arch. Gen. Psych.* 35: 176–84.

CAIN, A.C., FAST, I., and ERICKSON, M.E. 1964. Children's disturbed reactions to the death of a sibling. *Am. J. Orthopsychiat.* 34: 741–52.

CAIRNS, N.U., CLARK, G.M., SMITH, S.D., and LANSKY, S.B. 1979. Adaptation of siblings to childhood malignancy. *Pediat.* 95(3): 484–87.

CALDWELL, B. 1972. What does research tell us about daycare: For children under 3? *Child. Today* 1(1): 6–12.

CALDWELL, B.M. 1964. The effects of infant care. In *Review of child development research,* Vol. 1. ed. M.L. Hoffman and L.W. Hoffman, pp. 9–87. New York: Russel Sage Foundation.

CALL, J.D. 1980. Attachment disorders of infancy. In *Comprehensive textbook of psychiatry,* 3d ed. ed. H.I. Kaplan et al., pp. 2586–97. Baltimore: Williams & Wilkins.

CAMERON, P., KLINE, S., KORENBLUM, M., SELTZER, A.G., and SMALL, F. 1978. A method of reporting formulation. *Can. Psychiat. Assn. J.* 23: 43–50.

CAMPBELL, M. 1973. Biological interventions in psychoses of childhood. *J. Aut. & Child. Schiz.* 3: 347–73.

CAMPBELL, M. 1976a. Children's personal data inventory (additional items) early clinical drug evaluation unit program (ECDEU). *Intercom.* 5: 12–21.

———. 1976b. Pharmacotherapy. In *Autism: A reappraisal of concepts and treatment,* ed. M. Rutter and E. Schopler, pp. 337–55. New York: Plenum Press.

———, ANDERSON, L.T., MEIER, M., COHEN, I.L., SMALL, A.M., SAMIT, C., and SACHAR, E.J. 1978. A comparison of haloperidol and behavior therapy and their interaction in autistic children. *J. Am. Acad. Child Psychiat.* 17: 640–55.

CAMPBELL, M., FISH, B., DAVID, R., SHAPIRO, T., COLLINS, P., and KOH, C. 1972. Response to triiodothyronine and dextroamphetamine: A study of preschool schizophrenic children. *J. Aut. & Child Schiz.* 2: 343–58.

CAMPBELL, M., FISH, B., KOREIN, J., SHAPIRO, T., COLLINS, P., and KOH, C. 1972. Lithium and chlorpromazine: A controlled crossover study in hyperactive severely disturbed young children. *J. Aut. Child Schiz.* 2: 234–63.

References

CAMPBELL, M., FISH, B., SHAPIRO, T. et al. 1971. Imipramine in preschool autistic and schizophrenic children. *J. Aut. & Child. Schiz.* 1: 267–82.

CAMPBELL, M., FISH, B., SHAPIRO, T., and FLOYD, A., Jr. 1971. Study of molindone in disturbed preschool children. *Cur. Therap. Res.* 13: 28–33.

CAMPBELL, M., SCHULMAN, D., and RAPOPORT, J.L. 1978. The current status of lithium therapy in child and adolescent psychiatry: A report of the committee on biological aspects of child psychiatry of the American academy of child psychiatry. *J. Am. Acad. Child Psychiat.* 17: 717–20.

CAMPBELL, S., SCHLEIFER, M., and WEISS, G. 1978. Continuities in maternal reports and child behaviors over time in hyperactive and comparison groups. *J. Abnorm. Child Psychol.* 6: 33–45.

CAMPBELL, S.B. 1975. Mother–child interaction: A comparison of hyperactive learning disabled and normal boys. *Am. J. Orthopsychiat.* 45: 51–57.

CANNON-BONVENTRE, K., and KAHN, J. 1979. Interviews with adolescent parents. *Child. Today,* 8(5): 17–19, 41.

CANTWELL, D. 1975a. Genetic studies of hyperactive children: Psychiatric illness in biologic and adopting parents. In *Genetic research in psychiatry,* ed. R. Fieve, D. Rosenthal, and H. Brill, Baltimore: Johns Hopkins Univ. Press.

———. (ed.) 1975b. *The hyperactive child: Diagnosis, management, current research.* New York: Spectrum Publications.

CANTWELL, P., BAKER, L., and MATTISON, R.E. 1979. The prevalence of psychiatric disorders in children with speech and language disorder: An epidemiologic study. *J. Am. Acad. Child Psychiat.* 18: 450–61.

CANTWELL, D.P. 1972. Psychiatric illness in the families of hyperactive children. *Arch. Gen. Psychiat.* 27: 414–17.

———. 1974. Prevalence of psychiatric disorder in a pediatric clinic for military dependent children. *J. Pediat.* 85: 711–14.

———. 1976. Genetic factors in the hyperkinetic syndrome. *J. Am. Acad. Child Psychiat.* 15: 214–23.

———, MATTISON, R., RUSSELL, A.T., and WILL, L. 1979a. A comparison of DSM-II and DSM-III in the diagnosis of childhood psychiatric disorders. IV. Difficulties in use, global comparison and conclusions. *Arch. Gen. Psychiat.* 36: 1227–28.

CANTWELL, D.P., RUSSELL, A.T., MATTISON, R., and WILL, L. 1979b. A comparison of DSM-II and DSM-III in the diagnosis of childhood psychiatric disorders. I. Agreement with expected diagnosis. *Arch. Gen. Psychiat.* 36: 1208–13.

CAPLAN, G. 1964. *Principles of preventive psychiatry.* New York: Basic Books.

———. 1976. The family as a support system. In *Support systems and mutual help: Multidisciplinary explorations,* ed. G. Kaplan and M. Killilea, pp. 19–26. New York: Grune & Stratton.

———. 1980. An approach to preventive intervention in child psychiatry. *Can. J. Psychiat.* 25(8): 671–82.

———, and KILLILEA, M. (eds.) 1976. *Support systems and mutual help: Multidisciplinary explorations.* New York: Grune & Stratton.

CARANDANG, M.L.A., FOLKINS, C.H., HINES, P.A., and STEWARD, M.S. 1979. The role of cognitive level and sibling illness in children's conceptualization of illness. *Am. J. Ortho psychiat.* 49(3): 474–81.

CARD, J., and WISE, L., 1978. Teenage mothers and teenage fathers: The impact of early child bearing on the parents' personal and professional lives. *Fam. Plan. Persp.* 11(4): 199–205.

CARLSON, G.A., and CANTWELL, D.P. 1979. A survey of depressive symptoms in child and adolescent psychiatric population. *J. Am. Acad. Child Psychiat.* 18:587–99.

———. 1980. Unmasking masked depression in children and adolescents. *Am. J. Psychiat.* 137: 445–49.

CARTER, E.A., and McGOLDRICK, M. (eds.) 1981. *The family life cycle: A framework for family therapy.* New York: Gardner Press.

CASSELL, S. 1965. Effects of brief puppet therapy upon the emotional responses of children undergoing cardiac catheterization. *J. Cons. Psychol.,* 29: 1–8.

CAUTLEY, P., and ALDRIDGE, M. 1973. *Predictors of success in foster family care.* Madison, Wisc: Department of Health and Social Services.

CAVALLIN, H. 1966. Incestuous fathers: A clinical report. *Am. J. Psychiat.* 122(10): 1132–38.

CECI, S.J., RINGSTROM, M., and LEA, S.E.G. 1981. Do language-learning disabled children have impaired memories? In search of underlying processes. *J. Learn. Disab.* 14(3): 159–62.

References

CHAPMAN, J.W., and BOERSMA, F.J. 1979. Academic self-concept in elementary learning disabled children: A study with the student's perception of ability scale. *Psychol. in the Schools,* 16(2): 201–206.

CHESS, S. 1971. Autism in children with congenital rubella. *J. Aut. & Child. Schiz.* 1: 33–47.

———. 1979. Developmental theory revisited: Findings of longitudinal study. *Can. J. Psychiat.* 24: 101–112.

———, and HASSIBI, M. 1970. Behavior deviations in mentally retarded children. *J. Am. Acad. Child Psychiat.* 9: 282–97.

———. 1978. *Principles and practice of child psychiatry.* New York: Plenum Press.

CHURCHILL, S.R. 1965. Social group work: A diagnostic tool in child guidance. *Am. J. Orthopsychiat.* 35: 581–88.

CLAMPIT, M.K. 1981. Residual attentional deficits in adolescence, *J. Learn. Disab.* 14(4): 218–19.

CLEMENTS, D.A. 1971. Psychological problems in adopted children: A review of the literature and some critical comments. Diss. submitted for fulfillment of the requirement for the Diploma Course in Child Psychiatry, University of Toronto, March, 1971.

CLIFFORD, H. Reprinted 1973. *Current trends and issues in day care in Canada; Status of day care in Canada.* Health and Welfare Canada.

CLINE, F.W., and ROTHENBERG, M.B. 1974. Preparation of a child for major surgery: A case report. *J. Am. Acad. Child Psychiat.* 13: 78–94.

COATES, J. 1970. Obstetrics in the very young adolescent. *Am. J. Ob. Gyn.* 108(1): 68–72.

COELHO, G.V., and STEIN, J.J. 1977. Coping with the stresses of an urban planet: Impacts of uprooting and overcrowding. *Habitat,* 2: 379–90.

COHEN, D., JOHNSON, W., and CAPARULO, B. 1976. Pica and elevated blood lead level in autistic and atypical children. *Am. J. Dis. Child.* 130: 47–48.

COHEN, D.J., SHAYWITZ, B.A., YOUNG, J.G., CARBONARI, C.H., NATHANSON, J.A., LIEBERMAN, B.S., BOWERS, M.B., and MAAS, J.W. 1979. Central biogenic amine metabolism in children with the syndrome of chronic multiple tics of Gilles de la Tourette. *J. Am. Acad. Child Psychiat.* 18: 320–41.

COHEN, D.J., and YOUNG, J.G. 1977. Neurochemistry and child psychiatry. *J. Am. Acad. Child Psychiat.* 16: 353–411.

COHEN, N.J., SULLIVAN, J., MINDE, K., NOVAK, C., and HELWIG, C. 1981. Evaluation of the relative effectiveness of methylphenidate and cognitive behavior modification in the treatment of kindergarten-aged hyperactive children. *J. Abnorm. Child Psychol.* 9(1): 43–54.

COHEN, P.C. 1962. The impact of the handicapped child on the family. *Soc. Casework* 43: 137–42.

COHEN, R.L. 1979a. Case formulation and treatment planning. In *Basic handbook of child psychiatry,* Vol. 1. ed. J.D. Call, pp. 633–640. New York: Basic Books.

COHEN, R.L. 1979b. The approach to assessment. In *Basic handbook of child psychiatry,* Vol. 1 ed. J.D. Call, pp. 485–504. New York: Basic Books.

COHEN, S. 1981a. Cocaine: Gift of the sun god or third scourge of mankind. *Drug Ab. & Alcohol. Newsletter* 10(7) (Vista Hill Foundation, San Diego).

———. 1981b. *The substance abuse problems.* New York: Haworth Press.

———. 1982. Therapeutic communities for substance abusers. *Drug ab. & Alcohol. Newsletter* 9(2) (Vista Hill Foundation, San Diego).

COHEN, S.A. 1971. Dyspedagogia as a cause of reading retardation: Definition and treatment. In *Learning disorders,* Vol. 4. ed. B.D. Bateman. Seattle: Special Child Publications.

COLEMAN, J.C. 1980. *The nature of adolescence.* London, New York: Methuen.

COLEMAN, R.W., and PROVENCE, S. 1957. Environmental retardation (hospitalism) in infants living in families. *Pediat.* 19: 285–92.

COLODNY, D., and KURLANDER, L.F. 1970. Psychopharmacology as a treatment adjunct for the mentally retarded: Problems and issues. In *Psychiatric approaches to mental retardation,* ed. F.L. Menolascino. New York: Basic Books.

COMPTON, R. Speech before the symposium on the Relationship of Delinquency to Learning Disabilities Among Youth. Little Rock, Ark., December, 1974.

CONDON, W.S. 1975. Multiple responses to sound in dysfunctional children. *J. Aut. & Child. Schiz.* 5(1): 37–56.

CONNELL, H.M. 1972. Attempted suicide in school children. *Med. J. Austr.* 59: 686–90.

CONNERS, C. 1967. The syndrome of minimal brain dysfunction: Psychological aspects. *Pediat. Clin. N. Am.* 14: 749–66.

691

CONNERS, C.K. 1969. A teacher rating scale for use in drug studies with children. *Am. J. Psychiat.* 126: 884–88.

——. 1971. Recent drug studies with hyperkinetic children. *J. Learn. Disab.* 4: 476–83.

——. 1973. Rating scales for use in drug studies with children. In *Pharmacotherapy of children,* pp. 24–28. (Special Issue of *Psychopharmacol. Bull.*)

——. 1979. Rating scales. In *Basic handbook of child psychiatry,* Vol. 1. ed. J.D. Call, pp. 675–89. New York: Basic Books.

——, GOYETTE, C.H., SOUTHWICK, D.A., LEES, J.M., and ANDRULONIS, P.A. 1976. Food additives and hyperkinesis: A controlled double-blind experiment. *Pediat.* 58: 154–66.

CONWAY, F., and SEIGELMAN, J. 1978. *Snapping: America's epidemic of sudden personality change.* New York: Delta.

COOLIDGE, J.C., WILLER, M.L., TESSMAN, E., and WALDFOGEL, S. 1960. School phobia in adolescence: A manifestation of severe character disturbance. *Am. J. Orthopsychiat.* 30: 599–607.

COOPER, J.D. 1978. *Patterns of family placement: Current issues in fostering and adoption.* London: National Children's Bureau.

CORMIER, B., KENNEDY, M., and SANGOWICZ, J. 1962. Psychodynamics of father–daughter incest. *Can. Psychiat. Assn. J.* 7:203–17.

COWIE, J., COWIE, V.A., and SLATER, E.T.O. 1968. *Delinquency in girls.* New York: Humanities Press.

CRAIN, A.J., SUSSMAN, M.B., and WEIL, W.B., Jr. 1966. Effects of a diabetic child on marital integration and related measures of family functioning. *J. H. & Soc. Behav.* 7:122–27.

CREAK, M. 1961. The schizophrenic syndrome in childhood: Progress report of a working party. *Brit. J. Med.* 2: 889–90.

——. 1963. Childhood psychosis: A review of 100 cases. *Brit. J. Psychiat.* 109: 84–89.

——. 1964. The schizophrenic syndrome in childhood—Further progress report of a working party. *Dev. Med. Child. Neurol.* 6: 530–35.

CRELLIN, E., KELLMER-PRINGLE, M.L., and WEST, P. 1974. *Born illegitimate, social and educational implications: A report by the national children's bureau.* Windsor: NFER.

CREWS, F.T., and SMITH, C.B. 1978. Presynaptic alpha–receptor subsensitivity after long-term antidepressant treatment. *Science* 202: 322–24.

CRISP, A.H. 1981. Therapeutic outcome in anorexia nervosa. *Can. J. Psychiat.* 26: 232–35.

——, PALMER, R.L., and KALUCY, R.S. 1976. How common is anorexia nervosa? A prevalence study. *Brit. J. Psychiat.* 128: 549–54.

CRITCHLEY, E.M.R. 1968. Reading retardation, dyslexia and delinquency. *Brit. J. Psychiat.* 114: 1537–47.

CROCKER, E. 1978. Play programs in pediatric settings. In *Psychosocial aspects of pediatric care,* ed. E. Gellert, 95–110. New York: Grune & Stratton.

——. 1980. Preparation for elective surgery: Does it make a difference? *J. Assn. Care Child. in Hosp.* 9(1): 3–11.

CROOK, T., and ELIOT, J. 1980. Parental death during childhood and adult depression: A critical review of the literature. *Psychol. Bull.* 87(2): 252–59.

CROOKE, W.I. 1975. *Can your child read? Is he hyperactive?* pp. 144–55. Jackson, Tenn.: Pedicenter Press.

CROSS, T.G. 1977. Mother's speech adjustments: The contribution of selected child listener variables. In *Talking to children: Language input and acquisition,* ed. C. Snow and C. Ferguson, pp. 151–89. Cambridge, England: Cambridge Univ. Press.

CUNNINGHAM, C.F., and BARKLEY, R.A. 1978. The role of academic failure in hyperactive behavior. *J. Learn. Disab.* 11: 274–80.

CUNNINGHAM, L., CADORET, R.J., LOFTUS, R., and EDWARDS, J.E. 1975. Studies of adoptees from psychiatrically disturbed biological parents: Psychiatric conditions in childhood and adolescence. *Brit. J. Psychiat.* 126: 534–49.

CUTRIGHT, P. 1971. Income and family events: Marital stability. *J. Marr. & Fam.* 33: 291–306.

CYTRYN, L., GILBERT, A., and EISENBERG, L. 1960. The effectiveness of tranquilizing drugs plus supportive psychotherapy in treating behavior disorders in children: A double blind study of 8 out-patients. *Am. J. Orthopsychiat.* 30: 113–28.

CYTRYN, L., and LOURIE, R.S. 1967. Mental retardation. In *Comprehensive textbook of psychiatry,* ed. A.M. Freedman and H.I. Kaplan. Baltimore: Williams & Wilkins.

CYTRYN, L., and McKNEW, D.H. 1979. Affective disorders. In *Basic handbook of child psychiatry,* Vol. 2, *Disturbances in development.* ed. J.D. Call, pp. 321–40. New York: Basic Books.

References

CYTRYN, L., McKNEW, D.H., LOGUE, M., and DESAI, R.B. 1974. Biochemical correlates of affective disorders in children. *Arch. Gen. Psychiat.* 31: 659–61.

DaCOSTA, G.A. Clinical aspects of long parent–child separation and reunion. Paper presented at the Ontario Psychiatric Association meeting in Toronto, January, 1975.

DAHL, V. 1976. A follow-up study of a child psychiatric clientele with special regard to the diagnosis of psychosis. *Acta Psychiat. Scand.* 54: 106–12.

DANILOWICZ, D.A., and GABRIEL, H.P. 1971. Postoperative reactions in children: "Normal" and abnormal responses after cardiac surgery. *Am. J. Psychiat.* 128: 185–88.

DARE, C. 1977. Dynamic treatments. In *Child psychiatry: Modern approaches,* ed. M. Rutter and L. Hersov, pp. 949–66. Oxford: Blackwell Scientific Pub.

DAVANLOO, H. 1978. *Basic principles and techniques in short-term dynamic psychotherapy.* New York: S.P. Medical & Scientific Books.

DAVID, O.J., HOFFMAN, P., SVERD, J., and CLARK, J. 1977. Lead and hyperactivity: Lead levels among hyperactive children. *J. Abnorm. Child Psychol.* 5: 405–16.

DAY, G. 1951. The psychosomatic approach to pulmonary T.B. *Lancet,* 1:1025–28.

DeFRANCIS, V. 1971. Protecting the child victims of sex crimes committed by adults. *Fed. Prob.* 35: 15–20.

DELAMATER, A.M., LAHEY, B.B., and DRAKE, L. 1981. Toward an empirical subclassification of "learning disabilities": A psychophysiological comparison of "hyperactive" and "nonhyperactive" subgroups. *J. Abnorm. Child Psychol.* 9(1): 65–77.

DELL, G.A. 1963. Social factors and school influence in juvenile delinquency. *Brit. J. Educ. Psychol.* 33: 312–22.

DeLONG, G.R. 1978. Lithium carbonate treatment of select behavior disorders in children suggesting manic-depressive illness. *J. Pediat.* 93(4): 689–94.

DEMB, N., and RUESS, A.L. 1967. High school drop-out rates for cleft palate children and their siblings. *Cleft Pal. J.* 4: 327–33.

DEMBINSKI, R.J., and MAUSER, A.J. 1977. What parents of the learning disabled really want from professionals. *J. Learn. Disab.* 10(9) (November): 578–84.

DEMYER, M., WARD, S., and LINTZENICH, J. 1968. Comparison of macronutrients in the diets of psychotic and normal children. *Arch. Gen. Psychiat.* 18: 584–90.

DEMYER, M., et al. 1971. Free fatty acid response to insulin and glucose stimulation in schizophrenic, autistic and emotionally disturbed children. *J. Aut. & Child Schiz.* 1: 436–52.

DEMYER, M.K., ALPERN, G.D., BARTON, S., DEMYER, W.E., CHURCHILL, D.W., HINGTGEN, J.N., BRYSON, C.Q., PONTIUS, W., and KIMBERLIN, C. 1972. Imitation in autistic, early schizophrenic and non-psychotic subnormal children. *J. Aut. & Child Schiz.* 2(3): 264–87.

DENCKLA, M.B., BEMPORAD, J.R., and MacKAY, M.C. 1976. Tics following methylphenidate administration: A report of 20 cases. *J. Am. Med. Assn.,* 235: 1349–51.

DENHOFF, E. 1973. The natural life history of children with minimal brain dysfunction. *Ann. N.Y. Acad. Sci.* 205: 188–205.

DeQUIROS, J.B., and SCHRAGER, O.L. 1979. *Neuropsychological fundamentals in learning disabilities.* rev. ed. Novato, Calif.: Academic Therapy Pubs.

DERDEYN, A.P. 1975. Child custody consultation. *Am. J. Orthopsychiat.* 45(5): 791–801.

———. 1976a. Child custody contests in historical perspective. *Am. J. Psychiat.* 133(12) 1369–76.

———. 1976b. A consideration of legal issues in child custody contests. *Arch. Gen. Psychiat.* 33(2): 165–71.

———. 1977. A case for permanent foster placement of dependent, neglected and abused children. *Am. J. Orthopsychiat.* 47 (October): 604–14.

DESMOND, M.M., WILSON, G.S., VERINAUD, W.M., MELNICK, J.L., and RAWLS, W.E. 1970. The early growth and development of infants with congenital rubella. *Adv. Teratol.* 4: 39–63.

DESPERT, J.L. 1946. Psychosomatic study of fifty stuttering children. *Am. J. Orthopsychiat.* 16:100–113.

DeWALD, P.A. 1969. *Psychotherapy: A dynamic approach.* New York: Basic Books.

DICKS, H.V. 1967. *Marital tensions: Clinical studies towards a psychological theory of interaction.* London: Routledge & Kegan Paul.

DIEPOLD, J., and YOUNG, R. 1979. Empirical studies of adolescent sexuality: A critical review. *Adol.* 14:47.

DiLEO, J. 1977. *Child Development: Analysis and synthesis.* New York: Brunner/Mazel.

693

DILLER, L. 1972. Psychological aspects of physically handicapped children. In *Manual of child psychopathology*, ed. B.B. Wolman, pp. 591–623. New York: McGraw-Hill.

DIMASCIO, A. 1970. Behavioral toxicity. In *Clinical handbook of psychopharmacology*, ed. A. Dimascio and R. Shader, pp. 185–93. New York: Science House.

———, SHADER, R.I., and GILLER, D.R. (1970) Behavioral toxicity. Part III: Perceptual–cognitive functions. And Part IV: Emotional (mood) states. In *Psychotropic drug side effects* ed. R.J. Shader, A. Dimascio and Associates, pp. 124–41. Baltimore: Williams & Wilkins.

DIMASCIO, A. SOLTYS, J.J., and SHADER, R.I. 1970. Psychotropic drug side effects in children. In *Psychotropic drug side effects*, ed. R.I. Shader, A. Dimascio, & Associates, pp. 235–60. Baltimore: Williams & Wilkins.

DINGMAN, H.F., and TARJAN, G. 1960. Mental retardation and the normal distribution curve. *Am. J. Ment. Def.* 64: 991–94.

D'IORIO, M., and STEINHAUER, P. Seeking out one's birth parents: Acting out a fantasy of reattachment. Presentation at Current Issues in Child Psychiatry, Geneva Park, Ontario, June 15, 1978.

DIXON, K.N., et al. 1978. "Father-Son Incest." *Amer. J. Psychiat.* 135(7): 835–38.

DIXON, S.D., YOGMAN, M., and BRAZELTON, T.B. et al. 1981. Early infant social interaction with parents and strangers. *J. Am. Acad. Child Psychiat.* 20: 32–52.

DOHRENWEND, B.S., and DOHRENWEND, B.P. 1970. Class and race as status-related sources of stress. In *Social stress*, ed. S. Levine and N.A. Scotch, pp. 111–40. Chicago: Aldine.

DOLL, E.A. 1941. The essentials of an inclusive concept of mental deficiency. *Am. J. Ment. Def.* 46: 214–19.

DOMINIAN, J. 1968. *Marital breakdown.* Plymouth: Penguin.

DONALDSON, J. 1981. The visibility and image of handicapped people on television. *Except. Child.* 47(6): 413–16.

DORPAT, T.L., JACKSON, J.K., and RIPLEY, H.S. 1965. Broken homes and attempted and complete suicides. *Arch. Gen. Psychiat.* 12: 213–66.

DOUGLAS, J.W.B. 1975. Early hospital admissions and later disturbances of behavior and learning. *Dev. Med. Child. Neurol.* 17: 456–80.

DOUGLAS, V.I. 1976. Effects of medication on learning efficiency: research findings, review, and synthesis. In *Learning disability/minimal brain dysfunction syndrome: Research perspectives and applications*, ed. R.P. Anderson and C.G. Halcomb. Springfield, Ill.: Chas. C Thomas.

DOUGLAS, V.I., PARRY, P., MARTON, P., and GARSON, C. 1976. Assessment of a cognitive training program for hyperactive children. *J. Abnorm. Child Psychol.* 4: 389–410.

DROSKE, S.C. 1978. Children's behavioral changes following hospitalizations: Have we prepared the parents? *J. Assn. Care Child. in Hosp.*, 7(2): 3–7.

DROTAR, D., DOERSHUK, C.F., STERN, R.C., BOAT, T.F., BOYER, W., and MATTHEWS, L. 1981. Psychological functioning of children with cystic fibrosis. *Pediat.* 67(3): 338–43.

DUBERMAN, L. 1975. *The reconstituted family.* Chicago: Nelson-Hall.

DUBOIS, P.M. 1980. *The hospice way of death.* New York: Human Sciences Press.

DUGDALE, R.L. 1975. *The jukes: A study in crime, pauperism, disease and heredity.* Reprint of 1877 ed. New York: Putnam.

DULING, F., EDDY, S., and RISKO, V. 1970. Learning disabilities and juvenile delinquency. Unpublished paper prepared at the Robert F. Kennedy Youth Center, Morgantown, W. Va.

DUNN, L. 1973. An overview. In *Exceptional children in the schools: Special education in transition*, 2d ed. ed. L. Dunn, pp. 3–62. New York: Holt Rinehart & Winston.

DUPLESSIS, J.M., and LOCHNER, L.M. 1981. The effects of group psychotherapy on the adjustment of four 12-year-old boys with learning and behavior problems. *J. Learn. Disab.*, 14(4): 209–12.

DUPONT, R.Z., GOLDSTEIN, A., and O'DONNELL, J. (eds.) 1979. *Handbook on drug abuse.* Washington, D.C.: U.S. Government Printing Office.

DZIK, D. 1966. Vision and the juvenile delinquent. *J. Am. Optomet. Assn.* 37: 461–68.

EARLS, F. 1980. Epidemiologic methods for research in child psychiatry. In *Studies of children.* ed. F. Earls, pp. 1–33. New York: Prodist.

———. 1980*b.* "The prevalence of behavior problems in 3-year-old children: A cross-national replication." *Arch. Gen. Psychiat.* 37: 1153–1157.

EASSON, W.M. 1968. Care of the young patient who is dying, *J. Am. Med. Assn.* 205(4): 203–207.

———. 1969. *The severely disturbed adolescent.* New York: International Universities Press.

694

References

EASTMAN, K. 1979. The foster family in a systems theory perspective. *Child Wel.* 58: 564–70.
EDGERTON, R.B. 1967. *The cloak of competence: Stigma in the lives of the mentally retarded.* Berkeley, Calif.: Univ. of California Press.
EIDUSON, B.T. 1976. The commune reared child. In *Basic handbook of child psychiatry,* Vol. 1. *Normal Development.* ed. J.D. Call, pp. 406–12. New York: Basic Books.
———, and ALEXANDER, J.W. 1978. The role of children in alternative family styles, ed. N. Feschbach and S. Feschbach. *J. Soc. Iss.* 34(2): 149–67.
EIDUSON, B.T., COHEN, J., and ALEXANDER, J. 1973. Alternatives in child rearing in the 1970's. *Am. J. Orthopsychiat.* 43: 720–31.
EISENBERG, L. 1956. The autistic child in adolescence. *Am. J. Psychiat.* 112: 607–12.
———. 1961. The strategic deployment of the child psychiatrist in preventive psychiatry. *J. Child Psychol. Psychiat.* 2(4): 229–41.
———. 1966. The management of the hyperkinetic child. *Dev. Med. Child Neurol.* 8: 593–632.
———, ASCHER, E., and KANNER, L. 1959. A clinical study of Gilles de la Tourette's disease (Maladie des Tics) in children. *Am. J. Psychiat.* 115(8): 715–23.
EISENBERG, L., and KANNER, L. 1956. Childhood schizophrenia. Paper presented at Symposium 1955, Early Infantile Autism, 1943–55. *Am. J. Orthopsychiat.* 26: 556–66.
EISENBERG, W. 1962. The sins of the fathers: Urban decay and social pathology. *Am. J. Ortho-psychiat.* 32: 5–17.
EISLER, R.M., and HERSEN, M. 1973. Behavioral techniques in family-oriented crisis intervention. *Arch. Gen. Psychiat.* 28: 111–16.
EKSTEIN, R. 1964. On the acquisition of speech in the autistic child. *Reiss-Davis Bull.* 1: 63–79.
ELDRED, C.A., ROSENTHAL, D., WENDER, P.H., KETY, S., SCHULSINGER, F., WELNER, J., and JACOBSEN, B. 1976. Some aspects of adoption in selected samples of adult adoptees. *Am. J. Orthopsychiat.* 46(2) (April): 279–90.
ELLERSTEIN, N.S., and CANAVAN, J.W. 1980. Sexual abuse of boys. *Am. J. Dis. Child.* 134: 255–57.
ELLIOT, D.S., and VOSS, H.L. 1974. *Delinquency and dropout.* Lexington, Mass.: Lexington Books.
EMDE, R.N., and ROBINSON, J. 1979. The first two months: Recent research in developmental psychobiology and the changing view of the newborn. In *Basic handbook of child psychiatry,* Vol. 1, *Normal development,* ed. J.D. Call. New York: Basic Books.
EMLEN, A., et al. 1976. *Barriers to planning for children in foster care.* Portland, Oregon: Regional Research Institute for Human Services, Portland State University.
EMLEN, A., LAHTI, J., DOWNS, G., McKAY, A., and DOWNS, S. 1978. *Overcoming barriers to planning for children in foster care.* Washington, D.C.: Department of Health, Education and Welfare, publication no. (OHDS) 78-30138.
ENGEL, G. 1968. A life setting conducive to illness—The giving up/given up complex. *Ann. Intern. Med.* 69: 293–300.
ENGELHARDT, D.M. CNS consequences of psychotropic drug withdrawal in autistic children: A follow-up report. Paper Presented at the Annual ECDEU Meeting, National Institute of Mental Health (NIMH), Key Biscayne, Florida, May 23–25, 1974.
———, POLIZOZ, P., WAIZER, J., and HOFFMAN, S.P. 1973. A double blind comparison of fluphenazine and haloperidol. *J. Aut. & Child Schiz.* 3: 128–37.
ENROTH, R.M. 1977. *Youth, brainwashing, and the extremists cults.* Grand Rapids, Mich.: Zondervan Corp.
ENZER, N.B. 1979. Preschool children. In *Basic handbook of child psychiatry,* Vol. 3. ed. S.L. Harrsion New York: Basic Books.
EPSTEIN, M.H. et al. 1980. Understanding children with learning disabilities. *Child Wel.* 59(1): 2–14.
EPSTEIN, N.B., and BISHOP, D.S. 1981. Problem-centered systems therapy of the family. In *Handbook of family therapy,* ed. A.S. Gurman and D.P. Kniskern, pp. 444–82. New York: Brunner/Mazel.
EPSTEIN, N.B., LEVIN, S., and BISHOP, D.S. 1976. The family as a social unit. *Can. Fam. Physician.* 22: 1411–13.
EPSTEIN, N.B., SIGAL, J.J., and RAKOFF, V. 1968. Family categories schema. Monograph prepared in the Family Research Group of the Department of Psychiatry, Jewish General Hospital, Montreal: In collaboration with The McGill University Human Development Study: revised, 1968.
ERIKSON, E.H. 1959. *Identity and the life cycle.* New York: International Universities Press.
———. 1963. *Childhood and society.* 2d ed. New York: W.W. Norton.

——. 1968. *Identity, youth and crisis.* New York: W.W. Norton.

——. 1972. Play and actuality. In *Play and development,* ed. M.W. Piers, pp. 127–67. New York: W.W. Norton.

Escalona, S., Leitch, M., et al. 1952. Early phases of personality development. *Mono. Soc. Res. Child Dev.* Serial no. 54, 17(1).

Esman, A. 1977. Nocturnal enuresis: Some current concepts. *J. Am. Acad. Child Psychiat.* 16:150–58.

Evans, R.G., and Robinson, G.C. 1980. Surgical day care: Measurements of the economic payoff. *Can. Med. Assn. J.* 123: 873–80.

Eymann, R.K., and Padd, W.S. 1980. Epidemiology of aggression. In *Aggression, mental illness and mental retardation,* London, Ontario: C.M. Hincks Lectures, Ontario Mental Health Foundation, Univ. Western Ontario Press.

Falk, W.E. 1981. Steroid psychosis: Diagnosis and management. In *Psychiatric medicine update,* ed. T. Manschrek. New York: Elsevier.

Fanshel, D., and Shinn, E.B. 1978. *Children in foster care: A longitudinal investigation.* New York: Columbia Univ. Press.

Fantz, R.L. 1956. A method for studying early visual development. *Percept. & Mot. Skills.* 6: 13–15.

Farber, B. 1959. Effects of a severely mentally retarded child on family integration. *Mono. Soc. Res. Child Devel.* 24(2).

Faretra, G., Dooher, L., and Dowling, J. 1970. Comparison of haloperidol and fluphenazine in disturbed children. *Am. J. Psychiat.* 126: 1670–73.

Farley, G.K., Eckhardt, L.O., and Hebert, F.B. 1979. *Handbook of child and adolescent psychiatric emergencies.* New York: Medical Examination.

Farran, D., and Ramey, C. 1977. Infant day care and attachment behavior toward mothers and teachers. *Child Devel.* 48(3): 1112–17.

Feifel, H. (ed.) 1959. *The meaning of death.* New York: McGraw-Hill.

——. 1963. Death. In *Taboo topics,* ed. N.L. Farberow, pp. 8–21. New York: Atherton Press.

——, and Hanson, S. 1967. *Physicians consider death.* Proceedings of the Seventh Annual Convention, American Psychological Assn.

Fein, E., Davies, L.J., and Knight, G. 1979. Placement stability in foster care. *Soc. Work.* 24: 156–57.

Feinberg, J., and Carroll, B.J. 1979. Effects of dopamine agonists and antagonists in Tourette's disease. *Arch. Gen. Psychiat.* 36: 979–85.

Feingold, B.F. 1975. *Why your child is hyperactive.* New York: Random House.

Feinstein, S.C., and Miller, D. 1979. Psychoses of adolescence. In *Basic handbook of child psychiatry,* Vol. 2, *Disturbances of Development.* ed. J.D. Call, pp. 708–22. New York: Basic Books.

Feldhusen, J.F. et al. Prediction of social adjustment over an eight year period; correlates and long-range implications of classroom aggression; prediction of academic achievement of children who display aggressive–disruptive classroom behavior. Papers presented at the American Educational Research Assn. Convention, New York, February 1971.

Felice, M. 1978. Follow-up observations of adolescent rape victims. *Clin. Pediat.* 17: 311–17.

Ferri, E. 1976. *Growing up in a one parent family: A long-term study of child development.* National Foundation for Educational Research. Atlantic Highlands, N.J.: Humanities Press.

Feuerstein, R., Krasilowsky, D., and Rand, Y. 1974. Innovative educational strategies for integration of high risk adolescents in Israel. *Phi Delta Kappan* 55(8): 556–58.

Finkelstein, N.E. 1980. Children in limbo. *Soc. Work* 25: 100–105.

Firestone, P., Peters, S., Rivier, M., and Knights, R. 1978. Minor physical anomalies in hyperactive, retarded and normal children and their families. *J. Child Psychol. & Psychiat.* 19: 155–60.

Fisch, R. O., Bilek, M. K., Deinard, A. S., and Di-Nian, C. 1976. Growth, behavioral and psychologic measurements of adopted children: The influences of genetic and socioeconomic factors in a prospective study. *J. of Pediat.* 89: 494–500.

Fish, B. 1959. Longitudinal observations of biological deviations in a schizophrenic infant. *Am. J. Psychiat.* 116: 25–31.

——. 1960. Drug therapy in child psychiatry: Pharmacological aspects. *Compreh. Psychiat.* 1: 212–27.

References

————. 1975. Biologic antecedents of psychosis in children. In *The biology of the major psychoses: A comparative analysis*, ed. D.X. Freedman 54: 49–80. Assn. for Research in Nervous and Mental Disease. New York: Raven Press.

————. 1976. Unpublished analysis of data from Fish *et al.* 1958, and the next 20 psychotic children admitted to the nursery.

————. 1977. Neurobiological antecedents of schizophrenia in children: Evidence for an inherited, congenital neurointegrative defect. *Arch. Gen. Psychiat.* 34: 1297–1313.

————, and RITVO, E.R. 1979. Psychoses of childhood. In *Basic handbook of child psychiatry*, Vol. 2, *Disturbances of development.* J.D. Call, pp. 249–304. New York: Basic Books.

FISH, B., and SHAPIRO, T. 1964. A descriptive typology of children's psychiatric disorders, II: A behavioral classification. *Psychiat. Res. Rep. Am. Psychiat. Assn.* 18: 75–90.

————, CAMPBELL, M., and WILE, R. 1968. A classification of schizophrenic children under five years. *Am. J. Psychiat.* 124: 1415–23.

FISH, B., SHAPIRO, T., HALPERN, F., and WILE, R. 1965. The prediction of schizophrenia in infancy, III: A ten-year follow-up report of neurological and psychological development. *Am. J. Psychiat.* 121: 768–75.

FISHER, C., KAHN, E., EDWARDS, A., and DAVIS, D.M. 1973. A psychophysiological study of nightmares and night terrors. *Arch. Gen. Psychiat.* 28: 252–59.

FISHER, L. 1976. Dimensions of family assessment: A critical review. *J. Marr. & Fam. Counsel.*, 2: 67–82.

FITZHARDINGE, P.M., and RAMSAY, M. 1973. The improving outlook for the small prematurely born infant. *Develop. Med. Child. Neurol.* 15: 447–59.

FOGARTY, T. 1976. *On emptiness and closeness.* Part I and Part II New Rochelle, N.Y.: Center for Family Learning.

FOLEY, J.M. 1979. Effect of labelling and teacher behaviour on children's attitudes. *Am. J. Ment. Def.* 83(4): 380–84.

FORD, F.R., and HERRICK, J. 1974. Family rules: Family life styles. *Am. J. Orthopsychiat.* 44(1): 61–69.

FOSTER CARE COMMITTEE 1972. *Report on child foster care.* Edmonton, Alta.: Queen's Printer.

FOTHERINGHAM, J.B., and MORRISON, M. 1976. *Prevention of mental retardation.* Toronto: N.I.M.R., Mental Retardation Supplement.

FOTHERINGHAM, J.B., SKELTON, M., and HODDINOTT, B.A. 1972. The effects on the family of the presence of a mentally retarded child. *Can. Psychiat. Assn. J.* 17: 283–98.

FOWLE, A. 1968. Atypical leukocyte patterns of schizophrenic children. *Arch. Gen. Psychiat.* 8: 666–80.

FOX, J.R. 1962. Sibling incest. *Brit. J. Sociol.* 13: 128–50.

————. 1980. *The red lamp of incest.* New York: Dutton.

FOX, M. Predictive neurology or clinical mythology. Paper presented at the Canadian Psychiatric Research Institute Symposium on Early Diagnosis, London, Ontario, May 31, 1978.

FRAIBERG, S. 1959. *The magic years.* New York: Scribners.

————. 1968. Parallel and divergent patterns in blind and sighted infants. *Psych. Quart.* 23: 264–300.

————. 1971. Intervention in infancy: A program for blind infants. *J. Am. Acad. Child Psychiat.* 10: 381–405.

FRAMO, J.L. 1981. The integration of marital therapy with sessions with family of origin. In *Handbook of family therapy*, ed. A.S. Gurman and D.P. Kniskern, pp. 133–58. New York: Brunner/Mazel.

FRANK, G. 1980. Treatment needs of children in foster care. *Am. J. Orthopsychiat.* 50: 256–63.

FRANKLIN, D.S., and MASSARIK, F. 1969. The adoption of children with medical conditions: I: Process and outcome. *Child Wel.* 46(8): 459–67; II: The families today *Child Wel.* 46(9): 533–39; III: Discussions and conclusions *Child Wel.*, 46(10): 595–601.

FREEDMAN, A.M., HELME, W., HAVEL, J., EUSTIS, M.J., RILEY, C., and LANGFORD, W.S. 1957. Psychiatric aspects of family dysautonomia. *Am. J. Ortho. Psychiat.*, 27: 96–106.

FREEDMAN, D.A. 1981. The effect of sensory and other deficits in children on their experiences with people. *J. Am. Psychoanal. Assn.* 29: 831–38.

FREEDMAN, M. 1971. A reliability study of psychiatric diagnosis in childhood and adolescence. *J. Child Psychol. Psychiat.* 12: 43–54.

FREEDMAN, R.D. 1967. Emotional reactions of handicapped children. *Rehab. Lit.*, 28: 274–82.

————. 1970. Psychopharmacology and the retarded child. In *Psychiatric approaches to mental retardation,* ed. F.J. Menolascino, pp. 294–368. New York: Basic Books.

————. 1976. Minimal brain dysfunction, hyperactivity and learning disorders: epidemic or episode? *School Rev.* 85: 5–30.

FREIBERGS, V., and DOUGLAS, V.I. 1969. Concept learning in hyperactive and normal children. *J. Abnorm. Psychol.* 74: 388–95.

FREUD, A. 1946. *The ego and the mechanisms of defence.* New York: International Universities Press.

————. 1952. The role of bodily illness in the mental life of children. *The Psychoanal. Stud. of the Child,* 7: 69–81.

————. 1960. Discussion of Dr. John Bowlby's paper. *Psychoanal. Stud. Child.* 15: 53–62.

————. 1962. Assessment of childhood disturbances. In *The psychoanalytic study of the child,* Vol. 17. ed. R. Eissler, pp. 149–58. New York: International Universities Press.

————. 1965. *The psychoanalytic treatment of children.* New York: International Universities Press.

————, and BURLINGHAM, D.T. 1943. *War and children.* New York: Medical Warbooks.

FREUD, S. 1896. The aetiology of hysteria. In The Standard Edition of *The complete psychological works of Sigmund Freud,* Vol. 3. ed., trans. J. Strachey. London: Hogarth Press (1962).

————. 1905. Three essays on sexuality. In The Standard Edition of *The complete psychological works of Sigmund Freud,* Vol. 7. ed. trans. J. Strachey. London: The Hogarth Press and the Institute of Psychoanalysis (1953).

————. 1913. Totem and taboo. In The Standard Edition of *The complete psychological works of Sigmund Freud,* Vol. 13. ed., trans. J. Strachey. London: The Hogarth Press and The Institute of Psychoanalysis (1953).

————. 1917. Lecture XXIV, introductory lectures. In The Standard Edition of *The complete psychological works of Sigmund Freud,* Vol. 16. ed., trans. J. Strachey. London: The Hogarth Press and The Institute of Psychoanalysis (1953).

————. 1938. Splitting of the ego in the defensive process. *Collected Papers,* Vol. 5. New York: Basic Books (1950), pp. 372–75.

FREUDENBERGER, H.J., and RICHELSON, G. 1980. *Burn out: The high cost of high achievement.* Garden City, N.Y.: Doubleday.

FREUND, V.W. 1976. Evaluation of a self-approval method for inducting foster parents. *Smith Coll. Stud. in Soc. Work.* March: 114–26.

FRIEDMAN, R. 1975. The vicissitudes of adolescent development and what it activates in adults. *Adol.* 10: 520–26.

FRIEDMAN, S.B. 1964. The child with leukemia and his parents. *Cancer,* 4:73.

————. 1967. Care of the family of the child with cancer. *Pediatrics* 40:498.

FROESE, A.P. KAMIN, L.E., and LEVINE, C.A. 1976. Teamwork: A multidisciplinary pediatric-liaison service. *Int. J. Psychiat.* 7(1): 47–56.

FROMMER, E.A. 1967. Treatment of childhood depression with antidepressant drugs. *Brit. Med. J.* 1: 729–32.

FROYD, H. 1973. Counselling families of severely visually handicapped children. *New Outlook for the Blind.* 67(6): 251–57.

FULTON, R. 1979. Anticipatory grief, stress and the surrogate griever. In *Cancer, stress and death,* ed. J. Tache, H. Selye and S.B. Day, pp. 87–93. New York: Plenum.

FURMAN, E. 1974. *A child's parent dies.* New Haven, Conn.: Yale University Press.

————. 1979. Filial therapy. In *Basic handbook of child psychiatry,* Vol. 3, ed. S.L. Harrison. New York: Basic Books.

FURSTENBURG, F., Jr. 1976. The social consequences of teenage parenthood. *Fam. Plan. Perspect.* 8(4): 148–64.

GAENSBAUER, T., and HARMON, R. 1981. Clinical assessment in infancy utilizing structural playroom situation. *J. Am. Acad. Child Psychiat.* 20: 264–80.

GALENSON, E., and ROIPHE, H. 1971. The impact of early sexual discovery on mood, defensive organization and symbolization. *Psychoanal. Stud. Child.* 26: 195–216.

GALENSON, E., VOGEL, S., BLAU, S., and ROIPHE, H. 1975. Disturbance in sexual identity beginning at 18 months of age. *Int. Rev. Psychoanal.* 2: 389–97.

GARDNER, R.A. 1968. Psychogenic problems of brain-injured children and their parents. *J. Am. Acad. Child Psychiat.* 7: 471–91.

————. 1976. *Psychotherapy with children of divorce.* New York: Jason Aronson.

————. 1977. *The objective diagnosis of minimal brain dysfunction.* N. J.: Creative Therapeutics.

References

GARDNER, W.I. 1970. Use of behavior therapy with the mentally retarded. In *Psychiatric approaches to mental retardation,* ed. F.J. Menolascino. New York: Basic Books.

———, CROMWELL, R.L., and FOSHEE, J.G. 1959. Studies in activity level II: Effects of distal visual stimulation in organics, familials, hyperactives, and hypoactives. *Am. J. Ment. Def.* 63: 1028–33.

GARFINKEL, B.D. Suicidal behaviour in a paediatric population. *Proceedings Communications, 10th International Congress for Suicide Prevention and Crisis Intervention,* Ottawa, Canada, June 17–20, 1979.

———, and GOLOMBEK, H. 1974. Suicide and depression in children and adolescents. *Can. Med. Assn. J.* 110: 1278–81.

GARFINKEL, P.E. 1981. Some recent observations on the pathogenesis of anorexia nervosa. *Can. J. Psychiat.* 26: 218–23.

———, BROWN, G.M., STANCER, H.C., and MOLODOFSKY, H. 1975. Hypothalmic-pituitary function in anorexia nervosa. *Arch. Gen. Psychiat.* 32: 739–44.

GARFINKEL, P.E., MOLDOFSKY, H., and GARNER, D.M. 1980. The heterogeneity of anorexia nervosa. *Arch. Gen. Psychiat.* 37: 1036–40.

GARNER, D.M., and GARFINKEL, P.E. 1978. Sociocultural factors in anorexia nervosa. *Lancet.* 2: 674.

———, P.E., and BEMIS, K.M. 1982. A multidimensional psychotherapy for anorexia nervosa. *Int. J. Eat. Disord.* 1: 3–46.

GARDNER, R.A. 1971. *Therapeutic communication with children.* New York: Science House.

GARRARD, S.E., and RICHMOND, J.B. 1963. Psychological aspects of the management of chronic disease and handicapping conditions in childhood. In *The psychological basis of medical practice.* ed. H.I. Lief, V.F. Lief, and N.R. Lief, pp. 370–403. New York: Harper & Row.

———. 1978. Mental retardation without biological manifestations. In *Medical aspects of mental retardation,* 2d ed. ed. C.H. Carter. Springfield, Ill.: Chas. C Thomas.

GATH, A. 1977. The impact of an abnormal child upon the parents. *Brit. J. Psychiat.* 130: 405–10.

GAYTON, W.F., FRIEDMAN, S.B., TAVORMINA, J.F., and TUCKER, F. 1977. Children with cystic fibrosis. I: Psychological test findings of patients, siblings and parents. *Pediat.* 59(6): 888–94.

GEISER, R.L. 1979. *Hidden victims: The sexual abuse of children.* Boston: Beacon Press.

GEIST, R.A. 1977. Consultation on a pediatric surgical ward: Creating an empathic climate. *Am. J. Orthopsychiat.* 47(3): 432–44.

———. 1979. Onset of chronic illness in children and adolescents: Psychotherapeutic and consultative intervention. *Am. J. Orthopsychiat.* 49(1): 4–23.

GELLES, R.J. 1973. Child abuse as psychopathology: A sociological critique and reformulation. *Am. J. Orthopsychiat.* 43: 611–21.

———. 1979. Violence toward children in the United States. In *Critical perspectives on child abuse,* ed. R. Bourne and E.H. Newberger. Lexington, Mass.: Lexington Books.

GERHARD, P.H., GAGNON, J.H., POMEROY, W.N., and CHRISTENSON, C.V. 1965. *Sex offenders: An analysis of types.* New York: Harper & Row.

GIARETTO, H. 1976. The treatment of father–daughter incest. *Child. Today.* 5: 2–5.

———. Pro-train seminar on incest, for the Children's Aid Society, Toronto, February 16–17, 1981.

———, GIARETTO, A., and SGROI, S.M. 1978. Co-ordinated community treatment of incest. In *Sexual assault of children and adolescents,* ed. A.W. Burgess *et al.,* pp. 231–40. Lexington, Mass.: Lexington Books.

GIL, D.G. 1973. *Violence against children: Physical abuse in the United States.* Boston: Harvard Univ. Press.

GILMAN, A.G., GOODMAN, L.S., and GILMAN, A. 1980. *Pharmacological basis of therapeutics.* New York: Macmillan.

GINOTT, H.G. 1961. *Group psychotherapy with children.* New York: McGraw-Hill.

GIOVACCHINI, P.L. 1976. Symbiosis and intimacy. *Int. J. Psychoanal. & Psychother.* 5: 413–36.

GITTELMAN, R. 1980. Indications for the use of stimulant treatment in learning disorders. *J. Am. Acad. Child Psychiat.* 19: 623–36.

GITTELMAN-KLEIN, R. 1975. *Recent advances in child psychopharmacology.* New York: Human Sciences Press.

———. 1978. Psychopharmacological treatment of anxiety disorders, mood disorders and Tourette's disorder in children. In *Psychopharmacology: A generation of progress.* ed. M.A. Lipton, A. DiMascio, and K.F. Killan. New York: Raven Press.

———, and KLEIN, D. 1973. School phobia: Diagnostic considerations in the light of imipramine effects. *J. Nerv. Ment. Dis.* 156(3): 199–215.

GITTELMAN-KLEIN, R., and KLEIN, D.F. 1976. Methylphenidate effects in learning disabilities. *Arch. Gen. Psychiat.* 33: 655–64.

GITTELMAN-KLEIN, R., KLEIN, D.G., KATZ, S., SARAF, K., and POLLACK, E. 1976. Comparative effects of methylphenidate and thioridazine in hyperkinetic children. *Arch. Gen. Psychiat.* 33: 1217–31.

GITTELMAN-KLEIN, R., SPITZER, R.L., and CANTWELL, D.P. 1978. Diagnostic classifications and psychopharmacological indications. In *Pediatric psychopharmacology: The use of behaviour modifying drugs in children.* ed. J. Werry. New York: Brunner/Mazel.

GLASER, K. 1967. Masked depression in children and adolescents. *Am. J. Psychother.* 21: 565–74.

GLASSER, P.H., and GLASSER, L.N. (eds.) 1970. *Families in crisis.* New York: Harper & Row.

GLICK, P.C. 1955. Life cycle of the family. *J. Marr. & Fam. Liv.* 17: 3–9.

———, and NORTON, A.J. 1977. Marrying, divorcing and living together in the U.S. today. *Pop. Bull.* 32(5): 1–41.

GLUCK, M.R. 1977. Psychological intervention with pre-school age plastic surgery patients and their families. *J. Pediat. Psychol.* 2(1): 23–25.

GODDARD, H.H. 1912. *The Kallikak family.* New York: Macmillan.

GOFFMAN, E. 1963. *Stigma.* Englewood Cliffs, N.J.: Prentice-Hall.

GOGAN, J.L., O'MALLEY, J.E., and FOSTER, D.J. 1978. Treating the pediatric cancer patients: A review. *J. Pediat. Psychol.* 2(2): 42–48.

GOLD, P., and BERK, R.A. 1979. Prediction of the academic success of children with suspected neurological impairment. *J. Clin. Psychol.* 35(3): 505–09.

GOLDBERG, B. 1975. Comprehensive community programming revisited. *Can. Psychiat. Res. Inst. Mono.* (May). London, Ont.: Canadian Psychiatric Research Institute.

———. 1977. *The role of father.* London, Ont.: Canadian Psychiatric Research Institute.

———. 1979. Historical, scientific and social aspects of sterilization of the mentally retarded. In *Options on medical consent: Part I.* Toronto: Government Printing Office.

———. 1980a. *Ethics of mental health administration.* London, Ont.: Canadian Psychiatric Research Institute (July).

———. 1980b. Rights of the developmentally handicapped. In *Proceedings, St. Lawrence Regional Centre Second Annual Spring Conference, March 5–7, 1980,* Brockville, Ontario.

GOLDBERG, F.H., LESSER, S.R., and SCHULMAN, R. 1966. A conceptual approach and guide to formulating goals in child guidance treatment. *Am. J. Orthopsychiat.* 36: 125–33.

GOLDBERG, S. 1978. Prematurity: Effects on parent–infant interaction. *J. Ped. Psychol.* 3: 137–44.

GOLDEN, G.S. 1978. Tics and Tourette's: A continuum of symptoms. *Ann. Neurol.* 4: 145–48.

———. 1979. Tics and Tourette syndrome. *Hosp. Pract.* 14 (November) 91–100.

GOLDEN, M., and BIRNS, B. 1976. Social class and infant intelligence. In *Origins of intelligence,* ed. M. Lewis, pp. 299–352. New York: Plenum Press.

GOLDEN, M., et al. 1978. *The New York City infant day care study.* New York: Medical & Health Research Association of New York City Inc.

GOLDFARB, W. 1943. The effects of early institutional care on adolescent personality. *J. Exper. Educ.* 12: 106–29.

———. 1955. Emotional and intellectual consequences of psychologic deprivation in infancy: A re-evaluation. In *Psychopathology of childhood.* ed. P.M. Hoch, and J. Zubin, pp. 105–19. New York: Grune & Stratton.

———. 1956. Receptor preferences in schizophrenic children. *Arch. Neurol. Psychiat.* 76: 643–52.

———. 1961. *Childhood schizophrenia.* Cambridge, Mass.: Harvard Univ. Press.

———, BRAUNSTEIN, P., and LORGE, S. 1956. Childhood schizophrenia symposium, 1955: A study of speech patterns in a group of schizophrenic children. *Am. J. Orthopsychiat.* 26: 544–55.

GOLDFARB, W., GOLDFARB, N., and POLLACK, R.C. 1969. Changes in IQ of schizophrenic children during residential treatment. *Arch. Gen. Psychiat.* 21: 673–90.

GOLDMAN, J., and COANE, J. 1977. Family therapy after divorce: Developing a strategy. *Fam. Process* 16(3): 357–62.

GOLDSTEIN, J., FREUD, A., and SOLNIT, A. 1973. *Beyond the best interests of the child.* New York: The Free Press.

GOLOMBEK, H. 1969. The Therapeutic Contract With Adolescents, *Can. Psychiat. Assn. J.* 14: 497–502.

References

————, and GARFINKEL, B.D. 1981. *The adolescent and mood disturbance.* New York: International Universities Press.

GOODE, W.J. (ed.) 1971. *The contemporary American family.* Chicago: Quadrangle Books.

GOODMAN, J., and SOURS, J. 1967. *The child mental status examination.* New York: Basic Books.

GOODMAN, J.D., SILBERSTEIN, R.M., and MANDELL, W. 1963. Adopted children brought to child psychiatric clinics. *Arch. Gen. Psychiat.* 9: 451–56.

GOODSITT, A. 1977. Narcissistic disturbances in anorexia nervosa. In *Adolescent Psychiatry,* Vol. 5. ed. S.C. Feinstein and P. Giovacchini, pp. 304–12. New York: Jason Aronson.

GOODWIN, J., SIMMS, M., and BERGMAN, R. 1979. Hysterical seizures: A sequel to incest. *Amer. J. Orthopsychiat.* 49: 698–703.

GORDON, H. 1973. Abortion as a method of population regulation: The problems. *Brit. J. Hosp. Med.* 9: 303–306.

GOTTESMAN, I.I., and SHIELDS, J. 1972. *Schizophrenia and genetics: A twin study vantage point.* New York: Academic Press.

GOTTLIEB, M.I., ZINKUS, P.W., and BRADFORD, L.J. 1979. *Current issues in developmental pediatrics: The learning disabled child.* New York: Grune & Stratton.

GOUGH, D. 1966. The very young mother. In *Pregnancy in adolescence.* London: National Council for the Unmarried Mother and Her Child.

GOULD, M.S., WUNSCH-HITZIG, R., and DOHRENWEND, B. 1981. Estimating the prevalance of childhood psychopathology: A critical review. *J. Am. Acad. Child Psychiat.* 20: 462–76.

GRAD, J., and SAINSBURY, P. 1966. Evaluating the community psychiatric service in Chichester: Results. *Milbank Mem. Fund Quart.,* 44: 146–78.

GRAHAM, P., and RUTTER, M. 1968. The reliability and validity of the psychiatric assessment of the child. II: Interview with the parents. *Brit. J. Psychiat.* 114: 581–92.

————. 1973. Psychiatric disorder in the young adolescent. *Proc. Roy. Soc. Med.* 66: 1226–29.

————, and GEORGE, S. 1973. Temperamental characteristics as predictors of behavior disorders in children. *Am. J. Orthopsychiat.* 43: 328–39.

GRAHAM, S., and SHEINKER, A. 1980. Creative capabilities of learning disabled and normal students. *Percept. & Motor Skills* 50(2): 481–82.

GRAM, L.F., and RAFAELSON, O.J. 1972. Lithium treatment of psychotic children: A controlled clinical trial. In *Depressive states in childhood and adolescence,* ed. A.L. Annek, pp. 488–90. Stockholm: Almquist & Wiksell.

GRANT, M.Q. 1961. *Interpersonal maturity level classification: Juvenile.* Sacramento, Calif.: Youth Authority.

GRAY, J.D., CUTLER, C.A., DEAN, J., and KEMPS, C.H. 1976. Prediction and prevention of child abuse. In the transcripts of the 1st International Congress of Child Abuse and Neglect. Geneva, 1976, p. 15.

GRAZIANO, A.M. 1971. *Behavior Therapy With Children.* Chicago: Aldine/Atherton.

GREBLER, A.M. 1952. Parental attitudes toward mentally retarded children. *Am. J. Ment. Def.* 56(3): 475–83.

GREEN, A.H. 1978. Self-destructive behavior in battered children. *Am. J. Psychiat.* 135: 579–82.

GREEN, M. 1976. *Care of the dying child.* New York: Appleton-Century Crofts.

GREEN, R. 1975. The significance of feminine behavior in boys. *J. Child Psychol. & Psychiat.* 16: 341–44.

————. 1979. Childhood cross-gender behavior and subsequent sexual preference. *Am. J. Psychiat.,* 136: 106–08.

————, R. 1979. Quoted in Children of gays. ed. R. Epstein *Christopher Street,* (June).

————. 1980. Gender identity disorders of childhood. In *Comprehensive textbook of child psychiatry.* Vol. 3, 3d ed. ed. H.I. Kaplan, A.M. Freedman, and B.J. Sadock, pp. 2774–80. Baltimore: Williams & Wilkins.

GREENACRE, P. 1971. The fetish and the transitional object. In *Emotional Growth,* Vol. 1. pp. 315–52. New York: International Univ. Press.

GREENBAUM, G.H. 1970. An evaluation of niacinamide in the treatment of childhood schizophrenia. *Am. J. Psychiat.* 127: 89–92.

GREENHILL, L., PUIG-ANTICH, J., CHAMBERS, W., RUBINSTEIN, B., HALPERN, F., and SACHAR, E.J. 1981. Growth hormone, prolactin and growth responses in hyperkinetic males treated with d-amphetamine. *J. Am. Acad. Child Psychiat.* 20: 84–103.

GREENLEE, W.E., and HARE, B. 1978. A closer look at learning disabilities. *Acad. Ther.* 13(3): 345–49.

701

GREY, E., and BLUNDEN, R.M. 1971 *A survey of adoption in Great Britain.* Home Office Research Studies. London: Her Majesty's Stationery Office.

GRILL, J.J. 1977. Identification of learning-disabled adolescents. *Acad. Ther.* 13(1): 23–28.

GROSS, P.K., and BUSSARD, F. 1970. A group method for finding and developing foster homes. *Child Wel.* 49: 521–24.

GROSSMAN, F.K. 1972. *Brothers and sisters of retarded children: An exploratory study.* Syracuse, N.Y.: Syracuse Univ. Press.

GROTH, A.N. 1978. Patterns of sexual assault against children and adolescents. In *Sexual assault of children and adolescents,* ed. A.W. Burgess, et al., pp. 3–24. Lexington, Mass.: Lexington Books.

GROUP FOR THE ADVANCEMENT OF PSYCHIATRY. 1966. *Psychopathological disorders in childhood: Theoretical considerations and a proposed classification.* Vol. 6. Report No. 62. New York: Jason Aronson.

GROUP FOR THE ADVANCEMENT OF PSYCHIATRY: Committee on Child Psychiatry. 1973. *From diagnosis to treatment: An approach to treatment planning for the emotionally disturbed child.* Vol. 8. Report No. 87, New York: Group for the Advancement of Psychiatry.

GRUBER, A.R. 1978. *Children in foster care: Destitute, neglected, betrayed.* New York: Human Sciences Press.

GRUNEBAUM, H., and CHASIN, R. 1980. Thinking like a family therapist. In *The challenge of family therapy: A dialogue for child psychiatric educators,* ed. K. Flomenhaft and A.E. Christ, pp. 55–74. New York: Plenum Press.

GRUNEWALD, K. 1979. Mentally retarded children and young people in Sweden: Integration into society: The progress in the last decade. *Acta. Paediatr. Scand.* (Supplement) 275: 75–84.

GUALTIERI, C.T., BARNHILL, J., McGIMSEY, J., and SCHELL, D. 1980. Tardive dyskinesia and other movement disorders in children treated with psychotropic drugs. *J. Am. Acad. Child Psychiat.* 19: 491–510.

GUERIN, P. 1976a. Evaluation of family system and genogram. In *Family Therapy,* ed. P. Guerin, pp. 450–64. New York: Gardiner Press.

———. 1976b. Theoretical aspects of clinical relevance of the multigenerational model of family therapy. In *Family therapy,* ed. P. Guerin, pp. 91–110. New York: Gardiner Press.

GUGGENHEIM, F., and UZOGARA, E. 1981. Understanding and treating obesity. In *Psychiatric Medicine Update,* ed. T.C. Manschreck. New York: Elsevier.

GULL, W.W. 1874. Apepsia hysterica: Anorexia nervosa. *Clin. Soc. Trans.* 7: 180–85.

GUNDERSON, J.G., and SINGER, M.T. 1975. Defining borderline patients: An overview. *Am. J. Psychiat.* 132: 1–10.

GUTHEIL, T.G., and AVERY, N.C. 1977. Multiple overt incest as family defense against loss. *Fam. Process* 16: 105–16.

GUYATT, D.E. 1980. Panel on adolescent pregnancy and motherhood. Presented at St. John's, Newfoundland, June 18, 1980. Toronto: Ontario Ministry of Community and Social Services.

HAKA-IKSE, K., and VANLEEUWEN, J.J. 1976. Care of the long-term hospitalized infant. *Clin. Ped.* 15(7): 585–88.

HALEY, J. 1978. *Problem solving therapy.* San Francisco: Jossey-Bass.

HALL, D., and STACEY, M. 1979. *Beyond separation.* London: Routledge & Kegan Paul.

HALLAHAN, D.P., and COHEN, S.B. 1977. Learning disabilities: Problems in definition. *Behav. Disord.* 2(3): 132–35.

HALLAHAN, D.P. and KAUFFMAN, J.M. 1976. *Introduction to learning disabilities: A psycho-behavioral Approach.* Englewood Cliffs, N.J.: Prentice-Hall.

HALLECK, S.L. 1962. The physician's role in management of sex offences. *J. Am. Med. Assn.* 180: 273–78.

HALMI, K.A. 1980. Eating disorders. In *Comprehensive textbook of psychiatry,* Vol. 3. 3 ed. ed. H.I. Kaplan, A.M. Freedman, and B.J. Sadock, pp. 2598–2605. Baltimore: Williams & Wilkins.

———, and BRODLAND, D. 1973. Monozygotic twins concordant and discordant for anorexia nervosa. *Psychol. Med.* 3: 521–24.

HALMI, K.A., and FALK, J.R. 1981. Common physiologic changes in anorexia nervosa. *Int. J. Eat. Disord.* 1(1): 16–27.

HALMI, K.A., and LARSON, L. 1977. Behavior therapy in anorexia nervosa. In *Adolescent psychiatry,* Vol. 5. ed. S.C. Feinstein and P.L. Giovacchini, pp. 323–51. New York: Jason Aronson.

References

HAMILTON, J.R., et al. 1979. Inflammatory bowel disease in children and adolescents. *Adv. in Pediat.*, 26: 311–41.

HAMPSON, R.B., and TAVORMINA, J.B. 1980. Feedback from the experts: A study of foster mothers. *Soc. Work* 25: 108–113.

HANDLERS, A., and AUSTIN, K. 1980. Improving attitudes of high school students toward their peers. *Except. Child.* 47(3): 228–29.

HANSEN, H., BELMONT, L., and STEIN, Z. 1980. Epidemiology. In *Mental retardation and developmental disabilities: An annual review,* Vol. 10. ed. J. Wortis, pp. 21–54. New York: Brunner/Mazel.

HANSON, D.R., and GOTTESMAN, I.I. 1976. The genetics, if any, of infantile autism and childhood schizophrenia. *J. Aut. & Child. Schiz.* 6:209–34.

HARE, E.H., LAURENCE, K.M., PAYNES, H., and RAWNSLEY, K. 1966. Spina bifida cystica and family stress. *Brit. Med. J.* 2: 757–60.

HARLEY, J.P., ROY, R.S., TOMASI, L., EICHMAN, P.L., MATTHEWS, C.G., CHUN, R., CLEELAND, C.S., and TRAISMAN, E. 1978. Hyperkinesis and food additives: Testing the Feingold hypothesis. *Pediat.* 61: 818–28.

HARLOW, H.F., HARLOW, M.K., DODSWORTH, R.O., and ARLING, G.L. 1966. Maternal behavior of rhesus monkeys deprived of mothering and peer associations in infancy. *Proc. Am. Phil. Soc.* 110 (1): 58–66.

HARRIS, P.W. 1978. The interpersonal maturity of delinquents and nondelinquents. Ph.D. diss. State University of New York at Albany.

HARRISON, S.I. 1978. Child psychiatry perspectives: Therapeutic choice in child psychiatry. *J. Am. Acad. Child Psych.* 17: 165–72.

HARVEY, D., and GREENWAY, P. 1982. How parent attitudes and emotional reactions affect their handicapped child's self-concept. *Psychol. Med.* 12: 357–70.

HARVEY, O.J., HUNT, D.E., and SCHRODER, H.M. 1961. *Conceptual systems and personality organization.* New York: Wiley.

HASTINGS, J.E., and BARKLEY, R.A. 1978. A review of psychophysiological research with hyperkinetic children. *J. Abnorm. Child Psychol.* 6: 413–47.

HATCHER, S. 1973. The adolescent experience of pregnancy and abortion: A developmental analysis. *J. Youth & Adol.* 2(1): 53–102.

HAUSER, S.L., DELONG, G.R., and ROSMAN, N.P. 1975. Pneumographic findings in the infantile autism syndrome: A correlation with temporal lobe disease. *Brain* 98: 667–88.

HAUSKNECHT, R.O. 1972. The termination of pregnancy in adolescent women. ed. A. Altched. *Pediat. Clin. N. Am.* 19(3): 803–11.

HAVELKOVA, M. 1968. Follow-up study of 71 children diagnosed as psychotic in preschool age. *Am. J. Orthopsychiat.* 38: 846–57.

HAWKE, W.A., and LESSER, S.R. 1977. The child with a learning disorder. In *Psychological problems of the child and his family,* ed. P.D. Steinhauer and Q. Rae-Grant. Toronto: Macmillan.

HAWORTH, M.R. (ed.) 1964. *Child psychotherapy.* New York: Basic Books.

HAYDEN, T.L. 1980. Classification of elective mutism. *J. Am. Acad. Child Psychiat.* 19(1): 118–33.

HAZEL, N., COX, R., and ASHLEY-MUDIE, P. 1977. *Second report of the special family project.* Maidstone, U.K.: Kent Social Services Dept.

HEAGARTY, M.C. 1978. Terminal and life-threatening illness in children. In *Psychosocial aspects of pediatric care,* ed. E. Gellert, pp. 65–73. New York: Grune & Stratton.

HEATHERINGTON, E.M. 1979. Divorce: A child's perspective. *Am. Psychol.* 34(10): 851–58.

———, COX, M., and COX, R. 1977. The aftermath of divorce. In *Mother–child, father–child relations,* ed. J.H. Stevens, Jr., and M. Matthews. Washington, D.C.: NAEYC.

———. 1979. Play and social interaction in children following divorce. *J. Soc. Iss.* 35(4): 26–49.

———. 1979. Family interaction and the social, emotional and cognitive development of children following divorce. In *The family: Setting priorities.* ed. V. Vaughn and T. Brazelton. New York: Science & Medicine.

HEBER, R. 1964. Personality. In *Mental retardation: A review of research,* ed. H.A. Stevens and R. Heber, pp. 143–74. Chicago: Univ. of Chicago Press.

HEBER, R.F. 1978. Sociocultural mental retardation: A longitudinal study. In *Primary prevention of psychopathology,* Vol. 2, *Environmental Influences,* ed. D.G. Forgays, pp. 39–62. Hanover, N.H.: Univ. Press of New England.

HEBER, R., GARBER, H., and FALENDER, C. The Milwaukee project: An experiment in the prevention of cultural familial retardation. Mimeograph (September, 1973.) Summarized in *Can. Psychiat. Res. Inst.* Mono. 6. London, Ontario: Canadian Psychiatric Research Institute.

HECHTMAN, L., WEISS, G., FINKELSTEIN, J., WERNER, A., and BENN, R. 1976. Hyperactives as young adults: Preliminary report. *Can. Med. Assn. J.* 115: 625–30.

HEINICKE, C.M., and WESTHEIMER, I.J. 1965. *Brief separations* New York: International Universities Press.

HELFER, R.E., and KEMPE, C.H. 1974. *The battered child.* Chicago: Univ. of Chicago Press.

HENDERSON, J.O. 1972. Incest: A synthesis of data. *Can. Psychiat. Assn. J.* 17: 299–313.

HENDERSON, L.J. 1913. *The fitness of the environment.* New York: Macmillan.

HENDERSON, P. 1968. Changing pattern of disease and disability in school children in England and Wales. *Brit. Med. J.* 2:329–34.

HENDERSON, S. The significance of social relationships in the etiology of neurosis. In *The place of attachment in human behavior,* ed. C.M. Parkes and J. Stevenson-Hinde. New York: Basic Books.

HENOCH, M.J., BATSON, J.W., and BAUM, J. 1978. Psychosocial factors in juvenile rheumatoid arthritis. *Arth. and Rheum.*, 21: 229–33.

HEPWORTH, H.P. 1980. *Foster care and adoption in Canada.* Ottawa: The Canadian Council on Social Development.

HERJANIC, B., and WILBOIS, R.P. 1978. Sexual abuse of children: Detection and management. *J. Am. Med. Assn.*, 239: 331–33.

HERMELIN, B. 1968. Measures of the occipital alpha rhythm in normal, subnormal and autistic children. *Brit. J. Psychiat.* 114: 603–610.

———, and O'CONNOR, N. 1970. *Psychological experiments with autistic children.* Oxford: Pergamon Press.

HERSOV, L. 1973. The psychiatrist and modern adoption practice. *Child Adopt.* 71: 17–31.

———. 1976. Faecal Soiling. In *Child psychiatry: Modern approaches,* ed. M. Rutter and L. Hersov, pp. 613–27. Oxford: Blackwell Scientific Publications.

———. 1977. Adoption. In *Child psychiatry: Modern approaches,* ed. M. Rutter and L. Hersov, pp. 136–62. Oxford: Blackwell Scientific Publications.

HERSTEIN, A., HILL, R.H., and WALTERS, F. 1977. Adult sexuality and juvenile rheumatoid arthritis. *J. Rheumatol.* 4(1): 35–39.

HERTZIG, M. Treatment and neurologic organization in prematurely born children. Paper presented at the 26th Annual Meeting of the American Academy of Child Psychiatry, Atlanta, October, 1979.

HERTZIG, M.E., and BIRCH, H.G. 1968. Neurological organization in psychiatrically disturbed adolescents. *Arch. Gen. Psychiat.* 19: 528–37.

HERTZIG, M.E., BORTNER, M., and BIRCH, H.G. 1969. Neurologic findings in children educationally designated as brain-damaged. *Am. J. Orthopsychiat.* 39: 437–46.

HESTON, L.L., and DENNY, D. 1968. Interaction between early life experience and biological factors in schizophrenia. In *The transmission of schizophrenia,* ed. D. Rosenthal and S.S. Kety, pp. 363–76. London: Pergamon Press.

HILL, R. 1965. Generic features of families under stress. In *Crisis intervention: Selected readings,* ed. H.J. Parad, pp. 32–52. New York: Family Service Assn. of America.

HIMWICH, H.E. 1960. Biochemical and neurophysiological actions of psychoactive drugs. In *Drugs and behavior,* ed. L. Uhr and J.G. Miller. New York: Wiley.

HINDE, R.A., SPENCER-BOOTH, Y., and BRUCE, M. 1966. Effects of six-day maternal deprivation on rhesus monkey infants. *Nature,* 210: 1021–23.

HINKLE, L.E., and WOLF, S. 1952. A summary of experimental evidence relating life stress to diabetes mellitus. *Mt. Sinai J. Med.* 19: 537–70.

HIRSCH, J.G. 1979. Helping the family whose child has a birth defect. In *Basic handbook of child psychiatry,* Vol. 4. ed. J.D. Noshpitz, pp. 121–28. New York: Basic Books.

HIRSCHOWITZ, R.G. 1973. Crisis theory: A formulation. *Psychiat. Ann.* 3:33.

HOAG, J.M., et al. 1971. The encopretic child and his family. *J. Am. Acad. Child Psychiat.* 10: 242–56.

HOBBEN, M. 1980. Toward integration in the mainstream. *Except. Child* 47(2): 100–05.

HOBBS, N. 1975. *The futures of children: Categories, labels and their consequences.* San Francisco: Jossey-Bass.

HOFFMAN, H. 1845. *Der Struwwelpeter: Oder lustige geschichten und drollige bilder.* Leipzig: Insel Verlag.

References

HOFFMAN, L. 1975. Enmeshment and the too richly cross-joined system. *Fam. Proc.* 14(4): 457–68.

HOGENSON, D.L. 1974. Reading failure and juvenile delinquency. *Bull. Orton Soc.* 24: 164–69.

HOHMAN, L.B. 1922. Post-encephalitic behavior disorders in children. *Johns Hopkins Hosp. Bull.* 380: 372–75.

HOLDEN, C. 1976. Massachusetts juvenile justice: De-institutionalization on trial. *Science,* 192: 447–51.

HOLLENBECK, A.R., SUSMAN, E.J., NANNIS, E.D., STROPE, B.E., HERSH, S.P., LEVINE, M.S., and PIZZO, P.A. 1980. Children with serious illness: Behavioral correlates of separation and isolation. *Child Psychiat. Hum. Dev.* 11(1): 3–11.

HOLLINGSWORTH, C.E., and PASNAU, R.O. 1977. *The family in mourning: A guide for health professionals.* Part of the *Seminars in Psychiatry.* M. Greenblatt (Series ed.). New York: Grune & Stratton.

HOLMES, D.J. 1964. *The adolescent in psychotherapy.* Boston: Little, Brown.

HOOD, E., and ANGLIN, J. 1979. *Clinical assessment in children's services.* Toronto: Ontario Ministry of Community and Social Services, Children's Services Division.

HOPKINS, J., PERLMAN, T., HECHTMAN, L., and WEISS, G. 1979. Cognitive style in adults originally diagnosed as hyperactives. *J. Child Psychol. & Psychiat.* 20: 209–16.

HOWARD, J. 1957. *The little victims: How America treats its children.* New York: MacKay.

HOWARD, M. 1971. Pregnant school-age girls. *J. School H.* 41(7): 361–64.

HOWELL, M.C., EMMONS, E.G., and FRANK, D.A. 1973. Reminiscences of runaway adolescents. *Am. J. Orthopsychiat.* 43: 840–53.

HOWELLS, J.G. (ed.) 1976. *Modern perspectives in the psychiatric aspects of surgery.* New York: Brunner/Mazel.

HOY, E., WEISS, G., MINDE, K., and COHEN, H. 1978. The hyperactive child at adolescence: Emotional and social cognitive functioning. *J. Abnorm. Child Psychol.* 6:311–24.

HSU, L.K.G. 1980. Outcome of anorexia nervosa: A review of the literature (1954–78). *Arch. Gen. Psychiat.* 37: 1041–46.

HUDGENS, R.W. 1974. Affective disorders and "psychosis" and the problem of schizophrenia. In *Psychiatric disorders in adolescents,* pp. 38–39, 108–31. Baltimore: Williams & Wilkins.

HUESSY, H.R., METOYER, M., and TOWNSEND, M. 1974. 8–10 year follow-up of 84 children treated for behavioral disorder in rural Vermont. *Acta Paedopsychiat.,* 40: 230–35.

HULL, C.L. 1943. *Principles of behavior: An introduction to behavior therapy.* New York: Appleton-Century.

HUMPHREY, M. 1969. *The hostage seekers.* New York: Humanities Press.

HUMPHREY, M.E., and OUNSTED, C. 1963. Adoptive families referred for psychiatric advice, I: The children. *Brit. J. Psychiat.* 109: 599–608.

———. 1964. Adoptive families referred for psychiatric advice, II: The parents. *Brit. J. Psychiat.* 110: 549–55.

HUMPHRIES, T., KINSBOURNE, M., and SWANSON, J. 1976. Hyperactive children as a function of environmental stimulation. *J. Consul. Clin. Psychol.* 44: 693–97.

———. 1978. Stimulant effects on cooperation and social interaction between hyperactive children and their mothers. *J. Child Psychol. & Psychiat.* 19: 13–22.

HUNT, D.D., and HAMPSON, J.L. 1980. Follow-up of 17 biologic male transsexuals after sex reassignment surgery. *Am. J. Psychiat.* 137(4): 432–38.

HUNTINGTON, D. 1979. Supportive programs for infants and parents. In *The handbook of infant development,* ed. J. Osofsky. New York: Wiley.

HURWITZ, J., BIBACE, R.M., WOLFF, P.H., and ROWBOTHAM, B.M. 1972. Neuropsychological function of normal boys, delinquent boys, and boys with learning problems. *Percep. & Motor Skills* 35(2): 387–94.

HUTCHINGS, B., and MEDNICK, S.A. (in press). Registered criminality in the adoptive and biological parents of registered male criminal adoptees. In *Genetics and psychopathology,* ed. R. Fieve and D. Rosenthal. Baltimore: Johns Hopkins University Press.

ILLINGWORTH, R. (The Association of British Adoption Agencies) 1968. Assessment for adoption. In *Genetic and psychological aspects of adoption.* Aberdeen: The University Press.

INGRAM, T.T.S. 1959. Specific developmental disorders of speech in childhood. *Brain* 82: 450–68.

ITARD, J.M.G. 1801. *Wild Boy of Aveyron* (trans.) New York: G. & M. Humphrey, Appleton-Century Crofts.

IVERSEN, S.D. 1980. Brain chemistry and behaviour. *Psychol. Med.* 10: 527–39.

JACKSON, D.D. 1957. The question of family homeostasis. *Psychiat. Quart. Suppl.* 31: 79–90.

———, BEAVIN, J.H., and WATZLAWICK, P. 1967. *Pragmatics of human communication.* New York: W.W. Norton.

JACKSON, K., WINKLEY, R., FAUST, O.A., and CERMAK, E.G. 1952. Problem of emotional trauma in hospital treatment of children. *J. Am. Med. Assn.* 149: 1536–38.

JACOB, R., O'LEARY, K., and PRICE, G. 1973. Behavioral treatment of hyperactive children: An alternative to medication. Unpublished paper.

JACOBS, M. 1980. Foster parent training: An opportunity for skills enrichment and empowerment. *Child Wel.* 59: 615–24.

JACOBSON, F.N. 1974a. Learning disabilities and juvenile delinquency: A demonstrated relationship. In *Handbook of learning disabilities: A prognosis for the child, the adolescent, the adult,* ed. R.E. Weber, pp. 189–216. Englewood Cliffs, N.J.: Prentice-Hall.

JACOBSON, F.N. The juvenile court judge and learning disabilities. Paper presented at the National Council of Juvenile Court Judges Graduate College. University of Nevada, Reno, 12 August and 11 November, 1974a.

JACOBSON, G., STRICKLER, M., and MORLEY, W. 1968. Generic and individual approaches to crisis intervention. *Am. J. Pub. H.* 58: 338–43.

JACOBSON, N.S. 1981. Behavioral Marital Therapy. In *Handbook of family therapy,* ed. A.S. Gurman and D.P. Kinskern pp. 556–91. New York: Brunner/Mazel.

JAFFEE, B., and FANSHEL, D. 1970. *How they fared in adoption: A follow-up study.* New York: Columbia Univ. Press.

JANOV, A. 1971. *The anatomy of mental illness.* New York: Berkley.

JENSEN, A. R. 1969. How much can we boost IQ and scholastic achievement? *Harvard Ed. Rev.* 39(1): 1–123.

JESNESS, C.F., DERISI, W., McCORMICK, P., and WEDGE, R. 1972. *The youth center research project: Final Report.* Sacramento: California Youth Authority and American Justice Institute.

JESSNER, L., BLOM, G.E., and WALDFOGEL, S. 1952. Emotional implications of tonsillectomy and adenoidectomy on children. *Psychoanal. Stud. Child.* 7:126–69.

JOHNSON, A.M. 1949. Sanctions for superego lacunae of adolescents. In *Searchlights on delinquency.* ed. K. R. Eissler, pp. 225–34. New York: International Universities Press.

JOHNSON, D., and JOHNSON, R. 1980. Integrating handicapped children into the mainstream. *Except. Child.* 47(2): 90–98.

JOHNSON, F.K., DOWLING, J., and WESNER, N. 1980. Notes on infant psychotherapy. *Inf. Ment. H. J.* 1(1): 19–33.

JOHNSON, L.C. 1978. *Taking care: A report of the project child care survey of care-givers in metropolitan Toronto.* Toronto: Social Planning Council of Metropolitan Toronto.

———, and DENINE, J. 1981. *The Kin trade: Day care crisis in Canada.* Toronto: McGraw-Hill Ryerson.

JOHNSON, V.S. 1977. An environment for treating youthful offenders: The Robert F. Kennedy youth center. *Off. Rehab.* 2(2): 159–72.

JOINT CUSTODY: *A Handbook for Judges, Lawyers and Counsellors.* 1979. Portland, Ore: Assn. of Family Conciliation Courts.

JORDON, D. 1974. Learning disabilities and predelinquent behavior of juveniles. Report on a project sponsored by the Oklahoma Assn. for Children With Learning Disabilities.

JOURNAL OF ABNORMAL CHILD PSYCHOLOGY. 1980. *Special issue on learning disabilities,* 8(1).

JOURNAL OF THE AMERICAN MEDICAL ASSOCIATION. 1973. Editorial, "Methaqualone" 224(11): 1521–22.

KADUSHIN, A. 1970. *Adopting Older Children.* New York: Columbia Univ. Press.

———, and SEIDL, F.W. 1971. Adoption failure: A social work postmortem. *Soc. Work,* 16(3): 32–38.

KAGAN, J., KEARSLEY, R., and ZELAZO, P.R. 1978. *Infancy: Its place in human development.* Cambridge, Mass.: Harvard Univ. Press.

KAGAN, J., LAPIDUS, D., and MOORE, M. 1979. Infant antecedents of cognitive functioning: A longitudinal study. *Child Dev.* 49: 1005–23.

706

References

KAGEN-GOODHEART, L. 1977. Re-entry: Living with childhood cancer. *Am. J. Orthopsychiat.* 47(4): 651–58.

KALES, A., and KALES, J.D. 1974. Sleep disorders: Recent findings in the diagnosis and treatment of disturbed sleep. *N. E. J. Med.,* 290: 487–97.

KALES, A., SOLDATOS, D.R., CALDWELL, A.B., KALES, J.D., HUMPHREY, F.J. II, CHARNEY, D.S., and SCHWEITZER, P.K. 1980. Somnambulism: Clinical characteristics and personality patterns. *Arch. Gen. Psychiat.* 37: 1406–10.

KALES, A., SOLDATOS, C.R., BIXLER, E.O., LADDA, R.L., CHARNEY, D.S., WEBER, G., and SCHWEITZER, P.K. 1980. Hereditary factors in sleepwalking and night terrors. *Brit. J. Psychiat.* 137: 111–18.

KALES, J.D., KALES, A., SOLDATOS, C.R., CALDWELL, A., CHARNEY, D.S., and MARTIN, E.D. 1980. Night terrors: Clinical characteristics and personality patterns. *Arch. Gen. Psychiat.* 37: 1413–17.

KALES, J.D., KALES, A., SOLDATOS, C.R., CHAMBERLIN, K., and MARTIN, E.D. 1979. Sleepwalking and night terrors related to febrile illness. *Am. J. Psychiat.* 136: 1214–15.

KALLMAN, F.J., and ROTH, B. 1956. Genetic aspects of preadolescent schizophrenia. *Am. J. Psychiat.* 112: 599–606.

KALNINS, I.V., CHURCHILL, M.P., and TERRY, G.E. 1980. Concurrent stresses in families with a leukemic child. *J. Ped. Psychol.* 5(1): 81–92.

KALTER, N. 1977. Children of divorce in an outpatient psychiatric population. *Am. J. Orthopsychiat.* 47(1): 40–51.

———, and RENBAR, J. 1981. The significance of a child's age at the time of divorce. *Am. J. Orthopsychiat.* 51(1): 85–100.

KANNER, L. 1944. Early infantile autism. *J. Pediat.* 25: 211–17.

———. 1948. Feeblemindedness: Absolute, relative and apparent. *Nerv. Child.* 7(4): 365–97.

———. 1953. To what extent is early infantile autism determined by constitutional inadequacies? *Proc. Assn. Res. Nerv. Ment. Dis.* 33: 378–85.

———. 1975. *Child Psychiatry.* 4th ed. Springfield, Ill.: Chas C Thomas.

———, and EISENBERG, L. 1955. Notes on the follow-up studies of autistic children. In *Psychopathology of childhood,* ed. P.H. Hoch and J. Zubin, pp. 117–129. New York: Grune & Stratton.

KANTOR, D. 1980. Critical identity image: A concept linking individual, couple and family development. In *Family therapy: Combining psychodynamic and family systems approaches,* ed. J. K. Pearce and L. J. Friedman, pp. 137–67. New York: Grune & Stratton.

———, and LEHR, W. 1975. *Inside the family.* San Francisco: Jossey-Bass.

KAPLAN, D.M., GROBSTEIN, R., and SMITH, A. 1976. Predicting the impact of severe illness in families. *H. & Soc. Work* 1(3): 72–82.

KAPLAN, D.M., SMITH, A. GROBSTEIN, R., and FISCHMAN, S.E. 1973. Family mediation of stress. *Soc. Work* 18(4): 60–69.

KAPLAN DE-NOUR, A. 1979. Adolescents' adjustment to chronic hemodialysis. *Am. J. Psychiat.* 136: (April): 430–33.

———, CZACKES, J.W., and LILOS, P. 1972. A study of chronic hemodialysis teams: Differences in opinions and expectations. *J. Chron. Dis.* 25 (August): 441–48.

KARPEL, M. 1976. Individuation: From fusion to dialogue. *Fam. Proc.* 15: 65–82.

KASANIN, J. 1929. Personality changes in children following cerebral trauma. *J. Nerv. Ment. Dis.* 69: 385.

KASHANI, J., HUSAIN, A., SHEKIM, W.O., HODGES, K.K., CYTRYN, L., and McKNEW, D.H. 1981. Current perspectives on childhood depression: An overview. *Am. J. Psychiat.* 138: 143–53.

KASLOW, F.W. and COOPER, B. 1978. Family therapy with the learning disabled child and his/her family. *J. Marr. & Fam. Counsel,* 4(1) (January): 41–49.

KATZ, S., SARAF, K.G., GITTLEMAN-KLEIN, R., and KLEIN, D.F. 1975. Clinical pharmacological management of hyperkinetic children. *Int. J. Ment. H.* 4: 157–81.

KATZ, S.N. 1976. The changing legal status of foster parents. *Child. Today.* 5(6) (November/December): 11–13.

KAUFMAN, I., PECK, A.L., and TAQUIRI, C. 1954. The family constellation and overt incestuous relations between father and daughter. *Am. J. Orthopsychiat.* 24: 266–79.

KEITH, D.V. 1974. Use of self: A brief report. *Fam. Proc.* 13: 201–206.

KEITH, P.R. 1975. Night terrors. *J. Am. Acad. Child Psychiat.* 14: 477–89.

KELLERMAN, J., RIGLER, D., SIEGEL, S.E., and KATZ, E.R. 1977. Disease-related communication and depression in pediatric cancer patients. *J. Ped. Psychol.* 2(2): 52–53.

KEMPE, C.H., and HELFER, R.E. 1972. *Helping the battered child and his family.* Philadelphia: J.B. Lippincott.

KEMPE, C.H., SILVERMAN, F.N., STEELE, B.F., DROEGEMUELLER, W., and SILVER, H.K. 1962. The battered child syndrome. *J. Am. Med. Assn.,* 181: 17–24.

KEMPE, R.S., and KEMPE, C.H. 1978. *Child Abuse.* Cambridge, Mass.: Harvard Univ. Press.

KENDALL, N., et al. 1973. Adolescents as mothers. *J. Youth Adol.,* 2: 233–49.

KENISTON, K. 1977. The transformation of the family. In *All our children: The American family under pressure.* New York: Harcourt Brace & Jovanovitch.

KEOGH, B.K., MAJOR, S.M., OMORI, H., GANDARA, P., and REID, H.P. 1980. Proposed markers in learning disabilities research. *J. Abnorm. Child Psychol.* 8(1): 21–31.

KERCKHOFF, A.C. 1974. The social context of interpersonal attraction. In *Foundations of interpersonal attractions,* ed. T. L. Huston, pp. 61–76. New York: Academic Press.

KERSHNER, J.R. 1978. Leeches, quicksilver, megavitamins and learning disabilities. *J. Spec. Ed.* 12(1) (Spring): 7–15.

KESSLER, J.W. 1972. Neurosis in childhood. In *Manual of child psychopathology,* ed. B.B. Wolman. New York: McGraw-Hill.

KESSLER, M., and ALBEE, G.W. 1977. An overview of the literature of primary prevention. In *Primary prevention of psychopathology,* Vol. 1, *Ths Issues.* ed. G.W. Albee and J. M. Jaffee, pp. 351–99. Univ. Press of New England.

KHAN, A.U. 1979. Coping with chronic illness; and facing a dying child and his family. In *Psychiatric emergencies in pediatrics,* ed. A. U. Khan, pp. 53–65, 195–208. Chicago: Year Book Medical Pub.

———. (ed.) 1979. *Psychiatric emergencies in pediatrics.* Chicago: Year Book Medical Pub.

KINARD, E.M., and KLERMAN, L.V. 1980. Teenage parenting and child abuse: Are they related? *Am. J. Orthopsychiat.* 50(3): 481–504.

KING, J., and ZIEGLER, S. 1981. The effects of hospitalization on children's behavior: A review of the literature. *J. Assn. Care Child. H.* 10(1): 20–28.

KINSBOURNE, M., and CAPLAN, P.J. 1979. *Children's learning and attention problems.* Boston: Little, Brown.

KINSEY, A.C., POMEROY, W.B., and MARTIN, C.E. 1948. *Sexual Behavior in the human male.* Philadelphia: W. B. Saunders.

KINSEY, A.C., AND THE STAFF OF THE INSTITUTE FOR SEX RESEARCH, INDIANA UNIVERSITY. 1953. *Sexual Behavior in the human female.* Philadelphia; W.B. Saunder.

KIRK, H.D. 1964. *Shared fate: A theory of adoption and mental health.* London: The Free Press of Glencoe.

KLAUS, M.H., and KENNELL, J.H. 1970. Mothers separated from their infants. *Ped. Clin. N. Am.* 17: 1015–37.

———. 1976. *Maternal–infant bonding.* St. Louis: C.V. Mosby.

———. 1981*a*. Labor, Birth and Bonding. In *Parent–infant bonding.* 2d ed. pp. 22–98. St. Louis: C.V. Mosby.

———. 1981*b*. *Parent–infant bonding.* 2d ed. St. Louis: C.V. Mosby.

KLEIN, D.F. 1977. Pharmacological treatment and delineation of borderline disorders. In *Borderline personality disorders: The concept, the syndrome, the patient,* ed. P. Hartocollis, pp. 365–83. New York: International Universities Press.

KLEIN, M. 1946. Notes on some schizoid mechanisms. *Int. J. Psychoanal.* 27: 99–110.

KLEIN, M., and STERN, L. 1971. Low birthweight and the battered child syndrome. *Amer. J. Dis. Child.* 122: 15–18.

KLEIN, R.S., ALTMAN, S.D., DREIZEN, K., FRIEDMAN, R., and POWERS, L. 1981. Restructuring dysfunctional parental attitudes toward children's learning and behavior in school: Family-oriented psycho-educational therapy, Part II. *J. Learn. Disab.,* 14(2): 99–101.

KLINE, F., ADRIAN, A., and SPEVAK, M. 1974. Patients evaluate therapists. *Arch. Gen. Psychiat.* 31: 113–16.

KLINE, S., and CAMERON, P. 1978. Formulation. *Can. Psychiat. Assn. J.* 23: 39–42.

KLUGER, J.M. 1979. The asthmatic child. In *Basic Handbook of child psychiatry,* Vol. 1. *Normal development.* ed. J. D. Call, pp. 436–41. New York: Basic Books.

KNAPP, P.H. 1960. Acute bronchial asthma: Psychoanalytic observations on fantasy, emotional arousal and partial discharge. *Psychosom. Med.* 22: 88–105.

KNIGHT, I. 1970. Placing the handicapped child. *Child Adopt.* 62: 27–35.

References

KNITZER, J., ALLEN, M.L., and McGOWAN, B. 1978. *Children without homes.* Washington, D.C.: Children's Defense Fund.

KNOBEL, M., and LYTTON, G. 1959. Diagnosis and treatment of behavior disorders in children. *Dis. Nerv. Syst.* 20: 334–40.

KNOBLOCH, H., and GRANT, D.K. 1961. Etiologic factors in "early infantile autism" and "Childhood Schizophrenia." *Am. J. Dis. Child.* 102: 535–36.

KNOBLOCH, H., and PASAMANICK, B. 1966. Prospective studies on the epidemiology of reproductive casualty: Methods, findings, and some implications. *Merrill-Palmer Quart.* 12: 27–43.

————. 1974. *Gessell and Amatruda's developmental diagnosis.* 3d ed. New York: Harper & Row.

————. 1975. Some etiologic and prognostic factors in early infantile autism and psychosis. *Pediat.* 55(2): 182–91.

KOHLBERG, L. 1969. *Stages in the development of moral thought and action.* New York: Holt, Rinehart & Winston.

KOHN, M.L. 1968. Social class and schizophrenia: A critical review. In *The transmission of schizophrenia,* ed. D. Rosenthal and S.S. Kety, pp. 155–73. London: Pergamon Press.

KOLATA, G.B. 1979. New drugs and the brain. *Science.* 205: 774–76.

KOLLER, M.R. 1974. *Families: A multigenerational approach.* New York: McGraw-Hill.

KOLODNY, E.H. 1972. Clinical and biochemical genetics of the lipidoses. *Semin. Hematol.* 9: 251–55.

KOLVIN, I., OUNSTED, C., HUMPHREY, M., and McNAY, A. 1971. Studies in the childhood psychoses, II: The phenomenology of childhood psychoses. *Brit. J. Psychiat.* 118: 385–95.

KOLVIN, I., OUNSTED, C., RICHARDSON, L.M., and GARSIDE, R.F. 1971. Studies in the childhood psychoses, III: The family and social background in childhood psychoses. *Brit. J. Psychiat.* 118: 396–402.

KOLVIN, I., OUNSTED, C., and ROTH, M. 1971. Studies in the childhood psychoses, V: Cerebral dysfunction and childhood psychoses. *Brit. J. Psychiat.* 118: 407–14.

KOLVIN, I., et al., 1971. Studies in the childhood psychoses, I–VI. *Brit. J. Psychiat.* 118: 381–419.

KOPPITZ, E.M. 1977. Strategies for diagnosis and identification of children with behavior and learning problems. *Behav. Disord.* 2(3): 136–40.

KOREIN, J., FISH, B., SHAPIRO, T., GERNER, E.W., and LEVIDOW, L. 1971. E.E.G. and behavioral effects of drug therapy in children: Chlorpromazine and diphenhydramine. *Arch. Gen. Psychiat.* 24: 552–63.

KORENBLUM, M.S. 1979. Diagnostic difficulties in adolescent psychiatry. Ph.D. diss., University of Toronto pp. 65–67.

KORNBERG, M.S., and CAPLAN, G. 1980. Risk factors and preventive intervention in child psychopathology: A review. *J. of Prev.* 1(2): 71–133.

KOVACS, M., and BECK, A.T. 1977. An empirical–clinical approach toward a definition of childhood depression. In *Depression in childhood,* ed. J.G. Schulterbrandt and A. Raskin, pp. 1–31. New York: Raven Press.

KRAGER, J.M., and SAFER, D.J. 1974. Type and prevalence of medication used in the treatment of hyperactive children. *N. E. J. Med.* 291: 1118–20.

KREINDLER, S. 1976. Psychiatric treatment for the abusing parent and the abused child. *Can. Psychiatric Assoc. J.* 21: 275–280.

KRUGMAN, S., and KATZ, S. 1981. *Infectious diseases of children.* 7th ed. St. Louis: C.V. Mosby.

KUBLER-ROSS, E. 1969. *On death and dying.* Toronto: Collier-Macmillan.

————. 1974. *Questions and answers on death and dying.* New York: Macmillan.

————. 1980. *Living with death and dying.* New York: Macmillan.

KUBO, S. 1959. Researches and studies on incest in japan. *Hiroshima J. Med. Sciences,* 8: 99–159.

KUGEL, R., SCHERZ, R.G., SEIDEL, H.M., McMAHON, J.L., RINKER, A., GARELL, D.C., VAN GELDER, D.W., ELLIS, E.O., KNUTTI, S.H., and PONCHER, J.R. 1978. (The Council on Child Health) Medication for hyperkinetic children. *Pediat.* 55: 560–62.

KUGEL, R.B., TREMBATH, J., and SGARA, S. 1968. Some characteristics of patients legally committed to a state institution for the mentally retarded. *Ment. Retard.* 6(4): 2–8.

KULKA, R.A., and WEINGARTEN, H. 1979. The long-term effects of parental divorce in childhood on adult adjustment: A twenty-year perspective. *American Sociological Assoc. Meeting.*

KUTNER, B. 1980. The social psychology of disability. In *Rehabilitation medicine,* ed. N.S. Neff. Washington, D.C.: American Psychological Association.

References

KUTTY, I.N., FROESE, A.P., RAE-GRANT, Q.A.F. 1979. Hare Krishna movement: What attracts the western adolescent? *Can. J. Psychiat.* 24: 604–09.

LABARRE, M. 1969. Motherhood. In *The double jeopardy, the triple crisis—illegitimacy today,* pp. 9–21. New York: The National Council on Illegitimacy.

LACK, S.A., and BUCKINGHAM, R.W. III 1978. *First american hospice: Three years of home care.* New Haven: Hospice Inc.

LAGRECA, A.M., and MESIBOV, G.B. 1981. Facilitating interpersonal functioning with peers in learning disabled children. *J. Learn. Disab.,* 14(4): 197–99, 238.

LAKIN, M. 1957. Personality factors in mothers of excessively crying (coliky) infants. *Soc. Res. Child Dev. Mono.* 22:1.

LAMBERT, N.M., and SANDOVAL, J. 1980. The prevalence of learning disabilities in a sample of children considered hyperactive. *J. Abnorm. Child Psychol.* 8(1): 33–50.

LANDIS, J.T. 1956. Experiences of 500 children with adult sexual deviation. *Psychiatric Quarterly,* 30 (Supplement): 91–109.

LANGHORNE, J.E., JR., LONEY, J., PATERNITE, C.E., and BECHTOLDT, H.P. 1976. Childhood hyperkinesis: A return to the source. *J. Abnorm. Psychol.* 85: 201–209.

LANGNER, T.S., HERSON, J.H., GREENE, E.L., JAMESON, J.D., and GOFF, J.A. 1970. Children of the city: Affluence, poverty and mental health. In *Psychological factors in poverty,* ed. V.L., Allen, pp. 185–209. Chicago: Markham.

LANGSLEY, D.G., and KAPLAN, D.M. 1968. *The treatment of families in crisis.* New York: Grune & Stratton.

LANSKY, S.B., CAIRNS, N.O., HASSANEIN, R., WEIR, J., and LOWMAN, J.T. 1978. Childhood cancer: Parental discord and divorce. *Pediat.* 62(2): 184–88.

LANSKY, S.B., CAIRNS, N.U., CLARK, G.M., LOWMAN, J., MILLER, L., and TRUEWORTHY, R. 1979. Childhood cancer: Nonmedical costs of the illness. *Cancer,* 43: 403–408.

LAPERRIERE, K. 1980. On children, adults and families: The critical transition from couple to parents. In *Family therapy: Combining psychodynamic and family systems approaches,* ed. J.K. Pearce and L.J. Friedman, pp. 81–92. New York: Grune & Stratton.

LAUFER, M. 1971. Long-term management and some follow-up findings on the use of drugs with minimal cerebral syndromes. *J. Learn. Disab.* 4:519–22.

———, and DENHOFF, E. 1957. Hyperkinetic behavior syndrome in children. *J. Pediat.* 50: 463–74.

LAUFER, M.W., LAFFEY, J.J., and DAVIDSON, R.E. 1974. Residential treatment for children and its derivatives. In *American handbook of psychiatry,* 2d ed. Vol. 2. ed. G. Caplan, pp. 193–210. New York: Basic Books.

LAVIE, P., GADOTH, N., GORDON, C.R., GOLDHAMER, G., and BECHAR, M. 1979. Sleep patterns in Klein-Levin syndrome. *Electroencephalog. Clin. Neurophysiol.* 47(3): 369–71.

LAVIGNE, J.V., and RYAN, M. 1979. Psychological adjustment of siblings of children with chronic illness. *Pediat.* 63(4): 616–27.

LAWRENCE, M.M. 1976. The appraisal of ego strength in evaluation, treatment and consultation: "Is this the one?" *J. Am. Acad. Child Psychiat.* 15: 1–14.

LAZARRE, A. 1981. Current concepts in psychiatry: Conversion symptoms. *N. E. J. Med.,* 305(13): 745–48.

LAZARUS, A.A., DAVISON, G.C., and POLEFKA, A. 1965. Classical and operant factors in the treatment of a school phobia. *J. Abnorm. Psychol.* 70: 225–30.

LEAVERTON, D.R. 1979. The child with diabetes mellitus. In *Basic handbook of child psychiatry,* Vol. 1., *Normal development* ed. J.D. Call, pp. 452. New York: Basic Books.

———, WHITE, C.A., McCORMICK, C.R., SMITH, P., and SHEIKHOLISLAM, B. 1981. Parental loss antecedent to childhood diabetes mellitus. *J. Am. Acad. Child Psychiat.* 19: 678–89.

LEBEL. J. ZUCKERMAN. B.S. 1981. Feeding problems, obesity, in *Behavioral Problems in Childhood: A Primary Care Approach.* S. Gabel ed. New York: Grune & Stratton.

LEBOVITZ, P.S. 1972. Feminine behavior in boys: Aspects of his outcome. *Am. J. Psychiat.* 128: 1283–89.

LEE, H. S. 1976. The psychological aspects of abusing parents. *Transcript of the First International Congress on Child Abuse and Neglect.* Geneva. p. 110.

LEFEBVRE, A., and BARCLAY, S. Psychosocial impact of craniofacial deformities before and after reconstructive surgery. Paper presented at the Canadian Psychiatric Association Annual Meeting, Toronto, October, 1980.

References

LEFEBVRE, A., and MUNRO, I. 1978. The role of psychiatry in a craniofacial team. *Plast. & Recons. Surg.* 61(4): 564–69.

LEIGHTON, D. 1971. The empirical status of the intergenerational–disintergenerational hypothesis. In *Psychiatric disorders and the urban environment,* ed. B. Kaplan, pp. 68–78. New York: Behavioral Pub.

LELAND, H., and SMITH, D.E. 1965. *Play therapy with mentally subnormal children.* New York: Grune & Stratton.

LELORD, G., et al. 1973. Comparative study of conditioning of averaged evoked responses by coupling sound and light in normal and autistic children. *Psychophysiol.* 10: 415–25.

LeMASTERS, E.E. 1970. *Parents in modern america: A sociological analysis.* Homewood, Ill.: Dorsey Press.

LESHAN, L. 1966. An emotional life history pattern associated with neoplastic disease. *Ann. N.Y. Acad. Sci.* 125: 780–93.

LESLIE, S.A. 1974. Psychiatric disorders in the young adolescents of an industrial town. *Brit. J. Psychiat.* 125: 113–24.

LESSE, S. 1981. Hypochondriachal and psychosomatic disorders masking depression in adolescence. *Am. J. Psychother.* 35(3): 356–67.

LESSER, R., and EASSER, B.R. 1972. Personality differences in the perceptually handicapped. *J. Am. Acad. Child Psychiat.* 11: 458–66.

LESTER, E.P. 1968. Brief psychotherapies in child psychiatry. *Can. Psychiat. Assn. J.,* 13: 301–309.

LEVIN, A.C. 1978. Forum of hyperkinesis. *Mod. Med.,* 46: 87–88.

LEVINE, S.V. 1974. Adolescents in alternative life styles. Paper presented to the American Orthopsychiatric Association, San Francisco, 1974, and the Association of Children with Learning Disabilities, London. 1974.

———. 1978. Fringe religions: Data and dilemmas. *Ann. Soc. Adol. Psych.* 6: 75–89.

———. 1979a. Adolescents, believing and belonging. *Ann. Adol. Psych.* 7: 41–53.

———. 1979b. Role of psychiatry in the phenomenon of cults. *Can. J. Psychiat.* 24: 593–603.

———. 1982. Alienation as an affect in adolescence. In *The adolescent and mood disturbance,* ed. H. Golombek and B. Garfinkel. New York: International Universities Press.

———, HORENBLAS, W., and CARR, R.P. 1972. The urban commune: Fact or fad, promise or pipe dream? *Am. J. Orthopsychiat.* 42(2): 295.

LEVINE, S.V., LLOYD, D.D., and LONGHON, W.H. 1972. The speed user: Social and psychological factors in amphetamines abuse. *Can. Psychiat. Assn. J.* 17(3): 229–41.

LEVINE, S.V., and SALTER, N.E. 1976. Youth and contemporary religious movements: Psychosocial findings. *Can. Psychiat. Assn. J.* 21: 411–20.

LEVINGER, G. 1965. Marital cohesiveness and dissolution: An integrative review. *J. Marr. & Fam.* 27: 19–28.

———. 1979. A social psychological perspective on marital dissolution. In *Divorce and separation,* ed. G. Levinger and O.C. Moles. New York: Basic Books.

LEVITT, E.E. 1971. Research on psychotherapy with children. In *Handbook of psychotherapy and behavior change: An empirical analysis.* ed. A.E. Bergin and S.L. Garfield, pp. 411–36. New York: Wiley.

LEVY, D.M. 1943. *Maternal overprotection.* New York: Columbia Univ. Press.

LEVY, F., DUMBRELL, S., HOBBES, G., RYAN, M., WILTON, N., and WOODHILL, J.M., 1978. Hyperkinesis and diet: A double blind crossover trial with tatrazine challenge. *Med. J. Aust.* 1: 61–64.

LEWIS, M. 1971. *Clinical aspects of child development.* Philadelphia: Lea & Febiger.

———. 1981. Child psychiatry perspectives: Child development research and child analysis. *J. Am. Acad. Child Psychiat.* 20: 189–99.

LEWIS, J.M., BEAVERS, W.R., GOSSETT, J.T., and PHILLIPS, V.A. 1976. *No single thread: Psychological health and family systems.* New York: Brunner/Mazel.

LICKORISH, J.R. 1971. The significance of intelligence ratings in adolescence. In *Modern perspectives in adolescent psychiatry,* Vol. 4. ed. J.G. Howells. Edinburgh: Oliver & Boyd.

LIDZ, T. 1963. Family organization and personality structure. In *The family and human adaptations.* ed. T. Lidz, pp. 39–76. New York: International Universities Press.

———. 1979. Family studies and changing concepts of personality development. *Can. Psychiat. Assn. J.* 24(7): 621–32.

711

————. 1980. The family and the development of the individual. In *Family evaluations and treatment,* ed. V.K. Hofling and J.M. Lewis, pp. 45–68. New York: Brunner/Mazel.

————, CORNELISON, A.R., FLECK, S., and TERRY, D. 1957. The intrafamilial environment of schizophrenic patients. 2: Marital schism and marital skew. *Am. J. Psychiat.* 114: 241–48.

LIDZ, T., FLECK, S., and CORNELISON, A. 1965. *Schizophrenia and the family.* New York: International Universities Press.

LIEBERMAN, M.A. 1979. Help seeking and self-help groups. In *Self-help groups for coping with crisis.* ed. M.A. Lieberman and L.D. Borman, et al., pp. 116–49. San Francisco: Jossey Bass.

LIGHTMAN, E.S., and SCHLESINGER, B. 1980. Maternity homes and single mothers. *J. Ontario Assn. Child. Aid Soc.* 23: 5–8.

LINDE, L.M., et al. 1979. The child with congenital heart disease. In *Basic handbook of child psychiatry,* Vol. 1, *Normal development.* ed. J.D. Call, pp. 447–52. New York: Basic Books.

LINDEMANN, E. 1944. Symptomatology and management of acute grief. *Am. J. Psychiat.* 101: 141–48.

LINDSAY, J., OUNSTED, C., and RICHARDS, P. 1979. Long-term outcome in children with temporal lobe seizures: I: Social outcome and childhood factors. *Dev. Med. Child Neurol.* 21: 285–98. II: Marriage, parenthood, and sexual indifference. *Dev. Med. Child Neurol.* 21: 433–40. III: Psychiatric aspects in childhood and adult life. *Dev. Med. Child. Neurol.* 21: 630–36.

LINDZEYN, G. 1967. Some remarks concerning incest, the incest taboo and psychoanalytic theory. *American Psychologist,* 22: 1051.

LINKS, P.S. 1982. Community surveys of the prevalence of childhood psychiatric disorders: A review. *Child Dev.* (in press).

LIPOWSKI, Z.J. 1968. Review of consultation psychiatry and psychosomatic medicine, III: Theoretical Issues. *Psychosom. Med.* 30(4): 395–422.

LITTNER, N. 1960. The child's need to repeat his past: Some implications for placement. *Soc. Serv. Rev.* 34(2): 118–48.

————. 1974. The challenge to make fuller use of our knowledge about children. *Child Wel.* 53(5): 287–94.

LIVINGSTON, S., PAULI, L.L., and PRUCE, I. 1980. Neurological evaluation of the child. In *Comprehensive textbook of psychiatry,* Vol. 3. 3d ed. ed. H.I. Kaplan, A.M. Freedman, and B.J. Sadock, pp. 2461–73. Baltimore: Williams & Wilkins.

LONEY, J. The hyperkinetic child grows up: Predictors of symptoms, delinquency and achievement at follow-up. Paper presented at the Annual Meeting of the American Association for the Advancement of Science, January 7, 1979.

————, KRAMER, J., and KOSIER, T. Medicated versus unmedicated hyperactive adolescents: Academic, delinquent, and symptomatological outcome. Paper presented at the Annual Meeting of the American Psychological Association, Los Angeles, 1981.

LONEY, J., PRINZ, R.J., MISHAHOW, J., and JOAD, J. 1978. Hyperkinetic/aggressive boys in treatment: Predictors of clinical response to methylphenidate. *Am. J. Psychiat.* 135: 1487–91.

LOOFF, D.H. 1976. *Getting to know the troubled child.* Knoxville, Tenn.: Univ. of Tennessee Press.

LOPATA, H.Z., 1978. *Family factbook.* Chicago: Marquis Academic Media.

LOPEZ, R.E. 1965. Hyperactivity in twins. *Can. Psychiat. Assn. J.* 10: 421–26.

LORANGER, A.W., and LEVINE, P.M. 1978. Age at onset of bipolar affective illness. *Arch. Gen. Psychiat.* 35: 1345–48.

LOTTER, V. 1966. Epidemiology of autistic conditions in young children. I: Prevalence. *Soc. Psychiat.* 1: 124–37.

————. 1967. Epidemiology of autistic conditions in young children, II: Some characteristics of the parents and children. *Soc. Psychiat.* 1: 163–73.

LOURIE, R.S. 1949. The role of rhythmic patterns in childhood. *Am. J. Psychiat.* 105(9): 653–60.

LOURIE, R.S. 1977. Introduction in *Psychopharmacology in childhood and adolescence,* ed. J. Weiner, pp. 3–6. New York: Basic Books.

LOURIE, R.S., LAYMAN, E.M., and MILLICAN, F.K. 1963. Why children eat things that are not food. *Children.* 10(4): 143–46.

LOVAAS, I., KOEGEL, R., SIMMONS, J.Q., and LONG, J.S. 1973. Some generalization and follow-up measures on autistic children in behavior therapy. *J. App. Behav. Anal.* 6: 131–66.

LOVE, W.C., and BACHARA, G.H. 1975. A diagnostic team approach for juvenile delinquents with learning disabilities. *Jun. Just.* 26(1): 27–30.

LOVELL, K., HOYLE, H.W., and SIDDALL, M.Q. 1968. A study of some aspects of the play and language of young children with delayed speech. *J. Child Psychol. & Psychiat.* 9: 41–50.

References

LOWENFELD, B. 1977. *Our blind children.* Springfield, Ill.: Chas. C Thomas.

LOWINSON, J.H., and RUIZ, P. (eds.) 1981. *Substance abuse: Clinical problems and perspectives.* Baltimore: Williams & Wilkins.

LOWIT, I.M. 1973. Social and psychological consequences of chronic illness in children. *Dev. Med. & Child Neurol.* 15: 75–77.

LUCAS, A., KRAUSE, E., and DOMINO, E. 1971. Biological studies in childhood schizophrenia: Plasma and RBC cholinesterase activity. *J. Aut. & Child Schiz.* 1: 72–81.

LUCAS, A.R., LOCKETT, H.J., and GRIMM, F. 1965. Amitriptylene in childhood depressions. *Dis. Nerv. Syst.* 26: 105–10.

LUCAS, A.R., and WEISS, M. 1971. Methylephenidate hallucinoisis. *J. Am. Med. Assn.* 217: 1079–81.

LUKIANOWICZ, N. 1972. Incest: paternal incest. *Brit. J. Pschiat.* 120: 301–313.

LUSTIG, N., DRESSER, J.W. SPELLMAN, S.W. and MURRAY, T.B. 1966. Incest: A family group survival pattern. *Arch. Gen. Psychiat.* 14: 31–40.

LYNCH, J. 1977. Statistics on living together and health. Appendix B. In *The broken heart: The medical consequences of loneliness,* New York: Basic Books.

LYNCH, M. and ROBERTS, J. 1976. Child abuse—early identification in the maternity hospital. *Transcript of the first International Congress on Child Abuse and Neglect,* Geneva. p. 13.

MAAS, H.S. 1960. The successful adoptive parent applicant. *Soc. Work.* 5:14–20.

————, and ENGLER, R.E., 1959. *Children in need of parents.* New York: Columbia Univ. Press.

McANARNEY, E.R. 1978. Adolescent pregnancy: A national priority. *Am. J. Dis. Child.* 132(2): 125–26.

————, PLESS, I.B., SATTERWHITE, B., and FRIEDMAN, S.B. 1974. Psychological problems of children with chronic juvenile arthritis. *Pediat.* 53: 523–28.

McANARNEY, E.R. ROGHMANN, K.J., ADAMS, B.N., TATAELBAUM, R.C., KASH, C., COULTER, M., PLUME, M., and CHARNEY, E. 1978. Obstetric, neo-natal and psychological outcomes of pregnant adolescents. *Pediat.* 61(2): 199–205.

McANDREW, J.B., CASE, Q., and TREFFERT, D. 1972. Effect of prolonged phenothiazine intake on psychotic and other hospitalized children. *J. Aut. Child. Schiz.* 2:75–91.

McCALL, R. 1979. The development of intellectual functioning in infancy and the prediction of later I.Q. In *The handbook of infant development,* ed. J. Osofsky. New York: Wiley.

McCOLLUM, A.T., and GIBSON, L.E. 1970. Family adaptation to the child with cystic fibrosis. *J. Pediat.* 77(4): 571–78.

McCONVILLE, B.J., BOAG, L.C., and PUROHIT, A.P. 1974. Three types of childhood depression. *Can. Psychiat. Assn. J.* 18: 133–38.

McDERMOTT, J.F. 1970. Divorce and its psychiatric sequelae in children. *Arch. Gen. Psychiat.* 23(11): 421–27.

————, TSENG, W.S., CHAR, W.F., and FUKUNAGA, C.S. 1978. Child custody decision making: The search for improvement. *J. Am. Acad. Child Psychiat.* 17(1): 104–16.

McDONALD, M. 1965. The psychiatric evaluation of children. *J. Am. Acad. Child. Psychiat.* 4:569–612.

MacFARLANE, J. 1975. Olfaction in the development of social preferences in the human neonate. In *Parent-infant interaction. Ciba foundation symposium 33.* pp. 103–113. Amsterdam: Elsevier.

MacFARLANE, J.W., ALLEN, L., and HONZIK, M.P. 1962. *A developmental study of the behavior problems of normal children.* Berkeley & Los Angeles: Univ. of California Press.

MacGREOGOR, F.C. 1979. *After plastic surgery: Adaptation and adjustment.* New York: A.O.F. Bergin.

McINTOSH, W.J., and DUNN, L.M. 1973. Children with specific learning disabilities. In *Exceptional children in the schools. special education in transition,* ed. L.M. Dunn. New York: Holt, Rinehart & Winston.

MacKAY, M.C., BECK, L., and TAYLOR, R. 1973. Methylphenidate for adolescents with M.B.D. *N.Y. State J. Med.* 73: 550–54.

McKEY, R.M., JR. 1973. Coping with a family-shattering disease. In *Psychosocial aspects of cystic fibrosis.* ed. P.R. Patterson, C.R. Denning, and A.H. Kutscher, pp. 93–96. New York: Columbia Univ. Press.

MacKINNON, R.A., and MICHELS, R. 1970. The role of the telephone in the psychiatric interview. *Psychiat.* 33: 82–93.

McKNEW, D.H., and CYTRYN, L. 1974. Urinary metabolites in chronically depressed children. *J. Am. Acad. Child. Psychiat.* 18: 608–15.

713

References

McCLURE, G.T. 1976. Sex role identification: Do boys need fathers and do girls need mothers? In *The single parent family: Proceedings of the changing family conference V, University of Iowa,* ed. S. Burden, P. Houston, E. Kripke, R. Simpson, and W.F. Stultz, pp. 48–54. Iowa City: Univ. of Iowa Press.

MacMILLAN, D.L., JONES, R.L., and ALORA, G.F. 1974. The mentally retarded label: A theoretical analysis and review of research. *Am. J. Ment. Def.* 79:241–61.

McNEESE, M.C., and HEBELER, J.R. 1979. The abused child—a clinical approach to identification and management. *Ciba Clinical Symposia.* 31(1): January.

McPHERSON, S.R., BRACKELMANNS, W.E., and NEWMAN, L.E. 1974. Stages in the family therapy of adolescents. *Fam. Proc.* 13:77–94.

MADDISON, D., and RAPHAEL, B. 1971. Social and psychological consequences of chronic disease in childhood. *Med. J. Aust.* 2: 1265–70.

MADDOX, B. 1975. *The half-parent.* New York: Evans.

MADISON, B., and SCHAPIRO, M. 1970. Permanent and long-term foster family care as a planned service. *Child Wel.* 49(March): 131–36.

MAHLER, M.S. 1952. On child psychosis and schizophrenia: Autistic and symbiotic infantile psychosis. *Psychoanal. Stud. Child* 7: 286–305.

———. 1961. On sadness and grief in infancy and childhood: Loss and restoration of the symbiotic love object. *Psychoanal. Stud. Child,* 16: 332–51.

———. 1965. On the significance of the normal separation–individuation phase with reference to research in symbiotic child psychoses. In *Drives, affects and behavior,* ed. K.M. Loewenstein. New York: International Universities Press.

———, PINE, F., BERGMAN, A. 1975. *The psychological birth of the human infant.* New York: Basic Books.

MAHRER, A.R., LEVINSON, J.R., and FINE, S. 1976. Infant psychotherapy: Theory, research and practice. *Psychotherapy: Theory, research and practice* 13(2): 131–40.

MAISCH, H. 1973. *Incest.* London: Andre Deutsch.

MALINOWSKI, B. 1953. *Sex and repression in savage society.* London: Routledge & Kegan Paul.

MALMQUIST, C.P. 1979. Development from thirteen to sixteen years. In *Basic handbook of child psychiatry,* Vol. 1. *Normal development* ed. J.D. Call pp. 205–13. New York: Basic Books.

MALMQUIST, C.P., KIRESUK, T.J. and SPANO, R.M. 1966. Personality characteristics of women with repeated illegitimacies: Descriptive aspects. *Amer. J. Ortho-psychiat.* 36: 476–484.

MALONE, A.J., and MASSLER, M. 1952. Index of nail-biting in children. *J. Abnorm. Psychol.* 47: 193.

MALUCCIO, A.N., FEIN, E., HAMILTON, J.L., KLIER, J., and WARD, D. 1980. Beyond permanency planning. *Child wel.* 59: 515–30.

MANNINO, F.V., and SHORE, M.F. 1974. Family structure, aftercare and post-hospital adjustment. *Am. J. Orthophychiat.* 44: 76–85.

MARCUS, J., and ROBINSON, H.B. (eds.) 1972. *Growing up in groups: The Russian day care center and the Israeli kibbutz.* New York: Gordon & Breach.

MARINELLI, R.R., and KELZ, J.W. 1975. Anxiety and attitudes towards visibly disabled persons. *Rehab. Counsel. Bull.* 16:197–205.

MARMOR, J. 1975. The nature of the psychotherapeutic process revisited, *Can. Psychiat. Assn. J.* 20(8):557–65.

MARSHALL, S., MARSHALL, H.H., and LYON, R.P. 1973. Enuresis: An analysis of various therapeutic approaches. *Pediat.* 51:813–17.

MARTIN, H.P. 1976. *The abused child—a multidisciplinary approach to developmental issues and treatment.* Cambridge, Mass.: Ballinger.

MARTIN, P.R., and LEFEBVRE, A.M. 1981. Surgical treatment of sleep apnea associated psychosis. *Can. Med. Assn. J.* 124: 978–80.

MARTINSON, I.M. 1978. Home care for the child with cancer. Paper presented at Association for the care of Children in Hospitals, 13th Annual Conference, pp. 83–89.

MARTY, P., and DE M'UZAN, M. 1963. Aspects fonctionels de la vie onirique: La "pensée" opératoire. *Rev. Franc. Psychoanal.* 27(Supplement 13): 61–64.

MASH, E.J., and DALBY, J.T. 1979. Behavioral intervention for hyperactivity. In *Hyperactivity in children: Etiology, measurement and treatment implications,* ed. R. Trites. Baltimore: University Park Press.

MASI, W. 1979. Supplement stimulation of the premature infant. In *Infants born at risk: Behavior and development,* ed. T.M. Field, pp. 367–388. Jamaica, N.Y.: Spectrum.

714

References

MASNICK, G., and BANE, M.J. 1980. *The nations' families 1960–1990.* Boston: Auburn House.

MASON, E.A. 1965. The hospitalized child: His emotional needs. *N. E. J. Med.* 272(8):406–14.

MASTERSON, J.F. 1967. The symptomatic adolescent five years later: He didn't grow out of it. *Am. J. Psychiat.* 123:1338–45.

———. 1972. *Treatment of the borderline adolescent: A developmental approach.* New York: Wiley.

———. 1980. *From borderline adolescent to functioning adult: The test of time,* pp. 5–28. New York: Brunner/Mazel.

MATAS, L., AREND, R.A., and SROUFE, L.A. 1978. Continuity of adaptation in the second year and the relationship between quality of attachment and later competence. *Child Dev.* 49:547–56.

MATHENY, A.P., JR., and VERNICK, J. 1969. Parents of the mentally retarded child: Emotionally overwhelmed or informationally deprived? *J. Pediat.* 74(6): 953–59.

MATTHEWS, C. (undated). A project to prevent school dropouts in the Quincy, Ill. public schools. Unpublished paper, Delinquency Study Project, Southern Illinois University.

MATTHEWS, D.E., VANLEEUWEN, J.J., and CHRISTENSEN, L. 1981. Psychosocial problems of young children and their families in a dialysis/transplant program. *Dial. & Trans.* 10(1):73–80.

MATTISON, R., CANTWELL, D.P., RUSSELL, A.T., and WILL, L. 1979. A comparison of DSM II and DSM III in the diagnosis of childhood psychiatric disorders. II. Interrater agreement. *Arch. Gen. Psychiat.* 36:1217–22.

MATTSSON, A. 1972. Long-term physical illness in childhood: A challenge to psychosocial adaptation. *Pediat.* 50(5): 801–811.

———, and GROSS, S. 1966. Adaptational and defensive behavior in young hemophiliacs and their parents. *Am. J. Psychiat.* 122:1349–56.

MATTSSON, A., SEESE, L.R., and HAWKINS, J.W. 1969. Suicidal behavior as a child psychiatric emergency: Clinical characteristics and follow-up results. *Arch. Gen. Psychiat.* 20: 100–109.

MAUSER, A. 1974a. Learning disabilities and delinquent youth. *Acad. Therap.* 9(6): 389–402.

———. 1974b. Learning disabilities and delinquent youth. In *Youth in Trouble, Proceedings of a Symposium, Dallas-Fort Worth Regional Airport, May, 1974,* ed. B. pp. Kratoville, 91–102. San Rafael, Calif.: Academic Therapy Pub.

MAY, P.R.A. 1976. Pharmacotherapy of schizophrenia in relation to alternative treatment methods. In *Antipsychotic drugs: Pharmacodynamics and pharmacokinetics,* ed. G. Sedvall, B. Urnas, and Y. Zotterman. New York: Pergamon.

———. 1981. Scizophrenia: A follow-up study of the results of five forms of treatment. *Arch. Gen. Psychiat.* 38:776–84.

MAYNARD, R. Omaha pupils given "behavior" drugs. *Washington Post* 29 June 1970.

MEAD, M. 1977. *Culture and commitment: The new relationships between the generations in the 1970's.* New York: Basic Books.

MEDLICOTT, R.W. 1967. Parent-child incest. *Aust. and New Zealand J. Psychiat.* 1:180–87.

MEEKS, J.E. 1971. *The fragile alliance.* Baltimore: Williams & Wilkins.

MEICHENBAUM, D.H. 1977. *Cognitive behavior modification: An integrative approach.* New York: Plenum.

———, and GOODMAN, J. 1971. Training impulsive children to talk to themselves: A means of developing self-control. *J. Abnorm. Psychol.* 77:115–26.

MEIER, J.H. 1976. *Developmental and learning disabilities: Evaluation, management and prevention in children.* Baltimore: University Park Press.

MEISELMAN, K.C. 1979. *Incest.* San Francisco: Jossey Bass.

MEISSNER, W.W. 1978. The conceptualization of marriage and family dynamics from a psychoanalytic perspective. In *Marriage and marital therapy: Psychoanalytic, behavioral and systems theory perspectives,* ed. T.J. Paolino and B.S. McCrady, pp. 25–88. New York: Brunner/Mazel.

MELAMED, B.G., and SIEGEL, L.J. 1975. Reduction of anxiety in children facing hospitalization and surgery by use of filmed modelling. *J. Cons. & Clin. Psychol.* 43:511–21.

MELTZOFF, A.N., and MOORE, M.K. 1977. Imitation of facial and manual gestures by human neonates. *Science,* 198:75–78.

MENDELSON, W., JOHNSON, N., and STEWART, M.A. 1971. Hyperactive children as teenagers: A follow-up study. *J. Nerv. Ment. Dis.* 153:273–79.

MENKEN, J. 1972. The health and social consequences of teenage childbearing. *Fam. Plan. Persp.* 4(3): 45–54.

MENKES, M., ROWE, J.S., and MENKES, J.H. 1967. A twenty-five year follow-up study on the hyperactive child with minimal brain dysfunction. *Pediat.* 39:393–99.

MENLOVE, F.L. 1965. Aggressive symptoms in emotionally disturbed adopted children. *Child. Dev.* 36:519–32.

MENOLASCINO, F.J. 1970. Psychiatry's past, current and future roles in mental retardation. In *Psychiatric approaches to mental retardation,* ed. F.J. Menolascino pp. 709–44. New York: Basic Books.

——, and EATON, L.F. 1980. Future trends in mental retardation. *Child Psychiat. & Hum. Dev.* 10(3): 156–68.

MERCER, C.D., ALGOZZINE, B., and TRIFILETTI, J.J. 1979. Early identification: Issues and considerations. *Except. Child* 46(1) (September):52–54.

MESSINGER, L., WALKER, K.N., and FREEMAN, S.J.J. 1978. Preparation for remarriage following divorce: The use of group technique. *Am. J. Ortho. Psychiat.* 48(2):263–72.

MEYER, J.E. 1980. The influence of adolescence on the clinical development of neuroses. (Germ.) *Praxis der Kinderpsychol. und Kinderpsychiat.* 29(4):115–17.

MEYEROWITZ, J.H., and KAPLAN, H.B. 1967. Familial responses to stress: The case of cystic fibrosis. *Soc. Sci. Med.* 1:249–66.

MEYERS, D., and GOLDFARB, W. 1962. Psychiatric appraisals of parents and siblings of schizophrenic children. *Am. J. Psychiat.* 118:902–908.

MIKKELSON, W.M. 1981. Twenty-fourth rheumatism review. *Arth. & Rheum.* 24(2):151–59.

MILICH, R., and LONEY, J. 1979. The role of hyperactive and aggressive symptomatology in predicting adolescent outcome among hyperactive children. *J. Ped. Psychol.* 4:93–98.

MILLAR, S. 1974. *The psychology of play.* New York: Jason Aronson.

MILLER, P., CHOQUETTE, J., KIRKPATRICK, P.T., MASTERS, L.E., ROWE, R., and DEAN, W. 1977. Adolescent pregnancy. *J. Fam. Prac.* 5(5):859–62.

MILLER, R. 1975. Child schizophrenia: A review of selected literature. In *Annual progress in child psychiatry and child development,* ed. S. Chess, and A. Thomas, pp. 357–401. New York: Brunner/Mazel.

MILLER, R.G., PALKES, N.S., and STEWART, M.A. 1973. Hyperactive children in suburban elementary schools. *Child Psychiat. Hum. Dev.* 4:121–27.

MILLER, W.H., and BERNAL, M.E. 1971. Measurement of the cardiac response in schizophrenic and normal children. *Psychophysiol.* 8:533–37.

MILLICHAP, J.G. 1973. Drugs in management of minmal brain dysfunction. *Ann. N.Y. Acad. Sci.* 205:321–34.

——. (Ed.) 1977. *Learning disabilities and related disorders: Facts and current issues.* Chicago: Year Book Med. Pub.

MINDE, K. 1976. *A parents' guide to hyperactivity in children.* Montreal: Quebec Assn. for Children with Learning Disabilities.

——. 1978. Coping styles of 34 adolescents with cerebral palsy. *Am. J. Psychiat.* 135(11):1344–49.

——. 1980a. Bonding of parents to premature infants: Theory and practice. In *Parents–infants relationships,* ed. P.M. Taylor, pp. 291–313. Monographs in Neonatology Series. New York: Grune & Stratton.

——. 1980b. Some thoughts on the social ecology of present day psychopharmacology. *Can. J. Psychiat.* 25(3):201–212.

——, and COHEN, N. 1977. Research. In *Experience and experiment,* ed. J. Shamsie, pp. 257–68. Toronto: Macdonald-Downie.

——. 1978. Hyperactive children in Canada and Uganda: A comparative evaluation. *J. Am. Acad. Child Psychiat.,* 17:476–87.

MINDE, K., FORD, L. CELHOFFER, L. and BOUKYDIS, C. 1975. Interactions of mothers and nurses with premature infants. *Can. Med. Assoc. J.* 113: 741–45.

MINDE, K., HACKETT, J.D., KILLOU, D., and SILVER, S. 1972. How they grow up: 41 physically handicapped children and their families. *Am. J. Psychiat.* 128(12):1554–59.

MINDE, K., LEWIN, D., WEISS, G., LAVINGNEUR, H., DOUGLAS, V., and SYKES, D. 1971. The hyperactive child in elementary school: A five year controlled follow-up. *Except. Child* 38:215–21.

MINDE, K., MARTON, P., MANNING, D., and HINES, B. 1980. Ch. 23. Some determinants of mother–infant interaction in the premature nursery: A controlled evaluation. *J. Am. Acad. Child Psychiat.* 19:1–21.

MINDE, K., PERROTTA, M., and CARTER, C. In press. The effect of neonatal complications in premature twins on their mother's preference. *J. Am. Acad. Child Psychiat.*

MINDE, K., SHOSENBERG, N., MARTON, P., THOMPSON, J., RIPLEY, J., and BURNS, M.A. 1980b. Ch.

References

23. Self-help groups in a premature nursery: A controlled evaluation. *J. Pediat.* 96(5)(May):933–40.

MINDE, K., WEBB, G., and SYKES, D. 1968. Studies on the hyperactive child, VI: Prenatal and paranatal factors associated with hyperactivity. *Dev. Med. Child Neur.* 10:355–63.

MINDE, K., WEISS, G., and MENDELSON, N. 1972. A five year follow-up study of 91 hyperactive school children. *J. Am. Acad. Child Psychiat.* 11:595–610.

MINEKA, S. and SUOMI, S.J. 1978. Social separation in monkeys. *Psychol. Bull.* 85(6):1376–1400.

MINISTRY OF HEALTH AND WELFARE CANADA. 1981. *Disabled persons in Canada.* Cassette Recording. Ottawa: Ministry of Health and Welfare Canada.

MINUCHIN, S. 1974. *Families and family therapy.* Cambridge, Mass: Harvard Univ. Press.

———. 1975. *Families of the slums.* New York: Basic Books.

———, BAKER, L., ROSMAN, B.L., LIEBMAN, R., MILMAN, L., and TODD, T.C. 1975. A conceptual model of psychosomatic illness in children. *Arch. Gen. Psychiat.* 32:1031–38.

MINUCHIN, S., and FISHMAN, C.H. 1981. *Family therapy techniques.* Cambridge, Mass.: Harvard Univ. Press.

MINUCHIN, S., ROSMAN, B.L., BAKER, L., and LIEBMAN, R. 1978. *Psychosomatic families: Anorexia nervosa in context.* Cambridge, Mass.: Harvard Univ. Press.

MOHR, J.W., TURNER, R.E., and Jerry, M.B. 1964. *Pedophilia and exhibitionism.* Toronto: University of Toronto Press.

MOLNAR, G. and CAMERON, P. 1975. Incest syndromes: Observations in a general hospital psychiatric unit. *Can. Psychiat. Assoc. J.,* 20: 373–377.

MONYAGU, A. 1962. *Prenatal influences.* Springfield, Ill.: Chas. Thomas.

MOORE, G.L. 1972. Nursing response to the long-term dialysis patient. *Nephron* 9:193–99.

MOORE, K., HOFFERTH, S., and WERTHEIMER, R. 1979. Teenage motherhood: Its social and economic costs. *Child. Today* 8(5):12–16.

MORGENSTERN, M. 1973. Community attitudes toward sexuality of the retarded. In *Human sexuality and the mentally retarded,* ed. F.F. de la Cruz, and G.D. La Veck, pp. 157–63. New York: Brunner/Mazel.

MORLEY, M.E. 1965. *The development and disorders of speech in childhood.* 2d ed. Edinburgh: E & S Livingstone.

MORRICE, J. 1976. *Crisis intervention: Studies in community care.* New York: Pergamon Press.

MORRISON, G.C. 1969. Therapeutic intervention in a child psychiatry emergency service. *J. Am. Acad. Child. Psychiat.* 8:452–558.

MORRISON, J.R., and STEWART, M.A. 1971. A family study of the hyperactive child syndrome. *Biol. Psychiat.* 3:189–95.

———. 1973. The psychiatric status of the legal families of adopted hyperactive children. *Arch. Gen. Psychiat.* 28:888–91.

MUIR, M. 1975. The consideration of emotional factors in the diagnosis and treatment of learning–disabled children. *J. Ped. Psychol.* 3(3):6–9.

MULLIGAN, W. 1969. A study of dyslexia and delinquency. *Acad. Ther. Quart.* 4(3):177–87.

———. 1972. Dyslexia, specific learning disability, and delinquency. *Juv. Just.* 23(3):20–25.

———. 1974. This side of the court. In *Youth in trouble, proceedings of a symposium, Dallas–Fort Worth Regional Airport, May, 1974,* ed. B. Kratoville, pp. 32–38. San Rafael, Calif.: Academic Therapy Pub.

MURDOCK, G.P. 1949. *Social structure.* New York: MacMillan.

———. 1960. The universality of the nuclear family. In *A modern introduction to the family,* ed. N.W. Bell, and E.F. Vogel, pp. 37–45. Glencoe: Free Press.

MURPHY, E., and BROWN, G.W. 1980. Life events, psychiatric disturbance and physical illness. *Brit. J. Psychiat.* 136:326–38.

MUSSEN, P.H., CONGER, J.J., and KAGAN, J. 1981. *Child development and personality.* 5th ed. New York: Harper & Row.

MYKLEBUST, H.R., and BOSHES, B. 1969. *Minimal brain damage in children.* Washington, D.C.: Department of Health, Education and Welfare, U.S. Public Health Service.

NAGERA, H. 1970. Children's reactions to the death of important objects: A developmental approach. *Psychoanal. Stud. Child.* 25: 360–400.

NAGY, M. 1959. The child's view of death. In *The meaning of death,* ed. H. Feifel. New York: McGraw-Hill.

NAKAGAWA, T., SUGITA, M., NAKAI, Y., and IKEMI, Y. 1979. Alexithymic features in digestive diseases. *Psychotherap. & Psychosom.* 32: 191–203.

NAKASHIMA, I.I. 1977. Teenage pregnancy: Its causes, costs and consequences. *Nurse Practit.* 2(7): 10–13.

NASJLETI, M. 1980. Suffering in silence: The male incest victim. *Child Wel.* 59: 269–75.

NATIONAL ADVISORY COMMITTEE ON HYPERKINESIS AND FOOD ADDITIVES. 1975. *Report to the nutrition foundation.* (M. Lipton, Committee Chairman). New York: The Nutrition Foundation.

NATIONAL CENTER FOR HEALTH STATISTICS. 1970. *Morality from selected census by marital status.* Series 20: 8A & 8B. Washington, D.C.: U.S. Government Printing Office.

———. 1970. *Selected symptoms of psychological distress.* U.S. Vital and Health Stats, Series 11:37. Washington, D.C.: U.S. Government Printing Office.

———. 1977. Summary Report, *Final Divorce Statistics 1975,* Monthly Vital Stats. Report, 26.2 Supplement. Washington, D.C.: U.S. Government Printing Office.

NATIONAL COMMISSION ON CHILDREN IN NEED OF PARENTS 1979. *Who knows? Who cares? Forgotten children in foster care.* Written by J.E. Persico. New York: National Commission on Children in Need of Parents.

NATIONAL CONFERENCE ON SOCIAL WELFARE. 1978. *The hospice as a social health care institution: Report of the pre-forum institute of the 105th annual forum of the national conference on social welfare.* Columbus, Ohio: National Conference on Social Welfare.

NATIONAL DAY CARE INFORMATION CENTRE. Canada Assistance Plan Directorate. 1973. *Status of day care in Canada: A review of the major findings of the national day care study, 1973.* Written by H. Clifford. Ottawa: Ministry of National Health and Welfare, Canada.

NATTERSON, J.M., and KNUDSON, A.G. 1960. Observations concerning fear of death in fatally ill children and their mothers. *Psychosom. Med.* 22: 456–65.

NELSON, K. 1973. Structure and strategy in learning to talk. *Mono. Soc. Res. Child. Dev.* 38: 1–2.

NELSON, W.E. 1975. *Textbook of pediatrics.* Philadelphia: W.B. Saunders.

NELSON, W.J., and BICKIMER, J.C. 1978. Role of self-instruction and self-reinforcement in the modification of impulsivity. *J. Cons. Clin. Psychol.* 46: 183–91.

NESSELROADE, J.R., and BALTES, P.B. 1974. Adolescent personality development and historical change: 1970–72. *Mono. Soc. Res. Child Dev.* 39(1), Serial No. 154. Chicago: Univ. of Chicago Press.

NEWBERGER, E.H. 1973. The myth of the battered child syndrome. *Curr. Med. Dial.* 20: 327–34.

———, and DANIEL, J. 1976. Knowledge and epidemiology of child abuse: A critical review of concepts. *Pediat. Ann.* 5(3): 140–44.

NEWMAN, L.E. 1970. Transsexualism in adolescence: Problems in evaluation and treatment. *Arch. Gen. Psychiat.* 23: 112.

1976 CENSUS OF CANADA. Vol. 9: *Supplementary bulletins: Housing and families.* Ottawa: Ministry of Supply and Services Canada.

NIRJE, B. 1976. The normalization principle. In *Changing patterns in residential services for the mentally retarded,* ed. R.B. Kugel and A. Shearer, pp. 231–40. Rev. ed. Washington, D.C.: U.S. Government Printing Office.

NISWANDER, K.R., FRIEDMAN, E.A., HOOVER, D.B., et al. 1966. Fetal morbidity following potentially anoxigenic obsetric conditions, I: Abruptio placenta. *Am. J. Obstet. Gyn.* 95: 838–45.

NORTH, A.F. Jr. 1976. When should a child be in the hospital? *Pediat.* 57(4): 540–43.

NORTON, A.J., and GLICK, P.C. 1979. Marital instability in America: Past, present, and future. In *Divorce and separation,* eds. Levinger and Moles, pp. 6–19. New York: Basic Books.

NOSHPITZ, J.D. 1975. Residential treatment of emotionally disturbed children. In *American handbook of psychiatry,* Vol. 5, ed. S. Arieti and G. Caplan, pp. 634–51. New York: Basic Books.

NOVER, R.A. 1973. Pain and the burned child. *J. Am. Acad. Child Psychiat.* 12: 499–505.

O'DELL, S. 1974. Training parents in behavior modification: A review. *Psychol. Bull.* 81: 418–33.

O'DONOHOE, N.V. 1979. *Epilepsies of childhood.* London: Butterworths.

OFFER, D. 1969. *The psychological world of the teenager,* chapter 2. New York: Basic Books.

OFFICE OF POPULATION CENSUSES AND SURVEYS MONITOR. 1976. FM3 76/3. London: Her Majesty's Stationery Office.

OFFORD, D.R. 1982. Primary prevention: Aspects of program design and evaluation. *J. Am. Acad. Child Psychiat.* 21(3): 225–30.

———, ABRAMS, N., ALLEN, N., and POUSHINSKY, B.A. 1979. Broken homes, parental psychiatric illness and female delinquency. *Am. J. Orthopsychiat.* 49(2): 252–64.

718

References

OFFORD, D.R., ALLAN, N., and ABRAMS, N. 1978. Parental psychiatric illness, broken homes and delinquency. *J. Am. Acad. Child Psychiat.* 17(2): 224–37.

OFFORD, D.R., APONTE, J.F., and CROSS, L.A. 1969. Presenting symptomatology of adopted children. *Arch. Gen. Psychiat.* 20: 110–16.

OFFORD, D.R., and WATERS, B.G.H. 1983. Socialization and its failure. In *Developmental behavioral pediatrics,* ed. M.D. Levine, W.B. Carey, A.C. Crocker, and R.T. Gross. Philadelphia: W.B. Saunders.

O'GORMAN, G. 1970. Childhood schizophrenia. In *The nature of childhood autism,* ed. G. O'Gormon, pp. 15–23. 2nd ed. London: Butterworths.

OLDHAM, D.G., LOONEY, J., and BLOTCKY, M. 1980. Clinical assessment of symptoms in adolescents. *Am. J. Orthopsychiat.* 50: 697–703.

O'LEARY, K.D., PELHAM, W.E., ROSENBAUM, A., and PRICE G.H. 1976. Behavioral treatment of hyperkinetic children: An experimental evaluation of its usefulness. *Clin. Pediat.,* 15:510–15.

OLSHANSKY, S. 1962. Chronic sorrow: A response to having a mentally defective child. *Soc. Casework,* 43: 191–93.

OLSON, L. 1980. Social and psychological correlates of pregnancy resolution among adolescent women: A review. *Am. J. Orthopsychiat.* 59(3): 432–45.

O'MALLEY, J.E., FOSTER, D., KOOCHER, G., and SLAVIN, L. 1980. Visible physical impairment and psychological adjustment among pediatric cancer survivors. *Am. J. Psychiat.* 137(1): 94–96.

ONTARIO CHILD ABUSE REGISTER. 1981. Confidential Provincial Government File.

ONTARIO MINISTRY OF COMMUNITY AND SOCIAL SERVICES: Children's Services Division. 1979. *Foster care: A discussion paper.* Toronto: Queen's Printer.

ONTARIO MINISTRY OF COMMUNITY AND SOCIAL SERVICES. 1981. *Report on the hard-to-serve child in Ontario.* Written by A.R.A. Consultants. Not yet a public document.

ORGUN, I. 1973. Playroom setting for diagnostic family interviews. *Am. J. Psychiat.* 130(5): 540–42.

ORNITZ, E.M. 1969. Disorders of perception common to early infantile autism and schizophrenia. *Comp. Psychiat.* 10: 259–74.

———. (In press). Neurophysiologic studies of autistic children. In *Autism: A reappraisal of concepts.* ed. M. Rutter and E. Schopler, pp. 117–40. New York: Plenum.

———, FORSYTHE, A.B., and TANGUAY, P.E. et al. 1974. The recovery cycle of the averaged auditory evoked response during sleep in autistic children. *Electroencephal. & Clin. Neurophysiol.* 37: 173–74.

ORNITZ, E.M., and RITVO, E.R. 1968. Perceptual inconstancy in early infantile autism. *Arch. Gen. Psychiat.* 18:76–98.

———. 1976. The syndrome of autism: A critical review. *Am. J. Psychiat.* 133(6): 609–21.

———, PANMAN, L.M., et al. 1968. The auditory evoked response in normal and autistic children during sleep. *Electroencephal. & Clin. Neurophysiol.* 25: 221–30.

ORNITZ, E.M., RITVO, E.R., and WALTER, R.D. 1965. Dreaming sleep in autistic twins. *Arch. Gen. Psychiat.* 12: 77–79.

ORNITZ, E.M., WECHTER, V., HARTMAN, D. et al. 1971. The E.E.G. and rapid eye movements during REM sleep in babies. *Electroencephal. & Clin. Neurophysiol.* 30: 350–53.

ORTON, S.T. 1925. Word blindness in school children. *Arch. Neur. Psychiat.* 14: 581–615.

ORY, M., and EARP, J. The influence of teenage childbearing on child maltreatment: The role of intervening factors. Presentation to the American Public Health Association, Los Angeles, 1978.

OSOFSKY, H., HAGEN, J., and WOOD, P. 1968. A program for pregnant school girls: Some early results. *Am. J. Ob. Gyn.* 100(7): 1020–27.

OSOFSKY, H.J., and OSOFSKY, J.D. 1970. Adolescents as mothers. *Am. J. Orthopsychiat.* 40(5): 825–34.

OVERTON, D.A. 1964. State-dependent as dissociated learning produced by phenobarbital. *J. Comp. Physiol. Psychol.* 57: 3–12.

OWEN, M. 1976. Pre- and perinatal factors in abnormal behavior. Course Paper, York University.

OZER, M.N. 1980. *Solving learning and behavior problems of children: A planning system. Integrating assessment and treatment.* San Francisco: Jossey-Bass.

PAKES, E.H. 1974. Child psychiatry and pediatric practice: How disciplines work together. *Ont. Med. Rev.* 41: 69–71.

————, and FLEMING, S. (In press). Psychotherapy and self-help: Similarities and differences. *Can. J. Psychiat.*

PAKES, E.H., KIKUCHI, J., DARTE, J.H.M. (Panelists) SONLEY, M.J. (Mediator) 1972. Psychiatric problems in the management of children with malignancy. In *Cancer in childhood,* ed. J. Gooden pp. 199–201. Toronto: The Ontario Cancer Treatment and Research Foundation.

PALAZZOLI, M.S., BOSCOLO, L., CECCHIN, G., and PRATA, G. 1978. *Paradox and counterparadox: A New Model in the Therapy of the Family in Schizophrenic Transaction.* New York: Jason Aronson.

PALMER, S. 1974. Children in long-term care: The worker's contribution. *J. Ont. Assn. Child. Aid Soc.* 17(4): 1–14.

PALMER, S.E. 1979. Predicting outcome in long-term foster care. *J. Soc. Ser. Res.* 3(2): 201–214.

PALMER, T. 1978. *Correctional intervention and research: Current issues and future prospects.* Lexington, Mass.: Lexington Books.

PAPPENFORT, D.M., and KILPATRICK, D.M. 1969. Child caring institutions, 1966: Selected findings from the first national survey of children's and residential institutions. *Soc. Ser. Rev.* 43: 448–59.

PARENS, H. 1968. On an early genital phase. *Psychoanal. Stud. Child.* 23: 348–65.

PARKES, C.M. 1972. *Bereavement.* New York: International Univ. Press.

PARMELEE, A.H., and HABER, A. 1973. Who is the "risk" infant? *Clin. Ob. Gyn.* 16: 376–87.

PARSONS, T. 1954. The incest taboo in relation to social structure and socialization of the child. *Brit. J. Sociol.* 5:101–117.

————, and BALES, R.B. 1955. *Family, socialization and interaction process.* Glencoe, Ill.: Free Press.

PASAMANICK, B., and KNOBLOCH, H. 1966. Retrospective studies on the epidemiology of reproductive casualty: Old and new. *Merrill-Palmer Quart.* 12(1): 7–26.

PASCARELLI, E.M. 1973. Methaqualone abuse, the quiet epidemic. *J.Am. Med. Assn.* 224(11): 1512–14.

PATTERSON, G.R. 1975. *Families.* Champagne, Ill.: Research Press.

————. 1977. Naturalistic observation in clinical assessment. *J. Abnorm. Child Psychol.* 5: 309–22.

————, and GULLION, M.D. 1968. *Living with children.* Champagne, Ill.: Research Press.

PATTERSON, L.L. 1956. Some pointers for professionals. *Children* 3(1): 13–17.

PATTERSON, P.R., DENNING, C.R., and KUTSHER, A.H. (Eds.) 1973. *Psychosocial aspects of cystic fibrosis.* New York: Columbia Univ. Press.

PAUKER, J.D., and HOOD, E. 1979. *A review of four systems for classifying the "Impossible" child and adolescent.* Toronto: Laidlaw Foundation.

PAULSON, M.J., STONE, D., and SPOSTO, R. 1978. Suicide potential and behavior in children ages 4 to 12. *Suicide & Life Threat. Behav.* 8: 225–42.

PAVENSTEDT, E. 1967. *The drifters: Children of disorganized lower class families,* Boston: Little, Brown.

PEARCE, J.K. 1980. Ethnicity and family therapy: An introduction. In *Family therapy: Combining psychodynamic and family systems approaches,* ed. J.K. Pearce and L.J. Friedman, pp. 93–116. New York: Grune & Stratton.

PEARSON, G.H.J. 1941. Effects of operative procedures on the emotional life of the child. *Am. J. Dist. Child.* 62(4): 716–29.

PEREZ-REYES, M.G., and FALK, R. 1973. Follow-up after therapeutic abortion in early adolescence. *Arch. Gen. Psychiat.* 28: 120–26.

PERLMAN, L.V., FERGUSON, S., BERGUM, K., ISENBERG, E.L., and HAMMARSTEN, J.F. 1971. Precipitation of congestive heart failure: Social and emotional factors. *Ann. Int. Med.* 75: 1–7.

PESIKOFF, R.B., and DAVIS, P.C. 1971. Treatment of pavor nocturnus and somnambulism in children. *Am. J. Psychiat.* 128: 778–81.

PETERS, J.J. 1976. Children who are victims of sexual assault and psychology of the offender. *Am. J. Psychother.* 3: 398–421.

PETERSON, M. 1971. Juvenile delinquency as a form of learning disability. *Conn. Teacher* 39(2): 11–14, 31.

PETRILLO, M., and SANGER, S. 1980. *Emotional care of hospitalized children: An environmental approach.* Philadelphia: J.B. Lippincott

PETTI, T.A. 1978. Depression in hospitalized child psychiatry patients: Approaches to measuring depression. *J. Am. Acad. Child Psychiat.* 17: 49–59.

————. 1981. Depression in children: A significant disorder. *Psychosom.* 22(5): 444–47.

PFEFFER, C.R. 1981. Suicidal behavior of children: A review with implications for research and practice. *Am. J. Psychiat.* 138: 154–59.

References

————, Conte, H.R., Plutchik, R., and Jerrett, I. 1979. Suicidal behavior in latency-age children: An empirical study. *J. Am. Acad. Child Psych.* 18: 679–92.

Philips, I. 1967. Psychopathology and mental retardation. *Am. J. Psychiat.* 124(1): 29–35.

Phillips, J. 1973. Syntax and vocabulary of mother's speech to young children: Age and sex comparisons. *Child Dev.* 44: 182–85.

Phipps-Yonas, S. 1980. Teenage pregnancy and motherhood: A review of the literature. *Am. J. Orthopsychiat.* 50(3): 403–431.

Piaget, J. 1952. *The origins of intelligence in children.* New York: International Univ. Press.

————. 1954. *The construction of reality in the child.* New York: Basic Books.

————. 1962. *Play dreams and imitation in childhood.* New York: W.W. Norton.

————, and Inhelder, B. 1958. *The growth of logical thinking from childhood to adolescence.* London: Routledge & Kegan Paul.

Pierce, C.M. 1980. Encopresis. In *Comprehensive textbook of psychiatry.* ed. H.J. Kaplan, A.M. Freedman, and B.J. Sadock, pp. 2788–90. Vol. 3. 3d ed. Baltimore: Williams & Wilkins.

Pierpaoli, W. 1981. Integrated phylogenetic and ontagenetic evolution of neuroendocrine and identity–defense immune functions. In *Psychoneuroimmunology,* ed. R. Ader, pp. 575–606. New York: Academic Press.

Pike, V., Downs, S., Emlen, A., Downs, G., & Case, D. 1977. *Permanent planning for children in foster care: A handbook for social workers.* Washington, D.C.: U.S. Department of Health, Education and Welfare, publication no. (OHDS) 78–30124.

Pinsoff, W.M. 1981. Family therapy process research. In *Handbook of family therapy.* ed. A.S. Gurman and D.P. Kniskern. New York: Brunner/Mazel.

Plank, E.N., and Plank, R. 1978. Children and death: As seen through art and autobiographies. In *Psych. Stud. Child.,* ed. R.S. Eissler, et al. Vol. 33. New Haven: Yale Univ. Press.

Platt, J.E., Campbell, M., and Cohen, I.L. 1981. Effects of lithium carbonate and haloperidol on cognition in aggressive, hospitalized school-age children. *Psychopharmacol. Bull.* 17(1): 123–25.

Pless, I.B., and Douglas, J.W.B. 1971. Chronic illness in childhood: I: Epidemiological and clinical characteristics. *Pediat.,* 47: 405–14.

Pless, I.B., and Pinkerton, P. 1975. *Chronic childhood disorder: Promoting patterns of adjustment.* London: Henry Kimpton.

Pless, I.B., and Roghmann, K.J. 1971. Chronic illness and its consequences: Observations based on three epidemiologic surveys. *J. Pediat.* 79(3): 351–59.

Polizos, P., Engelhardt, D.M., Hoffman, S.P., and Waizer, J. 1973. Neurological consequences of psychotropic drug withdrawal in schizophrenic children. *J. Aut. & Child Schiz.* 3: 247–53.

Pool, D., Bloom, W., Mielke, D.H., Roniger, J.J., and Gallant, D.M. 1976. A controlled evaluation of loxitane in seventy-five adolescent schizophrenic patients. *Curr. Ther. Res.* 19: 99–104.

Pope, H., and Mueller, C.W. 1979. The intergenerational transmission of marital instability: Comparisons by race and sex. In *Divorce and separation,* ed. G. Levinger and O.C. Moles, pp. 83–99. New York: Basic Books.

Population Reference Bureau. *New York Times,* 27 November 1977.

Poremba, C. 1974. As I was saying. . . . In *Youth in trouble. Proceedings of a symposium, Dallas–Forth Worth regional airport, May, 1974,* ed. B. Kratoville, 74. San Rafael, Calif.: Academic Therapy Pub.

Poremba, C.D. 1975. Learning disabilities, youth and delinquency: Programs for intervention. In *Progress in learning disabilities,* Vol. 3. ed. H.R. Myklebust, pp. 123–49. New York: Grune & Stratton.

Poznanski, E.O., Krahenbuhl, V., and Zrull, J.R. 1976. Childhood depression: A longitudinal perspective. *J. Am. Acad. Child Psychiat.* 15: 491–501.

Poznanski, E.O. and Zrull, J.P. 1970. Childhood depression: Clinical characteristics of overtly depressed children. *Arch. Gen. Psycit.* 23:8–15.

Pozsonyi, J. 1973. *A longitudinal study of unmarried mothers who kept their first-born children.* London, Ont.: Family & Children's Services of London and Middlesex.

Prechtl, H., and Stemmer, C. 1962. The choreiform syndrome in children. *Dev. Med. Child. Neurol.* 4: 119–27.

Preodor, D., and Wolpert, E.A. 1979. Manic-depressive illness in adolescence. *J. Youth & Adol.* 8(2): 111–30.

The President's Commission on Law Enforcement and Administration of Justice. 1967. *Task force* report: *Juvenile delinquency and youth crime: Report on juvenile justice and consultants' papers.* Washington, D.C.: Government Printing Office.

PRIGMORE, C.S., and DAVIS, P.R. 1973. Wyatt & Stickney: Rights of the committed. *Soc. Work* 18(4): 10–18.

PRINGLE, M.L., and FIDDES, D.O. 1970. *The challenge of thalidomide: A pilot sutdy of the educational needs of children in Scotland affected by the drug.* London: Longmans.

PRINZ, R., and LONEY, J. 1974. Teacher-rated hyperactive elementary school girls: An exploratory developmental study. *Child Psychiat. Hum. Dev.* 4: 246–57.

PRONOVOST, W., WAKESTEIN, M.P., and WAKESTEIN, D.J. 1966. A longitudinal study of the speech behavior and language comprehension of 14 children diagnosed atypical or autistic. *Except. Child.* 33: 19–26.

PROSKAUER, S. 1971. Focused time-limited psychotherapy with children. *J. Am. Acad. Child Psychiat.,* 10:619–39.

PROSSER, H. 1977. Social consequences of teenage childbearing. In *Social demography: The state of the art,* ed. W. Petersen and L. Day, Cambridge: Harvard Univ. Press.

———. 1978. *Perspectives on foster care: An annotated bibliography.* Windsor: National Foundation for Educational Research, Humanities Press.

PROVENCE, S., and LIPTON, R.C. 1967. *Infants in institutions.* New York: International Univ. Press.

PRUGH, D.G., STAUB, E.M., SANDS, H.H., KIRSCHBAUM, R.M., and LENIHAN, E.A. 1953. A study of the emotional reactions of children and families to hospitalization and illness. *Am. J. Orthopsychiat.* 23: 70–106.

PRUYSER, P.W. 1979. *The psychological examination.* New York: International Univ. Press.

PUIG-ANTICH, J. 1980. Affective disorders in childhood—A review and perspective. *Psychiat. Clin. N. Am.* 3: 403–24.

———, BLAU, S., MARX, N., GREENHILL, L.L., CHAMBERS, W. 1978. Prepubertal major depressive disorder: A pilot study. *J. Am. Acad. Child Psych.* 17:695–707.

PUIG-ANTICH, J., CHAMBERS, W., HALPERN, F. HANLON, C., and SACHAR, E.J. 1979. Cortisol hypersecretion in prepubertal depressive illness: A preliminary report. *Psychoneuroendocrinol.* 4(3): 191–97.

PUIG-ANTICH, J., GREENHILL, L.L., SASSIN, J., and SACHAR, E.J. 1978. Growth hormone prolactin, and cortisol responses and growth patterns in hyperkinetic children treated with dextroamphetamine: Preliminary findings. *J. Am. Acad. Child Psychiat.* 17: 457–75.

PUIG-ANTICH, J., PEREL, J.M., LAPATKIN, W. CHAMBERS, W.J., SHEA, C., TABRIZI, M.S., and STILLER, R.L. 1979. Plasma levels of imipramine and desmethylimipramine and clinical response in prepubertal major depressive disorder: A preliminary report. *J. Am. Acad. Child Psychiat.* 18: 616–27.

PUIG-ANTICH J., ORVASCHEL, H., TABRIZI, M., and CHAMBERS, W. Schedule for affective disorders and schizophrenia for school age children. (Kiddie-SADS) New York, 1980.

QUAY, H.C. 1977. Measuring dimensions of deviant behavior: The behavior problem checklist. *J. Abnorm. Child Psychol.* 5:277–87.

———. 1978. Classification. In *Psychopathological disorders of childhood,* 2nd ed. ed. H.C. Quay, and J.S. Werry, pp. 1–42. New York: Wiley.

QUINN, P.O., and RAPOPORT, J.L. 1974. Minor physical anomalies and neurologic status in hyperactive boys. *Pediat.* 53:742–47.

QUINTON, D., and RUTTER, M. 1976. Early hospital admissions and later disturbances of behavior: An attempted replication of Douglas' findings. *Dev. Med. Child. Neurol.* 18:447–59.

QUITKIN, F., RIFKIN, A., and KLEIN, D.F. 1976. Neurologic soft signs in schizophrenia and character disorders. Organicity in schizophrenia with premorbid asociality and emotionally unstable character disorders. *Arch. Gen. Psychi.* 33:845–53.

RABKIN, J.K., and STRUENING, E.L. 1976. Life events, stress, and illness. *Science* 194(4269):1013–20.

RACHMAN, S., and BERGER, M. 1963. Whirling and postural control in schizophrenic children. *J. Child. Psychol. Psychiat.* 4:137–55.

RAE, W.A. 1981. Hospitalized latency-age children: Implications for psychosocial care. *J. Assn. Care of Child. H.* 9(3) (Winter):59–63.

References

RAE-GRANT, N. 1978. But they didn't live happily ever after . . . *J. Ont. Assn. Child. Aid Soc.* 21:3–8.

RAE-GRANT, Q.; HOLLISTER, WILLIAM G. (January/February 1972). The Principles of Parsimony in Mental Health Centre Operations. *Canada's Mental Health,* 20:18–24.

RAIMBAULT, G. 1973. Psychological problems in the chronic nephropathies of childhood. In *The child in his family,* Vol. 2, *The impact of disease and death.* ed. E.J. Anthony and C. Koupernik. London: Wiley.

RAKOFF, V.M. 1980. History in adolescent disorders. In *Adolescent psychiatry,* ed. S.C. Feinstein, et al., pp. 85–99. Vol. 8. Chicago: Univ. of Chicago Press.

RAMEY, C., and SMITH, B. 1977. Assessing the intellectual consequences of early intervention with high-risk infants. *Am. J. Ment. Def.* 81:318–24.

RANK, B. 1963. Intensive study and treatment of preschool children who show marked personality deviations or "Atypical development" and their parents. *J. Child Psychol. Psychiat.* 4:137–55.

RAPHLING, D.L., CARPENTER, B.L., and DAVIS, A. 1967. Incest: A genealogical study. *Arch. Gen. Psychiat.* 16:505–11.

RAPOPORT, J.L., BUCHSBAUM, M.S., ZAHN, T.P., WEINGARTNER, H., LUDLOW, C., and MIKKELSEN, E.J. 1978. Dextroamphetamine: Cognitive and behavioral effects in normal prepubertal boys. *Science* 199:560–63.

RAPOPORT, J.L., MIKKELSEN, E.J., and WERRY, J.S. 1978. Antimanic, antianxiety, hallucinogenic and miscellaneous drugs. In *Pediatric psychopharmacology: The use of behavior modifying drugs in children,* ed. J. Werry, pp. 316–55. New York: Brunner/Mazel.

RAPOPORT, J.L., MIKKELSEN, E.J., ZAVADIL, A., NEE, L., GRUENAU, C., MENDELSON, W., and GILLIN, J.C. 1980. Childhood enuresis II Psychopathology, tricyclic concentration in plasma, and antienuretic effect. *Arch. Gen. Psychiat.* 37(10):1146–52.

RAPOPORT, J.L., and QUINN, P.O. 1975. Minor physical anomalies (stigmata) and early developmental deviation: A major biologic sub-group of "hyperactive children." *Int. J. Ment. H.* 4:212–22.

RASCHKE, H.J., and RASCHKE, V.J. Family conflict and children's self concept: A comparison of intact and single parent families. *J. Marr. and Family.* 41(2):367.

RAVENSCROFT, K. 1974. Normal family regression at adolescence. *Am. J. Psychiat.* 131:31–35.

REED, E.F. 1965. Unmarried mothers who kept their babies. *Children* 12(3):118–19.

REED, E.W., and REED, S.C. 1965. *Mental retardation: A family study.* Philadelphia: W.B. Saunders.

REES, L. 1956. Physical and emotional factors in bronchial asthma. *J. Psychosom. Res.* 1:98–114.

REES, W.L. 1971. Psychiatric and psychological factors in migraine. In *Background to migraine: Fourth migraine symposium, September 11, 1970,* ed. J.N. Cummings, pp. 45–54. London: Heineman.

———. 1976. Stress, distress and disease. *Brit. J. Psychiat.* 128:3–18.

REID, A.H. 1980. Diagnosis of psychiatric disorder in the severely and profoundly retarded patient. *J. Roy. Soc. Med.* 73:607–09.

REIDER, B., and PORTNOY, S. 1977. *Early intervention and day care: Research report of federation of day care services.* Philadelphia: Strahley & Horrocks.

REIMER, S. 1940. A research note on incest. *Am. J. Sociol.* 45:566–75.

REISER, D.E., and BROWN, J.L. 1964. Patterns of later development in children with infantile psychosis. *J. Am. Acad. Child Psychiat.* 3(4):650–67.

REISS, I.L. 1980. *Family systems in america.* 3d ed. New York: Holt Rinehart & Winston.

REKERS, G.A., WILLIS, T.J., YATES, C.E., ROSEN, A.C., and LOW, B.P. 1977. Assessment of childhood gender behavior change *J. Child Psychol. Psychiat.* 18:53–65.

REPORT OF THE COMMITTEE ON THE WORKING OF THE ABORTION ACT. 1974. Cmnd. 5579, London: Her Majesty's Stationery Office.

REYNOLDS, A.R. 1979. Some social effects of the mentally retarded child on the family: A third survey. *Austr. J. Ment. Retard.* 5(6):214–18.

REYNOLDS, C.F. 3rd., BLACK, R.S., COBLE, P., HOLZER, B., and KUPFER, D.J. 1980. Similarities in EEG sleep findings for Keline–Levin Syndrome and unipolar depression. *Am. J. Psychiat.* 137(1):116–18.

RICCIUTI, H. 1974. Fear and development of social attachments in the first year of life. In *The origins of fear,* ed. M. Lewis and L. Rosenblum, pp. 73–106. New York:Wiley.

RICH, J. 1968. *Interviewing children and adolescents.* London: Macmillan.

723

RICHARDSON, S.A. 1963. Some psychological consequences of handicapping. *Pediat.* 32:291–97.

RICHER, S., and GANTCHEFF, H. 1976. Is hospitalizing a young child always detrimental? *Union Med. Can.* 105(12):1866–71.

RICHMAN, L.C., and HARPER, C.D. 1980. Personality profiles of physically impaired young adults. *J. Clin. Psychol.* 36(3) (July):668–71.

RICHMAN, L.C., and LINDGREN, S.D. 1980. Patterns of intellectual ability in children with verbal deficits. *J. Abnorm. Child Psychol.* 8(1):65–81.

RICHMAN, N. 1977. Behaviour problems in preschool children: Family and social factors. *Brit. J. Psychiat.* 131:523–27.

RIE, H. 1966. Depression in childhood—A survey of some pertinent contributions. *J. Am. Acad. Child. Psychiat.* 5:653–85.

RIE, H.F., RIE, E.D., STEWART, S., and AMBUEL, J.P. 1976. Effects of ritalin on underachieving children: A replication. *Am. J. Orthopsychiat.* 46:313–22.

RILEY, T.L., and ROY, A. 1982. *Pseudoseizures.* Baltimore: Williams & Wilkins.

RIMLAND, B. 1964. *Infantile Autism.* New York:Appleton-Century Crofts.

RIMON, R., et al. 1977. Psychological aspects of juvenile rheumatoid arthritis. *Scand. J. Rheumatol.* 6:1–10.

RINSLEY, D.B. 1974. Residential treatment of adolescents. In *American Handbook of Psychiatry,* Vol. 2. ed. S. Arieti and G. Caplan, pp. 353–66. New York:Basic Books.

———. 1981. Dynamic and developmental issues in borderline and related "Spectrum" disorders. *Psychiat. Clin. N.Am.* 4(1):117–32.

RISCH, S., KALIN, N.H., and MURPHY, D.L. 1981. Neurochemical mechanisms in the affective disorders and neuro-endocrine correlates. *J. Clin. Psychopharm.* 1(4):180–85.

RITCHIE, J. 1977. Children's adjustive and affective responses in the process of reformulating a body image following limb amputation. *Mat.-Child. Nurse J.* 6(1):25–35.

RITVO, E.R. 1977. Biochemical studies of children with the syndromes of autism, childhood schizophrenia and related developmental disabilities: A review. *J. Child Psychol. Psychiat.,* 18(4) (September):373–79.

———, CANTWELL, D., and JOHNSON, E. et al. 1971. Social class factors in autism. *J. Aut. Child. Schiz.* 1:297–310.

RITVO, E.R., ORNITZ, E.M., GOTTLIEB, F., POUSSAINT, A.F., MARON, B.J., DITMAN, K.S., and BLINN, K.A. 1969. Arousal and nonarousal enuretic events. *Am. J. Psychiat.* 126:77–84.

RITVO, E.R., ORNITZ, E.M., WALTER, R.D., and HANLEY, J. 1970. Correlation of psychiatric diagnoses and EEG findings: A double-bind study of 184 hospitalized children. *Am. J. Psychiat.,* 126:988–96.

RITVO, E.R., YUWILER, A., GELLER, E., ORNITZ, E.M., SAEGER, K., and PLOTKIN, S. 1970. Increased blood serontonin and platelets in early infantile autism. *Arch. Gen. Psychiat.* 23:566–72.

ROBB, P. 1981. *Epilepsy: A manual for health workers.* Bethesda, Md.: U.S. Department of Health and Human Services, NIH Publication 82–2350.

ROBERTSHAW, C. 1981. *A discussion paper on child protection in Canada.* Ottawa: Department of National Health and Welfare, Canada.

ROBERTSON, J. 1970. *Young children in hospital.* London: Tavistock Pub.

ROBERTSON, J.A. 1952. *A two-year-old goes to hospital.* Film 16 mm., 45 min., sound. London: Tavistock Child Development Research Unit, New York University Film Library, United Nations, Geneva.

ROBERTSON, J. and ROBERTSON, J. 1971. Young children in brief separation: A fresh look. *Psychoanal. Stud. Child* 26:264–315.

ROBINS, L.N. 1966. *Deviant children grown up: A sociological and psychiatric study of sociopathic personality.* Baltimore: Williams & Wilkins.

———. 1970. The adult development of the antisocial child. *Sem. Psychiat.* 2:420–34.

———. 1974. Antisocial behavior disturbances of childhood: Prevalence, prognosis and prospects. In *The child in his family: Children at psychiatric risk,* Vol. 3. ed. E.J. Anthony and C. Konpernik. New York: Wiley.

———. 1978. Psychiatric epidemiology. *Arch. Gen. Psychiat.* 35:697–702.

———. 1979. Longitudinal methods in the study of normal and pathological development. In *Grundlagen und Methoden der Psychiatrie.* Vol. 1 ed. K.P. Kisker, J.E. Meyer, C. Müller, and E. Strömgren. Heidelberg: Springer-Verlag.

References

———, and LEWIS, R.G. 1966. The role of the antisocial family in school completion and delinquency: A three generation study. *Soc. Quart.* 7(4):500–514.

ROBINSON, G. 1972. Physical growth and development: Some socio-economic factors during prenatal and postnatal life. In *Poverty and the child: A Canadian study,* ed. T.J. Ryan, pp. 19–40. Toronto: McGraw-Hill Ryerson.

ROBINSON, G.C., and CLARKE, H.F. 1980. *The hospital care of children: A review of contemporary issues.* New York: Oxford University Press.

ROBINSON, H.B., and ROBINSON, N.M. 1976. *The mentally retarded child: A psychological approach.* 2d ed. New York:McGraw-Hill.

ROBSON, B. 1979. *My parents are divorced too: What teenagers experience, and how they cope.* Toronto: Dorset.

ROBSON, B.E. 1982. A developmental approach to the treatment of children of divorcing parents. In *Therapy with remarriage families. Family Therapy Collections.* Rockville, Md.:Aspen Publications.

ROCHLIN, G. 1959. The loss complex. *J. Am. Psychoanal. Assn.* 7:299–316.

ROIPHE, H., and GALENSON, E. 1973. Object loss and early sexual development. *Psychoanal. Quar.* 42:73–90.

ROMEDER, J.M. 1981. Self-help groups and mental health: A promising avenue. *Can. Ment. H.* 29(1):10–12.

RONAGHY, H., and HALSTED, J. 1975. Zinc deficiency occurring in females. *Am. J. Clin. Nut.* 28(8):831–36.

ROOSEVELT, R., and LOFAS, J. 1976. *Living in step.* New York: Stein & Day.

ROSBERG, G. 1971. Parental attitudes in pediatric hospital admissions. *Acta Pediat. Scand.* Supplement No. 210.

ROSE, F.C. (Ed.) 1979. *Paediatric neurology.* Oxford: Blackwell Scientific Pub.

ROSEN, B.M., BAHN, A.K., and KRAMER, M. 1964. Demographic and diagnostic characteristics of psychiatric clinics and outpatients in the U.S.A., 1961. *Am. J. Orthopsychiat.* 34(3):455–68.

ROSEN, B.M., REDICK, R.W., KRAMER, M., and WILLNER, S.G. 1968. *Utilization of psychiatric facilities by children: Status, trends, implications.* National Institute of Mental Health, Statistics Series B, No. 1. Washington, D.C.: U.S. Government Printing Office.

ROSENBAUM, A., O'LEARY, K.D., and JACOB, R.G. 1975. Behavioral intervention with hyperactive children: Group consequences as a supplement to individual contingencies. *Behav. Therap.* 6:315–23.

ROSENBAUM, J., and ROSENBAUM, V. 1978. *Stepparenting.* Corte Madera, Calif.: Dutton.

ROSENBAUM, J.F. 1982. "Current Concepts in Psychiatry: The Drug Treatment of Anxiety." *New Eng. J. Med.* 306(7):401–4.

ROSENBERG, J.B., and WELLER, G.M. 1973. Minor physical anomalies and academic performance in young school children. *Dev. Med. Child. Neur.* 15:131–35.

ROSENBLUM, B. 1977. *Foster homes and adolescents: A research report.* Hamilton, Ont.: Hamilton–Wentworth Children's Aid Society.

ROSENFELD, A.A. 1979. The clinical management of incest and sexual abuse of children. *J. Am. Med. Assn.* 242:1761–64.

ROSENTHAL, A.J., and LEVINE, S.V. 1971. Brief psychotherapy with children: Process of therapy. *Am. J. Psychiat.* 128:141–46.

ROSENTHAL, D. 1970. *Genetic theory and abnormal behavior.* New York: McGraw-Hill.

ROSENTHAL, J.H. 1973. Neurophysiology of minimal cerebral dysfunctions. *Acad. Therap.* 8:291–94.

ROSKIES, E., BEDARD, P., GAUVREAU-GUILBAUT, H., and LAFORTUNE, D. 1975. Emergency hospitalization of young children: Some neglected psychosocial considerations. *Med. Care* 13(7) (July 7):570–81.

ROSS, A.O. 1976. *Psychological aspects of learning disabilities and reading disorders: The unrealized potential.* New York: McGraw-Hill.

ROSS, D.M., and ROSS, S.A. 1976. *Hyperactivity: Research, theory and action,* p. 32. New York: Wiley.

ROTHENBERG, M.B. 1968. Child psychiatry–pediatrics liaison: A history and commentary. *J. Am. Acad. Child Psychiat.* 7:492–509.

ROUTH, D.K., and ROBERTS, R.D. 1972. Minimal brain dysfunction in children: Failure to find evidence for a behavioral syndrome. *Psychiat. Reports,* 31:307–14.

ROWE, J., and LAMBERT, L. 1973. *Children who wait.* London: Association of British Adoption Agencies.

RUBIN, A.L., and RUBIN, R.L. 1980. The effects of physician counselling technique on parent reactions to mental retardation diagnosis. *Child Psychiat. & Hum. Dev.* 10(4) (Summer):213–21.

RUESCH, J., and BATESON, G. 1951. *Communication: The social matrix of psychiatry* New York: W.W. Norton.

RUOPP, R., BACHE, W.L. 3rd., O'NEIL, C., SINGER, J. et al. 1979. *Children at the center: Summary findings and their implications.* Cambridge, Mass.: Abt Books. (Single copies available free from the Daycare Division, Administration for Children, Youth and Families, P.O. Box 1182, Washington, D.C., 20013)

RUSH, D. 1974. Examination of the relationship between birthweight, cigarette smoking during pregnancy, and maternal weight gain. *Brit. J. Ob. Gyn.* 81:746–52.

RUSH, F. 1980. *The best kept secret: Sexual abuse of children.* Englewood Cliffs, N.J.: Prentice-Hall.

RUSSEL, G. 1977. General management of anorexia nervosa and difficulties in assessing the efficacy of treatment. In *Anorexia nervosa,* ed. R. Vigersky, pp. 277–89. New York: Raven Press.

RUSSELL, A.T., CANTWELL, D.P., MATTISON, R., and WILL, L. 1979. A comparison of DSM-II and DSM-III in the diagnosis of childhood psychiatric disorders. III. Multiaxial features. *Arch. Gen. Psychiat.* 36:1223–26.

RUTTER, M. 1965. The influence of organic and emotional factors on the origins, nature and outcome of childhood psychosis. *Dev. Med. Child. Neur.* 7:518–28.

———. 1967. A children's behavior questionnaire for completion by teachers: Preliminary findings. *J. Child. Psychol. Psychiat.* 8:1–11.

———. 1970. Psychological development: Predictions from infancy. *J. Child Psychol. Psychiat.* 11:49–62.

———. 1972a. Childhood schizophrenia reconsidered. *J. Aut. Child Schiz.* 2:315–37.

———. 1972b. *Maternal deprivation reassessed.* Hamondsworth, Middlesex, U.K.:Penguin Books.

———. 1973. Why are London children so disturbed? *Proc. Roy. Soc. Med.* 66:1221–25.

———. 1974a. The development of infantile autism. *Psychol. Med.* 4:147–63.

———. 1974b. Emotional disorder and educational underachievement. *Arch. Dis. Child.* 49:249–56.

———. 1974c. Epidemiological strategies and psychiatric concepts in research on the vulnerable child. In *The child in his family,* ed. E.J. Anthony and C. Koupernik. Vol. 3, *Children at psychiatric risk.* New York: Wiley.

———. 1975. Underachievement, learning inhibitions and other problems. In *Helping troubled children,* New York: Plenum.

———. 1977a. Brain damage syndromes in childhood: Concepts and findings. *J. Child. Psychol. Psychiat.* 18:1–21.

———. 1977b. Classification. In *Child psychiatry: Modern approaches,* ed. M. Rutter and L. Hersov pp. 359–84. Oxford: Blackwell Scientific Pub.

———. 1977c. Sociocultural influences. In *Child psychiatry: Modern approaches,* ed. M. Rutter and L. Hersov. Oxford: Blackwell Scientific Pubs.

———. 1978. Diagnostic validity in child psychiatry. *Adv. Biol. Psychiat.* 2:2–22.

———. 1979. Protective factors in children respond to stress and disadvantage. In *Primary prevention of psychopathology.* Vol. III *Social Competence in children,* ed. M.W. Kent and J.E. Rolf, Hanover: University Press of New England.

———. 1979a. Invulnerability, or why some children are not damaged by stress. In *New directions in children's mental health,* ed. S.J. Shamsie. New York: S.P. Medical & Scientific Books.

———. 1979b. Maternal deprivation, 1972–1978: New findings, new concepts, new approaches. *Child Dev.* 50:283–305.

———. 1980a. School influences on children's behavior and development: The 1979 Kenneth Blackfan lecture, Children's Hospital Medical Center, Boston. *Pediat.* 65:208–20.

———. 1980b. Attachment and the development of social relationships. In *Scientific foundations—Developmental psychiatry,* ed. M. Rutter pp. 267–279. London: Heinemann.

———. 1981b. The city and the child. *Am. J. Orthopsychiat.* 51:610–25.

———. 1981c. Psychological sequelae of brain damage in children. *Am. J. Psychiat.* 138:1533–44.

———. 1982. Syndromes attributed to "Minimal Brain Dysfunction" in childhood. *Am. J. Psychiat.* 139(1):21–33.

———, BIRCH, H., THOMAS, A., and CHESS, S. 1964. Temperamental characteristics in infancy and the later development of behaviour disorders. *Brit. J. Psychiat.* 110:651–61.

References

RUTTER, M., COX, A., TUPLING, C., BERGER, M., and YULE, W. 1975. Attainment and adjustment in two geographical areas: 1—The prevalence of psychiatric disorder. *Brit. J. Psychiat.* 126:493–509.

RUTTER, M., GRAHAM, P. 1966. Psychiatric disorders in 10-and 11-year-old children. *Proc. Roy. Soc. Med.* 59:382.

———. 1968. The reliability and validity of the psychiatric assessment of the child: I: Interview with the child. *Brit. J. Psychiat.* 114:563–79.

———, CHADWICK, O., and YULE, W. 1976. Adolescent turmoil—fact or fiction. *J. Child Psychol. Psychiat.* 17:35–56.

RUTTER, M., GREENFIELD, D., and LOCKYER, L. 1967. A five to fifteen year follow-up study of infantile psychosis: II: Social and behavioural outcome. *Brit. J. Psychiat.* 113:1183–99.

RUTTER, M., LEBOVICI, S., EISENBERG, L., SNEZNEVSKIJ, A.V., SADOUN, R., BROOKE, E., and LIN, T-Y. 1969. A tri-axial classification of mental disorders in childhood. *J. Child Psychol. Psychiat.* 10:41–61.

RUTTER, M., and LOCKYER, L. 1967. A five to fifteen year study of infantile psychosis, I: Description of the sample. *Brit. J. Psychiat.* 113:1169–82.

RUTTER, M., MAUGHAN, B., MORTIMER, P., and OUSTON, J. 1979. *Fifteen thousand hours: Secondary schools and their effects on children.* Cambridge, Mass.: Harvard Univ. Press.

RUTTER, M., and MITTLER, P. 1972. Environmental influences on language development. In *The child with delayed speech,* ed. M. Rutter, and J.A.M. Martin *Clin. in Dev. Med.* No. 43, pp. 52–67. London: Spastics International Medical Publications.

RUTTER, M., and SHAFFER, D. 1980. DSM-III : A step forward or back in terms of the classification of child psychiatric disorders? *J. Am. Acad. Child. Psychiat.* 19:371–94.

———, and SHEPHERD, M. 1975. *A multi-axial classification of child psychiatric disorders.* Geneva: World Health Organization.

RUTTER, M., TIZARD, J., GRAHAM, P., and WHITMORE, K. 1976. Isle of Wight studies, 1964–1974. *Psychol. Med.* 6(2):313–32.

RUTTER, M., TIZARD, J., and WHITMORE, K. 1970. *Education, health and behaviour.* London: Longman.

RUTTER, M., YULE, B., QUINTON, D., ROWLANDS, O., YULE, W., and BERGER, M. 1975. Attainment and adjustment in two geographical areas—Some factors accounting for area differences. *Brit. J. Psychiat.* 126:520–33.

RYAN, T.J. 1972. *Poverty and the child: A Canadian study.* Toronto: McGraw-Hill Ryerson.

SACKIN, H.D., and MEYER, A.D. 1976. In-patient care for disturbed children: Criteria for admission. Paper presented at the Annual Meeting of the American Academy of Child Psychiatry, Toronto.

SAFER, D., ALLEN, R., and BARR, E. 1972. Depression of growth in hyperactive children on stimulant drugs. *N.E.J.M.* ed. 287 (5): 217.

SAFER, D.J. 1973. A familial factor in minimal brain dysfunction. *Behav. Genet.* 3: 175–87.

———, and ALLAN, R.P. 1976. *Hyperactive children: Diagnosis and management,* pp. 7–9. Baltimore: University Park Press.

SALADINO, C., and SIVA-SANKAR, D. 1969. Studies on Erythrocyte magnesium and potassium levels in childhood schizophrenia and growth. *Behav. Neuropsychiat.* 10: 24–28.

SAMEROFF, A.J. 1975. Early influences on development: Fact or fancy? *Merrill-Palmer Quart.* 21(4): 267–94.

———. 1977. Concepts of humanity. In *Primary prevention of psychopathology,* ed. G. Albee and J.M. Joffe, pp. 42–63. Vol. 1. Hanover, N.H: Univ. Press of New England.

———, and CHANDLER, M.J. 1975. Reproductive risk and the continuum of caretaking casualty. In *Review of child development research,* ed. F.D. Horowitz, pp. 187–244. Vol. 4. Chicago: Univ. of Chicago.

SANDBERG, S.T., RUTTER, M., and TAYLOR, E. 1978. Hyperkinetic disorder in psychiatric clinic attenders. *Dev. Med. Child Neurol.* 20: 279–99.

SANDBERG, S.T., WEISELBERG, M., and SHAFFER, D. 1980. Hyperkinetic and conduct problem children in a primary school population: Some epidemiological considerations. *J. Child. Psychol. Psychiat.* 21(4): 293–311.

SANDER, L. 1964. Adaptive relationships in early mother–child interaction. *J. Am. Acad. Child Psychiat.* 3:231–64.

SANDLER, J., and JOFFE, W.G. 1965. Notes on childhood depression. *Int. J. of Psychoanal.* 46: 88–96.

SANTIAGO, L.P.R. 1973. *The children of Oedipus: Brother–Sister incest in psychiatry, literature, history and mythology.* Roslyn Heights, N.Y.: Libra Pubs.

SARAF, K.R., KLEIN, D.F., GITTLEMAN, R., GOOTMAN, N., and GREENHILL, P. 1978. E.K.G. effects of imipramine treatment in children. *J. Amer. Acad. Child Psychiat.* 17(1):60–69.

SARLES, R.M., and FRIEDMAN, S.B. 1979. Pediatric behavioral services. *Psychiat. Clin. of N. Am.* 2(2): 265–76.

SARNOFF, C. 1976. *Latency,* pp. 39–69. New York: Jason Aronson.

SATIR, V. 1967. *Conjoint family therapy.* Palo Alto: Science & Behavior Books.

SATTERFIELD, J.H., and BRALEY, B.W. 1977. Evoked potentials and brain maturation in hyperactive and normal children. *Electroencephal.* 43: 43–51.

SATTERFIELD, J., CANTWELL, D.P., and SATTERFIELD, B.T. 1964. Pathophysiology of the hyperactive child syndrome. *Arch. Gen. Psychiat.* 31(6):839–44.

SATTERFIELD, J.H., CANTWELL, D.P., SCHELL, A., and BLASCHKE, T. 1979. Growth of hyperactive children treated with methylphenidate. *Arch. Gen. Psychiat.* 36: 212–17.

SATTERFIELD, J.H., and DAWSON, M.E. 1971. Electrodermal correlates of hyperactivity in children. *Psychophysiol.* 8: 191–97.

SAUBER, M., and CORRIGAN, E.M. 1970. *The six-year experience of unwed mothers as parents.* New York: Community Council of Greater New York.

SAWYER, M.G. 1980. The burned child: Scarred for life? Diss. for Diploma of Child Psychiatry, University of Toronto.

SAXE, D.B. 1975. Some reflections on the interface of the law and psychiatry in child custody cases. *J. Psychiat. Law* 3(4): 501–514.

SCALLY, B.G. 1973. Marriage and mental handicap: Some observations in Northern Ireland. In *Human sexuality and the mentally retarded,* ed. F.F. de la Cruz and G.D. La Veck pp. 186–95. New York: Brunner/Mazel.

SCARR-SALAPATEK, S., and WILLIAMS, M.L. 1973. The effects of early stimulation of low birth weight infants. *Child Dev.* 44: 94–101.

SCHACHAR, R., RUTTER, M., and SMITH, A. 1981. The characteristics of situationally and pervasively hyperactive children: Implications for syndrome definition. *J. Child Psychol. Psychiat.* 22(4): 375–92.

SCHAFFER, H.R., and CALLENDER, W.M. 1959. Psychologic effects of hospitalization in infancy. *Pediat.* 24: 528–39.

SCHAFFER, H.R., and EMERSON, P.E. 1964. The development of social attachments in infancy. *Mono. Soc. Res. Child Dev.* Vol. 29, Series No. 94.

SCHAIN, R.J., and REYNARD, C.L. 1975. Observations on effects of central stimulant drug (methylphenidate) in children with hyperactive behavior. *Pediat.* 55: 709–16.

SCHAIN, R., and YANNET, H. 1960. Infantile autism: An analysis of 50 cases and a consideration of certain relevant neurophysiological concepts. *J. Pediat.* 57: 560–67.

SCHECHTER, M.D. 1960. Observations of adopted children. *Arch. Gen. Psychiat.* 3: 21–32.

———, CARLSON, P.V., SIMMONS, J.Q., and WORK, H.H. 1964. Emotional problems in the adoptee. *Arch. Gen. Psychiat.* 10: 109–18.

SCHECHTER, M.D., and HOLTER, F.R. 1979. The child amputee. In *Basic handbook of child psychiatry,* Vol. 1, *Normal development.* ed. J.D. Call, pp. 427–32 New York: Basic Books.

SCHEFLEN, A. 1978. Susan smiled: On explanation in family therapy. *Fam. Proc.* 17: 59–68.

SCHERE, R.A., RICHARDSON, E., and BIALER, I. 1980. Toward operationalizing a psychoeducational definition of learning disabilities. *J. Abnorm. Child Psychol.* 8(1): 5–20.

SCHERZ, F.H. 1971. Maturational crises and parent–child interaction. *Soc. Casework* 52: 362–70.

SCHERZER, L.N., and PADMA, L. 1980. Sexual offenses committed against children. *Clin. Ped.* 19: 679–85.

SCHICKLER, I. 1981. Early identification: The challenges. *Ont. Pub. School Man Teachers Fed. News* (November): 5–7.

SCHIELE, B.C., GALLANT, D., SIMPSON, G., GARDNER, E.A., and COLE, J.O. 1973. Tardive dyskinesia. *Am. J. Orthopsychiat.* 43: 506–688.

SCHIFFER, M. 1969. *The therapeutic play group.* New York: Grune & Stratton.

SCHLEIFER, M., WEISS, G., COHEN, N., ELMAN, M., CUEJIC, H., and KRUGER, D. 1975. Hyperactivity in preschoolers and the effect of methylphenidate. *Am. J. Orthopsychiat.* 45: 38–50.

SCHLESINGER, H.S. 1979. The deaf child. In *Basic handbook of child psychiatry,* Vol. 1, *Normal Development* ed. J.D. Call, pp. 421–27. New York: Basic Books.

References

Schmitt, B.D. 1980. The prevention of child abuse and neglect: A review of the literature with recommendations for application. *Intl. J. Child Ab. & Neg.* 4: 171–77.

———, and Kempe, C.H. 1975. Neglect and abuse of children. In *Nelson textbook of pediatrics,* ed. V.S. Vaughan and R.J. MacKay. 10th ed. Philadelphia: W.B. Saunders.

Schneer, H.I., Kay, P., and Brozovsky, M. 1961. Events and conscious ideation leading to suicidal behavior in adolescence. *Psychiat. Quart.* 35: 507–15.

Schneidman, E. 1973. Crisis intervention: Some thoughts and perspectives. In *Crisis intervention,* ed. G. Specter and W. Claiborn. New York: Behavioral Pub.

Schoettle, U.C., and Cantwell, D.P. 1980. Children of divorce: Demographic variables, symptoms and diagnoses. *J. Am. Acad. Child Psychiat.* 19(3): 453–75.

Scholom, A., and Schiff, G. 1980. Relating infant temperament to learning disabilities. *J. Abnorm. Child Psychol.* 8(1): 127–32.

Schopler, E. 1965. Early infantile autism and receptor processes. *Arch. Gen. Psychiat.* 13: 327–35.

———, and Reichler, R.J. 1971. Parents as cotherapists in the treatment of psychotic children. *J. Aut. & Child Schiz.* 1:87–102.

Schowalter, J. 1979. The chronically ill child. In *Basic handbook of child psychiatry,* ed. J.D. Call, Vol. 1, *Normal development.* New York: Basic Books.

Schowalter, J.E. 1970. Death and the pediatric house officer. *J. Pediat.* 76(5): 706–10.

———. 1971. The utilization of child psychiatry on a pediatric adolescent ward", *J. Am. Acad. Child Psychiat.* 10: 684–99.

———. 1977. Psychological reactions to physical illness and hospitalization in adolescence: A survey. *J. Am. Acad. Child Psychiat.* 16:500–516.

———, Ferholt. J.B., and Mann, N.M. 1973. The adolescent patient's decision to die. *Pediat.* 51(1): 97–103.

Schowalter, J.E., and Solnit, A.J. 1966. Child psychiatry consultation in a general hospital emergency room. *J. Am. Acad. Child Psychiat.* 5: 534–51.

Schull, W.J., and Neel, J.V. 1965. *The effects of inbreeding on Japanese children.* New York: Harper & Row.

Schwarz, J.C. 1972. Effects of peer familiarity on the behavior of preschoolers in a novel situation. *J. Pers. & Soc. Psychol.* 24(2): 276–84.

Schwartz, L.L., and Kaslow, F.W. 1979. Religious cults, the individual and the family. *J. Mar. & Fam. Therap.,* 5(2)(April):15–26.

Schwitzgebel, R.K., and Klob, D.A. 1974. *Changing human behavior.* New York: McGraw-Hill.

Scott, P.D., and Kahn, J. 1968. An XYY patient of above average intelligence as a basis for review of the psychopathology, medico-legal implications of the syndrome, and possibilities for prevention. In *Psychopathic offenders,* ed. D.J. West. Cambridge, U.K.: University of Cambridge, Institute of Criminology.

Scranton, T.R., Hajicek, J.O., and Wolcott, G.J. 1978. The physician and teacher as team: Assessing the effects of medication. *J. Learn Disab.,* 11(4)(April): 205–09.

Seeman, M.V. 1981. Pharmacologic features and effects of neuroleptics. *Can. Med. Assn. J.* 125(8): 821–26.

Seeman, P., Sellers, E.M., and Roschlau, W.H.E. 1980. *Principles of medical pharmacology.* 277. 3d ed. Toronto: Univ. of Toronto Press.

Seglow, J., Pringle, M.L., and Wedge. P 1972. *Growing up adopted: A long-term national study of adopted children and their families.* Windsor, Ont.: Nat. Found. Ed. Res.

Seidel, U.P., Chadwick, O.F.D., and Rutter, M. 1975. Psychological disorders in crippled children: A comparative study with and without brain damage. *Dev. Med. & Child Neurol.* 17: 563–73.

Seidl, A.H., and Altshuler, A. 1979. Interventions for adolescents who are chronically ill. *Child. Today* (November/December): 16–19.

Seignot, J. 1961. A case of the syndrome of tics of Gilles de la Tourette controlled by R 1625. *Ann. Med. Psychiat.* 119: 578–79.

Seligman, R. 1974. A psychiatric classification system for burned children. *Am. J. Psychiat.* 131: 41–46.

Selvini-Palazzoli, M.P. 1974. *Self starvation: From the intrapsychic to the transpersonal approach to anorexia nervosa.* London: Chaucer.

Selye, H. 1956. *The stress of life.* New York: McGraw-Hill.

SENN, M., and SOLNIT, A. J. 1968. *Problems in Child Behavior and Development.* Philadelphia: Lea and Febiger.

SEVERY, L.J., and DAVIS, K.E. 1971. Helping behavior among normal and retarded children. *Child Dev.* 42: 1017–31.

SGROI, S.M. 1978. Comprehensive examination for child sexual assault: Diagnostic therapeutic and child protection issues. In *Sexual assault of children and adolescents,* ed. A.W. Burgess, A.N. Goth, L.L. Holmstrom, and S.M. Sgroi. Lexington, Mass.: Lexington Books.

SHADER, R.E., and DIMASCIO, A. (eds.) 1970. *Psychotropic drug side effects.* Baltimore: Williams & Wilkins.

SHAFFER, D. 1974. Suicide in childhood and early adolescence. *J. Child Psychol. Psychiat.* 15: 275–91.

———. 1977. Enuresis. In *Child psychiatry: Modern approaches,* ed. M. Rutter and L. Hersov, pp. 581–612. Oxford: Blackwell Scientific Publications.

———. 1978. "Soft" neurological signs and later psychiatric disorders—A review. *J. Child Psychol. Psychiat.* 19:63–65.

SHAMES, G.H. 1968. Dysfluency and stuttering. *Ped. Clin. N. Am.* 15(3): 691–704.

SHAMSIE, S.J. 1981a. Antisocial adolescents: Our treatments do not work: Where do we go from here? *Can. J. Psychiat.* 26(5): 357–64.

———. 1981b. . *Family changes and their impact on children's mental health.* Unpublished manuscript.

SHAPIRO, E.R., ZINNER, J., SHAPIRO, R.L., and BERKOWITZ, P.A. 1975. The influence of family experience on borderline personality development. *Int. Rev. Psychoanal.* 2:399–411.

SHAPIRO, T., BURKES, L., PETTI, T.A., and RANZ, J. 1978. The consistency of "non-focal" neurological signs. *J. Am. Acad. Child Psychiat.* 17(1): 70–79.

SHAPIRO, T., and FISH, B. 1969. A method to study language deviation as an aspect of ego organization in young schizophrenic children. *J. Am. Acad. Child Psychiat.* 8: 36–56.

———, and GINSBERG, G.L. 1972. The speech of a schizophrenic child from two to six. *Am. J. Psychiat.* 128: 1408–14.

SHAPIRO, T., ROBERTS, A., and FISH, B. 1970. Imitation and echoing in young schizophrenic children. *J. Am. Acad. Child Psychiat.* 9: 548–67.

SHAW, C.R., and SCHELKUN, R.F. 1965. Suicidal behavior in children. *Psychiat.* 28: 157–68.

SHEAGREN, T.G., MANGURTEN, H.H., BREA, F., and LUTOSTANSKI, S. 1980. Rumination—A new complication of neonatal intensive care, *Pediat.* 66(4): 551–55.

SHEARD, M.H. MARINI, J.L., BRIDGES, C.I., and WAGNER, E. 1976. The effect of lithium on impulsive–aggressive behavior in man. *Am. J. Psychiat.* 133(12): 1409–13.

SHELTON, M.N. 1977. Affective education and the learning disabled student. *J. Learn. Disab.,* 10(10) (December): 618–29.

SHEPHERD, M. 1980. Psychotropic drugs and taxonomic systems. *Psychol. Med.,* 10(1): 25–33.

SHERE, E., and KASTENBAUM, R. 1966. Mother–child interaction in cerebral palsy: Environmental and psychosocial obstacles to cognitive development. *Genet. Psychol. Mono.* 73: 255–335.

SHERMAN, E.A., NEUMAN, R., and SHYNE, A. 1973. *Children adrift in foster care.* New York: Child Welfare League of America.

SHETTY, T., and CHASE, T. 1976. Central monoamines and hyperkinesis of childhood. *Neurology.* 26(10): 1000–1002.

SHORE, M.F., and GOLDSTON, S.E. 1978. Mental health aspects of pediatric care—Historical review and current status In *Psychological management of pediatric problems,* Vol. 2. ed. P.R. Magrab. Baltimore: Univ. Park Press.

SHULMAN, J.C. 1976. *Coping with tragedy: Successfully facing the problem of a seriously ill child.* Chicago: Follett.

SIEBEN, R.L. 1977. Controversial medical treatment of learning disabilities. *Acad. Ther.* 13(2) (November): 133–47.

SIEGEL, L.J. 1976. Preparation of children for hospitalization: A selected review of the research literature. *J. Ped. Psychol.* 1(4): 26–30.

SIEVER, L.J., and GUNDERSON, J.G. 1979. Genetic determinants of borderline condition. *Schiz. Bull.* 5(1): 59–86.

SIFNEOS, P.E. 1967. Two different kinds of psychotherapy of short duration. *Am. J. Psychiat.* 123: 1069–74.

———. 1973. The prevalence of alexithymic characteristics in psychosomatic patients. *Psychother. Psychosom.* 22: 255–62.

References

SIGAL, J.J., CHAGOYA, L., VILLENEUVE, C., and MAYEROVITCH, J. 1973. Later psychosocial sequelae of early childhood illness (severe group). *Am. J. Psychiat.* 130: 786–89.

SILBERSTEIN, R.M., BLACKMAN, S., and MANDELL, W. 1966. Autoerotic head banging: A reflection on the opportunism of infants. *J. Am. Acad. Child Psychiat.* 5:235–42.

SILLENCE, D.O., SENN, A., and DANSK, D.M. 1979. Genetic heterogeneity in osteogenesis imperfecta. *J. Med. Genet.* 16: 101–116.

SILVER, L.B. 1980. Stereotyped movement and speech disorders of childhood and adolescence. In *Comprehensive textbook of psychiatry,* Vol. 3. 3d ed. H. I. Kaplan, A.M. Freedman, and B.J. Sadock. pp. 2571–79. Baltimore: Williams & Wilkins.

SILVERMAN, P.R. 1978. *Mutual help groups: A guide for mental health workers.* Wash., D.C.: National Institute of Mental Health (DHEW Publication No. (AOM) 78–646).

SIMEONSSON, R.J., BUCKLEY, L., and MONSON, L. 1979. Conceptions of illness causality in hospitalized children. *J. Ped. Psychol.* 4(1) (March): 77–84.

SIMMONS, J.E. 1974. *Psychiatric examination of children.* 2nd ed. Philadelphia: Lea & Febiger.

———, TEN EYCK, R.L., McNABB, R.C., COLEMAN, B.S., BIRCH, B., and PARR, M. 1981. Parent treatability: What is it? *J. Am. Acad. Child Psychiat.* 20:792–809.

SIMON, A.W. 1964. *Stepchild in the family.* New York: Odyssey Press.

SIPERSTEIN, G.N., BOPP, M.J., and BAK, J.J. 1978. Social status of learning disabled children. *J.Learn.Disab.,* 11(2) (February): 98–102.

SITLINGTON, P.L. 1981. Vocational and special education in career programming for the mildly handicapped adolescent. *Except. Child.* 47(8) (May): 592–98.

SIVA SANKAR, D. 1970. Biogenic amine uptake by blood platelets and RBC in childhood schizophrenia. *Acta Paedopsychiat.* 37: 174–82.

SKIPPER, J.K., and LEONARD, R.C. 1968. Children, stress and hospitalization: A field experiment. *J. H. & Soc. Behav.* 4: 275–87.

SKLAR, L.S., and ANISMAN, H. 1980. Social stress influences tumor growth. *Psychosom. Med.* 42(3): 347–65.

SKYNNER, A.C.R. 1969. A group-analytic approach to conjoint family therapy. *J. Child Psychol. Psychiat.* 10: 81–106.

SLADE, C.I., REIDL, C.J., and MANGURTEN, H.H. 1977. Working with parents of high-risk newborns. *J. Ob. Gyn. Neonat. Nurs.* 6(2):(March/April)21–26.

SLATER, E., and COWIE, V. 1971. *The genetics of mental disorders.* London: Oxford Press.

SLATER, E., and SHIELDS, J. 1969. Genetical aspects of anxiety. In *Studies of anxiety. Brit. J. Psychiat. Spec. Pub. #3,* ed. M.H. Lader, pp. 62–71. Ashford, Kent: Headley Bros.

SLEATOR, E.K., and VON NEUMANN, A.W. 1974. Methylphenidate in the treatment of hyperkinetic children. *Clin. Pediat.* 13: 19–24.

———, and SPRAGUE, R.L. 1974. Hyperactive children: A continuous long-term placebo-controlled follow-up. *J. Am. Med. Assn.* 229: 316–17.

SLIPP, S. 1980. Interactions between the interpersonal in families and individual intrapsychic dynamics. In *Family therapy: Combining psychodynamic and family systems approaches,* ed. J.K. Pearce and L.J. Friedman, pp. 117–35. New York: Grune & Stratton.

SLIVKIN, S.E., and BERNSTEIN, N.R. 1968. Goal directed group psychotherapy for retarded adolescents. *Am. J. Psychother.* 22: 35–45.

SLOANE, P., and KARPINSKI, E. 1942. Effects of incest on the participants. *Am. J. Orthopsychiat.* 12: 666–73.

SMALL, J.G. 1971. Sensory evoked responses of autistic children. In *Infantile autism,* ed. D.W. Churchill, G.D. Alpern, and M.K. Meyer, pp. 224–39. Springfield, Ill.: Chas. C. Thomas.

———, DEMYER, M.K., and MILSTEIN, V. 1971. CNV responses of autistic and normal children. *J. Aut. & Child. Schiz.* 102: 215–31.

SMITH, D.A., and WILBORN, D.L. 1977. Specific predictors of learning difficulties. *Acad. Therap.* 11(4)(Summer): 471–77.

SMITH, S.M. 1975. *The battered child syndrome.* Toronto: Butterworth Pub.

SOLNIT, A.J. 1978. Child abuse: The problem. In *Family violence: An international and interdisciplinary study,* ed. J.M. Eekelaar and S.N. Katz. Toronto: Butterworth Pub.

———, and GREEN, M. 1959. Psychologic considerations in the management of deaths on pediatric hospital services. I: The doctor and the child's family. *Pediat.* 24: 106–12.

SOLNIT, A.J. and STARK, M.H. 1961. Mourning and the birth of a defective child. *Psychoanal. Stud. Child.* 16: 523–37.

731

SOLOMONS, G. 1979. Child abuse and developmental disabilities. *Dev. Med. Child Neurol.* 21(1): 101–108.

SOLOW, R.A., and ADAMS, P.L. 1977 Custody by agreement: Child psychiatrist as child advocate. *J. Psychiat. Law* 5(1): 77–100.

SONIS, W.A., and COSTELLO, A. 1981. Evaluation of differential data sources. *J. Am. Acad. Child Psychiat.* 20(3): 597–610.

SOROSKY, A.D., BARAN, A., and PANNOR, R. 1975. Identity conflicts in adoptees. *Am. J. Orthopsychiat.* 45(1): 18–27.

———. 1976. The effects of the sealed record in adoption. *Am. J. Psychiat.* 133(8): 900–904.

SOSA, R., KENNELL, J.H., KLAUS, M., ROBERTSON, S., and URRUTIA, J. 1980. The effect of a supportive companion on perinatal problems, length of labor and mother–infant interaction. *N. E. J. Med.* 303(11) (September): 597–600.

SPERLING, E. 1978. Psychological issues in chronic illness and handicap. In *Psychosocial aspects of pediatric care.* ed. E. Gellert, pp. 51–63. New York: Grune & Stratton.

SPERLING, M. 1949. The role of the mother in psychosomatic disorders in children. *Psychosom. Med.* 11(6): 377–85.

———. 1960. Symposium on Disturbances of the Digestive tract, II: Unconscious fantasy life and object relationships in ulcerative colitis. *Int. J. Psychoanal.* 41 (July–October): 450–55.

SPIEGEL, L. 1959. The self, the sense of self and perception. In *Psychoanal. Stud. Child.* 14:81–109.

SPINETTA, J.J. 1977. Adjustment in children with cancer. *J. Pediat. Psychol.* 2(2): 49–51.

SPITZ, R.A. 1945. Hospitalism: An inquiry into the genesis of psychiatric conditions in early childhood. *Psychoanal. Stud. Child* 1:53–74.

———. 1946a. Anaclitic depression: An inquiry into the genesis of psychiatric conditions in early childhood, II. *Psychoanal. Stud. Child.* 2:313–41.

———. 1946b. Hospitalism: A follow-up report. *Psychoanal. Stud. Child* 2:113–17.

———. 1965. *The first year of life.* New York: International Univ. Press.

SPITZER, R.L., and CANTWELL, D.P. 1980. The DSM-III classification of the psychiatric disorders of infancy, childhood and adolescence. *J. Am. Acad. Child Psychiat.* 19: 356–70.

SPIVACK, G., and SWIFT, M. 1977. The Hannemann high school behavior (HHSB) rating scale. *J. Abnorm. Child Psychol.* 5: 299–307.

SPOCK, B.M. 1968. *Baby and child care.* New York: Meredith Press.

SPRAGUE, R. 1976. Overview of psychopharmacology for the retarded in the U.S. *The use of psychopharmacological agents in mental retardation.* (R.L. Sprague, Chair.) Symposium presented at the Fourth International Congress of the International Assn. for the Scientific Study of Mental Deficiency, Washington, D.C.

———. 1977. Psychopharmacotherapy in children. In *Child psychiatry: Treatment and research.* ed. M. McMillan and S. Henao. New York: Brunner/Mazel.

———, COHEN, M.N., and EICHLSEDER, W. Are there hyperactive children in Europe and the South Pacific? Presented to the American Psychological Association symposium on the Hyperactive Child: Fact, Fiction and Fantasy (R. Halliday, Chair.), San Francisco, 1977.

SPRAGUE, R., and SLEATOR, E.K. 1977. Methylphenidate in hyperkinetic children: Differences in dose effects on learning and social behavior. *Science* 198(4323): 1274–76.

SPRAGUE, R.L., and SLEATOR, E.K. 1973. Effect of psychopharmacologic agents on learning disorders. *Pediat. Clin. N. Am.* 20: 719–35.

SROLE, L., LANGNER, T.S., MICHAEL, S.T., OPLER, M.K., and RENNIE, T.A.C. 1962. *Mental health in the Metropolis.* New York: McGraw-Hill.

SROUFE, L.A. 1975. Drug treatment of children with behavior problems. In *Review of child development research,* Vol. 14. ed. F.D. Horowitz. Chicago: Univ. of Chicago Press.

———. 1979. The coherence of individual development: Early care, attachment, and subsequent developmental issues. *Am. Psychol.* 34: 834–41.

STABENAU, J.R., and POLLIN, W. 1967. Early characteristics of monozygotic twins discordant for schizophrenia. *Arch. Gen. Psychiat.* 17: 723–34.

STANTON, H.E. 1981. A therapeutic approach to help children overcome learning difficulties. *J. Learn. Disab.* 14(4)(April): 220–37.

STARFIELD, B. 1972. Enuresis: Its pathogenesis and management. *Clin. Pediat.* 11: 343–50.

STATISTICS CANADA. 1979. Canada Year Book 1978–9. Ottawa: Information Canada.

STAYTON, D.J., and AINSWORTH, M.D.S. 1973. Individual differences in infant responses to brief, everyday separation as related to other infant and maternal behaviors. *Dev. Psychol.* 9:226–35.

References

STECHLER, G. 1980. Facing the problem of the sexually abused child. *N.E.J.Med.* 302: 348–49.

STEIN, S., and CHARLES, E. 1971. Emotional factors in juvenile diabetes mellitus: A study of early life experiences of adolescent diabetes. *Am. J. Psychiat.* 128: 700–705.

STEINBERG, D. 1980. The use of lithium carbonate in adolescence. *J. Child Psychol. Psychiat.* 21(3): 263–71.

STEINHAUER, P.D. 1968. Reflections on criteria for selection and prognosis in family therapy. *Can. Psychiat. Assn. J.* 13: 317–22.

———. 1974. Abruptio familiae: The premature separation of the family. In *Beyond clinic walls,* ed. A.B. Tulipan, C.L. Attneave, and E. Kingstone, pp. 204–11. Univer. of Alabama Press.

———. 1977. Visits of foster children with natural families. *Hops, Steps and Jumps,* June, 1977. Children's Welfare Assn. of Victoria, Australia.

———. 1978. The Laidlaw workshop on "the impossible child": An overview. *Can. Psychiat. Assn. J. Spec. Supp.* 23: 5561–74.

———. 1980. How to succeed in the business of creating psychopaths without even trying. Vol. 2 and 4, *Training resources in understanding, supporting and treating abused children.* Foster parents training program for Children's Aid Societies, Toronto: Ministry of Community and Social Services, Children's Services Division, Section 9, 239–328, December, 1980.

———. 1981. Assessing for parenting capacity. In *Plenary Session Papers:* Ontario Family Court Clinic Conference, Toronto, May, 1981.

———. 1982a. The courts from the children's perspective. Presented at Family Law and Social Policy Workshop Series, Faculty of Law, University of Toronto, March 11, 1982.

———. 1982b. Youth in the '80s. Abridged in Children's Services Division, *Training Program for Children's Aid Societies,* pp. 1–15. Vol. 5. Toronto: Ministry of Community and Social Services.

———, LEVINE, S.V., and DaCOSTA, G.A. 1971. Where have all the children gone? Child psychiatric emergencies in a metropolitan area. *Can. Psychiat. Assn. J.* 16: 121–27.

STEINHAUER, P.D., SANTA-BARBARA, J., and SKINNER, H.A. The process model of family functioning. In *The process model of family functioning: Theory, research and clinical applications.* (in press).

———. 1982. Advantages of the process model of family functioning. Submitted for publication.

STEINHAUSEN, H.C., and KRUEZER, E.M. 1981. Learning in hyperactive children: Are there stimulant-related and state-dependent effects? *Psychopharmacol.* 74: 389–90.

STEINMAN, S. 1981. The experience of children in a joint custody arrangement: A report of the study. *Am. J. Orthopsychiat.* 51(3): 403–414.

STENGER, M. 1975. Frequency of learning disabilities in adjudicated delinquents. Master's thesis, University of Missouri–Kansas City, Kansas City, Mo.

STERLING, P. 1979. Psychiatry's drug addiction. *New Republic,* 181:14–18.

STERN, P.N. 1978. Step-father families: Integration around discipline. *Iss. Ment. H. Nurs.* 1(2): 50–56.

STEVENS, A. 1975. Attachment and polymatric rearing. Thesis for D.M., University of Oxford.

STEVENS, M. 1949. Visitors are welcome on the pediatric ward. *Am. J. Nurs.* 49: 233–35.

STEVENS, J.R., SACHDEV, K., and MILSTEIN, V. 1968. Behavior disorders of childhood and the electroencephalogram. *Arch. Neurol.* 18: 160.

STEWART, M.A., and OLDS, S.W. 1973. *Raising a hyperactive child.* New York: Harper & Row.

STEWART, M.A., PITTS, F., CRAIG, A.G., and DIERUF, W. 1966. The hyperactive children syndrome. *Am. J. Orthopsychiat.* 36: 861–67.

STEWART, M.A., THACH, B.T., and FREIDIN, M.R. 1970. Accidental poisoning and the hyperactive child syndrome. *Dis. Nerv. Syst.* 31:403–407.

STIERLIN, H., and RAVENSCROFT, K. Jr. 1972. Varieties of adolescent separation conflicts. *Brit. J. Med. Psychol.* 45:299–313.

STONE, M.H. 1979. Contemporary shift of the borderline concept from a subschizophrenic disorder to a sub-affective disorder. *Psychiat. Clin. N. Am.* 2(3) (December): 577–94.

STONER, C., and PARKE, J.A. 1977. *All God's children: The cult experience.* Radnor, Pa.: Chilton.

STORES, G. 1978. School children with epilepsy at risk for learning and behavior problems. *Dev. Med. Child. Neur.* 20(4):502–508.

STORES, G. 1978. Antiepileptics. In *Pediatric psychopharmacology: The use of behavior modifying drugs in children,* ed. J. Werry. New York: Brunner/Mazel.

733

STOTT, D.H. 1973. Follow-up study from birth of the effects of prenatal stresses. *Dev. Med. Child Neur.* 15:770–87.

STRAUSS, A.A., and LEHTINEN, L.E. 1947. *Psychopathology and education of the brain injured child.* New York: Grune & Stratton.

STRECKER, E.A., and EBAUGH, F.J. 1924. Neuropsychiatric sequelae of cerebral trauma in children. *Arch. Neur. Psychi.* 12:443–53.

STRIDER, F.D., and MENOLASCINO, F.J. 1979. Counselling parents of mentally retarded infants. In *Modern perspectives in the psychiatry of infancy,* ed. J.G. Howells. New York: Brunner/Mazel.

STUART, R.B. 1971. Behavioral contracting within the families of delinquents. *J. Behav. Therap. Exp. Psychiat.* 2:1–11.

SUGAR, M. 1976. At risk factors for the adolescent mother and her infant. *J. Youth Adol.* 5(3):251–70.

SULSER, F. 1979. New perspectives on the mode of action of antidepressant drugs. *Trends. Pharmacol. Sci.* 1:92–94.

SURAN, B.G., and RIZZO, J.V. 1979. *Special children: An integrative approach.* Glenview, Ill.: Scott, Foresman.

SUSSMAN, M.B. (Ed.) 1972. *Non-traditional family forms in the 1970's.* National Council on Family Relations.

SWANSON, J.M., and KINSBOURNE, M. 1976. Stimulant related state dependent learning in hyperactive children. *Science* 192:1354–57.

————. 1980. Food dyes impair performance of hyperactive children on a laboratory learning test. *Science* 207:1485–87.

————. ROBERTS, W., and ZUCKER, K. 1978. A time response analysis of the effect of stimulant medication on the learning ability of children referred for hyperactivity. *Pediat.* 61:21–29.

SWANSON, L. 1979. Comparison of normal and learning disabled children on short-term memory recall and selective attention. *J. Genet. Psychol.* 135:155–56.

SWARTZBERG, M., LIEB, J., and SCHWARTZ, A.H. 1973. Methaqualone withdrawal. *Arch. Gen. Psychiat.* 29:46–47.

SWYER, P.R. 1970. The regional organization of special care for the neonate. *Pediat. Clin. N. Am.,* 17:761–76.

SZYMANSKI, L.S. (Ed.) 1980. *Emotional disorders of mentally retarded persons.* Baltimore: Univ. Park Press.

TAFT, L.T., and GOLDFARB, W. 1964. Prenatal and perinatal factors in childhood schizophrenia. *Dev. Med. Child. Neur.* 6:32–43.

TALLMAN, I. 1970. The family as a small problem group. *J. Marr. & Fam.* 32:94–104.

TANGUAY, P. 1976. Clinical and electrophysiological research. In *Autism: Diagnosis, current research and management.* E.R. Ritvo, pp. 75–84. New York: Spectrum.

TANNER, J.M. 1962. *Growth at adolescence.* Oxford: Blackwell.

TARJAN, G., and KEERAN, C.V. 1974. An overview of mental retardation. *Ped. Ann.* 4(2):6–21.

TARJAN, G., LOWERY, V.E., and WRIGHT, S.W. 1957. Use of chlorpromazine in two hundred seventy-eight mentally deficient patients. *J. Dis. Child.* 94:194–300.

TARJAN, G., TIZARD, J., RUTTER, M., BEGAB, M., BROOKE, E.M., DE LA CRUZ, F., LIN, T.-Y., MONTENEGRO, H., STROTZKA, H., and SARTORIUS, N. 1972. Classification of mental retardation issues arising in the fifth WHO seminar on psychiatric diagnosis, classification and statistics. *Am. J. Psychiat.* Supp. 128(11) (May):34–45.

TARJAN, G., WRIGHT, S.W., EYMAN, R.K., and KEERAN, C.V. 1973. Natural history of mental retardation: Some aspects of epidemiology. *Am. J. Ment. Def.* 77:369–79.

TARNOPOL, L. et al. 1977. Learning disabilities in minority adolescents. *Bull. Orton Soc.* 27:132–48.

TAYLOR, G., DOODY, K., and NEWMAN, A. 1981. Alexithymic characteristics in patients with inflammatory bowel disease. *Can. J. Psychiat.* 26(November):470–74.

TAYLOR, G.J. 1975. Separation–Individuation in the psychotherapy of symbiotic states. *Can. Psychiat. Assn. J.* 20:521–26.

TEICHER, J.D. 1979. Suicide and suicide attempts. In *Basic handbook of child psychiatry.* ed. J.D. Noshpitz, pp. 685–97. Vol. 2 New York: Basic Books.

TENANT, C. et al. 1980. Parental death in childhood and risk of adult depressive disorders: A review. *Psychol. Med.* 10(2):289–99.

TERKELSON, K.G. 1980. Toward a theory of the family life cycle. In *The Family Life Cycle: A*

References

Framework for Family Therapy, ed. Carter and McGoldrick, pp. 21–52. New York: Gardner Press.

TESSMAN, L.H. 1978. *Children of parting parents.* New York: Jason Aronson.

THARP, R.G. 1963. Psychological patterning in marriage. *Psychol. Bull.* 60:97–117.

THOMAS, A. 1981. Current trends in developmental theory. *Am. J. Orthopsychiat.* 51(4)(October):580–609.

———, and CHESS, S. 1977. *Temperament and development.* New York: Brunner/Mazel.

———, and BIRCH, H.G. 1969. *Temperament and behavior disorders in children.* New York: New York Univ. Press.

THURSTON, D.L., MIDDLEKAMP, J.N., and MASON, E. 1955. The late effects of lead poisoning. *J. Pediat.* 47:413–23.

TILLELI, J.A., TUREK, D., and JAFFEE, A.C. 1980. Sexual abuse of children: Clinical findings and implications for management. *N. E. J. Med.* 302:319–23.

TINBERGEN, E.A., and TINBERGEN, N. 1976. The Aetiology of Childhood Autism: A Criticism of the Tinbergens' Theory: A Rejoinder. *Psychol. Med.* 6:545–49.

TIZARD, B. 1977. *Adoption: A second chance.* London: Open Books.

———, and HODGES, J. 1978. The effect of early institutional rearing on the development of eight-year-old children. *J. Child Psychol. Psychiat.* 19:99–118.

TIZARD, B., and REES, J. 1975. The effect of early institutional rearing on the behavior problems and affectional relationships of four-year-old children. *J. Child Psychol. Psychiat.* 16:61–73.

TIZARD, J. 1970. The role of social institutions in the causation, prevention and alleviation of mental retardation. In *Social–cultural aspects of mental retardation: Proceedings of the Peabody–N.I.M.H. Conference,* ed. H.C. Haywood, pp. 281–340. New York: Appleton-Century Crofts.

TOFFLER, A. 1970. *Future shock,* New York: Random House.

TOLPIN, M. 1970. The infantile neuroses, a metaphysical concept of a paradigmatic case history. *Psychoanal. Stud. Child* 25:273–305.

TOOLAN, J.M. 1975. Suicide in children and adolescents. *Am. J. Psychother.* 29:339–44.

———. 1981. Depression and suicide in children: An overview. *Am. J. Psychother.* 35(3) (July): 311–22.

TOOLEY, K. 1976. Antisocial behavior and social alienation post divorce: The "man of the house" and his mother. *Am. J. Orthopsychiat.* 46(1):33–42.

TOOLEY, K.M. 1978. Irreconcilable differences between parent and child: A case report of interactional pathology. *Am. J. Orthopsychiat.* 48(4):703–716.

TOPPER, A.B. 1979. Options in big brothers involvement in incest. *Child Ab. & Neg.* 3(1):291–96.

TORREY, E.F., HERSH, S.P., and McCABE, K.D. 1975. Early childhood psychosis and bleeding during pregnancy: A prospective study of gravid women and their offspring. *J. Aut. Child. Schiz.* 5:287–97.

TRAVIS, G. 1976. *Chronic illness in children: Its impact on child and family.* Stanford, Calif.: Stanford Univ. Press.

TREFFERT, D.A. 1970. Epidemiology of infantile autism. *Arch. Gen. Psychiat.* 22:431–38.

TRISELIOTIS, J. 1970. *Evaluation of adoption policy and practice.* Edinburgh: Univ. of Edinburgh.

———. 1973. *In search of origins: The experiences of adopted people.* London: Routledge & Kegan Paul.

TSAI, M., and WAGNER, N.N. 1978. "Therapy Groups for Women Sexually Molested as Children." *Arch. Sex. Beh.* 7:417–527.

TU, J.-B. 1981. Neuropsychotropic drug treatment in the mentally handicapped. *Can. Ment. H.* 29(2):14–17.

TYHURST, J. 1957. The role of transition states including disasters in mental illness. Symposium on Preventive and Social Psychiatry, Walter Reed Army Institute of Research, Washington, D.C.

UMPHRESS, A., MURPHY, S., NICKOLS, J., and HAMMAR, S. 1970. Adolescent enuresis, a sociological study of family interaction. *Arch. Gen. Psychiat.* 22:237–44.

U.S. BUREAU OF THE CENSUS. 1972. *1970 census of population marital status.* First Report PC(2)-4C, Washington, D.C.: U.S. Government Printing Office.

———. 1973. *1970 census of population age at first marriage.* Final Report PC(2)-4C, Washington, D.C.: U.S. Government Printing Office.

U.S. CONGRESSIONAL COMMITTEE ON EDUCATION AND LABOR. Subcommittee on Select Education 1978. *Adolescent pregnancy: Hearings before the subcommittee on select education of the committee on education and labor, House of Representatives, 95th Congress. 2nd session on H.R. 12146 . . . July 24, 1978.* Washington, D.C.: U.S. Government Printing Office.

VACHON, M.L.S. 1982. Staff stress in hospice care: A theoretical model. In *The hospice: Development and administration.* 2d ed. ed. G.W. Davidson, Washington, D.C.: Hemisphere Pub.

———, and PAKES, E.H. 1982. Staff stress in the care of the critically ill and dying child. In *Childhood and death,* ed. H. Wass and C. Corrs, Washington, D.C.: Hemisphere Pub.

VAN EYS, J. 1977. *The truly cured child: The challenge of the child with cancer.* Baltimore: University Park Press.

VAN LEEUWEN, J.J. Providing psychological services for patients and families with muscular dystrophy. Paper presented at the American Association of Psychological Services for Children, November 1979.

———, and MATTHEWS, D.E. 1975. Comprehensive mental health care in a pediatric dialysis–transplantation program. *Can. Med. Assn. J.* 113:959–62.

VANCE, J.C. et al. 1980. Effects of nephrotic syndrome on the family: A controlled study. *Pediat.* 65(5)(May):948–55.

VANIER, J. 1969. *The evolution of the family and the modern crisis.* Ottawa: The Vanier Institute of the Family.

VARDI, J., FLETCHER, S., TUPILSKY, M., RABEY, J.M., CARASSO, R., and STREIFLER, M. 1978. Kleine–Levin syndrome with periodic apnea during hypersomnic stages "EEG study." *J. Neur. Trans.* 43(2):121–32.

VARSAMIS, J., and MACDONALD, S.M. 1972. Manic–depressive disease in childhood. *Can. Psychiat. Assn. J.* 17:279–81.

VAUGHAN, G.F., and LOND, M.B. 1957. Children in hospital. *Lancet* 1:1117–20.

VERNICK, J. 1973. Meaningful communication with the fatally ill child. In *The child in his family,* Vol. 2, *The impact of disease and death.* ed. E.J. Anthony, and C. Koupernik, pp. 105–19. New York: Wiley.

VERNON, D.T.A., SCHULMAN, J.L., and FOLEY, J.M. 1966. Change in children's behavior after hospitalization. *Am. J. Dis. Child.* 3:581–93.

VESTERDAL, J. 1978. Psychological mechanisms in child abusing parents. In *Family violence: An international and Interdisciplinary Study,* ed. J.M. Eekelaar and S.N. Katz, Toronto: Butterworth Pub.

VINCENT, C.E. 1961. *Unmarried mothers.* New York: Free Press of Glencoe.

VINCENT, M.O. 1971. The doctor's life and practice. The doctor's marriage and family. *Nova Scot. Med. Bull.* 50:139–46.

VISHER, E.B., and VISHER, J.S. 1979. *Step-families: A guide to working with stepparents and stepchildren.* New York: Brunner/Mazel.

VISINTAINER, M.A., and WOLFER, J.A. 1975. Psychological preparation for surgical pediatric patients: The effects on children's and parents' stress responses and adjustment. *Pediat.* 56(2) (August):187–202.

VOGEL, E.F., and BELL, N.W. 1960. The emotionally disturbed child as a family scapegoat. *Psychoanal.* 47:21–42.

WALDROP, M.F., and GOERING, J.D. 1971. Hyperactivity and minor physical anomalies in elementary school children. *Am. J. Orthopsychiat.* 42:602–607.

WALDROP, M.F., and HALVERSON, C.F. 1971. Minor physical anomalies and hyperactive behavior in young children. In *Exceptional infant,* Vol. 2. ed. J. Hellmuth, New York: Brunner/Mazel.

WALKER, A. 1977. Incidence of minor physical anomaly in autism. *J. Aut. Child. Schiz.* 7:165–76.

WALKER, S. 1975. Drugging the American child: We're too cavalier about hyperactivity. *J. Learn. Disab.* 8:354–58.

WALLERSTEIN, J.S., and KELLY, J.B. 1980. *Surviving the breakup: How children and parents cope with divorce.* New York: Basic Books.

WALLIN, P., and CLARK, A.L. 1958. Marital satisfaction and husbands' and wives' perception of similarity in their preferred frequency of coitus. *J. Abnorm. Soc. Psychol.* 47:370–73.

WALLINGA, J.V. 1979. The hospitalized child: Intervention and prevention. In *Basic handbook of child psychiatry,* Vol. 4, *Prevention and current issues.* ed. I.N. Berlin and L.A. Stone, pp. 128–35. New York: Basic Books.

736

References

WALSH, B.T. 1980. The endocrinology of anorexia nervosa. *Psychiat. Clin. N. A.* 3(2)(August):299–312.

WARD, A.J. 1970. Early infantile autism: Diagnosis, etiology and treatment. *Psychol. Bull.* 73:350–62.

WARD, F., and BOWER, B.D. 1978. A study of certain social aspects of epilepsy in childhood. Supp. No. 39 to *Dev. Med. & Child Neurol.* 20(1).

WARNICK, L. 1969. The effect upon a family of a child with a handicap. *New Outlook for The Blind* 63:299–304.

WARREN, M.Q. 1978. The impossible child, the difficult child and other assorted delinquents: Etiology, characteristics and incidence. *Can. Psychiat. Assn. J.* 23 (December):SS41–60.

————, AND THE COMMUNITY TREATMENT STAFF. 1966. *Interpersonal maturity level classification: Juvenile: diagnosis of low, middle and high maturity delinquents* Sacramento, Calif.: California Youth Authority.

WARREN, R. 1978. The female offender. In *The psychology of crime and criminal justice,* ed. H. Tock New York: Holt Rinehart & Winston.

WATSON, A.S. 1969. The children of Armageddon: Problems of custody following divorce. *Syracuse Law Rev.* 1:55–86.

WATT, S. 1971. Adolescent medical care: A legal denial of a basic human right. *Ont. Med. Rev.* 38:623–27.

WATZLAWICK, P. 1963. A review of the double bind theory. *Fam. Proc.* 2:132–53.

————, BEAVIN, J., and JACKSON, D. 1967. *Pragmatics of human communication* New York: W.W. Norton.

WATZLAWICK, P., BEAVIN, J., SIKORSKI, L., and MECIA, B. 1970. Protection and scapegoating in pathological families. *Fam. Proc.* 9(1): 27–39.

WEALE, J., and BRADSHAW, J. 1980. Prevalence and characteristics of disabled children: Findings from the 1974 general household survey. *J. Epidem. Comm. H.* 34:111–18.

WECHSLER, D., and JAROS, E. 1965. Schizophrenic patterns on the W.I.S.C. *J. Clin. Psychol.* 21:288–91.

WEINBERG, K.S. 1955. *Incest Behavior.* New York: Citadel Press.

WEINBERG, N., and SANTANA, R. 1978. Comic books: Champions of the disabled stereotype. *Rehab. Lit.* 39(11–12):327–31.

WEINBERG, W.A., RUTMAN, J., SULLIVAN, L. et al. 1973. Depression in children referred to an educational diagnostic center: Diagnosis and treatment. *J. Ped.* 83:1065–72.

WEINER, H. 1977. *Psychobiology and human disease.* New York: Elsevier.

WEINER, I.B. 1962. Father–daughter incest: A clinical report. *Psychiat. Quart.* 36:607–32.

————. 1970. Psychological disturbance in adolescents. In *Psychotherapy,* Wiley Series on Psychological Disorders. New York: Wiley.

————. 1975. *Principles of psychotherapy.* New York: Wiley.

————. 1980. Psychopathology in adolescence. In *Handbook of adolescent psychology,* ed. J. Adelson, pp. 447–71. New York: Wiley Interscience.

WEINER, J.M. 1970. Attitudes of pediatricians toward the care of fatally ill children. *J. Pediat.* 76: 700–705.

WEISNER, T.S., and EIDUSON, B. 1978. Alternate family styles: Effects on young children. In *Mother–child, father–child relationships,* ed. J. Stevens and M. Mathews, pp. 197–221. Washington, D.C.: National Association for the Education of Young Children.

WEISS, G. 1981. Controversial issues of the pharmacotherapy of the hyperactive child. *Can. J. Psychol.* 26:(6) 385–92.

————, HECHTMAN, L., and PERLMAN, T. 1978. Hyperactives as young adults: School, employer, and self-rating scales obtained during 10-year follow-up evaluation. *Am. J. Orthopsychiat.* 48: 438–45.

————, HOPKINS, J., and WENER, A. 1979. Hyperactives as young adults: A controlled prospective 10-year follow-up. *Arch. Gen. Psychiat.* 36: 675–81.

WEISS, G., KRUGER, E., DANIELSON, U., and ELMAN, M. 1975. Effect of long-term treatment of hyperactive children with methylphenidate. *Can. Med. Assn. J.* 112: 159–65.

WEISS, G., MINDE, K., WEERY, J., DOUGLAS, U., and NEMETH, E. 1971. Studies of the hyperactive child, VIII: Five-year follow-up. *Arch. Gen. Psychiat.* 24: 409–14.

WEISS, R.S. 1979. The emotional impact of marital separation. In *Divorce and separation,* ed. G. Levinger and O.C. Moles, pp. 184–201. New York: Basic Books.

WENAR, C., and RUTTENBERG, B. 1976. The use of BRIAC for evaluating therapeutic effectiveness. *J. Aut. & Child Schiz.* 6: 175–91.

WENDER, P.H. 1971. *Minimal brain dysfunction in children,* p. 18 New York: Wiley,

————. 1973. Minimal brain dysfunction in children: Diagnosis and management. *Pediat. Clin. N. Am.* 20(1): 187–202.

————. 1977. The contribution of adoption studies to an understanding of the phenomenology and etiology of borderline schizophrenia. In *Borderline personality disorders: The concepts, the syndrome, the patient,* ed. P. Hartocollis, pp. 255–69. New York: International Univer. Press.

————, ROSENTHAL, D., KETTY, S.S., SCHULSINGER, F. and WELNER, J. 1974. Cross-fostering: A research strategy for clarifying the role of genetic and experimental factors in the etiology of schizophrenia. *Arch. Gen. Psychiat.* 30:121–28.

WERKMAN, S.L. 1965. The psychiatric diagnostic interview with children. *Am. J. Orthopsychiat.* 35: 764–71.

————. 1974. Psychiatric disorders of adolescence. In *American Handbook of psychiatry,* Vol. 2. 2d ed. ed. G. Caplan, pp. 223–33. New York: Basic Books.

WERNER, E.E., and SMITH, R.S. 1979. "An epidemiological perspective on some antecedents and consequences of childhood mental health problems and learning disabilities: A report from the Kauai longitudinal study." *J. Amer. Acad. Child Psychiat.* 18: 292–306.

WERRY, J.S. 1968. Studies on the hyperactive child, IV: An empirical analysis of the minimal brain dysfunction syndrome. *Arch. Gen. Psychiat.* 19: 9–16.

————. 1977. The use of psychotropic drugs in children. *J. Am. Acad. Child Psychiat.* 16: 446–68.

————, and AMAN, M.G. 1975. Methylphenidate and haloperidol in children. *Arch. Gen. Psychiat.* 32: 790–95.

————, and DIAMOND, E. 1980. Imipramine and methylphenidate on hyperactive children. *J. Child Psychol. Psychiat.* 21: 27–35.

WERRY, J.S., DOWRICK, P.W., LAMPEN, E.L., and VAMOS, M.J. 1975. Imipramine in enuresis: Psychological and physiological effects. *J. Child Psychol. Psychiat.* 16: 289–99.

WERRY, J.S., MINDE, K., GURZMAN, A., WEISS, G., DOGAN, K., and HOY, E. 1972. Studies on the hyperactive child. VII: Neurological status compared with neurotic and normal children. *Am. J. Orthopsychiat.* 42(3): 441–51.

WERRY, J.S., and SPRAGUE, R.L. 1972. Psychopharmacology. In *Mental retardation: An annual review,* Vol. 4. ed. J.A. Wortis New York: Grune & Stratton.

————. 1974. Methylphenidate in children: Effect of dosage. *Austr. & N. Z. J. Psychiat.* 8: 9–19.

————, and COHEN, M.N. 1975. Conners' teacher rating scale for use in drug studies with children. *J. Abnorm. Child Psychol.* 3: 217–29.

WERRY, J.S., SPRAGUE, R.L., WEISS, G., and MINDE, K. 1970. Some clinical and laboratory studies of psychotropic drugs in children: An overview. In *Drugs and cerebral function,* ed. W.L. Smith, pp. 134–44. Springfield, Ill.: Chas. C Thomas.

WERRY, J.S., WEISS, G., and DOUGLAS, V. 1964. Studies on the hyperactive child. I: Some preliminary findings. *Can. Psychiat. Assn. J.* 9: 120–30.

WERRY, J.S., and WOLLERSHEIM, J.P. 1967. Behavior therapy with children: A broad overview. *J. Am. Acad. Child Psychiat.* 6: 346–70.

WESSEL, M.A., COBB, J.C., JACKSON, E.B., HARRIS, G.S., and DETWILER, A.C. 1954. Paroxysmal fussing in infancy, sometimes called colic. *Pediat.* 14: 421–35.

WEST, R. 1958. An agnostic's speculations about stuttering. In *Stuttering: A symposium,* ed. J. Eisenson, pp. 167–222. New York: Harper.

————, and ANSBERRY, M. 1957. *The rehabilitation of speech.* 3d ed. New York: Harper.

WESTLEY, W.A., and EPSTEIN, N.B. 1970. *The silent majority.* San Francisco: Jossey, Bass.

WESTMARCK, E.A. 1921. *The history of human marriage.* 5th ed. London: Macmillan.

WHALEN, C.K., and HENKER, B. 1976. Psychostimulants and children: A review and analysis. *Psychol. Bull.* 83: 1113–30.

————. 1980. The social ecology of psychostimulant treatment: A model for conceptual and empirical analysis. In *Hyperactive child: The social ecology of the identification and treatment,* ed. C.K. Whalen and B. Henker, pp. 3–51. New York: Academic Press.

————, COLLINS, B.E., MCAULIFFE, S., and VAUX, A. 1979. Peer interaction in a structured communication task: Comparisons of normal and hyperactive boys and of methylphendiate (ritalin) and placebo effects. *Child Dev.* 50: 388–401.

738

References

WHITAKER, C.A., and KEITH, D.V. 1981. Symbolic–experimental family therapy. In *Handbook of family therapy*, ed. A.S. Gurman and D.P. Kinskern. New York: Brunner/Mazel.

WHITAKER, C.A. and MILLER, M.H. 1969. A re-evaluation of "Psychiatric Help" when divorce impends. *Am. J. Psychiat.* 126(5): 611–18.

WHITE, B.L. 1978. *Experience and the environment.* Vol. 2, *Major influences on the development of the young child.* Englewood Cliffs, N.J.: Prentice-Hall.

————, KABAN, B. et al. 1977. Competence and experience. In *The structuring of experience*, ed. I.C. Uzgiris and F. Weizmann, pp. 115–152. New York: Plenum.

WHITE, J. 1980. Psychopharmacology in childhood: Current status and future prospectives. *Psychiat. Clin. N. Am.* 3(3): 443–54.

WHITE, J.H. 1977. *Pediatric psychopharmacology: A practical guide to clinical application.* Baltimore: Williams & Wilkins.

WHITE, L.A. 1948. The definition and prohibition of incest. *Am. Anthrop.*, 50: 416–35.

WHITELAW, A., MINDE, K., BROWN, J., and FITZHARDINGE, P. 1981. The effect of complications in premature infants on early parent–infant interaction. Submitted for publication.

WIDELITZ, M., and FELDMAN, W. 1969. Pink spot in childhood schizophrenia. *Behav. Neuropsychiat.* 1: 29–30.

WILKES, J.R. 1979. The stresses of fostering. Part I: On the fostering parents. *J. Ont. Assn. Child. Aid Soc.* 22 (November): 1–8.

WILLER, B.S., INTAGLIATA, J.C., and ATKINSON, A.C. 1979. Crises for families of mentally retarded persons, including the crisis of deinstitutionalization. *Brit. J. Ment. Subnorm.* 25(48): 38–49.

WILLERMAN, L. 1973. Activity levels and hyperactivity in twins. *Child Dev.* 44: 288–94.

WILLIAMS, J.I., CRAM, D.M., TANSIG, F.T., and WEBSTER, E.T. 1978. Relative effects of drug and diet on hyperactive behaviors: An experimental study. *Pediat.* 61: 811–17.

WILLIAMS, J.R., and GOLD, M. 1972. From delinquent behavior to official delinquency. *J. Soc. Prob.* 20(2): 209–29.

WILTSE, K.T. 1976. Decision-making needs in foster care. *Child. Today* 5(6): 2–5.

————. 1979. Foster care in the 1970's: A decade of change. *Child. Today* 8(3): 10–14.

WING, J.K., O'CONNOR, N., and LOTTER, V. 1967. Autistic conditions in early childhood: A survey in Middlesex. *Brit. J. Med.* 2: 389–92.

WINN, D., and HALLA, R. 1966. Observations of children who threaten to kill themselves. *Can. Psychiat. Assn. J.* II: Spec. Supp. S-283-294.

WINNICOTT, D.W. 1953. Transitional objects and transitional phenomena: A study of the first not-me possession. *Int. J. Psychoanaly.* 24(2): 89–97.

————. 1957. *The child and the outside world.* London: Tavistock Pub.

————. 1958. Psychoanalysis and the sense of guilt. In *Psychoanalysis and contemporary thought*, ed. J.D. Sutherland, London: Hogarth Press.

————. 1964. *The child, the family and the outside world.* Harmondsworth, Middlesex, U.K.: Penguin Books.

————. 1965. The mentally ill in your caseload. In *The maturational processes and the facilitating environment: Studies in the theory of emotional development*, pp. 217–229. New York: International Univ. Press.

————. 1971. *Therapeutic consultations in child psychiatry.* New York: Basic Books.

————. 1976. The capacity to be alone. In *The maturational processes and the facilitating environment: Studies in the theory of emotional development.* New York: International Univ. Press.

WINSBERG, B.G., and YPES, L.E. 1978. Antipsychotics. In *Pediatric psychopharmacology: The use of behavior modifying drugs in children*, ed. J. Werry, 234–73. New York: Brunner/Mazel.

WOLFF, S. 1969. *Children under stress.* 2d ed. Harmondsworth, Middlesex, U.K.: Penguin Books.

————. 1978. A bell for Roseto: Town loses immunity to stress. *Brain/Mind Bull.* 3(17)(July): 2.

————, and CHESS, S. 1965. An analysis of the language of fourteen schizophrenic children. *J. Child Psychol. Psychiat.* 6: 29–41.

WOLFENSBERGER, W., and MENOLASCINO, F.J. 1970. A theoretical framework for the management of parents of the mentally retarded. In *Psychiatric approaches to mental retardation*, ed. F.J. Menolascino. New York: Basic Books.

WOLFENSTEIN, M. 1966. How is mourning possible? *Psychoanal. Stud. Child.* 21: 93–123.

WOLINS, M. 1963. *Selecting foster parents: The ideal and the reality.* New York: Columbia Univ. Press.

WOLKIND, S., and RUTTER, M. 1973. Children who have been "in care"—An epidemiological study. *J. Child Psychol. Psychiat.* 14: 97–105.

WOLPERT, A., HAGAMEN, M.B., and MERLIS, S. 1967. A comparative study of thiothixene and trifluoperazine in childhood schizophrenia. *Curr. Therap. Res.* 9: 482–85.

WOLPERT, E.A. 1975. Manic–depressive illness as an actual neurosis. In *Depression and human existence,* ed. E.J. Anthony and T. Benedek, pp. 199–221. Boston: Little, Brown.

WOLRAICH, M., DRUMMOND, T., KERNER SALOMON, M., O'BRIEN, M., and SIVAGE, C. 1978. Effects of methylphenidate alone and in combination with behavior modification procedures on the behavior and academic performance of hyperactive children. *J. Abnorm. Child. Psychol.* 6: 149–61.

WOOD, D.R., REIMHERR, F.W., WENDER, P.H., and JOHNSON, G.E. 1976. Diagnosis and treatment of minimal brain dysfunction in adults. *Arch. Gen. Psychiat.* 33 (December): 1453–60.

WOODS, G. 1975. *The handicapped child: Assessment of management.* Philadelphia: Blackwell Scientific Pub.

WORLAND, J. 1976. Effects of positive and negative feedback on behavioral control in hyperactive and normal boys. *J. Abnorm. Child Psychol.* 4: 315–26.

WORLD HEALTH ORGANIZATION 1962. *Deprivation of maternal care: A reassessment of its effects.* World Health Organization, Public Health Papers, No. 14, Geneva.

————. 1965. *International statistical classification of diseases, injuries and causes of death.* 8th rev. Geneva: World Health Organization.

————. 1977. *Manual of the international statistical classification of diseases, injuries, and causes of death.* 9th rev. (ICD-9). Geneva: World Health Organization.

WRIGHT, B.A. 1960. *Physical disability: A psychological approach.* New York: Harper & Row.

WURTMAN, R.J., and FERNSTROM, J.D. 1976. Control of brain neurotransmitter synthesis by precursors availability and nutritional state. *Biochem. Pharmacol.* 25: 1691–96.

WYNN, A., and WYNN, M. 1976. *Prevention of handicap of perinatal origin: An introduction to French policy and legislation.* London: Foundation for Educational Research in Childbearing.

————. Characteristics of cost effective maternal and child helath care. Address presented at the Canadian Association for Young Children Conference in Winnipeg, Manitoba, 13 October 1978.

WYNNE, L.C. RYCKOFF, I.M., DAY, J., and HIRSCH, S.I. 1958. Pseudomutuality in the family relations of schizophrenics. *Psychiat.* 21: 205–220.

WYNNE, L.C., and SINGER, M.T. 1963. Thought disorder and family relations of schizophrenics. *Arch. Gen. Psychiat.* 9: 191–98.

YARROW, L.J. 1967. The development of focused relationships during infancy. In *Exceptional infant, Vol. 1: The normal infant,* ed. J. Hellmuth Seattle, Wash.: Special Child Publication.

YATES, A.J. 1958. The application of learning theory to the treatment of tics. *J. Abnorm. Psychol.* 56: 175.

YELLOLY, M.A. 1965. Factors relating to an adoption decision by the mothers of illegitimate infants. *Sociol. Rev.* 13: 5–14.

YOUNG, D. (Ed.) 1972. *The modern american family.* New York: Arno Press.

YOUNG, D.R., NELSON, R.R., ZAMOFF, R.B., JACKSON, E.L., LYLE, J.R., and KRASHINSKY, M. 1973. *Public policy for day care of young children: Organization, finance and planning.* Lexington, Mass.: Lexington Books.

YOUNGERMAN, J., and CANINO, I.A. 1978. Lithium carbonate use in children and adolescents: A survey of the literature. *Arch. Gen. Psychiat.* 35: 216–24.

ZEIDEL, A. 1973 Problems of emotional adjustment in juvenile diabetes. In *The child in his family,* Vol. 2, *The impact of disease and death.* E.J. Anthony and C. Koupernik. New York: Wiley.

ZELNIK, M., and KANTNER, J. 1974. The resolution of teenage first pregnancies. *Fam. Plan. Persp.* 6(2): 74–80.

ZENTALL, S. 1975. Optimal stimulation as theoretical basis of hyperactivity. *Am. J. Orthopsychiat.* 45: 549–63.

ZENTALL, S.S., and ZENTALL, T.R. 1976. Activity and task performance of hyperactive children as a function of environmental stimulation. *J. Cons. Clin. Psychol.* 44: 693–97.

ZINKUS, P.W. 1979. Behavioral and emotional sequelae of learning disorders. In *Current issues in developmental pediatrics: The learning–disabled child,* ed. M.I. Gottlieb, P.W. Zinkus, and L.J. Bradfore. New York: Grune & Stratton.

GLOSSARY

ADDISON'S DISEASE—Adrenal insufficiency results in anemia, general langor and debility, feebleness of heart action, irritability of the stomach, and a color change in the skin.

AFFECT/AFFECTIVE—Affect: An immediately expressed and observed emotion. A feeling state becomes an affect when it is observable, for example as overall demeanor, or tone and modulation of voice. Affect is to be distinguished from mood, which refers to a pervasive and sustained emotion. Affect is to mood as weather is to climate.

AFFECTIVE DISORDER(s)—Disorders of mood, including depression and mania.

AGNOSIA—Lack or loss of the ability to understand the meaning or to recognize the importance of various types of stimuli, especially in the nonlanguage field.

AKATHISIA—Motor restlessness and, specifically, a feeling of muscular quivering; one of the possible complications of treatment with phenothiazines. The symptoms often make it difficult for patients to remain still day or night.

ALLERGENS—Substances to which the body is allergic and will react if sufficient antibodies are formed by the body's immune system.

AMBIVALENCE—The simultaneous occurrence of two strong but opposite feelings.

AMENHORRHEA—Absence or cessation of the menses, or menstrual periods. Also called Amensia.

AMENTIA—(Feeblemindedness, mental retardation, hypophrenia, oligophrenia, oligergasia.) Subnormal development of the mind, with particular reference to intellectual capacities, present from birth or from the early months of life.

AMNIOCENTESIS—The removal of fluid from the amniotic sac, a process useful in diagnosing many fetal deformities.

ANAL-SADISTIC—Relating to the aggression, destructiveness, negativism, and externally directed rage that are typical components of the second portion of the anal stage of development and its holdovers in later life.

ANOREXIA/ANOREXIC—Loss of appetite.

ANOREXIA NERVOSA—A psychiatric syndrome usually occurring in young women. The cardinal features are self-imposed reduction of food intake, severe weight loss, and amenorrhea.

ANTIEMETIC—A drug that prevents or alleviates nausea and vomiting.

ANTIMETABOLITES—Drugs which interfere with the normal metabolic process of cell division. They are used in the treatment of malignancies (cancer) and are being used in some chronic inflammatory conditions such as inflammatory bowel disease.

ANTISOCIAL—Opposed or antagonistic to accepted societal values. Generally used to describe behavior or personalities that actively contravene society's laws and behavioral codes.

ANXIOLYTIC DRUGS—One of the five groups of psychotrophic drugs. Also known as *minor tranquilizers*, or *psycholeptics*. They reduce pathologic anxiety, tension, and agitation without therapeutic effects on disturbed cognitive or perceptual processes. They may lower the

741

convulsive threshold and have a high potential for drug dependency. Included in this group are meprobamate and derivatives, diazepoxides, and benzodiazapines.

APPERCEPTION—Conscious realization; the awareness of the significance of what is perceived, especially through relating percepts to similar, already existing knowledge.

ARTERIOSCLEROSIS—A group of diseases characterized by thickening and loss of elasticity of arterial walls.

ASOCIAL—Indifferent to, or unaffected by, accepted societal expectations, codes, and values.

ASYMPTOMATIC—Showing or causing no symptoms.

ATAXIA/ATAXIC—Absence or lack of order. Refers in neurology to inability to maintain balance or unstreadiness in gait.

ATHETOID—Resembling athetosis.

ATHETOSIS—Repeated slow, writhing, involuntary movements, especially of the fingers and hands.

ATTENTION DEFICIT DISORDER—See chapter 10.

ATTENTION SPAN—The length of time that the individual can fix his/her attention on a given activity without losing interest or being distracted.

AUTOSOMAL CHROMOSOME—One of the pairs of ordinary chromosomes (as opposed to the sex chromosomes) composed of genes which carry the genetic code.

AUTOEROTIC (EROTISM)—Spontaneous sexual emotion generated in the absence of an external stimulus proceeding directly or indirectly from another person. Common usage has made autoeroticism synonymous with masturbation, but masturbation is just one common form of autoerotic activity.

AUTOIMMUNE MECHANISMS—The body reacts to some of its own tissues as if they were a foreign protein and develops an immune response directed against its own tissues. (See also immune mechanisms)

AUTONOMIC NERVOUS SYSTEM—The autonomic nervous system, at times called the vegetative nervous system, is that part of the nervous system that regulates those bodily activities that are carried out usually outside conscious awareness. The beating of the heart and circulation of the blood, breathing, digestion, and temperature regulation are examples of bodily processes under the control of the autonomic nervous system. (See biofeedback mechanism.)

AUTOSOMAL DOMINANTS (GENES)—A gene on an autosomal chromosome which, if present, will assert itself over a recessive gene received from the other parent

AUTOSOMAL RECESSIVE GENE—A gene on an autosomal chromosome which, if present, will assert itself only if the same recessive gene is received from the other parent. If the other parent has a contrasting dominant gene, the recessive gene will not be expressed in the offspring, though it may be transmitted to the offspring who are then termed *carriers* of the trait or quality in question.

BARBITURATES—A group of drugs commonly prescribed as sedatives which depress the central nervous system causing first disinhibition and then drowsiness. As street drugs, they are known as "downers." (See also anxiolytic drugs.)

BASAL GANGLIA—Specific interconnected gray masses deep in the cerebral hemispheres and in the upper brainstem; they are involved in motor coordination.

BEHAVIORAL DEFENSES—Behavior which serves as a defense against psychological conflict.

BELL-SHAPED CURVE—The normal distribution curve.

BIOFEEDBACK MECHANISM—Biofeedback is the physiological mechanism whereby an individual can control certain bodily functions such as heart rate, basal metabolic rate, blood pressure, and so forth, which were until recently thought to be totally under the control of the autonomic system. Since people can be trained to develop a greater degree of control over these autonomic functions, they can thereby achieve concomitant changes in mood such as tranquility, relaxation, the inducement of a dreamlike state, etc.

BIOPSY—A section of tissue taken for microscopic examination to reach a diagnosis.

BRONCHIAL TREE—The bronchial tubes through which air passes to reach the air spaces in the lung.

BONDING—The formation of long-lasting attachments between individuals or groups, for example, early infant–mother bonding, marital bonding.

BUCCAL SMEARS—Smears from the lining of the cheek that are viewed microscopically to detect chromosomal (i.e., genetic) abnormalities.

Glossary

CAROTENE PIGMENTED SKIN—A yellowing of the skin, resembling jaundice, resulting from the presence of excessive carotene in the blood. Carotene is a chromolipoid hydrocarbon found in carrots, sweet potatoes, leafy vegetables, milk fat, and egg yolk as well as body fat.

CACHEXIA—Malnourishment resulting in weight loss, usually from a chronic disease process.

CAT SCAN—Computerized axial tomography scan; a scan involving x-rays which give a display of the body in cross section on a cathode ray tube.

CATARACTS—A loss of transparency of the lens of the eye.

CATATONIA (Catatonic Schizophrenia)—A form of schizophrenia characterized by extreme negativism, phases of stupor or excitement, impulsive posturing, and stereotyped and highly ritualistic behavior.

CENTRAL NERVOUS SYSTEM—The brain and spinal cord together constitute the central nervous system.

CEREBELLUM—The posterior mass of the brain, concerned primarily with coordination of movement. The main symptom of cerebellar dysfunction is incoordination.

CEREBRAL DOMINANCE—If the left hemisphere of the cerebrum is dominant, the individual will be right handed and vice versa.

CEREBRUM—The principal part of the brain, occupying most of the skull. Disturbed functioning of its outer layer (the cerebral cortex) results in intellectual dysfunctioning and confusion.

CEREBRAL PALSY—See chapter 22 for definition.

CHOREA—A disorder characterized by multiple, irregular, spasmodic involuntary movements of the limbs or facial muscles.

COREIC/CHOREIFORM—Resembling chorea.

CHROMOSOMAL TRANSLOCATIONS—The situation when part of a chromosome, split off from where it belongs, has become attached to another chromosome where it may be responsible for genetic malfunctioning.

CHRONIC PANCREATITIS—Chronic disease of the pancreas.

CLEFT LIP AND PALATE—A congenital deformity in which the right and left sides of the lip and/or palate fail to join in the midline, leaving a variable gap between them.

COELIAC DISEASE—A disease of infants and young children in which an inability to digest gluten (in wheat flour) results in impaired absorption of ingested foods with resultant diarrhea and interference with growth.

COGNITIVE/COGNITION—Referring to the set of mental processes involved in gaining or integrating knowledge, and in problem solving. The processes involved—discrimination, judgement, remembering, and reasoning—are based on sensory perception.

COLIC—Spasmodic contractions of smooth muscles or ducts; infant colic, often occurring in the first 4 months of life, refers to recurrent episodes of intestinal colic and the associated pain and irritability.

COLLAGEN—A protein present in connective tissue, bone, and cartilage.

COLOSTOMY—A surgical opening of the large bowel (colon) onto the abdominal wall, performed because of chronic disease of the lower bowel or rectum.

COMMUNITY CARE—Care for retarded or handicapped individuals in their own homes, foster homes, or group homes, assisted by a variety of specialized community services, rather than in large institutions separated from the community.

CONDUCT DISORDER—See chapter 13 for definition.

CONFLICT RESOLUTION—Ability to resolve conflict. Failure of conflict resolution usually results in chronic tension.

CONGENITAL RECEPTIVE DYSPHASIA—An inherited impairment in the ability to understand speech.

CONSTITUTION—The relatively constant physiological composition and biological makeup of a person, resulting largely from inherited tendencies but to some extent modified by past environmental experiences whose effects have permanently influenced the individual.

CONVERSION DISORDERS—See chapter 12 for definition.

COPROLALIA—The involuntary uttering of vulgar or obscene words.

COPROPHAGIA—The eating of feces.

CORTISOL HYPERSECRETIONS—An oversecretion of hormones of the adrenal cortex, one of the endocrine glands.

COUNTERTRANSFERENCE—One aspect of the professional's emotional reaction to his/her patient (client). While at times triggered by the patient's behavior or the ongoing interaction between them, countertransference results from the often unrecognized influence of the vulnerabilities, attitudes, and conflicts derived from the therapist's past life which are still very much operative in the present. For example, a therapist may believe that a child's refusal to cooperate is the source of his/her frustration, not realizing that it is really the therapist's discomfort with his/her own inability to control the situation, and to be successful in his/her attempts to help that child, that is accounting for the extreme annoyance.

COVERT CONFLICT—Conflict that is masked from others and carried on despite a facade of amiability.

CRANIAL MALFORMATION—A malformation of the bones of the skull.

CRANIAL SUTURES—The junction points where the separate bones which together make up the skull meet and fuse.

CROHN'S DISEASE—A chronic inflammatory disease of the bowel, particularly affecting the small intestine.

CUSHING'S SYNDROME—A complex condition resulting from oversecretion or overadministration of the hormones of the cortex of the adrenal gland. Cushinoid (Cushing-like) signs such as obesity of the head and neck (moon face) and increased facial acne are common complications of the corticosteroids used to treat many chronic inflammatory diseases.

CYANOSIS/CYANOTIC—A bluish coloring of the skin and mucous membranes which results from insufficient oxygen supply to the tissues.

CYSTIC FIBROSIS—A congenital chronic disease which features widespread changes in the mucus secreting glands of the body leading to eventual destruction of the pancreas and repeated respiratory infections. Until recently, few children who had the disease survived into adolescence. Improved treatment has allowed many sufferers to survive at least into young adulthood.

CYTOMEGALOVIRUS—A rare viral disease, affecting multiple organ systems, one of which can be the brain, which can be severely damaged. Least uncommon in newborn infants.

DECEREBRATE—Removal of the brain, either surgically or as a result of an injury which severs the nerve pathways connecting brain and spinal cord. In either case, because of the lack of connection, the organism is deprived of the highly complex and sophisticated functions normally controlled by the cerebral cortex (e.g., speech, hearing, vision, thought, voluntary movements, etc.) and so exists at a brainstem level (i.e., with respiration, circulation of the blood, temperature control, digestion, elimination, and some reflex activities remaining,) but no more.

DECIBELS—A measure of the intensity of sound, often used to indicate the level at which the individual can hear.

DECOMPENSATION—Breakdown or failure in the functioning of the defense system, such as occurs in relapses in schizophrenic patients, which leads to a deterioration of the customary level of adjustment.

DEEP CIRCULAR CONSTRICTION—Congenital narrowing of a limb at any point without complete amputation.

DEEP TENDON REFLEXES—Involuntary muscular contractions following percussion of a tendon or bone (e.g., the knee jerk). Increased, decreased, or unequal reflexes can indicate disease of the nervous and/or muscular systems.

DEFENSE MECHANISM, DEFENSES—See chapter 12 for definition.

DENIAL—A defense mechanism which consists of a refusal to admit the truth or any unpleasant reality, even to oneself.

DEGENERATIVE MYOPATHY—A disease in which muscle tissue is destroyed.

DERMATOMYOSITIS—An inflammatory and degenerative disease of the muscles followed by swelling, hardening, and calcium.

DEVELOPMENTAL CRISIS—Symptoms of a brief and transient nature related to, and arising from, periods of temporarily increased anxiety generated by the process of normal development.

DEVELOPMENTAL DEVIATIONS—Those deviations in development which may be considered abnormal in that they occur at a time, in a sequence, or to a degree not expected for a given age-level or stage of development.

DIABETES MELLITUS—A disease resulting from failure to produce sufficient insulin, a hormone essential to the successful utilization of sugars by the body; can be controlled but not cured by the right combination of diet, exercise, and, if necessary, daily insulin injections.

DIATHESIS—A constitutional state predisposed to any disease or group of diseases—for example, epileptic diathesis—a predisposition to epilepsy.

DISPLACEMENT—A defense mechanism in which strong feelings are shifted or transferred from the original ideas or people to whom they were attached. For example, a child with school phobia may not recognize how angry he/she is at the mother because he/she has displaced the anger to his/her teacher, whom he/she must then avoid.

DIZYGOTIC—Derived from two separate fertilized ova, for example, fraternal, as opposed to identical, twins.

DOPAMINE SYSTEM—See chapter 29 for definition.

DOPAMINERGIC—A substance acting upon the dopamine system.

DOUBLE BLIND STUDY—An experimental study in which neither the subject nor the experimenter is aware of which subjects are receiving treatment and which are being given placebo. By minimizing subjective influences, by both subject and experimenter, a double blind study gives a truer picture of the pharmacologic effect of the drug being tested.

DRIVES—Strong biological or social pressures experienced by the individual which demand relief. Common biological drives include hunger, thirst, elimination, sex. Common social drives include the drive for attachment, the need for companionship, and so forth.

DYSARTHRIA—Imperfect articulation of speech.

DYSGRAPHIA—A disturbance in handwriting originating from a dysfunction affecting those areas of the brain which govern the act of writing.

DYSLEXIA—Disturbance in learning to read, due to dysfunction or a lesion affecting those areas of the brain governing the act of reading.

DYSPHAGIA—Difficulty in swallowing.

DYSPHASIA—Impairment of speech due to a lesion in the dominant hemisphere of the cerebral cortex. This results in a lack of coordination and an inability to combine words for effective speech.

DYSRHYTHMIA—Defective rhythm.

DYSTHMIC—Pertaining to disorders of feeling, particularly depression.

DYSTONIA MUSCULORUM—A progressive syndrome of involuntary choreoathetoid movements involving most muscle groups, causing peculiar, grotesque, twisting movements of the entire body.

ECHOLALIA—The meaningless repetition of words or phrases.

EEG SCAN (ELECTROENCEPHALOGRAM)—The graphic record of the electrical activity of the brain, usually obtained by means of electrodes attached to the scalp. The regular, spontaneous oscillations of the electrical potential of the brain are amplified and recorded on an oscillograph. Characteristic changes in the type, frequency, and potential of the brain waves occur in various intercranial lesions.

EGO—A theoretical construct used to refer to one of the psychic structures or systems within the mental apparatus; the "executive" portion of the personality, which perceives, discriminates, and integrates stimuli from the external world and from within. The ego employs thought processes, communication, defenses, tension regulation, and other devices in achieving adaptation to reality.

EGO-ALIEN—Anything that is unacceptable to the ego. Its opposite is ego-syntonic.

EGOCENTRIC—Concerned excessively with oneself. The term should not be used synonymously with narcissistic.

ELECTROCONVULSIVE THERAPY—A form of somatic treatment for certain psychiatric conditions—mania, depression, and some cases of schizophrenia—which uses an electrical stimulus to the central nervous system in order to influence the course of the condition.

ELECTROLYTE DEPLETION—Excessive loss of ions from the body, leading to disturbances of acid-base balance or electrical conduction.

ELECTROMYOGRAM, ELECTROMYOGRAPHY—A graphic record of the electric currents through the muscles. The process of obtaining electromyograms.

ENDOCRINE SYSTEM—The system of the ductless glands, which produces hormones that govern many aspects of growth and metabolism.

ENDOGENOUS—Internally caused, in contrast with exogenous (i.e., externally caused).

ETIOLOGY/AETIOLOGY—The study of the cause of a disease.

EUGENICS—The systematically organized efforts of preventive medicine to improve average human qualities through (a) encouraging reproduction by persons biologically most highly qualified, and (b) preventing parenthood among those least qualified physically and mentally.

EUTHANASIA—Artificially putting an end to someone's life in cases of incurable or painful disease.

EXTRAPYRAMIDAL TRACT—Those nerve tracts whose main action is concerned with automatic movements involved in postural adjustment and with autonomic regulation. Disorders of the extrapyramidal system may occur either from damage to the nervous system (e.g., cerebral palsy) or as a side effect of certain medications (e.g., phenothiazines).

EPIGENETIC—A theory which holds that development proceeds in an orderly, steplike manner through a series of stages, each of which represents a higher level of function than its predecessors.

ESOTROPIA—Deviation of a visual axis toward that of the other eye when fusion is a possibility, as in cross-eyes or squint.

ESSENTIAL HYPERTENSION—See Hypertension/Essential Hypertension.

ENURESIS—Defined in chapter 9.

ENMESHMENT—Defined in chapter 3.

FAMILY SYSTEM—See chapter 3 for definition.

FEBRILE—Having a fever.

FETAL ANOXIA—Distress of the fetus resulting from lack of oxygen. If severe and/or prolonged, may cause permanent damage, especially to the brain.

FETISH—A part of the body or some object associated with a loved person that replaces and substitutes for the loved person. Although sexual activity with the loved person may occur, gratification is possible only in the presence of the fetish, or, at least, if it is fantasied during such activity. Typically, the fetishist can obtain sexual gratification from the fetish alone, in the absence of the person for whom it substitutes.

FINE AND GROSS MOTOR COORDINATION—Gross coordination refers to the coordination of major movements and large muscle groups, in contrast with fine muscle coordination which deals with smaller movements (e.g., those of the finger) which require more precision.

FLEXOR PLANTAR RESPONSES—A reflex: the normal downward curling of the toes evoked by stroking the sole of the foot. Its opposite, an extension of the great toe and fanning of the toes occurs normally in infants less than 1 year old, but thereafter in a number of conditions all of which indicate serious neurological disease.

FUNCTIONAL DISORDERS—A disturbance in the functioning of one or more organs, but without any accompanying lesion or change in structure. Usually used to indicate the absence of organic disease.

FUGUE STATE—A condition in which the patient suddenly leaves his or her previous activity and begins to wander, or goes on a journey which has no apparent relation to what he or she has been doing and for which he has amnesia afterwards. Fugues may occur with epilepsy (twilight state), as a form of catatonic excitement, or as a form of conversion hysteria (dissociative reaction).

GENERIC AGENCIES—Agencies providing a broad range of services, as opposed to one providing only highly specialized services within a more limited range.

GENETICS—The science of natural development and the laws of heredity (as opposed to eugenics, which is the science of development through artificial selection).

GENOTYPE—The genetic inheritance; the sum total of the physical and psychological characteristics carried in the chromosomes.

GESTALT—The total quality of the image perceived (i.e., the overall perceptual experience) is more than just the sum of the various stimuli presented. Rather the total response is a pattern (i.e., a gestalt) which differs from the original stimulus in that it is organized and modified by the past experience and integrative mechanisms of the individual exposed to the perception. For example, someone who becomes violently ill whenever he/she tastes

Glossary

seafood will have a very different response to a broiled lobster than will someone for whom lobster is a favorite food, although what is seen and smelled is the same.

GLIOSIS—Overgrowth or tumor of the neuroglia (the supporting structure of the nerves).

GROWTH—Increase in size and weight, resulting from an increase in the number and size of the cells.

GUILT—A feeling of regret or self-recrimination for having done a wrong (or unworthy or evil) thing, experienced by a person who has a basic feeling of self-worth or self-respect. (See also Shame.)

GYNECOMASTIA—Breast enlargement in a male.

HEMANGIOMA—A tumor composed of multiplied and dilated blood vessels.

HALOPERIDOL—See chapter 29 for definition.

HERITABILITY—A general genetic term synonymous with inheritability.

HIRSUTISM—Having an excessive growth of body and facial hair.

HOMEODYNAMIC—See Homeostasis.

HOMEOSTASIS—The tendency of an organism to maintain a constancy and stability of its internal environment; the result of the various automatic mechanisms which adjust and adapt the organism to changes in the external or internal environment.

HOSPITALISM—The condition of physical and psychological disturbance and retardation, increased susceptibility to illness, apathy, and profound sadness occurring in children confined to prolonged institutional care, whether in hospitals or orphanages, where physical needs are met and emotional needs ignored.

HYDROCEPHALUS—A usually congenital condition which causes excessive accumulation of fluid in the cerebral ventricles. These are dilated, compressing and damaging the cerebral cortex, separating the cerebral sutures, and enlarging the head if not adequately treated.

HYPERACTIVITY/HYPERKINESIS—Excessive muscular activity; exaggerated motility.

HYPERREFLEXIA—A condition in which the deep tendon reflexes are exaggerated.

HYPERSOMNIA—Excessive need for sleep.

HYPERTELORISM—Having an unusually broad space between the eyes.

HYPERTENSION/ESSENTIAL HYPERTENSION—High arterial blood pressure. Essential hypertension—hypertension without any known cause.

HYPERTHYROIDISM—An abnormality of the thyroid gland in which thyroid secretion is usually increased and is no longer under the regulatory control of hypothalamic-pituitary centers.

HYPERVENTILATION—Overventilation, overbreathing; increased alveolar ventilation relative to metabolic carbon dioxide production so that alveolar carbon dioxide pressure tends to fall below normal. Can cause dizziness and fainting.

HYPNAGOGIA—Disorders of perception occurring just as the individual is falling asleep or awakening.

HYPOACTIVE—Less than usually active.

HYPOGLYCEMIA—Abnormally low level of blood sugar, usually due to excessive levels of insulin and/or excessive exercise balanced by too little food. If severe, may lead to coma and/or death.

HYPOMANIA—Elevation of mood, increased activity, sense of exaggerated well-being and impaired judgment, short of degree of impairment seen in fully developed mania.

HYPOTHALAMIC-ADRENAL AXIS—The influence of the hypothalamus (part of the pituitary system) on the function of the adrenal gland, mediated by specific hormone output.

HYPOTHALAMIC-OVARIAN AXIS—The influence of the hypothalamus (part of the pituitary system) on the function of the ovarian glands mediated by specific hormone output.

HYPOTHYROIDISM—Syndrome resulting from lack of sufficient thyroid hormone, which causes marked lowering of the metabolism.

IATROGENIC DISEASE—Caused by a physician; a condition resulting from inappropriate treatment by a physician or other member(s) of the "helping" or health professions.

IDENTITY FORMATION—The process by which an individual develops a sense of himself/herself as a distinct/unique person with qualities of his/her own.

ILEOSTOMY—An opening of the small bowel (ileum) onto the abdominal wall, sometimes necessary to bypass (and allow a chance to rest) a chronically inflamed section of the small bowel.

IMMUNE MECHANISMS—The mechanisms by which the body mobilizes to defend itself against the intrusion of/invasion of proteins (i.e., allergens) it recognizes as abnormal. (See also autoimmune mechanisms).

IMMUNOLOGICAL REACTIVITY—The capacity of the immune system to defend via an immune response to invasion by an allergen (foreign protein).

INFANTILE AUTISM—The most severe form of psychosis of childhood, whose cardinal features are extreme withdrawal and failure to respond to others, gross deficits in language development and onset before 30 months. See also chapter 15.

INSOMNIA—Excessive wakefulness; the inability to fall asleep in the absence of external interferences.

INTENTION TREMOR—A tremor that is aggravated when the individual attempts a voluntary movement.

INTRACRANIAL VASCULAR LESIONS—An abnormality of the blood vessels inside the skull.

INTRAPSYCHIC—Refers to sensations, feelings or thoughts occurring within the psyche or mental apparatus of the individual.

IQ—Intelligence Quotient. Measure of performance on a standardized test of intellectual functioning.

IRRITABLE COLON SYNDROME—Sometimes termed spastic colon, this syndrome consists of crampy abdominal pain and diarrhea with mucus in the stools resulting from overactivity of the bowel. Emotional tension is considered a frequent cause or contributor.

KAYSER-FLEISCHER RING—A yellow-green pigmented ring around the cornea of the eye; characteristic of Wilson's Disease.

KERNICTERUS—Staining of the basal ganglia of the brain by bile pigments associated with jaundice of the newborn. At one time, was a common cause of cerebral palsy.

LABILITY/LABILE—Free and uncontrolled expression of the emotions (suggests instability).

LATENCY—A psychoanalytic term denoting the period of life extending from the end of the infantile to the beginning of the adolescent stage, i.e., about age 5 to puberty.

LATENT—Not visible or apparent; dormant, quiescent.

LATERALITY—Handedness; right or left dominance of the cerebral cortex.

LEAD ENCEPHALOPATHY—The brain damage resulting from the absorption of lead.

LESION—A wound, injury, or site of pathological change in the body.

LOBOTOMY—Division of the nerve tracts of the cerebral cortex, usually in the prefrontal area of the brain, as a surgical treatment for mental illness. Lobotomized: one who has had a lobotomy.

LONG-TERM MEMORY—The ability to store and recall information from the recent or distant past. Information received is first stored in short-term memory where it decays in a matter of seconds unless it is moved into long-term memory by means of rehearsal.

LONG-TERM VISUAL SEQUENTIAL MEMORY—The ability to remember what a sequence of letters or words looks like for an extended period of time. A defect in this causes major difficulty in spelling and reading.

LUMBOSACRAL REGION—The region of the lumbar spine and the sacrum; that is, the lower back, just above the buttocks.

LUTEINIZING HORMONES—A glycoprotein hormone stimulating the final ripening of the follicles and the secretion of progesterone by one of them, their rupture to release the egg, and the conversion of the ruptured follicle into the corpus luteum.

MANIC-DEPRESSIVE—A severe form of affective disorder in which periods of mania alternate with periods of severe depression—bipolar affective disorder (see chapter 14).

MASKED—Concealed, or finding alternative representation; for example, masked depression showing as hyperactivity and irritability rather than as sadness.

MASOCHISTIC PERSONALITY—A person with a recurrent need to expose himself/herself to pain or punishment.

MENINGITIS—An inflammation of the coverings of the brain (the meninges).

METASTASIZE—The process by which a disease (especially a malignant tumor) invades or spreads to other parts of the body.

METABOLISM—Tissue change; the sum of chemical changes occurring in tissue, consisting of anabolism—those reactions which convert small molecules into large, and catabolism—those reactions that convert large molecules into small.

Glossary

MICROCEPHALY—Abnormal smallness of the head, usually resulting from premature closure of the cranial sutures and associated with compression damage to the brain.

MINIMAL BRAIN DAMAGE—A formerly used diagnostic category in which there was a postulated but not clearly determined neurological impairment to account for such clinical pictures as attention disorders and autism. (See chapter 10)

MIXED LATERALITY—Instead of one cerebral hemisphere being clearly dominant, functioning suggests that both hemispheres are incompletely dominant, leading to ambidexterity (or ambilaterality).

MODALITIES—Methods of therapeutic intervention, for example, group, individual, family, and so forth.

MONOZYGOTIC—Denoting twins derived from a single fertilized ovum (identical twins). In contrast to dizygotic—twins derived from two fertilized ova (fraternal twins).

MORBIDITY—Sickness; suffering.

MOTOR CORTEX—That part of the cerebral cortex which mediates motor activities.

MULTIFACTORIAL—More than one factor acting together is needed to produce a common result.

MYASTHENIA GRAVIS—A severe, chronic disease characterized by abnormal fatiguability of skeletal muscles which ultimately proves fatal, often after a number of remissions and exacerbations.

MYELOMENINGOCELE—Failure of fusion of the spine in the midline (i.e., spina bifida) with protrusion of the spinal cord and its coverings, the meninges.

NARCISSISTIC—Preoccupied with self; ignoring the needs of others.

NEOPLASMS—Tumor (literally "new growth").

NEPHROTIC SYNDROME—Nephritis—infection of the kidneys: Nephrotic syndrome—a chronic illness characterized by excessive swelling of the lower parts of the body caused by excessive loss of proteins in the urine and lower levels of proteins in blood plasma due to disease of the kidneys.

NEURODERMATITIS—Inflammation of the skin of nervous or psychogenic origin.

NEUROFIBROMATOSIS—The occurrence of multiple tumors resulting from localized proliferation of the fibrous structure of the nerves.

NEUROGENIC—Caused by the nerves, the nervous system.

NEURONS—Nerve cells.

NEUROPHYSIOLOGY—Normal physiology of the nervous system.

NEUROTIC DEFENSES—See chapter 12 for definition.

NIGHT TERRORS—See chapter 9 for definition.

NORMALIZATION PRINCIPLE—Any individual is best served when living in as close to normal a situation as possible.

NORMAL STATISTICAL CURVE—Expected distribution of a characteristic above and below the mean.

NYSTAGMUS—Rhythmical oscillation of the eyeballs, either horizontal, vertical, or circular.

OBJECT PERMANENCE—The ability of a child to retain a mental image of an object even when it is no longer present.

OBSESSIVE–COMPULSIVE—See chapter 12 for definition.

OBSESSIVE PERSONALITY TYPES—See chapter 12 for definition.

OCCIPITAL—Related to the occiput, the posterior portion of the cranium.

OLIGROPHRENIA—Feeble mindedness, mental weakness.

OPISTHOTONUS—A prolonged muscular spasm causing marked arching of the body which is bowed backward, resting on the head and on the heels.

OPTIC ATROPHY—Wasting of the optic nerve which supplies the retina and is essential for vision.

OPTIC FUNDI—The back wall of the eye, as seen through an ophthalmoscope.

ORAL–SADISTIC—A psychoanalytic term used to characterize the second 6 months of life, emphasizing the exploratory activities and at times the hurtful element (biting).

ORGANIC ILLNESS (SYMPTOMS)—Organic symptoms result from a change in the structure as well as the function of one or more organs, in contrast with functional conditions, in which the change in function is not accompanied by a change in structure.

OTITIS—Inflammation of the ear.

PALLIATIVE—Intended to reduce the severity of symptoms, not cure the disease.

PARAESTHAESIAS/PARESTHESIA—Abnormal sensations; that is, numbness, tingling, burning, and the like.

PARANOID—Unduly suspicious of being watched, followed, harassed, or persecuted.

PARENTERAL—By injection.

PAROXYSMAL, INAPPROPRIATE DISCHARGES OF IMPULSE—Irregular, abnormal discharges.

PATHOGENS/PATHOGENESIS—Pathogenesis: The process of development of disease. Pathogens: Any substances (e.g., bacterium, virus, other) which cause a disease.

PATHOGNOMIC—Characteristic of a particular disease.

PATHOLOGICAL—Pertaining to, or derived from, an illness or disorder.

PATHOPHYSIOLOGY—The physiology of the disordered function.

PEPTIC ULCER—Ulceration of the lining of the stomach or duodenum.

PERINATAL—Occurring in the period shortly before, during, or after birth.

PERIPHERAL VASODILATATION—Dilatation (expansion) of the blood vessels at the outer or distant parts of the body.

PERSONALITY DISORDERS—See chapter 12 for definition.

PERSONALITY INTEGRATION—The development of a harmonious relationship between cognitive, personal and affective components of an individual's personality that leads to effective social functioning.

PERVASIVE DEVELOPMENTAL DISORDER—See chapter 15 for definition.

PHENOMENOLOGY—The study and description of signs and symptoms of the various diseases.

PHENOTHIAZINES—Group of major tranquilizers. (See chapter 29.)

PHOBIA—A fixed, irrational fear of a specific object or situation despite the realization that this fear is unwarranted.

PLACENTA PRAEVIA—Frequent cause of severe hemorrhage and fetal distress in the final third of pregnancy which results from the placenta being attached to the wall of the uterus near and obstructing the cervix instead of well back in the fundus.

PLANTAR RESPONSE—The reflex action obtained by stroking the sole of the foot, which is altered in some forms of neurological injury or disease.

PNEUMOENCEPHALOGRAMS—A form of X ray of the central nervous system in which the cerebro-spinal fluid which normally surrounds the brain and spinal cord is replaced by air to increase the contrast.

POLYMYOSITIS—Inflammation of many muscles simultaneously.

POSITIVE SHAPING—Using behavior therapy to encourage desired forms of behavior.

POSTPRANDIAL BLOATING—Bloating subsequent to a meal.

POSTTRAUMATIC NEUROSIS—A pattern of characteristic symptoms following a traumatic event, for example; rape, natural disaster, car accident, physical injury. Characteristic symptoms are numbing of responsiveness to the external world and reexperiencing of the traumatic event.

PREMORBID—Present before the development of disease, as in "premorbid personality."

PRESENILE DEMENTIAS—Deterioration of the brain (and subsequent confusion and growing intellectual impairment) occurring before the age at which this could be expected on the basis of senility.

PRIMARY PREVENTION—See chapter 17 for definition.

PSEUDOMATURE—Appearing more mature than is actually the case.

PSYCHODYNAMIC—Relating to theories of how the mind operates and of the interplay between internal forces, defenses, and the reactions to environmental stresses and demands.

PSYCHOGENIC—Psychologically caused.

PSYCHOLOGICAL DECOMPENSATION—Deterioration from usual level of functioning which interferes with the individual's capacity to carry out the usual and expected personal and social tasks.

PSYCHOMETRIC—Measurement of psychological functioning.

PSYCHONEUROTIC/PSYCHONEUROSIS—That group of disorders not dependent on any evident neurological lesion, in which an emotional conflict which remains unconscious is masked and replaced by symptoms resulting from the excessive use of defense mechanisms. (see chapter 12).

PSYCHOPATHOLOGY—Disease or disturbance of the mind, behavior, or psychic process.

PSYCHOPHYSIOLOGICALLY—Changes in bodily functions that result from the mind and its functioning.

Glossary

PSYCHOSEXUAL—the influence of the mind on sexual functioning: the mental (i.e., emotional) component of sexual development.

PSYCHOSOMATIC—See chapter 16 for definition.

PSYCHOSOMATOGENIC—Factors contributing to psychosomatic reaction.

PSYCHOSURGERY—Neurosurgical intervention to treat a mental disorder for which no organic pathological cause can be determined.

PSYCHOTIC/PSYCHOSIS—Gross impairment in reality testing. The term may describe an individual's behavior at a given time, or a mental disorder during the course of which all individuals with the disorder display gross impairment on reality testing.

PSYCHOTROPIC—Drugs with an effect on psychic function, behaviour, or experience (see chapter 29.)

PUBERTY—That period of development marked by physical growth spurt and acquisition of secondary sexual characteristics.

PUBESCENCE—The onset of the process of sexual maturation.

PYRAMIDAL TRACT—A massive bundle of brain fibers the interruption of which causes impairment of movement which is especially strong in the arm and leg opposite to the side of this interruption; muscular weakness, spasticity and hyperreflexia, and impairment of finger and hand movements.

PYLORIC STENOSIS—A disease in newborn boys in which overdevelopment and blockage of the pyloric valve between stomach and duodenum causes repeated projectile vomiting.

REACTION–FORMATION—A form of defense against urges which are unacceptable to the ego; consists of the development of conscious, socialized attitudes and interests which are the direct opposite of repressed and unsocialized trends which continue to exist in the unconscious. An example is overprotection as a reaction–formation to unconscious hate or rejection.

REITER'S SYNDROME—A combination of arthritis, conjunctivitis, and urethritis, all nongonorrheal.

REM LATENCIES—The period between the onset of sleep and the period of rapid eye movement sleep.

RENAL CLEARANCE FUNCTION—A test of the capacity of the kidneys to carry out their elimination and excreting functions.

REPRESSION—A defense mechanism involving the automatic removal of unacceptable thoughts, memories, or feelings from conscious awareness; contrasts with *suppression* which is a conscious exclusion of unacceptable thoughts, memories, and feelings.

REPRODUCTIVE CASUALTIES—Children who have experienced malnutrition or other damage during the course of pregnancy and delivery. This results in varying degrees of handicap on a continuum from retardation, to cerebral palsy, minimal brain damage, and behavioral disorders.

RETINITIS PIGMENTOSA—A chronic, progressive inflammation of the retina with atrophy and pigmentary infiltration of the inner layers.

RETINOBLASTOMA—A retinal tumor; occurring often bilaterally, usually before the fourth year and exhibiting a familial tendency.

RETROLENTAL FIBROPLASIA—An abnormal growth of fibrous tissue behind the lens of the eye; a cause of blindness.

RHEUMATOID ARTHRITIS—A chronic infectious inflammatory disease affecting the structure of one or more of the joints, producing deformity and loss of function.

RUBELLA—German measles.

SCHIZOPHRENIA—One of the major mental illnesses characterized by lack of contact with reality, disturbed interpersonal relationships, thought disorder, and specific delusional systems.

SECONDARY ACIDOSIS—An increase in the acidity of the circulating blood consequent on diabetes, respiratory problems, and renal disorders.

SECONDARY SEXUAL CHARACTERISTICS—The physical changes that occur in adolescence, for example, breast development, growth of sexual organs, characteristic weight and height patterns, and distribution of hair.

SEDIMENTATION RATE—The rate with which red cells sink and form a sediment in a mass of drawn blood.

Glossary

SEQUELAE—Consequences or later effects.

SERIOUS ENVIRONMENTAL DEPRIVATION—Absence or major diminution of normal visual, auditory, or interpersonal experiences required for healthy growth.

SEROTONIN—A potent inhibitor of the passage of cerebral nerve impulses; normally active in the regulation of centres in the brain concerned with wakefulness, temperature and blood pressure regulation, and various other autonomic functions.

SHAME—Feelings of humiliation and embarrassment for having made oneself or being made to feel rediculous or for having contravened roles of decency, modesty or acceptable behavior.

SHORT-TERM MEMORY—The ability to store and recall information that has been received in the past few seconds. Without rehearsal, information can be stored in short-term memory only for a few seconds before it decays. Rehearsal allows for the establishment of memory traces. The information then goes into long-term memory storage.

SIBSHIP—Relationships between individuals of a family of the same generation.

SIGMOIDOSCOPY—Inspection, through a speculum, of the interior of the sigmoid colon (the lower curved portion of the digestive tract above the rectum).

SKIN LESIONS—Individual points or patches of a disease of the skin.

SLEEP APNEA—Periods of cessation of breathing during sleep.

SOMATIC—Relating to the organic tissues of the body. At times, the terms psyche and soma are employed as if they were opposites rather than inseparable constituents of the total person.

SOMATOFORM DISORDERS—A mental disorder characterized by physical symptoms but no organic cause. The production of the symptoms is linked to psychological factors or conflicts but is not under voluntary control.

SOMATOSENSORY SYSTEM—That part of the central nervous system concerned with vision, hearing, and touch.

SPASTICITY—A state of muscular rigidity and spasm with exaggeration of the reflexes.

SPECIFICITY—The phenomenon of heightened reactivity to stress in that organ system in which a psychosomatic patient's symptoms are localized.

SPINA BIFIDA—A limited defect in the spinal column, consisting of an absence of the vertebral arches, through which the spinal membrane with or without spinal cord tissue protrudes.

STEROIDS—Biochemical substances (hormones) excreted by such glands as the adrenal and the pituitary. Also used in the treatment of various conditions.

STURM UND DRANG—Noise and chaos.

SUBSYSTEM—A discrete but interrelated component within an overall system.

SURGENT—Pertaining to periods of intense developmental change.

SYMBOLIC COMMUNICATION—Communication utilizing mechanisms of similarity in association to protect from anxiety attached to the original idea.

SYMPATHOMIMETIC—Denoting simulating action of the central nervous system (the part of the nervous system which supplies the visceral and arterial muscles and regulates glandular activity).

SYMPTOMATIC—Indicative of underlying pathology.

SYNDROME—A constellation of symptoms and signs constituting a recognizable condition. Less specific than *disorder* or *disease*. Disease generally implies a particular etiology or pathophysiological process.

SYSTEMIC—Literally, relating to a system, but generally used to mean the somatic system, that is, the entire organism, as distinguished from any of its individual parts.

TARDIVE DYSKINESIA—A late appearing syndrome associated with antipsychotic drug use, characterized by stereotyped involuntary dyskinetic movements.

TAY-SACHS DISEASE—A congenital condition characterized by disorders of the fat storage system giving rise to major and rapid neurological deterioration including hypotonia, regression of development, and blindness, usually fatal by age 3.

TEMPOROMANDIBULAR JOINT—The point where the mandible or lower jaw meets the skull.

TERATOGENESIS—The origin or mode of production of a severely malformed fetus.

TETANIC—Relating to or marked by tetanus, an infectious disease involving painful tonic muscular contractions.

THOUGHT BROADCASTING—A delusion that the individual's thoughts are being broadcast and received by other people.

752

Glossary

THOUGHT CONTROL—The delusion that external agencies are controlling one's internal thoughts.

THOUGHT INSERTION—The delusion that thoughts are inserted into one's mind from the outside that are not one's own.

THROMBOCYTOPENIA—A condition marked by deficiency of thrombocytes or blood platelets.

THYROTOXICOSIS—Poisoning by an excess of toxic secretion.

TOXEMIA—Blood poisoning; the presence in the blood of poisonous products of any pathogenic microorganism.

TOXIC PSYCHOSIS—Pattern of organic psychosis resulting from physical illness of an infectious nature or from external ingested substances, for example, drugs.

TOXOPLASMOSIS—Infection with the protozoan parasite *toxoplasma*. May cause hydrodephaly or microcephaly, mental retardation, and cerebral calcification in the newborn and acute encephalitis in children.

TRAUMA—In psychiatry, a significant, upsetting experience or event that may precipitate or aggravate a mental disorder.

ULCERATIVE COLITIS—Inflammation of the mucous membrane of the colon (part of the large intestine) causing ulceration.

URINARY METABOLITES—The final end products of the body's metabolism, hormones or drugs administered that appear in the urine and are used to measure levels of function.

VASCULAR ACCIDENT—Rupture or blockage of a blood vessel, usually in the head, resulting in a stroke and consequent neurological damage.

VEGETATIVE—Growing or functioning involuntarily or unconsciously after the assumed manner of vegetable life; resting, not active.

VERTIGO—Dizziness, giddiness, a sensation of irregular or whirling motion.

VIREMIA—The presence of a virus in the bloodstream.

WHITE BLOOD CELLS—Those cells in the blood concerned with immunity and fighting infection, raised or lowered in various diseases.

NAME INDEX

Name Index

Ferri, E., 104
Feurstein, R., 267
Fiddes, D. O., 482, 496
Fine, S., 158, 165
Finkelstein, N. E., 89, 93
Firestone, P., 207
Fisch, R. O., 78, 133
Fish, B., 293, 294, 295, 296, 298, 300, 301, 316, 317, 318, 319, 325, 326
Fisher, L., 135
Fishman, C. H., 64
Fitzhardinge, P. M., 206
Fleck, S., 60
Fleming, S., 534
Fogarty, T., 60, 65
Foley, J. M., 365, 458, 510, 519
Ford, F. R., 50
Foshie, J. G., 201
Fotheringham, J. B., 384, 401, 599
Fowle, A., 318
Fox, J. R., 555, 562
Fox, M., 599
Fraiberg, S., 15, 156, 163
Framo, J. L., 60, 63
Frank, G., 90, 93n, 96
Franklin, D. S., 83
Freeman, R. D., 197, 411, 463, 480, 482
Freeman, 120
Freibergs, V., 200
Freidin, M. R., 203
Freud, A., 5, 61n, 70, 71, 73, 74, 86n, 87, 93n, 133n, 461, 515, 520, 521, 531, 553, 554, 576, 581
Freud, S., 61n, 65
Freudenberger, H. J., 540
Freund, V. W., 80n
Friedman, R., 36, 38
Friedman, S. B., 336, 461, 524
Froese, A. P., 172, 524
Frommer, E. A., 282, 652, 655
Froyd, H, 493
Fulton, R., 542
Furman, E. 71, 280, 629
Furstenberg, F., Jr., 105n

Gabriel, H. P., 466, 515
Gaensbauer, T., 136n
Galenson, E., 234
Gantcheff, H., 519
Garber, H., 391
Garfinkel, B. D., 36, 287, 288, 290, 291
Garfinkel, P. E., 421, 422

Gardner, R. A., 222
Gardner, W. I., 201, 411
Garner, D. M., 421, 422
Garrard, S. E., 399, 457, 470
Gath, A., 486
Gayton, W. F., 469
Geiser, R. L., 555, 561
Geist, R. A., 461, 463, 470, 472
Gelles, R. J., 545, 546, 549
George, S., 14
Gerhard, P. H., 555, 556
Giaretto, A., 554, 560, 561
Giaretto, H., 554, 555, 560, 561
Gibson, L. E., 462
Gil, D. G., 546
Gilbert, A., 210
Giller, D. R., 327
Gilman, A., 642, 646
Gilman, A. G., 642, 646
Giovacchini, P. L., 61
Gittelman-Klein, R., 209, 637n, 639, 648n, 652, 654, 656, 657, 660
Glaser, K., 278
Glasser, L. N., 533
Glasser, P. H., 533
Glick, P. C., 50, 103
Glick, P. J., 566n
Gluck, M. R., 461
Goddard, H. H., 390
Goering, J. D., 207
Goffman, E., 482, 486
Gogan, J. C., 472n
Golberg, S., 386
Gold, M., 265, 266
Gold, P., 371
Goldberg, B., 409
Goldberg, F. H., 143n, 163
Golden, G. S., 188, 190
Golden, M., 110
Goldfarb, N., 298
Goldfarb, W., 23, 298, 301, 316, 317, 318, 319, 325
Goldstein, A., 430, 576, 581
Goldstein, J., 70, 73, 86n, 87, 93n
Goldston, S. E., 605
Golombek, H., 36, 287, 288, 290, 291
Goodman, J., 136n, 211, 557
Goodman, L. S., 642, 646
Goodsitt, A., 423
Gordon, H., 79
Gottesman, I. I., 317
Gottlieb, M. I., 351, 352, 353, 360, 379
Gough, D., 79
Gould, M. S., 124, 125

Grad, J., 570
Graham, P., 14, 132, 136, 255, 267, 415
Graham, S., 353, 364
Gram, L. F., 326
Grant, D. K., 316
Grant, M. Q., 262
Gray, J. D., 552
Grebler, A. M., 401
Green, A. H., 288
Green, M. 461, 467, 528n
Green, R., 105, 195
Greenacre, P., 234, 235
Greenbaum, G. H., 326
Greenfeld, D., 298, 317, 320, 325
Greenhill, L., 648, 654n
Greenway, P., 484
Grey, E., 80
Grimm, F., 282
Gross, P. K., 80n, 98
Grossman, F. K., 401
Groth, A. N., 553n, 554, 555, 561
Gruber, A. R., 89, 93, 93n, 95n
Grugett, A. E., Jr., 294, 317
Grunebaum, H., 55
Grunewald, K., 391
Gualtieri, C. T., 651
Guerin, P., 133n
Guggenheim, F., 343
Gunderson, J. G., 417, 418
Guthiel, T. G., 555, 556
Guyatt, D. E., 77, 78, 79

Haber, A., 593
Hagamen, M. B., 326
Haka-Ikse, K., 520, 524
Haley, J., 133n, 134
Hall, D., 517
Halla, R., 289
Hallahan, D. P., 352
Halleck, S. L., 554, 558
Halmi, K. A., 174
Halsted, J., 175, 422, 425
Halverson, C. F., 207
Hamilton, J. R., 337
Hamilton, M. W., 78
Hammond, G. M., 104
Hampson, R. B., 96, 98
Handlers, A., 492
Hansen, H., 390
Hanson, D. R., 317
Hanson, S., 528
Hare, E. H., 497
Harley, J. P., 212
Harlow, H. F., 70

Name Index

Harmon, R., 136*n*
Harper, C D., 483
Harris, P. W., 263
Harrison, S. I., 636
Hartner, M. S. S., 600
Harvery, D., 484
Harvey, O. J., 264
Hassibi, M., 136*n*, 361
Hastings, J. E., 201
Hauser, S. L., 318, 319
Hausknecht, R. O., 77, 81
Havelkova, M., 294, 298, 316, 320, 321, 325
Hawke, W. A., 380
Hawkins, J. W., 289, 290, 291, 441, 441*n*, 445, 448
Hazel, N., 92, 98, 99
Hayden, T. L., 188
Heagarty, M. C., 461
Heatherington, E. M., 573, 574, 575
Heber, R. F., 391, 405, 601
Hebert, F. B., 449, 452
Hechtman, L., 206
Heinicke, C. M., 70
Helfer, R. E., 546, 547, 548, 549, 551, 552
Helme, W. H., 295, 296
Henderson, J. O., 554, 556
Henderson, L. J., 202
Henderson, S., 240, 442
Henker, B., 200, 209, 213
Hehoch, M. J., 502
Hepworth, H. P., 76, 77, 78, 83, 89, 90, 105
Herjanic, B., 560
Hermelin, B., 297, 298, 299, 319
Herrick, J., 50
Hersen, M., 245, 454
Herstein, A., 502
Hersov, L., 76, 77, 81, 183
Hertzig, M. E., 207, 319, 597
Heston, L. L., 317
Himwich, H. E., 326
Hinde, R. A., 70
Hinkle, L. E., 334
Hirsch, J. G., 479, 485
Hirshowitz, R. G., 447
Hoag, J. M., 183
Hobben, M. 491
Hobbs, N., 137, 147, 592
Hoddinott, B. A., 401
Hodges, J., 23
Hofferth, S., 105*n*
Hoffman, L., 61, 64
Hogenson, D. L., 367
Hohman, L. B., 198, 211
Holden, C., 632
Hollenbeck, A. R., 459

Hollingsworth, C. E., 534
Hollister, W. G., 676
Holmes, D. J., 137
Holter, F. R., 504, 505
Honzik, M. P., 192
Hopkins, J., 206
Hood, E., 133, 263, 264, 265
Horenblas, W., 106
Howard, J., 554, 556
Howells, J. G., 511
Hoy, E., 205, 206
Hoyle, H. W., 17
Hsu, L. K. G., 426
Hudgens, R. W., 435
Huessy, H. R., 204
Humphrey, M. E., 79, 80, 82
Humphries, T., 209*n*
Hunt, D. E., 264
Huntington, D., 156
Hurwitz, J., 367
Hutchings, B., 268

Illingworth, R., 83
Ingram, T. T. S., 186
Inhelder, B., 14, 30
Intagliata, J. C., 400

Jackson, D. D., 50, 53, 55, 135
Jackson, J. K., 289
Jackson, K., 511, 523
Jacob, R. G., 210, 211
Jacobs, M., 92, 98
Jacobson, F. N., 367
Jacobson, G., 445
Jacobson, N. S., 51
Jaffee, A. C., 555, 559, 560
Jaffee, B., 81, 83, 84, 85, 87
Janov, A., 315
Jerry, M. B., 553*n*, 555
Jesness, C. F., 264
Jessner, L., 510, 515, 519
Joffe, W. G., 278
Johnson, A. M., 269
Johnson, F. K., 166
Johnson, D., 491, 492
Johnson, L. C., 110
Johnson, N., 204
Johnson, R., 491, 492
Johnson, V. S., 264
Johnson, W, 318
Jones, R. L., 388

Kadushin, A., 79, 81, 82, 86, 87

Kagan, J., 111, 155, 601
Kahn, J., 111, 155, 601
Kahn, J., 105*n*, 270
Kales, A., 176, 177, 181
Kales, J. D., 176, 177, 178, 181
Kalin, N. H., 652
Kallinan, F. J., 317
Kalnins, I. V., 467
Kalter, N., 572
Kamin, L. E., 524
Kandel, H. J., 211
Kane, S. P., 105
Kanner, L., 188, 190, 219, 293, 294, 296, 317, 318, 325, 387
Kantor, D., 135, 441
Kaplan, D. M., 454, 461, 527
Kaplan, H. B., 458
Karpel, M., 61, 64
Karpinski, E., 562
Kasanin, J., 198
Kasiow, L. L., 108, 109
Kastenbaum, R., 469, 486
Katz, S. N., 19, 89, 98, 210
Kauffman, J. M., 352
Kaufman, I., 555, 557, 558, 562
Kay, P., 288
Kearsley, R., 111, 155, 601
Keeran, C. V., 387, 398, 411
Keith, D. V., 443, 454
Keith, P. R., 177
Kellerman, J., 472
Kelly, J. B., 573, 574
Kelly, R. 104
Kelz, J. W., 487
Kempe, C. H., 545, 546, 547, 548, 549, 551, 552
Keniston, K., 102
Kenna, G. C., 78
Kennedy, M., 557, 558
Kennell, J. H., 19, 162, 520, 546, 600
Kerckhoff, A. C., 567
Kershner, J. R., 380
Kessler, M., 598
Khan, A. U., 441, 441*n*, 449, 463, 464, 470, 528*n*
Killilea, M., 534
Kilpatrick, D. M., 632
Kinard, E. M., 105
King, J., 515
Kinsbourne, M., 201, 209*n*, 210, 212, 352, 353, 367, 377, 380
Kinsey, A. C., 553*n*
Kiresuk, 554, 558
Kirk, H. D., 81, 83

759

Name Index

Patterson, P. R., 472
Pauker, J. D., 263, 264, 265
Pauli, L. L., 193, 216
Paulson, M. J., 288
Pavenstedt, E., 50
Pearce, J. K., 50, 52
Pearson, G. H. J., 511
Peck, A. L., 555, 557, 558, 562
Pentti, R., 338
Perez-Reyes, M. G., 79
Perlman, L. V., 334
Perlman, T., 206
Pesikoff, R. B., 178
Peters, J. J., 555, 557, 562
Petrillo, M., 521
Petti, T. A., 278, 279, 281
Pfeffer, C. R., 287, 288
Philips, I., 405, 407
Phillips, J., 18, 22
Phipps-Yonas, S., 104
Piaget, J., 5, 14, 30, 34, 154
Pierce, C. M., 181, 184
Pierpaoli, W., 336
Pike, V., 94
Pine, F., 25, 61n, 234
Pinkerton, B., 457, 461
Plank, E. N., 529n
Plank, R., 529n
Platt, J. E., 654n
Pless, I. B., 336, 457, 461, 479
Polefka, A., 245
Polizos, P., 327
Pollack, R. C., 298
Pollin, W., 317
Pomeroy, W. B., 553n
Pool, D., 326
Pope, H., 569
Poremba, C. D., 367
Portnoy, S., 375
Poznanski, E. O., 277
Pozsonyi, J., 78
Praedor, D., 435
Prechtl, H., 207
Price, G., 210
Prigmore, C. S., 384
Pringle, M. L., 482, 496
Prinz, R., 201
Pronovost, W., 301
Prosser, H., 89, 92, 104
Provence, S., 317, 509, 511
Pruce, I., 193, 216
Prugh, D. G., 510, 511
Pruyser, P. W., 136n
Puig-Antich, J., 210, 279, 281, 282, 652, 654
Purohit, A. P., 278, 280

Quay, H. C., 132, 264
Quinn, P. O., 207
Quinton, D., 70, 510
Quitkin, F., 207

Rabkin, J. K., 542
Rachman, S., 296
Rae, W. A., 511
Rae-Grant, N., 79, 86n, 87n, 676
Rae-Grant, Q. A. F., 80n, 172
Rafaelson, O. J., 326
Raimbault, G., 461, 468
Rakoff, V. M., 51, 54, 606
Ramey, C., 110, 111
Ramsey, M., 206
Rand, Y., 267
Rank, B., 293
Raphael, B., 71, 458, 465
Raphling, D. L., 554, 555, 556
Rapoport, J. L., 183, 207, 209, 210, 436, 654, 657, 660
Raschke, H. J., 104
Ravenscroft, K., 36, 38
Ravenscroft, K., Jr., 131
Rayner, R., 617
Reed, E. F., 78
Rees, J., 73, 81, 224, 341
Reid, A. H., 409
Reider, B., 375
Reidl, C. J., 520
Reiser, D. E., 317
Reiss, I. L., 102
Rekers, G. A., 195
Renbar, J., 572
Reynard, C. L., 203, 209
Reynolds, A. R., 401
Reynolds, C. F., 179
Ricciuti, H., 111
Rich, J., 133n
Richards, P., 219
Richardson, S. A., 483
Richelson, G., 540
Richer, S., 519
Richman, L. C., 364, 483
Richman, N., 17
Richmond, J. B., 399, 457, 470
Rie, H. F., 199
Rifkin, A., 207
Riley, T. L., 220, 221
Rimland, B., 296
Rimon, R., 502
Rinsley, D. B., 418, 632
Ripley, H. S., 289
Risch, S., 652
Ritchie, J., 504, 505
Ritvo, E. R., 181, 293, 294,

295, 296, 298, 300, 316, 318, 319, 660
Rizzo, J. V., 352
Robb, P., 216n, 220
Roberts, A., 301
Roberts, J., 546
Roberts, R. D., 205
Robertshaw, C., 546
Robertson, J., 70, 510, 511, 515, 516
Robertson, J. A., 516
Robins, L. N., 122, 128, 259, 265, 266, 267, 268, 591
Robinson, G. C., 510, 511, 514, 520, 521, 597
Robinson, H. B., 106, 390, 400, 405, 406
Robinson, J., 15
Robinson, N. M., 390, 400, 405, 406
Robson, B., 104
Rochlin, G., 280
Roghmann, K. J., 104, 336, 458
Roiphe, H., 234
Romeder, J. M., 602
Ronaghy, H., 175
Roosevelt, R., 581
Rosberg, G., 466
Roschlau, W. H. E., 642
Rose, F. C., 223
Rosen, B. M., 232, 258
Rosenbaum, A., 211
Rosenbaum, J., 581, 584
Rosenbaum, J. F., 672
Rosenbaum, V., 581, 584
Rosenberg, J. B., 207
Rosenblum, B., 92
Rosenfeld, A. A., 560
Rosenthal, D., 317
Rosenthal, J. H., 201
Roskies, E., 523
Rosman, N. P., 318
Ross, A. O., 367, 371, 374, 376, 377
Ross, D. M., 203
Ross, S. A., 203
Roth, B., 317
Roth, M., 316
Rothenberg, M. B., 466, 524
Rowe, J. S., 78, 81, 199, 205
Routh, D. K., 205
Roy, A., 220, 221
Rubin, A. L., 402
Rubin, R. L., 402
Ruess, A. L., 469, 486
Ruesch, J., 50
Ruiz, P., 433
Rush, D., 19
Rush, F., 554, 562

Name Index

Name Index

SUBJECT INDEX

406; symptomatic treatment of, 454; *see also* Attention deficit disorder
Hyperammonemia, 394
Hyperkinesis, *see* Attention deficit disorder; Hyperactivity
Hypertelorism, 498
Hyperthyroidism, 333, 424
Hypnosis: for elective mutism, 188; for stuttering, 187
Hypochondriasis, 347; depression and, 278
Hypoglycemic coma, 221
Hypomania, 278, 282
Hypothalamic tumors, 424
Hypothyroidism, 341, 424, 656; congenital, 394
Hysterical gaits, 223
Hysterical neurosis, conversion type, 247–48
Hysterical symptoms, 208

Identification: in adolescence, 34, 436; of adopted children, 85; in conduct disorders, 270; conscience formation and, 75; depression and, 284; in early childhood, 15; with same-sex parent, 28; with scapegoat, 63
Identity disorder of childhood and adolescence, 253, 414–16; in borderline syndrome, 417
Identity transformation in adolescence, 34, 37–38
I-Levels, 263–64
Illegitimacy, 76–79, 84
Illingworth test, 399
Illinois Test of Psycholinguistic Abilities (ITPA), 372, 400
Imaginary playmates, 26
Imipramine, 178, 183, 209, 286, 453, 654, 657, 660
Immigrant families, 603–4, 630
Immune system, effects of stress on, 331, 336
Impulsivity, 75; in attention deficit disorder, 199–200, 211; in borderline syndrome, 416, 417; convulsive disorders and, 218, 219; learning disorders and, 364
Inborn errors of metabolism, 393
Incest, 553, 555–56, 562
Incidence of disorders, 123
Incontinence in spina bifida, 496, 497
Independence: in adolescence, 37–39, 44; of toddler, 25; *see also* Dependency
Indirect communication, 54
Indirect treatment of infants, 166
Individual psychotherapy, 623; for anorexia nervosa, 425; for borderline syndrome, 419, 420; for depression, 284–86; family and, 622–23; for learning disorders, 379; for psychosis, 321, 324–25
Individuation, 16; in adolescence, 44–45; boundaries and, 60–61

Infancy: attention deficit disorder in, 202–3; blindness in, 493–94; day care and, 110, 111; deafness in, 494; disorders of, 156–64; hospitalization in, 512, 515–16, 520; intervention during, 601–2; mental retardation in, 388, 405–6; migraine in, 224; physical handicaps in, 485; psychosis in, 294, 296, 298, 302
Infant development programs, 595
Infant psychiatry, 153–66; for developmental disorders, 159–61; diagnosis in, 164–65; for eating disorders, 158–59; history of, 153–55; for physiological problems of psychological origin, 161–62; for psychological disturbances with physical origin, 162–64; for reactive attachment disorders, 157–58; role of, 155–56; treatment approaches in, 165–66
Infantile autism, *see* Autism
Infections, mental retardation caused by, 396–97
Inflammatory bowel disease, 333, 337–40; alexithymia and, 335; immune mechanisms in, 336
Injury, handicaps caused by, 480, 500
Insight model, 133
Insomnia, 176
Institutional placements, 90; *see also* Residential treatment
Instrumental communication, 50, 54
Insulin, 461, 465
Intellectual deficits, mild, 353–54
Intellectual retardation, deprivation and, 70
Intelligence tests for mentally retarded, 387–88
Intensive psychotherapy, 623–24; supportive psychotherapy compared with, 625
Internal role consistency, 53
International Statistical Classification of Diseases, Injuries, and Causes of Death: Eigth Revision (ICD-8), 118, 119; Ninth Revision (ICD-9), 119–20, 122, 146, 200, 232, 264
Interpersonal level of equilibrium, 58, 59
Interviews: with children, 136; content and process in, 134–35; family diagnostic, 135; structure of, 134
Intracranial vascular lesions, 221
Intrafamilial adoption, 76, 77, 79
Intrapsychic level of equilbirium, 58, 59
Introjection, 61, 62
Irritable colon syndrome, 335
Isolation in chronic illness, 460

Jaundice, 651
Jehovah's Witnesses, 466
Joint custody, 579–80

distinguished from, 417, 419; conduct disorders and, 259, 271–74; crises precipitated by, 445; custody and, 578; in mentally retarded, 407; prognosis for, 255; referral for, 673; treatment for, 256; *see also* Anxiety disorders
Neurosyphilis, 315
Neurotic symptoms, 236, 237; as expression of family dysfunction, 65–66
Neurotransmitters, 638–41; major pathways of, 643; postulated excess and deficiency states, 644–45
Neutral communication, 54
Neutropenia, 651
Newborns, behavioral repertoire of, 15, 19
Nicotine, 427, 432
Night terrors, 176–78, 227, 332; migraine and, 226
Nightmares, 175–77
Nocturnal fears, 175–77
No-fault divorce, 568
Nonaggressive conduct disorder, 261
Norms, family, 50
Novelty shock, 400
Nuclear family, transformation of, 102–3
Nurses, mental health role of, 675
Nutritional deficits: fetal effects of, 396; learning disorders and, 355

Obesity, 341–43; amphetamines for, 431; fear of, in anorexia nervosa, 421
Object permanence, 20, 234
Object relationships, 25
Objectivity in work with adolescents, 43
Obsessions in borderline syndrome, 417
Obsessive-compulsive disorder, 249–50 in mentally retarded, 407
Occupational therapists, 675
Oculogyric crisis, 651
Oedipal period, 27–28, 235
Oligophrenia, 387
Olympics for the Disabled, 492
On-site assessment, 133
Operant conditioning, 410, 618; for attention deficit disorder, 210–11; for school refusal, 245
Opiates, 430; during pregnancy, 19
Oppositional personality disorder, 255; conduct disorder and, 259, 262; enuresis and, 181
Organic brain syndrome, 313; borderline syndrome distinguished from, 419; psychosis and, 318, 320
Organic factors: in attention deficit disorders, 205–7; in borderline syndrome, 418; in conduct disorders, 267; in psychosis, 293, 294, 316–18
Osteogenesis imperfecta, 480, 502

Overinvolvement in work with adolescents, 43–44

Pain: in chronic illness, 461, 464; hysterical, 247
Pancreatitis, 335
Panic disorder, 242
Paradox model, 133
Paradoxical communications, 55
Paralysis, hysterical, 247
Paranoia, parental, 233
Paranoid personality disorder, 252
Parens patriae, doctrine of, 576
Parent Teacher Questionnaire, 641
Parental rights, 592–93
Parenthood, developmental stage of, 18
Parents Anonymous, 549
Parkinsonism, 650
Parkinson's disease, 639
Partial seizures, 217
Passive/aggressive personality disorder, 255
Pavor nocturnus, 177; medication for, 656
PCP, 433
Peabody Picture Vocabulary Test, 400
Pedophilia, 555, 559
Peer group: chronic illness and, 461, 462, 472–73; crises precipitated by, 451; handicapped children and, 484; in middle childhood, 29, 30
Pemoline (Cylert), 648
Peptic ulcer, 333, 335
Perceptual function in psychosis, 296–98, 309
Perinatal period: interventions during, 600; mental retardation caused in, 396
Permanency planning, 94
Permanent detachment, 73–74
Personal-social development, *see* Social development
Personality disorders, 119, 237, 250–55; attachment and, 233; conduct disorders and, 259; conversion disorder and, 346; limited effectiveness of treatment of, 591; in mentally retarded, 407; school refusal and, 243
Pertusis, 205
Pervasive developmental disorders, 120–21, 309; atypical, 310; genetic factors in, 317; medication for, 660; organic factors in, 320
Petit mal, 217, 218, 220
Peyote, 431
"Phantom limb" sensations, 504
Phenobarbital, fetal effects of, 395
Phenothiazines, 198–99, 210, 324, 326, 327, 337, 648, 650, 651
Phenotype, 4
Phenylketonuria (PKU), 315, 393–94
Phenytoin, fetal effects of, 395
Phobic disorders, 242–43; behavior therapy